Pathology

for the Health-Related
Professions

Ivan Damjanov, MD, PhD

Professor
Department of Pathology and Laboratory Medicine
University of Kansas
School of Medicine
Kansas City, Kansas

Second Edition

Pathology

for the Health-Related Professions

W.B. Saunders Company
A Division of Harcourt Brace & Company
Philadelphia   London   Toronto
Montreal   Sydney   Tokyo

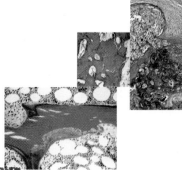

W.B. SAUNDERS COMPANY

A Division of Harcourt Brace & Company

The Curtis Center
Independence Square West
Philadelphia, Pennsylvania 19106

Library of Congress Cataloging–in–Publicaton Data

Damjanov, Ivan
    Pathology for the health-related professions / Ivan Damjanov.—
2nd ed.
        p.   cm.
    Includes index.
    ISBN 0–7216–8118–2
    1. Pathology. I. Title
    [DNLM: 1. Pathology. QZ 140 D161p 2000]
    RB25.D26   2000
    616.07—dc21
    DNLM/DLC   99–27976

Associate Editor: Shirley A. Kuhn

PATHOLOGY FOR THE HEALTH-RELATED PROFESSIONS   ISBN 0–7216–8118–2

Printed in the United States of America

Last digit is the print number: 9   8   7   6   5   4   3   2   1

To my agathodemons, Ivana and Milena,
with a quote from Gandhi:
"Almost anything you do will be insignificant,
but it is very important that you do it."
Of course, because the circle is never entirely round.

tata

Preface to the Second Edition

Almost four years have passed since the first edition of this book appeared in print. The book sales and the comments made by my colleagues and by students across the country indicate that it was well received. I was most gratified by this response, and I readily accepted the invitation from the publisher to prepare a Second Edition.

My task in revising the original work was facilitated by the input of "users"—that is, teachers and students who have sent me suggestions and have pointed out typos, misspellings and inaccuracies.

In addition to making the necessary corrections, I have updated the text to include new concepts and discoveries. At the suggestion of several teachers, I have inserted at the end of each chapter a new feature called *Review Questions.* These questions replace the clinicopathologic reviews that appeared in the First Edition. I hope that this new approach will be helpful to students and teachers alike.

With the generous support of the publisher, the artwork for the Second Edition was also spruced up, and virtually all of the illustrations now appear in color. Several new full-color drawings were added, replacing, for the most part, some of the more complex microphotographs.

I was reminded by a friend that good textbooks share some common features with the best Hollywood movies but differ from them in one important aspect: Textbook sequels are almost always better than the original. I hope that I have maintained this tradition. I also invite the users of this book to help me continue to improve it even more. I can be reached by e-mail **(idamjano@kumc.edu),** and I eagerly await your input.

Ivan Damjanov

Preface to the First Edition

The object of all science . . .
is to coordinate our experience
into a logical system.   Albert Einstein

I have written this book for students in allied health professions to provide them with an introductory textbook of pathology that is modern and up-to-date, both in content and presentation. I hope that students will find it an enticement for further studies and that the book will provide them with a solid foundation for future professional growth and a lifelong career in the health sciences.

The material is presented in a standard manner to enable students to study efficiently and gain knowledge systematically. The book is divided into 23 chapters grouped into two major sections: general pathology and organ system pathology. Emphasis is given to systemic pathology to meet the requirements of most curricula. Each chapter is a self-contained teaching unit. Each begins with an outline and a list of additional key terms and concepts. Learning objectives are provided to guide students and help them focus on the core material. Students should return to these opening pages for review after reading each chapter. Students who can discuss cogently, in their own words, all the learning objectives should be assured that they know the material.

At the beginning of each chapter, students are reminded that pathologic processes occur in organs and tissues that were normal before the disease began. A brief review of the normal structure and function of each organ is included to emphasize the most important aspects of normal anatomy, histology, and physiology that are essential to an understanding of pathology. Diagrams of the normal organs are also included, and these should help students refresh their knowledge of material that was covered in anatomy and physiology courses.

This book contains so many new facts and concepts that students might easily be lost in details. To enable students to keep their perspective, the beginning of each chapter on systemic pathology is devoted to an overview of major diseases and how they relate to the normal organ. The core information in each chapter is presented in these sections. Students are advised to keep these brief statements in mind as they study the material in greater detail later in the chapter. Students should spend as much time as possible thinking about these concepts because they are essential to an understanding of the details. These statements are the actual take-home messages that should remain with the student a long time after most of the minutiae are forgotten. Students should avoid at any cost memorizing details taken out of context. An understanding of general principles and concepts is encouraged.

Pathology is too vast a subject to be covered in one semester. In order to produce a book that could be read in a time frame mandated by most current curricula, I had to eliminate many diseases and concentrate on a few salient pathologic processes and entities that could serve as prototypes or instructional paradigms. These diseases, which are discussed in detail, were chosen either because they are common and thus frequently encountered in practice or because they illustrate important principles and thus provide significant insight into the reaction pattern of an injured organ. Understanding the principles of these paradigmatic diseases will facilitate the understanding of other similar or related disorders.

Each major disease is presented in a standardized format that includes, whenever feasible, a comprehensive **D**efinition or description of basic features of a disease; discussions on **E**tiology, **P**athogenesis, **P**athology, and **C**linical features; and a brief comment about **T**herapy or prognosis. I advise students to use this approach (which I call **DEPPICT**) in their studies of pathology, as well as in clinical medicine in general. It is a didactic approach that has repeatedly proven its validity and usefulness in practice.

As the students reading this text will practice clinical medicine rather than pathology, all the data presented here have a clinical slant and were included with the ultimate goal of preparing students for their work with living patients and enabling them to understand various clinical aspects of specific diseases. To this end, we have included a plethora of illustrations. Colorful diagrams and photographs of pathologic lesions contain important information, and students should spend time studying them. Illustrations can reinforce the written message, and often a concept can be made more vivid with figures than with words. To reinforce the message, at the end of each chapter, students will find reviews questions pertaining to the main topics covered in that chapter.

Students of pathology are asked to master a new vocabulary and memorize hundreds of new words. Most of these new pathologic terms are explained when they are first mentioned in the text. Additional definitions and explanations can be found in the glossary at the end of the book.

The contemporary layout and multicolor print were designed to facilitate reading and comprehension and to keep students' attention focused on important concepts during long hours of study. To enliven the text, material of human interest was inserted in boxes entitled "Did You Know?" The brief stories and curious facts presented here should serve as a reminder that, although pathology is a clinical discipline, the knowledge acquired from this book can be used not only in a medical setting but in everyday life as well.

Ivan Damjanov

Acknowledgments

Acknowledgments to the Second Edition

It is my pleasure to acknowledge the help of my secretaries Stephanie Yeager and Kathy Ulgener in Kansas City. Although my erstwhile editor, Selma Ozmat, became Ms. Kaszczuk and moved to Arizona, she still found time as a free-lance editor to guide me in the early stages of this project. Her place at W. B. Saunders was taken by Shirley Kuhn, who coordinated our later efforts flawlessly. My old friend Faith Voit, who is now also a free-lance editor, was available to help as well. Even though I felt guilty taking her away from her grandchildren, I greatly appreciate her support. With the help of all these wonderful people, the revision was completed more or less on time, and all that is left for me to say is *thank you all*.

Acknowledgments to the First Edition

When Napoleon signed edicts promoting his officers to the rank of general, he used to ask about each of them, "Is he lucky?" Although I never became a general, I am truly one of those lucky guys. Here I would like to take the opportunity to acknowledge that luck and the good fortune that allowed me to produce this book.

Ever since I was born 59 years ago in the Jewish Hospital of Subotica, a provincial town of the former Yugoslavia, my lucky star has shined over my head. It led me to Zagreb, Croatia, where I received my medical degree and learned how much fun and satisfaction one could derive from a life in medicine, from research, and from teaching. In Zagreb, I also met my future wife, Andrea, who, together with our three daughters, followed me to America, where we have lived happily ever after. During the past 20

years, I have been on staff at the University of Connecticut, Farmington, Connecticut; Hahnemann University and Thomas Jefferson University, Philadelphia, Pennsylvania; and the University of Kansas, Kansas City, Kansas.

In this acknowledgment section, which reads like an abbreviated autobiography, I must start with my mother, from whom I inherited a passion for dreams and storytelling or, as the German poet Goethe said of his mother, "die Lust zum Fabulieren." My grandmother, who spoiled me, taught me that you could love someone and still make him toil; for my grandmother, being idle was the greatest sin on earth and the source of most evils. My father strived all his life to be independent and urged me to do the same. Although it has been imposible for him to survive in war-torn Yugoslavia without my financial help, his ideals, which influenced me deeply, still hold true for both of us.

For the past 30 years, my wife, Andrea, has taken over the role of my guardian angel and has been a source of stability in my not-always-tranquil life. Finally, I should mention my daughters—Nevena, Ivana, and Milena—who are probably unaware of their contribution to my well-being and do not know how much they have inspired me. Were it not for their insistence, I would probably have dropped the "j" in my last name or Anglicized it to Damyanov to make it sound correct when read by Anglophones. My daughters helped me preserve my identity and integrity in more ways than one.

In the 1970s my lucky star brought me to Philadelphia, where I worked for 17 years with Emanuel Rubin, M.D., who was the chairman of the Department of Pathology at Hahnemann University School of Medicine for 9 years and is now the chairman of the Department of Pathology of the Jefferson Medical College, Thomas Jefferson University, Philadelphia. Dr. Rubin provided me with unconditional support and allowed me to devote myself to research, teaching, and writing as I pleased. There is no way for me to repay him for all he has done for me. A thank you seems perfunctory.

Through Dr. Rubin, I met Lisa Biello, under whose guidance I produced a book for medical students for another publisher. Lisa, who is now Vice President and Editor-in-Chief, Health-Related Professions, at W. B. Saunders, conceived this book, and the project was completed under the guidance of Selma Ozmat, Senior Editor, Health-Related Professions, and Faith Voit, Developmental Editor. Their help and support have been invaluable.

Jim Perkins, a talented artist from Atlanta, transformed my sketches and concepts into computer art. I consider him a magician. Peggy Gordon and her crew edited the text. One could almost say that they translated it into English from my mother tongue, officially known either as Croatian or Serbian, depending on which side of the front line in the former Yugoslavia you are standing on.

My acknowledgments would be incomplete without mentioning the extraordinary help of my secretaries, Sandra Dixon-Ross and Carla Aldi, Kathy Gordon in Philadelphia, and Cyndi Van Derbur in Kansas City. Their jobs, which defy description, included—among many other tasks—typing and retyping the lengthy manuscript.

Without the help and support of all those mentioned above, this project would not have come into being and could not have been completed. Again I must invoke my good luck and quote Dr. William Mayo:

We simply gather up good ideas . . .
put them together and tie a string around them.
All we can take credit for is the string.

Ivan Damjanov

Contents

Introduction

Welcome to the Wonderful World of Pathology!

In this book you will read about pathology—the basic medical science concerned with diseases.

The term pathology is derived from two Greek words: *pathos,* meaning disease, and *logos,* meaning science. Thus *pathology* is the science that studies diseases. It is also a medical specialty traditionally divided into anatomic and clinical pathology. Anatomic pathology—or, as the British like to call it, morbid anatomy—deals with the dissection and microscopic examination of human tissues removed from cadavers at postmortem autopsies or from biopsies taken of living patients to diagnose tumors and other diseases. Clinical pathology, on the other hand, is a vast field that includes medical chemistry, microbiology, immunopathology, hematopathology, and blood banking. It is, therefore, also called laboratory medicine. All of you will interact with and come to know pathologists, and some of you will work in pathology laboratories. To assist you in becoming knowledgeable of and conversant in pathology, this book is presented to you in the hope that it provides you with the medical knowledge essential for the understanding of diseases.

The primary goal of this book is to teach you the basic concepts underlying various pathologic processes. You will study the *pathogenesis* of diseases, learn their mechanisms, and understand how they develop. You will learn the *etiology* of pathologic changes and understand the causes of many diseases. However, it is important for you to know that, while many diseases are well delineated, such as cancer and AIDS, others are still shrouded in mystery and only poorly understood.

You will be shown gross and microscopic specimens of human organs and tissues affected by various diseases in order to visualize the *morphology* of various lesions. These pathoanatomic facts that you learn will be correlated with biochemical and immunologic findings, as well as with the clinical symptoms with which a specific disease presents in the living patient. Through *clinicopathologic* correlations, you will see how important the understanding of pathology is for your future medical practice.

Some of you will be caring for living patients and will encounter pathology every day in different guises. Others of you will be working in laboratories examining pathologic specimens on a daily basis. Nonetheless, all of you will be involved with people, and to understand and fully appreciate their problems, you will have to know pathology. Why? Because pathology is the basis of all medical practice. Dr. William Osler, the famous clinician who worked in the great hospitals of Baltimore, Philadelphia, and Boston at the turn of the century, noted that our clinical practice is only as good as our understanding of pathology. This adage is the motto of our textbook. Remember that you are laying the scientific foundations of your future medical career. Be sure that they are solid.

In the end, you will recall that the greatest pleasure from having done a job well stems from having done it at all. Nothing worthwhile ever comes easily. Persevere and your efforts will be rewarded.

Good Luck and Enjoy Your Studies!

Pathology

for the Health-Related Professions

Learning Objectives

After reading this chapter, the student should be able to:

1. Describe the essential components of a typical cell and their functions.
2. Explain how the functions of cells are coordinated and integrated and define homeostasis and steady state.
3. Define reversible cell injury.
4. Explain the cytoplasmic changes in reversible cell injury.
5. Define and describe the nuclear changes in irreversible cell injury.
6. List the most important causes of cell injury.
7. Describe three types of cell adaptations.
8. Explain atrophy and give three examples of this form of adaptation.
9. Define and explain hypertrophy and hyperplasia and give appropriate examples of each.
10. Define and explain metaplasia and dysplasia and give appropriate examples of each.
11. Discuss cellular aging.
12. Discuss the changing concepts of death.
13. Describe various forms of necrosis and give appropriate examples of each.

Additional Key Terms and Concepts

Calcification

Hemosiderin

Homeostasis

Hydropic degeneration

Lipid accumulation

Lipofuscin

Chapter Outline

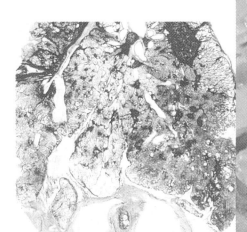

Cell Pathology
Chapter 1

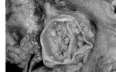

The foundation of modern pathology can be traced to the 19th century when German scientists realized that the cell represented the basic functional unit of the body and that all diseases could be related to disturbances in cell function. Rudolf Virchow (1821–1902), the scientist who introduced the concept of cellular pathology, is, thus, the father of pathology as we know it today.

The concepts of cellular pathology have been expanded and modified since Virchow's times, but most remain unchallenged. Today, we know that the cells consist of smaller functional units, cellular organelles, and that these comprise even smaller entities which can be further dissected by the techniques of molecular biology. These research endeavors are laying grounds for *molecular pathology,* a science that will encompass all living phenomena and provide explanations for pathologic processes at the level of the basic units of living nature, molecules, atoms, and their elementary particles. However, until this long-time goal of pathologists becomes a reality, we limit our discussions to cells (*cell pathology*), tissues (*histopathology*), and organs (*organ pathology*). At the same time, we should not forget that these are but parts of the human body, and that the main purpose of pathology is to gather knowledge about diseases and how these processes affect the human body, an integrated sum of all its anatomic parts.

Structure and Function of Normal Cells

All normal cells of the human body have some common features and consist of the same basic components. These include the nucleus, the cytoplasm, and the cell (plasma) membrane (Fig. 1-1).

Nucleus

The **nucleus** is the essential part of most living cells. It consists of nucleic acids, such as deoxyribonucleic acid (DNA) and ribonucleic acid (RNA), and nuclear proteins. In resting cells, these components are arranged into aggregates known as *chromatin,* and a specialized organelle composed primarily of RNA known as the *nucleolus.* In the dividing of cells—that is, during *mitosis*—the chromatin is restructured and the strands of DNA condense into *chromosomes.* The resting cells have a nuclear membrane, which delimits the nucleus from the cytoplasm. This membrane disappears in mitosis and reappears after cell division is completed.

The DNA of the nucleus contains essential genetic material that is identical for all cells of an individual body. This genetic material consists of genes which are, however, differentially expressed in various tissues and organs. Differential expression of

FIGURE 1-1

Normal cells have a nucleus and a cytoplasm. On the outside, the cell is delimited by a plasma membrane. In the cytoplasm, there are organelles, such as mitochondria, smooth and rough endoplasmic reticulum (SER and RER, respectively), Golgi apparatus, and lysosomes.

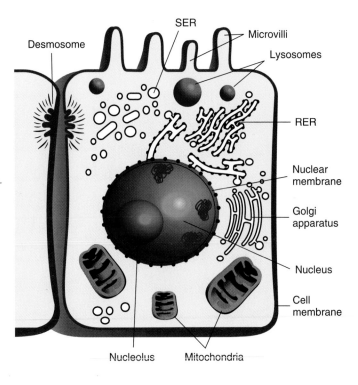

genes allows the cells to assume unique features in various tissues and organs and to perform specialized functions. Such cells are called *differentiated,* in contrast to embryonic cells, which have not undergone specialization and which are, therefore, termed *undifferentiated.*

The genetic information encoded in the DNA is transcribed into the nuclear RNA. From the nuclear RNA, the message is transmitted by transfer RNA (tRNA) and messenger RNA (mRNA) into the cytoplasm (Fig. 1-2). The ribosomal RNA (rRNA) serves as a template for translating the genetic messages into proteins. Protein synthesis is essential for the maintenance of life. Proteins are needed for cellular growth, replication, metabolism, respiration, and other essential functions. Proteins also act as structural elements, maintaining the cell's shape and the internal organization of the cytoplasm. None of these elementary functions (and many others which we shall mention later) would be possible without the nucleus, which acts as the main overseer of all critical cytoplasmic events. All human cells, except the red blood cells and platelets, need a nucleus for survival.

Cytoplasm

All cells have **cytoplasm.** However, the amount of cytoplasm and its structure vary from one cell to another. In embryonic cells, the cytoplasm is scant and contains few organelles. In specialized, highly differentiated cells, such as liver or kidney cells, the cytoplasm is more abundant and is replete with organelles. The ratio of the nucleus to the cytoplasm, the so-called nucleocytoplasmic (N:C) ratio, is high in undifferentiated embryonic cells and much lower in differentiated cells of adult tissues. As we shall see later, many tumor cells are also undifferentiated and have a high N:C ratio.

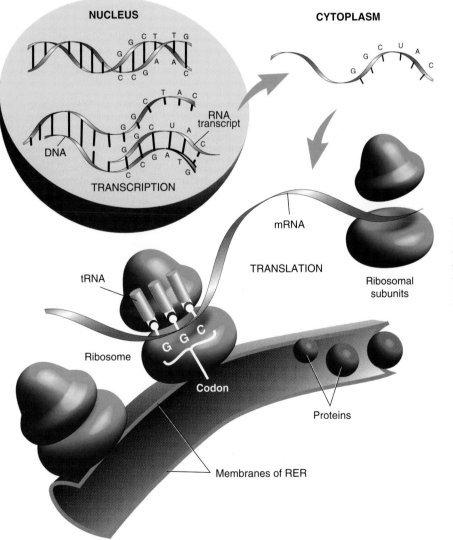

FIGURE 1-2
Transcription and translation by RNA of the genetic code stored in the DNA leads to protein synthesis on ribosomes. RER, rough endoplasmic reticulum; mRNA, messenger RNA; tRNA, transfer RNA.

The principal **cytoplasmic organelles** are the mitochondria, ribosomes, endoplasmic reticulum, Golgi apparatus, and lysosomes. In addition to these, some cells have organelles for specialized functions. For example, muscle cells have myofilaments composed of actin and myosin, which are essential for contraction; glandular cells have secretory granules, which contain enzymes or mucus destined for excretion. Furthermore, it is important to note that the cytoplasmic ground substance of all cells consists of an amorphous matrix called *hyaloplasm* and a fibrillar meshwork called *cytoskeleton.* Each cell is also enclosed by an outer *plasma membrane,* which forms the border between one cell and other cells or the extracellular spaces. This membrane, which is semipermeable, must remain intact to preserve the viability of the cell.

Mitochondria. *Mitochondria* are double-membrane–bound cytoplasmic organelles, involved primarily in the generation of energy (Fig. 1-3). Hence, mitochondria are rich in oxidative enzymes. These enzymes (e.g., cytochrome oxidase) are attached to the double membrane that encloses each mitochondrion and to the cristae that are seen by electron microscopy on the inside of cross-sectioned mitochondria. Energy generated by the mitochondria is essential for all other cellular functions. Cells with complex functions, like liver cells and nerve cells, require a considerable amount of energy and, therefore, contain numerous mitochondria. By comparison, undifferentiated cells, including many malignant tumor cells, have few mitochondria.

Ribosomes. *Ribosomes* are small granules composed of RNA. They may be arranged into aggregates that float freely in the cytoplasm, called *polysomes* or free ribosomes, or they may be attached to the membranes of the *rough endoplasmic reticulum* (RER). The ribosomes are involved in protein synthesis. Structural proteins and enzymes needed for the maintenance of basic cell functions ("proteins for internal purposes") are synthesized on the free ribosomes. Those intended for excretion ("export or luxury proteins") are synthesized on the RER and discharged from the cells through the cisternae lined by the membranes of the RER.

Endoplasmic Reticulum. The *endoplasmic reticulum* is a meshwork of membranes that are in continuity with the outer plasma membranes on one side and the nuclear membrane on the other (Fig. 1-4). By electron microscopy, one can distinguish two forms of endoplasmic reticulum: the RER and the smooth endoplasmic reticulum (SER). As stated earlier, the RER is the site of protein synthesis. SER has complex functions, the most important of which are the catabolism (i.e., metabolic degradation) of drugs, hormones, and various nutrients, and the synthesis of steroid hormones. SER is, therefore, most prominent in liver cells, known for their complex catabolic functions. The hormone-secreting gonadal cells of the testis and ovary and the adrenocortical cells that synthesize steroid hormones (e.g., estrogens, androgens, and corticosteroids) also have prominent SER.

Golgi Apparatus. The *Golgi apparatus* is a synthetic organelle adjacent to the nucleus (see Fig. 1-4). Its tubules and flattened cisternae, which are its main components, give rise laterally to vesicles. The vesicles arising from the concave side of the Golgi apparatus—the maturing surface—become secretory granules, lysosomes, and specialized structures, such as melanosomes. Melanosomes are the melanin-containing organelles of pigmented cells (melanocytes) in the skin and eye. The convex face is in continuity with the endoplasmic reticulum. Many proteins synthesized in the endoplasmic reticulum pass through the Golgi apparatus, where they are biochemically modified before being packaged into secretory granules or lysosomes. Glycoproteins and lipoproteins (i.e., proteins linked to a carbohydrate or lipid) are formed in the Golgi apparatus. These complex proteins are then incorporated into the internal cell membranes (e.g., endoplasmic reticulum) or the outer plasma membrane, or are secreted from the cell.

Lysosomes. *Lysosomes* are membrane-bound digestive cytoplasmic organelles that are rich in lytic enzymes. The lysosomes originate as small vesicles budding from enzymes on the maturing face of the Golgi apparatus (Fig. 1-5). These primary lysosomes contain acid hydrolases, which are digestive enzymes that are maximally active in an acidic milieu (i.e., at low pH levels). Under normal circumstances,

FIGURE 1-3
Mitochondrion. This organelle has a double membrane that unfolds and forms cristae. The membrane and cristae serve as attachment sites for oxidative enzymes.

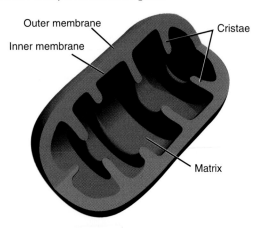

Outer membrane
Inner membrane
Cristae
Matrix

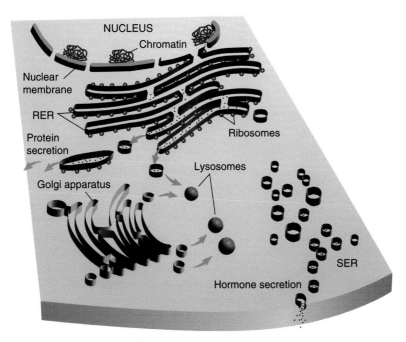

FIGURE 1-4
Endoplasmic reticulum. It consists of rough endoplasmic reticulum (RER) arranged into ribosome-studded cisternae and vesicles of smooth endoplasmic reticulum (SER).

the lytic enzymes are tightly enclosed by a lysosomal outer membrane and do not harm the cell. Even if some lysosomal content is spilled into the cytoplasm, the acid hydrolases would cause little damage in normal cytoplasm, which has a neutral pH. However, if the cell is injured and the pH of the cytoplasm becomes acidic, enzymes released from the lysosomes could cause damage.

The primary lysosomes fuse with other cytoplasmic vesicles to form secondary lysosomes. Typically, they fuse with the absorptive vesicles originating from the invaginated plasma membrane to form secondary lysosomes, which are also called *heterophago-*

somes. Secondary lysosomes that are involved in the autodigestion of a cell's own organelles are called *autophagosomes.* The digestive enzymes in secondary lysosomes degrade the material enclosed within its membrane. The metabolites obtained through this intracellular digestion are reutilized within the cell's cytoplasm. The undigested residues are extruded from the cytoplasm into the extracellular spaces by reverse endocytosis or exocytosis, a process that is colloquially known as "cellular defecation." Some of the undigested material, mostly complex lipids derived from cell membranes, may remain within the cytoplasm as "residual bodies." These residual bodies

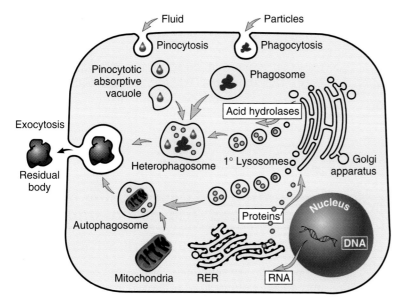

FIGURE 1-5
Lysosomes. Primary (1°) lysosomes, which originate from the Golgi apparatus, give rise to heterophagosomes and autophagosomes. Undigested material in phagosomes is extruded from the cell or remains in the cytoplasm as lipofuscin-rich residual bodies. RER, rough endoplasmic reticulum.

typically contain lipid-rich brown pigment known as *lipofuscin,* a term derived from the Greek word *lipos* (meaning fat) and the Latin word *fuscus* (meaning brown). Lipofuscin is also known as the "brown pigment of aging" because it is commonly found in cells of the elderly. With aging, all cellular processes become less efficient. Energy-dependent processes, like lysosomal digestion and exocytosis, are especially affected. The cells in an old organism, therefore, contain more lipofuscin than those in a metabolically active, more vigorous young body.

The **hyaloplasm,** which is the ground substance of the cytoplasm, has no distinct structure and appears as an "empty" space on electron microscopic studies. Biochemically, hyaloplasm consists predominantly of water, but it also contains minerals, proteins, carbohydrates, and lipids. The hyaloplasm is the fluid phase of the cell that contains the organelles. In between the organelles, the hyaloplasm is traversed by a network of filaments that form the **cytoskeleton.** Three types of filaments are recognized: **microfilaments,** composed of actin and myosin and measuring 5 nm in diameter, **microtubules,** which are 22 mm thick and composed of tubulin, and **intermediate filaments,** named so because their diameter (10 nm) is intermediate between that of microfilaments and microtubules.

In contrast to microfilaments and microtubules, which have the same biochemical composition in all cells, the **intermediate filament proteins** are cell-type–specific (Table 1-1). The intermediate filaments of epithelial cells contain *keratins,* mesenchymal cells contain *vimentin,* muscle cells contain *desmin,* glial cells contain *glial acidic fibrillary protein* (GAFP), and the neural cells contain *neurofilament* proteins. Intermediate filament proteins are useful markers for those cell types. Pathologists use antibodies to intermediate filaments for typing of tumors because tumor cells retain the same intermediate filament proteins as the normal cells from which they arise. For example, carcinomas, which are tumors involving epithelial cells, express keratin, whereas sarcomas, which are tumors of mesenchymal cells, express vimentin.

Table 1-1 Proteins of Cytoskeletal Filaments

Type of Filament	Diameter (nm)	Protein
Microfilaments	5	Actin, myosin
Intermediate filaments	10	Epithelial—keratins Mesenchymal—vimentin Muscle—desmin Glia—GFAP Nerve—neurofilaments
Microtubules	22	Tubulin

GFAP, glial fibrillary acidic protein

The function of the cytoskeleton is to maintain cell shape and to enable the cell to adapt to external mechanical pressure. Cytoskeletal filaments are also important for cell movement and the traffic of organelles in the cytoplasm. Microtubules also form the mitotic spindle during cell division.

Plasma Membrane

The **plasma membrane** forms the outer surface of the cell (Fig. 1-6). The plasma membrane is composed of proteins, lipids, and carbohydrates that are arranged in a polarized complex bilayer that has an internal and external surface. On the internal side, the plasma membrane is in continuity with the membrane of the endoplasmic reticulum. Invaginations of the plasma membrane give rise to endocytotic vesicles, which fuse with primary lysosomes to form heterophagosomes. The cytoplasmic surface of the cell membrane also serves as an anchorage site for cytoskeletal filaments. For example, intermediate filaments composed of keratin aggregate at the site of desmosomes, the typical intercellular bridges that interconnect epithelial cells of the skin (e.g., oral and vaginal mucosa). Microtubules are integral parts of cilia, which are specialized parts of the cell surface that have the ability to move and propel the cell (e.g., sperm) or to move the external secretions of the cell. For example, mucus is moved by the cilia of the bronchial ciliated cells; dysfunction of these cilia may predispose an individual to bronchial infection (bronchitis).

The external surface of the plasma membrane serves as the site of contact between the cell and the environment. This interaction between the cell and the environment is maintained through the action of specialized portions of the cell membrane that serve as receptors, adhesion molecules, transducers of signals, or metabolic channels. The complexity of the plasma membrane varies from one cell type to another.

The plasma membrane of cells is a living structure that is maintained by active expenditure of energy. The structural integrity of the plasma membrane is a prerequisite for the maintenance of all essential cellular functions. Rupture or major damage of the cell membrane that cannot be repaired invariably leads to cell death.

Integration and Coordination of Cell Functions and Response to Injury

Integration of Function of Normal Cells

Cells of the human body are arranged into tissue, and these tissues form organs. Organs are part of organ systems, all of which function in concert to

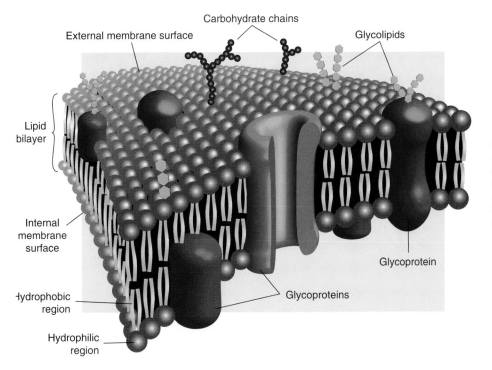

External membrane surface

Carbohydrate chains

Glycolipids

Lipid bilayer

Internal membrane surface

Hydrophobic region

Hydrophilic region

Glycoprotein

Glycoproteins

FIGURE 1-6
Plasma membrane. The bilipid layer also contains proteins and carbohydrates, which perform complex functions and serve as receptors, adhesion molecules, and transducers of signals.

meet the basic vital requirements of the body and to enable it to perform many complex functions. The integration of cells, tissues, and organs into functional units is achieved through several mechanisms, best illustrated by the response of cells to growth-stimulating factors (Fig. 1-7).

The simplest form of integration occurs at the level of single cells. For example, T lymphocytes secrete interleukin-2 (IL-2), a cytokine, which serves as lymphocytes' and some other cells' own growth factor. This self-stimulation, known as an *autocrine stimulation,* is feasible because T lymphocytes have surface receptors for their own secretory product. IL-2

FIGURE 1-7
Integration of cell functions occurs through interaction with other cells in the body. (A) Autocrine stimulation. Secretions from the cell may attach to the cell's own surface receptors, providing autocrine stimulation. (B) Paracrine stimulation. Closely adjacent cells act upon each other. (C) Endocrine stimulation. Hormones secreted by endocrine cells reach target cells via the blood.

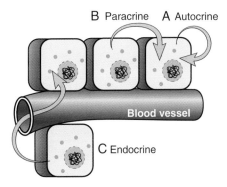

B Paracrine   A Autocrine

Blood vessel

C Endocrine

that is released from the cell binds to the surface of the same cells and stimulates its receptors to transmit signals for cell growth.

More complex integration of cells requires transmission of hormonal signals from one cell to another. This is done by the release of mediators from one cell and their uptake by another, a process called *paracrine stimulation.* Paracrine stimulation is typically mediated by biogenic amines (e.g., epinephrine) and neuropeptide hormones (e.g., glucagon, gastrin). The best example is the release of hydrochloric acid from chief gastric cells under the influence of gastrin. Gastrin is a hormone released from neuroendocrine G cells, which are located in the gastric mucosa, adjacent to the hydrochloric acid–secreting chief cells. Gastrin extruded from neuroendocrine cells attaches to receptors on the chief cells, triggering hydrochloric acid release.

Endocrine stimulation is achieved by hormones released into the blood circulation. This is clearly a higher form of integration of cell functions, as it may involve cells in several anatomically distinct organs. For example, insulin secreted by the islet cells of the pancreas affects the liver, muscle, fat cells, and many others. A similarly high level of integration of cell functions can be achieved by *neural stimulation.* The central and autonomic nervous systems are the ultimate coordinators of body functions. Without the central nervous system, humans would not be what they are.

From the point of view of cell pathology, each cell is best considered as a distinct functional unit in a defined *internal milieu* (from *milieu interieur,* the

French word for inside environment). In order to maintain its life and normal functions, the cell must be in *homeostasis* with its environment. **Homeostasis** (derived from the Greek words *homoios* [steady], and *stasis* [state]) is defined as state of balance between opposing pressures operating in and around a cell or tissue. From the environment, the cell receives nutrients, oxygen, water, and essential minerals. The cell generates energy by burning up some of the calories derived from the nutrients. This energy is used for the upkeep of the nucleus, and the integrity and function of the cytoplasm, cell organelles, and plasma membranes. By maintaining its own integrity, the cell contributes to the stability of the internal milieu. A normal internal milieu is essential for the normal function of the cell; likewise, the milieu remains normal only if all the cells are functioning properly. The cells and their internal milieu are interdependent.

The supply of essential minerals and water in which these minerals are dissolved is also of paramount importance for the maintenance of homeostasis. The essential minerals include sodium, chloride, potassium, calcium, and iron. Magnesium, zinc, copper, selenium—known as *oligominerals* because they are needed in minute amounts—are also required. The oligominerals are essential for the function of several important enzymes.

The cell is also critically dependent on a constant supply of oxygen and nutrients, provided to cells by circulation of the fluids that surround cells. At the same time, the circulating fluids carry away the degradation products of cellular metabolism.

When an equilibrium between the cells and their environment is achieved and maintained, the cells are said to be in a *steady state* (Fig. 1-8). External stimuli may alter this equilibrium. If the demands are increased, the cell may shift its metabolism to a higher level, achieving a new steady state. Similarly, the cell may shift to a lower steady state if the demands are decreased. In both instances, the adaptation is temporary, and the cell may revert to the original steady state after the external demands cease. However, if the demands exceed the capacity of the cell to adapt, a permanent disequilibrium may ensue. Like a pulled muscle that has exceeded its ability to stretch and has ruptured and cannot contract any more, the cell that has passed beyond the *point of no return* has been irreparably damaged and cannot return to the original steady state. Such a cell cannot maintain homeostasis and will die.

Reversible Cell Injury

If the adverse environmental influences evoke a cellular response that remains within the range of homeostasis, the changes produced are called *reversible cell injury*. Cessation of injury results in the return of the cell to the original steady state.

Reversible cell injury is typically mild or short-lived. It can be induced by exposure to toxins in low concentration. Brief hypoxia or anoxia (i.e., decreased oxygen supply or complete deprivation of oxygen) can induce the same changes, which are best described as swelling of the cytoplasm (Fig. 1-9).

Cellular swelling, known as *hydropic* or *vacuolar degeneration*, reflects an increased influx of water into the cytoplasm. The water crosses the plasma membrane and enters the hyaloplasm, but also accumulates within the mitochondria ("mitochondrial

FIGURE 1-8
Steady state. The range of the steady state is determined by the reactivity of each cell and the ability of the cells to respond to increased demands or stimuli. The increased or decreased functional adaptations are reversible. However, once response passes beyond the point of no return, the cell injury becomes irreversible.

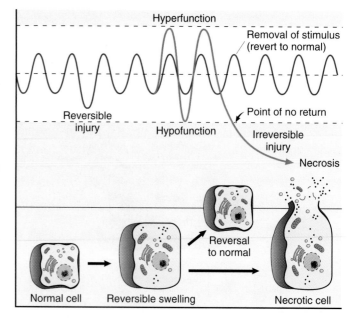

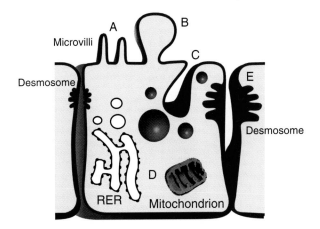

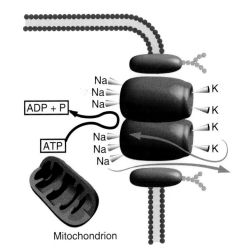

FIGURE 1-9
Cellular swelling. (A) Normal microvilli. (B) Swollen microvilli are the consequence of an influx of water in the cytoplasm. (C) Invagination of the cell membrane gives rise to fluid-filled cytoplasmic vacuoles which account, in part, for the changes known as "vacuolar degeneration." (D) Swollen mitochondria and dilated rough endoplasmic reticulum (RER) are also part of vacuolar degeneration. (E) Swollen cells lose contact with adjacent cells at the site of cell-to-cell junctions, like desmosomes.

FIGURE 1-10
Plasma membrane semipermeability is a function of the Na$^+$, K$^+$-ATPase pump. ADP, adenosine diphosphate; ATP, adenosine triphosphate; P, phosphorus.

swelling") and membrane-bound vacuoles formed from the invaginations of the plasma membrane and endoplasmic reticulum. This vacuolization of the cytoplasm is best appreciated by electron microscopy. After the insult is over, the cell recovers by pumping out the water, reverting from the state of vacuolar degeneration to the original steady state.

The pathogenesis of cellular swelling is relatively easy to explain in terms of altered permeability of the plasma membrane. The plasma membrane is a selectively permeable membrane that maintains gradient in the concentration of minerals—primarily, sodium (Na$^+$), potassium (K$^+$), and chloride (Cl$^-$)—inside and outside of the cell. This is achieved through the function of the Na$^+$, K$^+$-adenosine triphosphatase (ATPase) pump, which acts as a sodium pump, constantly pumping Na ions from the cytoplasm into the extracellular space (Fig. 1-10). Chloride generally follows Na ions, which are in counterbalance with K ions. Accordingly, the concentration of Na$^+$, Cl$^-$ is higher in the extracellular space than in the cytoplasm, whereas the concentration of K$^+$ is higher inside than outside the cell. Because the ATPase is fueled by high energy compounds like adenosine triphosphate (ATP), anoxia or any other form of energy deprivation will cause dysfunction of this enzyme. Without functioning ATPase, the cell membrane loses its capacity to maintain the gradient of intracellular and extracellular minerals. A high concentration of sodium in the extracellular space will result in an influx of sodium and chloride into the cell. This is followed by an influx of water and

concomitant cellular swelling. Once ATPase function is restored, the sodium and the water are pumped out of the cell and the swelling disappears.

Reversible cell injury is associated with many functional changes (Fig. 1-11). We will mention only the most important ones. Swollen mitochondria generate less energy. Instead of oxidative ATP production, the cell reverts to less efficient anaerobic glycolysis, which also results in excessive production of lactic acid. The pH of the cell becomes acidic, which further slows down the entire cell metabolism. The consequent dilatation and fragmentation of RER and the loss of membrane-attached ribosomes ("degranulation of the RER") result in decreased protein synthesis. Swollen organelles tend to disintegrate, and their membranes curl up into concentric bodies called myelin figures. If the hydrolytic lysosomal enzymes leak from overdistended phagosomes into the acidified cytoplasm, considerable damage may ensue. However, if the nucleus remains unscathed and if the energy source is restored or toxic injury is neutralized, the cell will revert to its normal state.

Irreversible Cell Injury

Cells exposed to heavy doses of toxins, severe hypoxia or anoxia, or other overwhelming insults cannot recover from the injury, hence the term **irreversible cell injury.** Morphologically, irreversible cell injury may be recognized by typical changes in the nucleus or by a loss of cell integrity and rupture of the cell membrane. Functional tests will show that the nuclear functions have been disrupted; the energy production within mitochondria has fallen below the essential minimum needed for cell func-

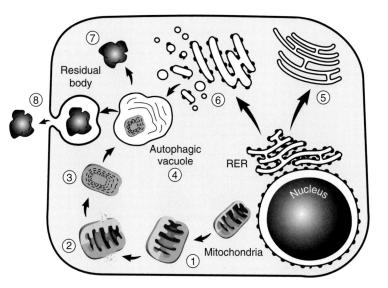

FIGURE 1-11
Cytoplasmic changes in reversible cell injury. Mito-chondria are swollen and some of them have rup-tured. The rough endoplasmic reticulum (RER) shows dilatation and degranulation. The number of phago-somes is increased. Myelin figures are formed from membranes of damaged organelles.

tion and cannot be restored to normal levels; and the plasma membrane functions are irrevocably lost.

Irreversible cell injury is characterized by typical ultrastructural changes, many of which can be recognized by light microscopy as well. The most characteristic are *nuclear changes;* clearly, without a viable nucleus, the cell cannot survive. Damage to the nucleus can present in three forms:

- *Pyknosis,* marked by condensation of the chromatin (*pyknos* means dense in Greek).
- *Karyorrhexis,* characterized by fragmentation into smaller particles, colloquially called "nuclear dust." (Karyorrhexis is a term derived from the Greek words *karyon,* meaning nucleus, and *rrhexis,* meaning disruption.)
- *Karyolysis,* which involves dissolution of nuclear structure and lysis of chromatin by enzymes, such as DNAase and RNAase (Fig. 1-12).

Dead cells release their contents into the extracellular fluid, whereby they reach the circulation and are washed away. Cytoplasmic enzymes, like aspartate aminotransferase (AST) or lactate dehydrogenase (LDH), which are released from damaged cells, can be measured in blood and are clinically useful signs of cell injury. Levels of AST and LDH are typically elevated in the serum of patients with myocardial infarct or viral hepatitis.

Causes of Cell Injury

Cell injury may be induced by numerous pathogenetic mechanisms, the most important of which are hypoxia, toxins, microbial pathogens, endogenous mediators of inflammation and immune reactions, and genetic/metabolic disturbances. Depending on the severity of the insult, the cell injury may be reversible or irreversible. The causes of cell injury

as they relate to pathogenesis are listed, together with clinical examples, in Table 1-2.

Hypoxia/Anoxia. *Hypoxia,* a reduced availability of oxygen, and *anoxia,* the complete lack of oxygen, are among the most important and most common causes of cell injury. Oxygen is essential for cellular respiration, and a lack of oxygen results in cessation of energy production. Without energy, the cell cannot survive. Short-term anoxia induces reversible cell injury. However, if the oxygen supply is interrupted for long periods of time, the injury becomes irreversible. Of course, not all cells respond the same way to injury, and the final outcome of anoxia will depend on many factors. For example, brain cells cannot survive without oxygen for more than a few

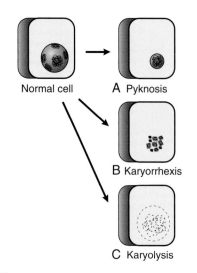

FIGURE 1-12
Nuclear changes in irreversible cell injury. (A) Pyknosis (condensation of chromatin). (B) Karyorrhexis (fragmentation of nucleus). (C) Karyolysis (lysis of chromatin).

Table 1-2 Major Causes of Cell Injury

Cause	Pathogenesis	Clinical Examples
Hypoxia/anoxia	Circulatory disturbances	Myocardial infarct
	Inadequate oxygen intake	Strangulation
Toxin	Direct toxicity	Mercury poisoning
	Indirect toxicity	Carbon tetrachloride poisoning
Microbes	Bacterial exotoxins	Food poisoning
	Direct (viral) cytopathic effect	Viral infection
	Indirect (immune-mediated cytotoxicity)	
Inflammation and immune reactions	Action of cytokines and complements	Autoimmune diseases
Genetic/metabolic disorders	Disruption of metabolic pathways	Lysosomal storage disease (e.g., Tay-Sachs disease)
	Abnormal metabolism	Diabetes

minutes, heart cells can survive 1 to 2 hours, and kidney cells can survive for several hours. Connective tissue cells are most resistant to anoxia; indeed, viable fibroblasts can be obtained from a cadaver even 1 day after death.

In clinical practice, hypoxia or anoxia may occur under many circumstances (Fig. 1-13), including (1) obstruction of the respiratory tubes (e.g., suffocation secondary to drowning); (2) inadequate transport of oxygen across the respiratory surfaces of the lung (e.g., pneumonia); (3) inadequate transport of oxygen in the blood (e.g., anemia); or (4) an inability of the cell to use oxygen for cellular respiration (e.g., cyanide poisoning). Cyanide inhibits oxidative enzymes in the cell and prevents oxidative phosphorylation.

Short-lived reversible cell injury secondary to hypoxia may be repaired completely upon reoxygenation. For example, a patient who suffers a heart block and loses consciousness as a result of brain anoxia can resume a normal life if resuscitation is timely and adequate. Ischemic myocardial injury caused by coronary artery thrombosis can be minimized, and sometimes even completely prevented, by the angioplastic removal of the thrombus with thrombolytic enzymes. However, reoxygenation of the tissue carries an additional risk because the oversupply of oxygen may have a deleterious effect on the reversibly damaged cells (Fig. 1-14). Oxygen toxicity results in such cases from activated *oxygen radicals*. These toxic compounds are formed in tissues in several ways from oxygen activated by ionized iron or in chemical reactions that produce hydrogen peroxide (H_2O_2) and superoxide (O_2^-). Under normal circumstances, these activated oxygen radicals are formed in small amounts and are inactivated by the cellular enzymatic scavenger mechanisms. However, if the oxygen consumption in the tissues is decreased and the scavenger enzyme systems (e.g., catalase or superoxide dismutase) are inoperational, excessive formation of oxygen radicals may result in additional tissue loss. In patients with myocardial infarction, this is called *post-perfusion myocardial injury*.

Toxic Injury. *Toxic injury* may be induced by substances known for their *direct* toxic effects on cells, as well as by those that are not directly toxic, but

FIGURE 1-13

The major causes of hypoxia-anoxia include (1) interruption of the oxygen supply; (2) inhibition of blood oxygenation in the lungs; (3) inadequate transport of oxygen in circulation; and (4) inhibition of cellular respiration.

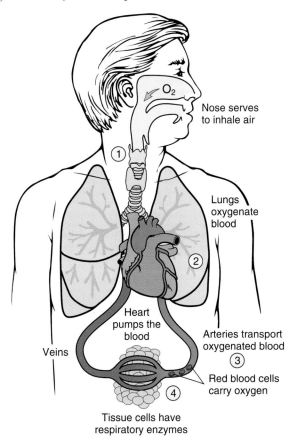

O_2

Nose serves to inhale air

①

Lungs oxygenate blood

②

Heart pumps the blood

Veins

Arteries transport oxygenated blood ③

Red blood cells carry oxygen

④

Tissue cells have respiratory enzymes

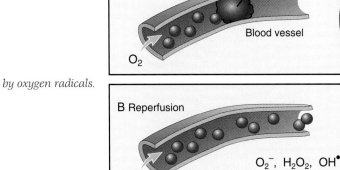

FIGURE 1-14
Post-perfusion injury by oxygen radicals.

must be metabolically activated to become toxins (*indirect toxicity*). Heavy metals, like mercury, are *directly* toxic because they inactivate cytoplasmic enzymes by disrupting the sulfhydryl (S-S) groups that hold the polypeptide chains of an enzyme together in an active state. Carbon tetrachloride (CCl_4), a component of commercial metal-cleaning solutions (metal polish), is the best studied *indirect* toxin. Upon ingestion, CCl_4 is metabolized to $CCl_3^{\cdot}$, which acts as a toxic free radical, damaging cell membranes.

Many drugs and their metabolites cause cell injury, especially if given in large amounts. Although the mechanism of cell injury varies from one drug to another, the end results are usually comparable. However, since various drugs affect various organs, the clinical presentations vary considerably. The effect of drugs is also dose-dependent. In large amounts, most drugs may be toxic and many are even lethal. Suicide by drug overdose is probably the best example of drug-induced toxicity.

Microbial Pathogens. *Microbial pathogens* cause cell injury in several ways. Bacteria most often produce *toxins,* which may inhibit various cell functions, such as respiration or protein synthesis. For example, food poisoning from spoiled, unrefrigerated, leftover food is caused by bacterial exotoxins.

Viruses that are directly cytopathic invade cells and "kill from within" by disturbing various cellular processes or by disrupting the integrity of the nucleus and/or plasma membrane (Fig. 1-15). Other viruses that are not directly cytopathic integrate themselves into the cellular genome. These viruses encode the production of foreign proteins, which are exposed on the cell surface and recognized by the body's immune cells, which react to any protein perceived as foreign. Viral antigens elicit an immune response that eventually kills the infected cells as if they were foreign to the body.

Mediators of Inflammatory and Immune Reactions. *Mediators of inflammation and immune reactions,* such as lymphokines, cytokines, or complement proteins, may injure cells in several ways. These biologically active substances are produced by the body in response to infection or in various immune reactions. Although such substances are valuable for eliminating the infectious agents, often, they kill not only the microbes, but the body's own cells as well. These substances are discussed in greater detail in Chapters 2 and 3.

Genetic/Metabolic Disturbances. *Genetic/metabolic disturbances* are important causes of cell injury. Many of the genetic inborn errors of metabolism cause disturbances of intermediate metabolism and subsequent accumulation of toxic metabolites in the

Did You Know?

Potassium cyanide is a potent toxin and has been used as a poison. In Germany, during World War II, many high-ranking Nazi officials carried a capsule of cyanide placed into a hole in their teeth which they could use for suicide in case they were captured by allied soldiers. As you know from history, however, for whatever reasons, the Nazi suicide plan was never implemented, and most such German officials were captured alive.

Cyanide is found naturally in fruit pits. Apricot seeds were used by quack doctors for production of an alleged anticancer drug called laetrile. Laetrile did not cure any cancers, and it is not known how many patients developed cyanide toxicity from this so-called treatment.

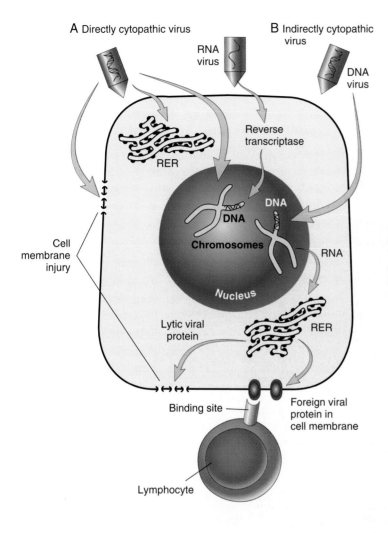

A Directly cytopathic virus

B Indirectly cytopathic virus

RNA virus

DNA virus

Reverse transcriptase

RER

DNA

DNA

Chromosomes

RNA

Nucleus

Cell membrane injury

Lytic viral protein

RER

Binding site

Foreign viral protein in cell membrane

Lymphocyte

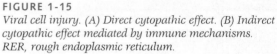

FIGURE 1-15
Viral cell injury. (A) Direct cytopathic effect. (B) Indirect cytopathic effect mediated by immune mechanisms. RER, rough endoplasmic reticulum.

cells. For example, in Tay-Sachs disease (a genetic deficiency of hexosaminidase A), gangliosides accumulate in the lysosomes of nerve cells and eyes. Severe mental deficiency and blindness develop, and the patients usually die in early childhood.

Metabolic disturbances of adulthood also may cause various forms of cell injury, some of which are direct and some of which are indirect. For example, diabetes mellitus, a disease caused by insulin deficiency, produces pathologic changes in the small blood vessels. Vessel wall injury leads to tissue ischemia and pathologic changes in many, if not all, organs of the body.

Cell Adaptations

Prolonged exposure of cells to adverse or exaggerated normal stimuli evokes various adaptations at the level of individual cells, tissues, or organs. Once the cause is removed, most cells that have adapted to chronic stimulation revert to normalcy again. However, some forms of adaptation, especially those associated with cell loss (e.g., bone loss in osteoporosis), are irreversible.

Atrophy

Atrophy denotes a decrease in the size of a cell, tissue, organ, or the entire body. Like all adaptations, atrophy can be classified as physiologic or pathologic.

Physiologic atrophy occurs with age and involves essentially the entire body. For example, in the brain, a certain number of cells is lost every day from birth onward; over the years, this results in a decrease in the entire brain. An atrophic brain has narrow gyri and widened sulci (Fig. 1-16). On cross sections, the ventricles appear to be dilated and contain more cerebrospinal fluid than normal (*hydrocephalus ex vacuo*), compensating for the loss of cerebral tissue. The atrophic bones of elderly people are thin and are thus more prone to fracture, and the atrophic muscles of this population are thin and weak.

Physiologic atrophy is not limited to very old age. The thymus undergoes physiologic atrophy during childhood, and only traces of thymic tissue are found after puberty. The ovaries, uterus, and breasts atrophy after menopause.

Pathologic atrophy typically occurs as a result of

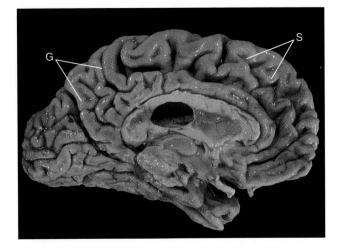

FIGURE 1-16
Atrophic brain. The gyri (G) are narrow and the sulci (S) are wide.

inadequate nutrition or stimulation. Ischemic organs are typically small, as, for example, kidneys affected by atherosclerosis (*nephroangiosclerosis*). Denervated muscles (e.g., leg muscles after spinal cord injury) are atrophic and flaccid. The general cachexia caused by cancer or malnutrition is marked by muscle wastage and atrophy of muscle fibers.

Atrophy causes functional deficits that are proportional to the degree of atrophy. Most serious con-

Did You Know?

We are all born with a finite number of nerve cells in our brains. It has been estimated that we lose thousands of nerve cells every day. Because nerve cells cannot regenerate, this loss results in gradual atrophy of the brain. But don't be concerned. Although many old people have "lost it" and are not as astute as when they were young, many others continue to function normally into their eighties and nineties.

Loss of brain substance does not leave holes in the head. Instead, the space formed by atrophy of the brain gyri is filled with cerebrospinal fluid (CSF) that normally bathes the brain. The lateral ventricles of the brain also dilate and contain increasing amounts of CSF, a phenomenon termed *hydrocephalus ex vacuo.* Physicians used to say that the "body abhors empty space," or in Latin, that there is a *horror vacui.* Increased amounts of CSF in the head of a person who has atrophy of the brain is just a compensatory mechanism, an expression of *horror vacui.*

Brain atrophy can be demonstrated by modern x-ray techniques using computed tomography, also known as CT scanning.

sequences are related to an irreversible loss of cells, as in the brains of elderly individuals. Brain atrophy often leads to senile dementia, which is clinically manifested in more than 50 percent of people older than 85 years of age.

Hypertrophy and Hyperplasia

Hypertrophy is an increase in the size of tissues or organs owing to an enlargement of individual cells. By contrast, *hyperplasia* is an increase in the size of tissues and organs caused by an increased number of cells (Fig. 1-17). Hypertrophy and hyperplasia are often combined. Pure hypertrophy occurs only in the heart and striated muscles, as these organs consist of cells that cannot divide.

Hypertrophy of the heart is a common pathologic finding that occurs as an adaptation of heart muscle to increased workload (Fig. 1-18). Hypertrophy of the left ventricle of the heart is a typical complication of hypertension. The increased pressure in the outflow side of the left ventricle requires more force to be overcome, and this is achieved by hypertrophy of muscle fibers. Similar hypertrophy can occur following narrowing of the aortic orifice (*aortic stenosis*) secondary to chronic valvular disease (*endocarditis*), which interferes with the normal flow of blood. Hypertrophic heart cells increase in size. Such cells contain more myofilaments, which allows them to contract more efficiently. *Hypertrophy of skeletal muscles* is commonly induced by exercise and is typically found in body builders.

Hypertrophy with hyperplasia occurs under a variety of conditions. For example, smooth muscle cells in the wall of the urinary bladder, when obstructed by a hyperplastic prostate, increase in size and number. This contributes to thickening of the wall of the urinary bladder (Fig. 1-19). Physiologic hypertrophy of uterine smooth muscle cells during pregnancy is also accompanied by hyperplasia.

Pure **hyperplasia** typically occurs as a result of hormonal stimulation. For example, when continuously stimulated by estrogen, the endometrium may become very thick (*endometrial hyperplasia*). Histologic examination reveals an increased number of glandular and stromal cells. In benign prostatic hyperplasia (a common cause of prostatic enlargement in the elderly which is also hormonally induced), hyperplasia of epithelial and stromal cells leads to the formation of grossly visible nodules.

Hyperplasia may also occur in response to chronic injury. In some cases, the cause is obvious. For example, tight shoes may cause chronic irritation of the skin. In such cases, the epidermal cells undergo hyperplasia and form a *callus* or corn. However, some hyperplastic lesions have no obvious cause and probably represent early neoplasia. Exam-

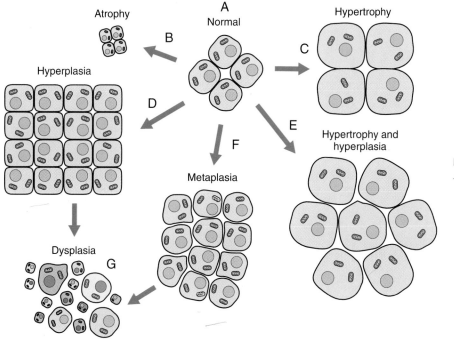

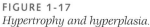

FIGURE 1-17
Hypertrophy and hyperplasia.

ples of such lesions are *hyperplastic polyps* of the large intestine and foci of *nodular hyperplasia* in the liver. Some forms of *endometrial hyperplasia* are also preneoplastic and, if left untreated, may progress to neoplasia.

Metaplasia

Metaplasia is a form of adaptation characterized by the change of one cell type into another. For example, columnar cells of the bronchial mucosa, when irritated by cigarette smoke, change into stratified squamous epithelium.

Metaplasia represents a reversible change. If the smoker stops smoking, the squamous epithelium will revert back to ciliated columnar cells. If the stimulus that has induced squamous metaplasia persists (i.e.,

if the smoker does not stop smoking), the squamous metaplasia may progress to *dysplasia*. In contrast to the regular layering of normal squamous cells that is typical of metaplasia, dysplasia is characterized by a disorderly arrangement of cells and nuclear atypia. Dysplasia may still be reversible if the stimulus is discontinued, but more often than not, it progresses to *neoplasia* (discussed in Chapter 4).

FIGURE 1-19
Hypertrophy and hyperplasia of the smooth muscle cells in an obstructed urinary bladder. The wall is thick and appears to be trabeculated because the smooth muscle bundles protrude into its lumen.

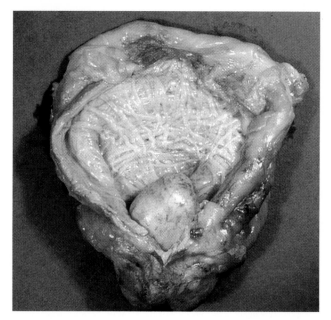

FIGURE 1-18
Hypertrophy of the left ventricle of the heart caused by hypertension.

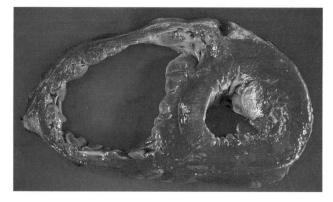

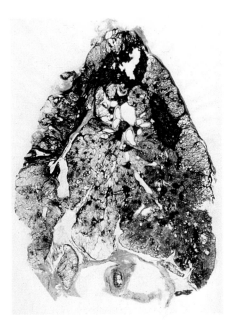

FIGURE 1-20
Anthracosis. The lung contains black pigment, mostly coal particles.

Intracellular Accumulations

Intracellular accumulations may occur as a result of an overload of various metabolites or exogenous material, or they may be attributable to metabolic disturbances that prevent excretion of metabolic by-products or normal secretions from cells. In most instances, the underlying mechanisms are complex and involve both an overload and underexcretion/underutilization.

Anthracosis (accumulation of coal particles) (Fig. 1-20) is the best example of exogenous material accumulation. Severe anthracosis is seen in the lungs of people who work in coal mines. Coal particles are released into the air from chimneys; in essence, any air pollution could cause anthracosis.

Hemosiderosis is an accumulation of blood-derived brown pigment called hemosiderin (derived from the Greek word *haima*, blood, and *sideros*, iron). Hemosiderin is usually derived from hemolyzed blood. Remember that red blood cells contain iron-rich hemoglobin which disintegrates into globin and heme. Heme gives rise to micelles of ferritin, which aggregate into hemosiderin. Iron in hemosiderin can be demonstrated in tissues with the so-called Prussian blue reaction.

Lipid accumulation in the liver is an example of intracellular accumulation of intermediate metabolites. Fat is normally stored in liver cells in the form of triglycerides. Obese people have fatty livers owing to an overload of fat. Fat accumulation in the liver is a typical finding in alcoholics.

As shown in Figure 1-21, alcohol stimulates accumulation of fat in the liver through several mechanisms. The fat is derived, in part, from free fatty acids mobilized from peripheral stores at an accelerated rate. Alcohol has a high caloric content and serves as a substrate for new fat formation in liver cells. It also inhibits several degradation enzymes and the utilization of internal fat. Finally, it inhibits protein synthesis and the export of fat from the liver in the form of lipoproteins.

The clinical consequences of cytoplasmic storage are variable. For example, fatty change of liver cells has almost no functional consequences, and the accumulation of carbon particles in the lung and lymph node cells in anthracosis is also innocuous. On the other hand, congenital lysosomal storage diseases

FIGURE 1-21
Pathogenesis of alcoholic fatty liver. Triglycerides (TG) in the liver cell are formed through several mechanisms, all of which contribute to the accumulation of fat. (1) Increased influx of free fatty acids (FFA) from peripheral stores. (2) Increased neolipogenesis from glucose, amino acids, and alcohol. (3) Decreased utilization of triglycerides because of the inhibition of enzymes. (4) Decreased synthesis of apoprotein, which is essential for the formation of lipoproteins, reduces export of lipids from the liver.

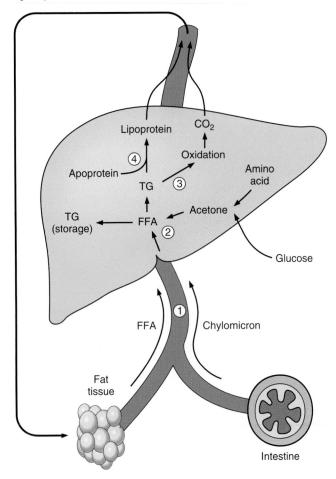

usually have serious and even lethal consequences. The neuronal changes induced by gangliosides in Tay-Sachs disease are irreversible and associated with profound mental retardation, neurologic symptoms, and death in infancy.

Aging

The aging of cells includes many complex adaptations and, unfortunately, many cellular events that are irreversible. Aging cannot be avoided or prevented, and the best we can do is to retard it or minimize its adverse effects on the body.

The process of aging is poorly understood. There are many theories of aging, none of which explains in full the essence of this complex biologic phenomenon. Everybody is aware of the remarkable differences between an old and a young person, but our understanding of these differences is still very shallow.

Scientists studying old age (gerontologists) favor two major hypotheses as an explanation for aging: the *wear-and-tear hypothesis* and the *genetic hypothesis.* Because cells represent the basic living units of all tissues and organs, it is thought that cellular aging represents the critical event in the aging of the organism, and that the decline of complex integrative and specialized functions of the body results from dysfunctions at the cellular level. In organs that are composed of cells that cannot regenerate, such as the brain and heart, the wear-and-tear hypothesis accounts, to a great extent, for the decline in function of these organs. However, as all people do not lose brain cells at the same speed, the genetic theory of aging also has merit. This hypothesis asserts that aging is a genetically predetermined process. Hormonal, immune, and neural theories that blame all the calamities of aging on the dysfunction of these integrative processes presently have few proponents.

Pathologic changes associated with aging vary from one individual to another. Overall, most organs undergo atrophy and have a reduced functional reserve. Resistance to infection declines with advancing age, whereas the incidence of cardiovascular diseases and cancer is increased. None of these changes is, however, unique to the elderly.

Death

Death, even more so than aging, is an inevitable feature of life. All the cells in the human body have a finite life span, and when it comes to an end, cells die. Some of the cells may be replaced from stem cells in that tissue, whereas others are irreplaceable. Heart cells belong to the latter category. However, even if all heart cells die, the life of a person can be ex-

Did You Know?

The Greek word *necros,* meaning dead, is also used to construct many other medical words. For example, the postmortem examination commonly performed by pathologists is called a *necropsy.* However, the same linguistic root can be found in other words as well. According to Greek mythology, *nectar,* sweet juice consumed by Greek gods, could bestow immortality. Nectarines, although good for our health are, unfortunately, not a remedy for our mortality.

tended today by heart transplantation. If the neural cells of the vital centers of the brain die, death is inevitable. Thus, we use the term *brain death* which, for legal purposes, means that a person cannot live any longer without artificial mechanical assistance provided by a respirator (artificial lung machine).

Cell Death

Cell death occurs in several forms. We have already mentioned that the irreversible cell injury caused by anoxia or toxins leads to cell death with typical nuclear changes (pyknosis, karyorrhexis, karyolysis), rupture of the cell membrane, and cessation of cellular respiration. This form of exogenously induced cell death is called *necrosis* (from the Greek term, *necros,* meaning dead). By contrast, *apoptosis* (Greek term for "dropping out") refers to endogenously programmed cell death. Necrosis and apoptosis represent the death of single cells or groups of cells within a living organism. Death of cells and tissues in a dead organism that occurs as a result of cessation of respiration and heart beat is called *autolysis* (from the Greek terms *autos,* meaning self, and *lysis,* meaning dissolution).

Necrosis

In contrast to autolysis, which is a postmortem event and is, therefore, of little significance for clinicians, **necrosis** is clinically important. It occurs in several forms: coagulative, liquefactive, caseous, and enzymatic fat necrosis.

Coagulative necrosis is the most common form of necrosis. It is called coagulative because the tissue appears like a solid mass of boiled meat in which the proteins are coagulated by heat. Coagulative necrosis is marked by rapid inactivation of cytoplasmic hy-

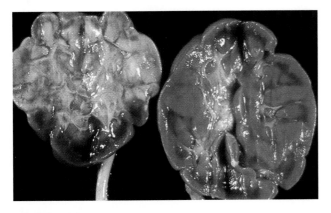

FIGURE 1-22
Coagulative necrosis of the kidney of an infant caused by ischemia. The necrotic area is pale yellow, in contrast to the normally perfused parenchyma of the kidney, which is reddish brown.

drolytic enzymes. This prevents lysis of tissues, which retain their original form and firm consistency. Coagulative necrosis typically involves solid internal organs such as the heart, liver, or kidneys (Fig. 1-22) and is most often caused by anoxia (e.g., myocardial infarct).

Liquefactive necrosis is characterized by the dissolution of tissues, which become soft and diffluent. It occurs most often in the brain. The brain cells lose their contours and are "liquefied" (i.e., transformed into semifluid mush). Liquefactive necrosis is typical of brain infarcts, which are usually soft and ultimately become transformed into a fluid-filled cavity (Fig. 1-23).

Coagulative necrosis may liquefy, usually through the action of leukocytes that invade the necrotic tissue to remove the dead cells. Leukocytes release lytic enzymes which, in turn, transform the solid tissue into liquid pus. Pus is a viscous yellow fluid composed of leukocytes and cell debris. Myocardial infarcts that initially show coagulative necrosis are invaded by leukocytes and undergo *secondary liquefaction,* usually 4 to 6 days after the blood vessel occlusion.

Caseous necrosis, which is typically found in tuberculosis, is a special form of coagulative necrosis with limited liquefaction. The center of a tuberculous granuloma becomes necrotic and the cells fall apart. The tissue is yellow-white and "cheesy," hence, the name caseous necrosis (in Latin, *caseum* means cheese). Caseous necrosis is not unique to tuberculosis, but may also be found in fungal infections, such as histoplasmosis.

Fat necrosis is a special form of liquefactive necrosis caused by the action of lipolytic enzymes. It is limited to fat tissue, usually around the pancreas. Pancreatic enzymes released into the adjacent fat tissue (e.g., after rupture of the pancreas caused by seat belt trauma following a traffic accident) degrade the fat into glycerol and free fatty acids. The free fatty acids rapidly bind with calcium, forming calcium soaps. The area of fat necrosis appears, therefore, like liquefied fat with whitish specks of calcium soap scattered throughout.

Necrotic tissue, especially that on extremities, may undergo secondary changes that produce specific morphologic features. Bacterial infection of coagulated tissue leads to inflammation and a secondary liquefaction that is clinically known as *wet gangrene.* If the necrotic tissue dries out, it becomes dark black and mummified, just as the ancient Egyptian mummies dried in the hot air of the sand desert. Such lesions are called *dry gangrene* (Fig. 1-24). Both forms of gangrene are most often seen on the toes and lower extremities and are usually caused by pe-

FIGURE 1-23
Cerebral infarct. The area of infarction is softened as a result of liquefaction necrosis.

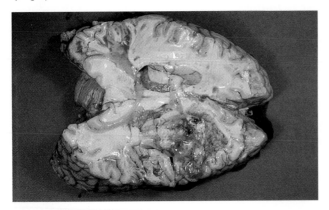

FIGURE 1-24
Dry gangrene of the toe.

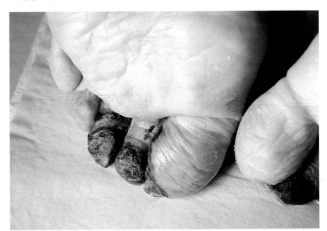

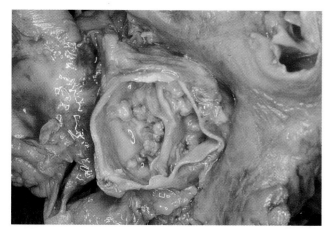

FIGURE 1-25
This calcified aortic valve is an example of dystrophic calcification.

ripheral vascular disease (atherosclerosis). Gangrene of the toes or the entire foot is especially common in diabetics.

Necrotic tissue attracts calcium salts and frequently undergoes calcification. Calcification of necrotic tissue is called *dystrophic calcification,* in contradistinction to *metastatic calcification,* which is typically a consequence of hypercalcemia. Dystrophic calcification is seen in atherosclerotic arteries, damaged heart valves (Fig. 1-25), or necrotic tumors. Metastatic calcification is a feature of metabolic hypercalcemia secondary to hyperparathyroidism or vitamin D toxicity. It most often involves the kidneys, presumably because the fluctuating pH levels in the renal parenchyma and the high concentration of calcium predispose the individual to deposition of calcium salts in the tissue.

Review Questions

1. What are the main components of the nucleus and the cytoplasm?
2. Which components of the cell contain RNA?
3. Compare mitochondria with endoplasmic reticulum and Golgi apparatus.
4. What is the difference between primary and secondary lysosomes, autophagosomes, and heterophagosomes?
5. Compare intermediate filaments with microfilaments and microtubules.
6. Explain autocrine, paracrine, and endocrine cell stimulation.
7. What is homeostasis?
8. How is cellular steady state maintained, and what does it mean when a cell reaches the point of no return?
9. Explain the pathogenesis of hydropic change and the role of Na^+, K^+-adenosine triphosphatase in cellular swelling.
10. What are the microscopic signs of irreversible cell injury?
11. Explain the pathogenesis of hypoxia or anoxia and give clinical examples of these conditions.
12. What are oxygen radicals and how do they damage cells?
13. How do toxins, microbes, and chemical mediators of inflammation kill cells?
14. Compare acute cell injury with cellular adaptations.
15. Compare atrophy with hypertrophy and hyperplasia and give clinical examples of each condition.
16. Explain the significance of smoking-induced metaplasia of the bronchial epithelium in the pathogenesis of bronchial neoplasia.
17. Compare anthracosis and hemosiderosis.
18. Explain the pathogenesis of fatty liver induced by alcohol.
19. Discuss the merits of the wear-and-tear and the genetic hypotheses of aging.
20. What is meant by the term brain death?
21. Compare the gross appearances of various forms of necrosis.
22. What is the difference between dry and wet gangrene?

Learning Objectives

After reading this chapter, the student should be able to:

1. Define inflammation.

2. List the main components of acute inflammation.

3. Describe the vascular changes in acute inflammation.

4. Describe the cellular events in acute inflammation.

5. Define the following terms pertaining to leukocytes involved in an inflammatory response: margination, diapedesis, emigration, exudation, chemotaxis, phagocytosis, and microbicidal substances.

6. List two cell-derived and three plasma-derived mediators of inflammation.

7. Explain the function of proteins of the complement system and the clotting system in inflammation.

8. Explain the role of arachidonic acid metabolites in inflammation.

9. Explain the main functions of cytokines released in inflammation.

10. Describe possible outcomes of acute inflammation.

11. Describe three pathogenetic pathways leading to chronic inflammation.

12. List the principal cells of acute and chronic inflammation.

13. Describe a granuloma and explain how it is formed.

14. Describe the typical complications of granulomatous inflammation.

15. Define the following pathologic terms: serous inflammation, fibrinous inflammation, purulent inflammation, abscess, ulcer, wound, scar, and keloid.

16. Describe the typical local and systemic symptoms of inflammation.

17. Explain the pathogenesis of fever.

18. Define healing and repair.

19. List three factors that may delay healing and repair.

20. List two complications of wound healing.

Additional Key Terms and Concepts

Abscess

Arachidonic acid

Chemotaxis

Complement

Granulation tissue

Granuloma

Pus

Scar

Ulceration

Chapter Outline

Inflammation
Chapter 2

Inflammation is a nonspecific but predictable response of living tissues, or the entire body, to injury. The injury may be caused by chemical agents, physical forces, living microbes, or many other physiologic or pathologic (exogenous or endogenous) stimuli that disturb the normal steady state. It is important to note the following with regard to inflammation:

- Inflammation includes a series of events that are interconnected, one with another. Thus, inflammation is a dynamic process, evolving through several phases which last from a few minutes to days or even months and years. Inflammation of sudden onset and short duration is characterized as *acute,* in contrast to *chronic* inflammation, which lasts a long time.
- Inflammation occurs only in multicellular organisms that are capable of mounting a neurovascular and cellular response to injury. Thus, in contrast to cell injury, which occurs at the level of single cells, inflammation is a coordinate reaction of the animal and human body, and it involves nerves, vessels, blood cells, and soluble mediators of inflammation.
- Inflammation has a *protective* role and is generally beneficial to the body. However, the side effects of inflammation may be *noxious.* For example, fever, which initially has a beneficial effect, may be so high that it may cause death. Sometimes the process may become *uncontrollable,* producing more harm than good. For example, pulmonary tuberculosis elicits a protective tissue reaction. This inflammatory response may erode pulmonary vessels and cause massive bleeding.
- Inflammation occurs only in living tissues. Necrotic or dead tissue cannot mount an inflammatory response. For example, a gangrenous foot cannot become inflamed. As the body cannot combat infection in necrotic tissue, a foot that is affected by gangrene must be amputated.

Did You Know?

A decomposing body of a child who froze to death in an unheated apartment was examined by a forensic pathologist. The skin showed numerous small holes. The forensic pathologist thought that these holes might have been caused by rats who tried to eat the dead body. Histologic examination showed signs of inflammation around every skin wound. The pathologist concluded that the animal bites must have occurred before death because inflammation is a "vital reaction," occurring only in living organisms.

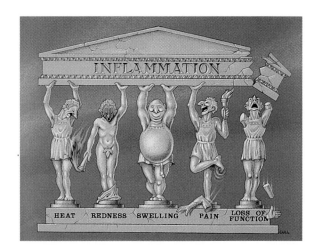

FIGURE 2-1
The cardinal signs of inflammation were described in Roman times. (Reprinted by permission of Professor Peter Cull, London University.)

From a forensic point of view, inflammation is considered to be a "vital reaction." If histologic signs of inflammation are found in tissues recovered at autopsy, this indicates that injury occurred before death, because inflammation cannot develop postmortem.

Signs of Inflammation

The Roman physician Celsus (~30 B.C. to 38 A.D.) described the four *cardinal signs* of inflammation: *calor* (heat), *rubor* (redness), *tumor* (swelling), and *dolor* (pain) (Fig. 2-1). Galen (130 A.D. to 200 A.D.), another Roman physician, is credited for adding *functio laesa,* or disturbed function, as the fifth classical symptom of inflammation. However, the pathology of inflammation remained poorly understood until the scientific advances of the 19th century made possible microscopic studies of inflamed tissues.

Today, we know that inflammation is a complex process that involves (1) changes in circulation of blood, (2) changes in vessel wall permeability, (3) a white blood cell response, and (4) the release of soluble mediators.

Pathogenesis of Inflammation

Circulatory Changes

Hemodynamic (vascular) changes—i.e., changes in blood flow—represent the body's first response to injury. The redness and swelling of the skin following a slap on the face or spanking are typical examples of such a vascular response. The mechanical

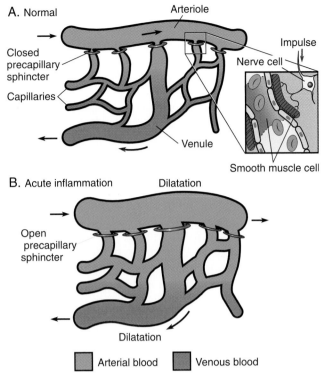

A. Normal

Arteriole

Closed precapillary sphincter

Capillaries

Venule

Impulse

Nerve cell

Smooth muscle cell

B. Acute inflammation

Dilatation

Open precapillary sphincter

Dilatation

Arterial blood

Venous blood

FIGURE 2-2

Circulatory changes in inflammation. Relaxation of the precapillary sphincter in the arterioles results in flooding of the capillary network and dilatation of capillaries and postcapillary venules.

is slow, which leads to *congestion* (the Latin root of which means "heaping together") and other hemodynamic changes. The sludged erythrocytes form stacks, called *rouleaux,* which impede the circulation even more, contributing to the turbulent flow of the blood. The white blood cells are marginalized and become attached to the endothelium, a phenomenon called *pavementing* (Fig. 2-3). These leukocytes develop elongated protrusions of their surface cytoplasm and become sticky, adhering to the endothelial cells lining the capillaries and particularly those of the postcapillary venules. This adhesion is accomplished by surface adhesion molecules, which are normally present on leukocytes and endothelial cells in an inactive form. During inflammation, the surface components of leukocytes and vascular cells are activated by soluble mediators of inflammation, the best known of which are the interleukins. Small amounts of interleukin are normally present in the blood. The concentration of interleukins is, however, increased at the site of inflammation. These mediators are derived in part from platelets and in part from leukocytes. The adhesion of leukocytes to the endothelial cells is one of the most common triggers for the release of mediators of inflammation. Platelets initiate clotting, which ultimately leads to formation of fibrin strands. These fibrin strands "anchor" the leukocytes to the vessel wall and prevent them from moving away.

stimulus stimulates nerves that transmit signals to smooth muscle cells on precapillary arterioles. The smooth muscle cells act as sphincters, regulating the inflow of blood into the capillaries (Fig. 2-2).

The relaxation of smooth muscle cells allows the blood to rush into the capillaries, and this accounts for the redness, swelling, and warmth of the tissue. The first response of arterioles to an injurious stimulus is vasoconstriction, which lasts only a few seconds. This is followed by vasodilatation (i.e., relaxation of the precapillary sphincter), which results in flooding of the capillary network with arterial blood, manifested by redness and mild swelling of the tissue engorged by blood. The arterial blood is warm, and because it is pumped into the area in large quantities, the inflamed tissue also becomes warm. This is called *hyperemia* (from Greek, meaning "too much blood"). The influx of blood dilates the capillaries, which consist only of endothelial cells and a basement membrane and thus cannot actively regulate blood flow. From the capillaries, the pressure is transmitted to venules, which also do not have a capacity to contract. Increased pressure in the capillaries and venules forces plasma filtration through the vessel wall, leading to edema.

The blood flow in dilated capillaries and venules

FIGURE 2-3

Cellular changes in inflammation. (1) Margination of neutrophils brings these inflammatory cells in close contact with the endothelium. (2) Adhesion of platelets results in the release of mediators of inflammation and coagulation. Fibrin strands are the first signs of clot formation. (3) Pavementing of leukocytes is mediated by adhesion molecules activated by the mediators of inflammation released from platelets and leukocytes. RBC, red blood cells.

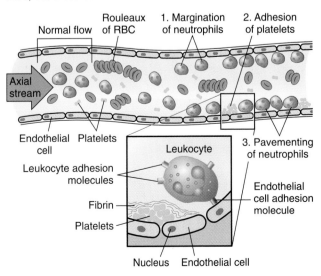

Normal flow

Rouleaux of RBC

1. Margination of neutrophils

2. Adhesion of platelets

Axial stream

Endothelial cell

Platelets

Leukocyte adhesion molecules

Fibrin

Platelets

Leukocyte

3. Pavementing of neutrophils

Endothelial cell adhesion molecule

Nucleus

Endothelial cell

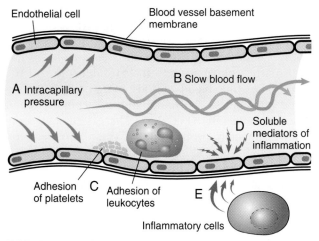

FIGURE 2-4
Increased permeability of blood vessels, the most important causes of which are increased intracapillary pressure (A), relative hypoxia secondary to slow blood flow (B), adhesion of leukocytes and platelets to endothelial cells (C), the action of soluble mediators of inflammation in the plasma (D), and mediators of inflammation released from inflammatory cells in the tissue surrounding the blood vessel (E).

Vessel Wall Changes

The permeability of the vessel wall of capillaries and postcapillary venules changes in response to inflammation owing to (1) increased pressure inside the congested blood vessels; (2) slowing of the circulation, which reduces the supply of oxygen and nutrients to endothelial cells; (3) adhesion of leukocytes and platelets to endothelial cells; and (4) the release of soluble mediators of inflammation from inflammatory cells, platelets, endothelial cells, and plasma (Fig. 2-4).

Mediators of Inflammation

The following brief summary contains three primary messages about the **chemical mediators of inflammation:**

1. The mediators of inflammation belong to two classes: plasma-derived and cell-derived substances. Plasma-derived mediators circulate in an inactive form and must be transformed into an active form by an activator. There are numerous specific and nonspecific activators. All activators have natural inactivators keeping them in balance. The cell-derived mediators may be preformed and stored in granules of platelets and leukocytes, or they may be synthesized *de novo* on demand. Preformed mediators (e.g., histamine) are released quickly, whereas the others require time to be produced and are released after a lag period.

2. Mediators of inflammation are biochemically heterogeneous. The most important are biogenic amines (e.g., histamine), peptides (e.g., bradykinin, complement), and arachidonic acid derivatives (e.g., prostaglandins).

3. Mediators of inflammation are multifunctional and thus have numerous effects on blood vessels, inflammatory cells, and other cells in the body. The most important effects relevant to an understanding of inflammation are vasodilatation or vasoconstriction, altered vascular permeability, activation of inflammatory cells, chemotaxis, cytotoxicity, degradation of tissue, pain, and fever.

Histamine. Early in inflammation, the vessels become leaky because of the action of biogenic amines, like histamine, and inflammatory polypeptides, like bradykinin. Histamine that is released from platelets and mast cells and basophils provokes a contraction of the endothelial cells of venules. This leads to formation of gaps, which increase blood vessel permeability and allow fluids and blood cells to exit into the interstitial spaces. This effect occurs quickly but lasts less than half an hour because histamine is rapidly inactivated by histaminase. It is, therefore, called an *immediate transient reaction.*

Bradykinin. Bradykinin, a plasma protein formed through the action of the enzyme kallikrein on its precursor kininogen, has effects similar to those of histamine, but these become evident at a slower pace (in Greek, *bradys* means slow, and *kinein* means acting). Bradykinin is formed in the plasma through the activation of Hageman factor, also known as coagulation factor XII. Hageman factor is also an activator of intravascular coagulation and plasminogen. The latter acts as a thrombolytic factor and also activates the complement system (Fig. 2-5). Apparently, this important initiator of inflammation leads to activation of several biological systems in the circulating blood, all of which may act on the wall of blood vessels, as well as the inflammatory cells, to amplify and sustain the response to injury. Finally, bradykinin is ca-

FIGURE 2-5
Activation of Hageman factor leads to increased vascular permeability, clotting, and thrombolysis.

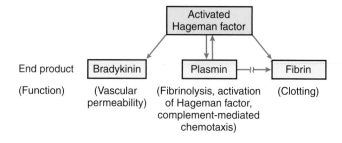

pable of inciting pain, and is one of the mediators of inflammation that account for *dolor,* the fourth cardinal sign of inflammation.

Complement System. Another important source of mediators of inflammation is the complement system, consisting of several proteins that are activated in a cascade, acting one upon another. These complement proteins are numbered from 1 to 9 (e.g., C1, C5, C9). Activation of the complement cascade can occur through two pathways. The *classical* pathway is typically activated by antigen-antibody complexes formed in immune reactions. It can also be initiated by some proteolytic enzymes, or by uric acid in gout. The *alternate* pathway is activated by bacterial endotoxins, fungi, snake venom, and some other substances. Both pathways converge toward a common terminal pathway (Fig. 2-6), which finally leads to the formation of the membrane attack complex (MAC). The MAC is enzymatically active and is able to destroy cells by literally boring holes in membranes. For example, in hemolytic anemia, MAC perforates the cell membrane of red blood cells and causes their lysis. Other biologically active complexes are formed along the common terminal pathway of complement cascade. These intermediate complexes also promote various aspects of inflammation. Furthermore, the activated complement compo-

nents are cleaved into fragments (labeled, for example, C3a or C5b), which are also biologically active. Intermediate complement complexes and fragments act on leukocytes and endothelial cells, the coagulation system, and plasminogen, and promote inflammation, as illustrated in Figure 2-6.

Arachidonic Acid Derivatives. Arachidonic acid metabolites represent an important group of mediators of inflammation. Arachidonic acid is derived from the phospholipids of cell membranes through the action of phospholipase. Once formed, it is further metabolized through one of two possible metabolic pathways (Fig. 2-7). The *lipoxygenase* pathway leads to the formation of leukotrienes, which are active in chemotaxis and which also increase vascular permeability. Leukotrienes are also known as the slow-reacting substances of anaphylaxis (SRS-A), and they cause bronchospasm in asthma and anaphylactic shock by contracting the smooth muscles in the bronchi. The *cyclooxygenase* pathway leads to formation of the prostaglandins, prostacyclin and thromboxane, which cause vasodilatation. Thromboxane promotes platelet aggregation and thrombosis, whereas prostacyclin counteracts this effect. These arachidonic acid derivatives are involved in all stages of inflammation, and are generated in large amounts from various sources. The process of prostaglandin synthesis can be blocked

FIGURE 2-6

Complement activation. Activation of the classical and alternative pathways leads to a common terminal pathway from C5 to C9. These complement components form the final membrane attack complex (MAC). Other intermediate complexes and fragments are also biologically active; opsonins facilitate phagocytosis, anaphylatoxins act on mast cells and mediate a release of histamine which acts on blood vessels, and chemotactic fragments and intermediate complexes attract leukocytes to the site of inflammation.

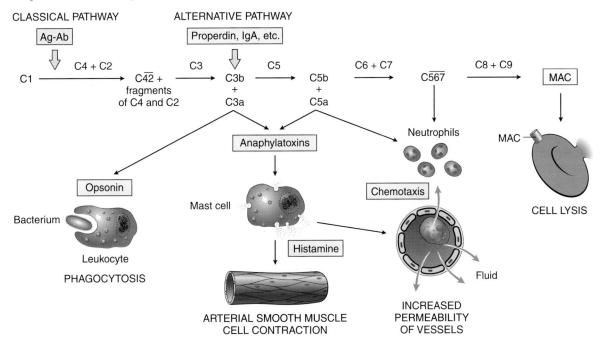

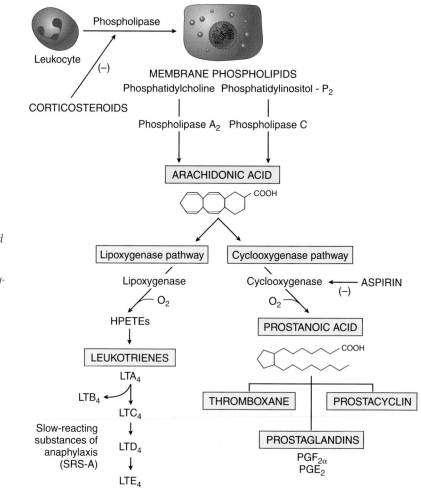

FIGURE 2-7
Arachidonic acid metabolism. Phospholipase from leukocytes acts on the phospholipids in cell membranes, forming the arachidonic acid pool. The cyclooxygenase and lipoxygenase pathway metabolites actively mediate all aspects of inflammation. HPETEs, hydroperoxy-eicosatetranoic acid compounds.

by aspirin, which is a potent inhibitor of cyclooxygenase. The anti-inflammatory effects of corticosteroid hormones are partially ascribed to their inhibitory effects on phospholipase and the inhibition of arachidonic acid formation.

Cellular Events in Inflammation

Emigration of Leukocytes

The increased permeability of the vessel walls of postcapillary venules and capillaries lasts from several hours to several days. It is usually accompanied by leakage of fluid from the vessels into the interstitial spaces. This process is called *transudation* and typically accounts for the formation of *edema,* which is rich in protein, but contains few cells. Emigration, or diapedesis, of cells across the vascular wall leads to the formation of *exudate.* Exudate contains much more protein than transudate and, in addition, contains inflammatory cells. In acute inflammation, most of these cells are polymorphonuclear leukocytes, also called polymorphonuclear neutrophils (PMNs).

As the inflammation evolves, PMNs are joined by other cells, such as monocytes and eosinophils, which become apparent in the exudate within the first 48 hours. As the inflammation proceeds into chronic stages, the PMNs, which have a life span of 2 to 4 days only, become less prominent and are replaced by macrophages, lymphocytes, and plasma cells.

The emigration of PNMs through the vessel wall

Did You Know?

Did the ancient Greeks use aspirin? Aspirin is a drug that was introduced in the 19th century. It contains acetylsalicylic acid, an inhibitor of cyclooxygenase that has anti-inflammatory properties. Today, it is used to treat headaches and fever. The ancient Greeks did not have the know-how to produce acetylsalicylic acid. However, they used the bark of the willow tree, which contains the same chemical, for medicinal purposes. Aspirin could, therefore, be considered one of the oldest medicinal substances still in use.

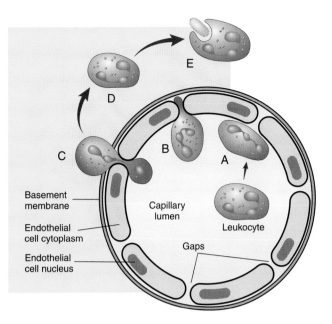

FIGURE 2-8

The emigration of leukocytes from blood vessels comprises several steps: adhesion (A), insertion of pseudopods between the endothelial cells (B), passage through the basement membrane (C), ameboid movement toward the source of chemotactic stimuli (D), and phagocytosis of bacteria that were the source of chemotactic stimuli (E).

is an active process that occurs in several phases. These phases include (1) adhesion of PMNs to the endothelial cells, (2) insertion of cytoplasmic pseudopods between the junctions of endothelial cells, (3) passage through the basement membrane, and (4) ameboid movement away from the vessel toward the cause of inflammation (e.g., bacteria) (Fig. 2-8).

Active movement of PMNs along a concentration gradient is called *chemotaxis* (in Greek, *taxis* means order). The chemoattractant is derived from bacteria or tissues destroyed by inflammation, or from activated complement. Chemotactic substances stimulate PMNs to move along a chemical concentration gradient until they reach its source or the site that has the highest concentration. In this respect, the movement of PMNs resembles the attraction that bees have for honey or that male insects have toward a sexually receptive female that is releasing pheromones.

Red blood cells do not migrate actively. Nevertheless, if the vascular wall defect is large enough, the red blood cells will be carried through it into the interstitial spaces. This is called *diapedesis* (in Greek, *dia* means through and *pedesis* means passage).

Phagocytosis

PMNs that reach the bacteria or other sources of chemotactic substances lose their mobility and begin acting as scavengers. This is accomplished through

phagocytosis (in Greek, *phagein* means to eat), or active uptake of bacteria and other cellular debris.

To illustrate phagocytosis, assume that a PMN has encountered a bacterium (Fig. 2-9). The bacteria are recognized as foreign particulate materials by the pseudopods extending from the surface of the PMN.

FIGURE 2-9

Phagocytosis of bacteria. (A) The bacterium that was opsonized (i.e., coated with IgG and complement [C3]) binds to the Fc and complement receptors on the surface of the leukocytes. (B) Engulfment of the bacterium into an invagination of surface membrane is associated with an oxygen burst and formation of oxygen radicals that are bactericidal and thus kill the bacterium. (C) Inclusion of the bacterium into a phagocytic vacuole is associated with the fusion of the vacuole with lysosomes and specific granules of the leukocyte. The contents of the lysosomes and specific granules are bactericidal and contribute to final inactivation and degradation of the bacterium in the heterophagosome. The cytoplasm of the leukocyte is, therefore, devoid of granules ("degranulation of leukocytes").

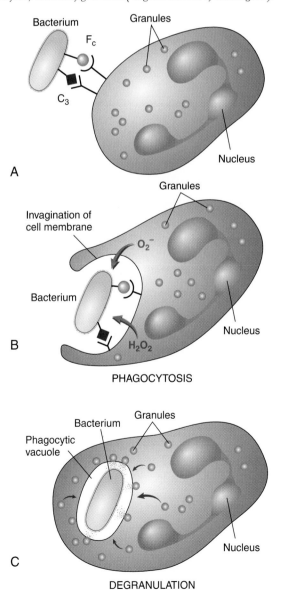

This recognition is followed by attachment of the cell membrane of the PMN to the bacterial wall. The attachment can be facilitated by immunoglobulin or complement, which may act like opsonins (derived from the Greek word for catering). Many leukocytes have receptors for C3 complement and the Fc portion of the immunoglobulin. These receptors mediate the contact of bacteria and leukocytes.

Engulfment of the bacterium is a process by which the cytoplasm of the PMN surrounds the foreign particle and encloses it into an invagination of the cell membrane. Inside the nascent vacuole, the bacterium is killed by bactericidal substances released from the cytoplasm of the PMN. The bacterium is internalized into a phagocytic vacuole, which fuses with lysosomes. The content of specific leukocytic granules and lysosomes is discharged into the lumen of this phagocytic vacuole. This *degranulation* of the PMN is the final step in the fight against bacteria. Lysosomal enzymes also kill bacteria that have survived earlier stages of phagocytosis. These lytic enzymes also digest bacteria and dissolve them into harmless elementary components.

Many PMNs die in their fight with bacteria. Dead and dying leukocytes, admixed with tissue debris and lytic enzymes released from their granules, form a viscous yellow fluid known as *pus*. Inflammations dominated by pus formation are called *purulent* or *suppurative*.

Cells of Inflammation

As stated before, PMNs are the primary mediators of acute inflammation caused by bacteria. Platelets are also present from the earliest stages of inflammation. Other cells are recruited shortly thereafter. These latecomers include eosinophils, macrophages, and lymphocytes.

Polymorphonuclear Neutrophils. PMNs are the most numerous **white blood cells** in the circulating blood, accounting for 60 percent to 70 percent of all white blood cells. They are the first cells to appear in acute inflammation. PMNs have a segmented nucleus and a well-developed cytoplasm filled with granules (Fig. 2-10). They are called PMNs because their nucleus may have one to five segments—i.e., it is polymorphous (variably shaped). Because the granules of PMNs stain with both hematoxylin and eosin, they are considered to be neutral. These cells are also known as neutrophilic granulocytes or, simply, neutrophils.

The most important features of PMNs include the following:

- *Mobility.* Because of their ability to form pseudopods used for ameboid movement, PMNs are

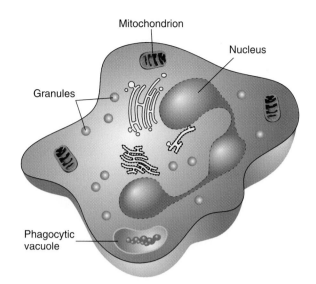

FIGURE 2-10

Diagram of a polymorphonuclear neutrophils. The nucleus has three segments and the cytoplasm contains the usual organelles, such as mitochondria, Golgi apparatus, endoplasmic reticulum, and lysosomes. There are also numerous, specific, membrane-bound granules and scattered phagocytic vacuoles. The cell surface extends into pseudopods, which enable the leukocyte to migrate.

highly mobile and are, therefore, the first cells to reach the site of inflammation. PMNs respond well to chemotactic substances.
- *Bactericidal activity.* PMNs are armed with specific granules that contain bacterial substances. They also can generate toxic oxygen radicals which can kill bacteria.
- *Phagocytosis.* PMNs are scavenger cells capable of ingesting bacteria and other cellular debris.
- *Cytokine production.* PMNs secrete and release various mediators of inflammation. These biologically active substances promote inflammation, recruit new leukocytes, and also cause systemic symptoms. For example, the release of interleukin-1 (IL-1) from PMNs serves as an endogenous *pyrogen,* which acts on the hypothalamic thermoregulatory centers and causes fever.

Eosinophils. Eosinophils, or eosinophilic leukocytes, account for 2 percent to 3 percent of circulating white blood cells. In the zone of inflammation, eosinophils appear 2 to 3 days after the PMNs. This is, in part, due to their slower mobility, as well as their comparatively slower reaction to chemotactic stimuli.

The term eosinophils is derived from their cytoplasmic granules, which stain pink with eosin. In many respects, eosinophils resemble PMNs. They are mobile, they can kill bacteria with reactive oxygen radicals, they phagocytose foreign material, and their granules are rich in lysosomal enzymes. In contrast to PMNs, however, eosinophils have a single nucleus, which is usually divided into two lobes located at opposite sides of the cytoplasm.

Eosinophils interact with basophils and are prominent in allergic reactions, such as hay fever and asthma. They also participate in the inflammatory response to parasitic infections. Eosinophils live longer than PMNs and are, therefore, present in chronic inflammations.

Basophils. Basophils account for less than 1 percent of circulating white blood cells. Nevertheless, these cells are important participants in inflammatory reactions and are most prominent in allergic reactions mediated by immunoglobulin E (IgE). Basophils have a bean-shaped, single nucleus and are somewhat larger than PMNs. Their cytoplasm contains granules rich in vasoactive substances, such as histamine. Basophils are precursors of *mast cells,* which have similar functions and are best considered as tissue basophils.

Macrophages. *Macrophages* are tissue mononuclear cells (histiocytes) derived from blood monocytes. They have a bean-shaped nucleus and are larger than PMNs. Macrophages appear at the site of inflammation 3 to 4 days after the onset of infection or tissue destruction. Macrophages are long-lived cells and, therefore, are typically present in chronic inflammation.

Macrophages, as their name implies, are capable of phagocytosis and are active in bacterial killing, albeit not as efficiently as the PMNs. Macrophages also secrete mediators of inflammation (cytokines) that act locally on other cells and the body as a whole.

Other Cells. *Lymphocytes and plasma cells* are components of chronic inflammation. However, because these cells have immune function, they will be described in greater detail in Chapter 3.

Platelets are fragments of cytoplasm released from megakaryocytes in the bone marrow (Fig. 2-11). They do not have a nucleus, and their cytoplasm contains vacuoles and three forms of granules: (1) dense granules, which are rich in histamine and adenosine diphosphate (ADP); (2) alpha-granules, which are rich in coagulation proteins and biologically active substances, such as platelet-derived growth factor (PDGF); and (3) lysosomes, which are rich in enzymes, such as acid hydrolases.

Platelets release their granules upon contact with extracellular matrix, endothelial cells, or thrombin formed in early thrombi. The release of histamine increases vascular permeability in the early stages of inflammation. Other substances released upon degranulation promote blood clotting. PDGF promotes the proliferation of connective tissue cells.

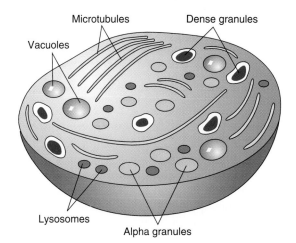

FIGURE 2-11
Diagram of a platelet as seen by electron microscopy. The platelet does not have a nucleus. The cytoplasm contains vacuoles, dense granules, alpha granules, and lysosomes. Its cytoskeleton consists of prominent microtubules that are instrumental in degranulation of the cytoplasm.

Classification of Inflammation

Inflammations can be classified in clinical practice according to four parameters. These include (1) duration, (2) etiology, (3) location, and (4) morphology, or pathologic characteristics.

Duration

Inflammation may last a short time or a long time. **Acute inflammation** lasts from a few hours to a few days. There are no exact definitions for it, nor is there a point at which it becomes chronic. Acute inflammation that occurs in bouts is considered to be recurrent. **Chronic inflammation** may become exacerbated and may be associated with recrudescences (i.e., intensification of symptoms).

Overall, chronic inflammation may represent (1) extension of an acute inflammation, (2) prolonged healing of an acute inflammation, or (3) persistence of causative agents. Some chronic inflammations evolve without a typical acute phase and represent slow-smoldering processes from their onset. For example, tuberculosis has a gradual onset and lasts a long time. Typically, patients complain of fatigue and have a low-grade fever. Frequently, they cannot pinpoint the exact onset of their symptoms and do not remember any acute phase of their disease.

Chronic inflammations also develop in response to foreign substances. For instance, foreign body granulomas will develop around thorns in subcutaneous tissue. Likewise, persons exposed to dust containing silica particles develop chronic lung silicosis, which does not have a recognizable acute phase. Autoimmune diseases, such as rheumatoid arthritis, also are characterized by a chronic course, although these diseases tend to have recrudescences and periodic exacerbations.

Etiology

Inflammations are caused by infectious pathogens or by chemical, physical, and immune factors. *Infections* are classified as bacterial, viral, protozoal, fungal, or helminthic. *Chemical causes* can be classified as organic or inorganic, industrial or medicinal, exogenous or endogenous. *Physical causes* of inflammation include foreign bodies, heat, irradiation, and trauma. The *immune causes* of inflammation are discussed in Chapter 3.

Many inflammations are multifactorial. For example, in the final analysis, many infectious inflammations are actually caused by chemicals released from the pathogens (e.g., bacterial toxins) or chemical mediators released from inflammatory cells. Infections often elicit an immune response as well, which may contribute to the pathogenesis of tissue damage. It is, therefore, important to keep all these facts in perspective and not be too dogmatic.

Location

Inflammation may be **localized** or **widespread.** For example, a boil or *furuncle* is a localized skin infection. Disseminated boils, a condition termed *furunculosis,* occur in people with a reduced resistance to bacterial infections. One such condition is called Job's syndrome, recalling the Biblical figure who was covered with numerous skin lesions. **Systemic inflammation** involving multiple organs is common in immunologically mediated diseases, such as systemic lupus erythematosus. Sepsis, characterized by a spread of bacteria through the blood, is also a systemic disorder. Nevertheless, it usually begins as a localized disease with a specific site of entry of bacteria into the blood.

Pathology of Inflammation

Several forms of inflammation can be recognized on gross examination of the affected tissues. These changes are readily seen in clinical practice. Physical examination of the patient may reveal typical signs of inflammation on the skin, eyes, oral mucosa, or genital organs. During surgery, it is possible to see the inflamed internal organs. These organs can also be visualized without surgery by using fiberoptic instruments, such as a laparoscope, which is used to inspect the abdominal cavity. Finally, in the autopsy room, various manifestations of inflammation can be observed in cadavers.

The terms for the various forms of inflammation are usually descriptive. Most terms are formed by adding a suffix *itis* to the Latin name for the organ. For example, hepatitis denotes inflammation of the liver, and appendicitis signifies inflammation of the appendix. Additional terms are used for greater precision. For example, post-transfusion viral hepatitis B indicates that the disease was acquired by transfusion and that it is caused by hepatitis B virus.

Serous Inflammation

Serous inflammation, considered to be the mildest form of inflammation, is characterized by the exudation of fluid that is clear, like serum (in Latin, *serum* means whey). Serous inflammation occurs in the early stages of most inflammations. In pneumonia, it can be recognized as a proteinaceous material inside the alveolar space that contains only a few inflammatory cells. As the inflammation progresses, these inflammatory cells proliferate in the fluid. However, if the disease is diagnosed early and the causative bacterium is eliminated, serous fluid is restored and the inflammation resolves.

Serous inflammation is typical of many viral infections. The skin vesicles caused by herpesvirus are, perhaps, the best examples of a serous inflammation. These vesicles are filled with proteinaceous fluid. Autoimmune diseases affecting serosal surfaces are also serous. Serous pericarditis, pleuritis, or peritonitis is characterized by an accumulation of clear, yellowish fluid in these cavities. Joint swelling secondary to fluid accumulation is typical of rheumatoid arthritis, the most common autoimmune disorder. Blisters of the skin caused by second-degree burns are yet another example of serous inflammation. The serous fluid is readily reabsorbed, and if the cause of the inflammation is eliminated, the lesions heal without any obvious consequences.

Fibrinous Inflammation

Fibrinous inflammation is characterized by an exudate that is rich in fibrin. Fibrin is formed from long strands of polymerized fibrinogen, which itself is one of the largest plasma proteins. In contrast to serous exudate, which contains predominantly albumin and immunoglobulins that have leaked from intact but permeable blood vessels or through small vascular defects, extravasation of fibrin occurs only through larger defects. Fibrinous exudate is, therefore, indicative of relatively severe inflammation.

Fibrinous inflammation is seen in many bacterial infections, such as "strep throat" or bacterial pneumonia. In bacterial pericarditis, the surface of the heart is covered with shaggy, yellowish layers of fibrin (Fig. 2-12).

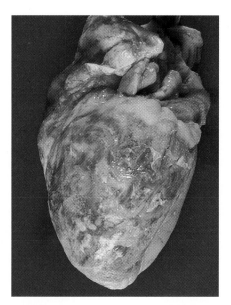

FIGURE 2-12
Fibrinous pericarditis. The epicardium is covered with a shaggy layer of fibrin.

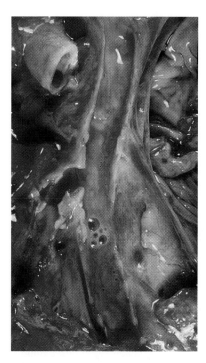

FIGURE 2-13
Purulent tracheobronchitis. The trachea is filled with pus, which appears as a turbid yellow exudate.

Fibrinous exudate does not resolve as easily as does serous exudate. Macrophages that invade the exudate have the capacity to lyse fibrin and thrombi. Blood vessels grow into the exudate, probably to provide a route for scavenger cells and the removal of the debris. These blood vessels fill the space occupied by fibrin and further obliterate it, a process termed *organization* of the exudate. Macrophages in the exudate also stimulate the ingrowth of fibroblasts, contributing further to formation of fibrous tissue. This fibrous tissue obliterates the cavities (e.g., organizing pneumonia). Adhesions form on the surface of organs that were previously smooth (e.g., adhesive pericarditis). Fibrous scarring of the pericardial sac may completely encase the heart and prevent its expansion in diastole (*constrictive pericarditis*).

Purulent Inflammation

Purulent inflammation is typically caused by pus-forming bacteria, such as streptococci and staphylococci. Pus is viscous yellow fluid composed of dead and dying PMNs and necrotic tissue debris. It is rich in lytic enzymes released from leukocytes, destroyed cells, and bacteria. Purulent exudate that is also rich in fibrin is said to be fibrinopurulent.

Pus may accumulate on the mucosa, skin, or in internal organs (Fig. 2-13). A localized collection of pus within an organ or tissue is called an *abscess* (Fig. 2-14). The central portion of an abscess is liquid or is composed of pus. In chronic abscesses, the wall of the cavity is composed of a capsule, which consists of

fibrotic granulation tissue. Abscesses do not heal spontaneously and must be evacuated surgically.

Large abscesses tend to rupture, forming a sinus or fistula (Fig. 2-15). A *sinus* is a cavity, usually occupied previously by an abscess that drains through a tract to the surface of the body. A *fistula* (in Latin, meaning tube) is a similar channel formed between two preexisting cavities or hollow organs and the surface of the body. A fistula may be formed, for exam-

FIGURE 2-14
Brain abscess.

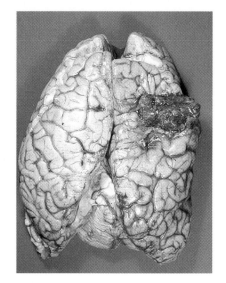

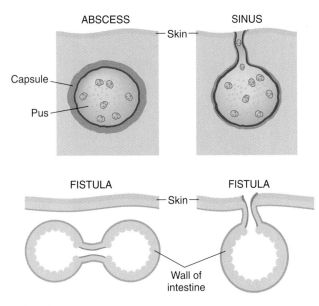

FIGURE 2-15

Diagram of an abscess, sinus, and fistula. (A) An abscess is a localized, purulent inflammation. Older abscesses are surrounded by a capsule that consists of granulation tissue. (B) A sinus forms a tract connecting the abscess with the skin. This allows the drainage of pus outside the body. (C) A fistula is an inflammatory tract that connects either two hollow organs or a hollow organ with the skin.

ple, between two loops of intestine that have been fused together by inflammation. Inflammatory cells create a hole in the intestinal wall, allowing the passage of pus and intestinal contents from one loop to another.

Accumulation of pus in a preformed cavity is called *empyema*. For example, empyema of the gallbladder occurs when drainage of pus from the gallbladder is obstructed by an impacted gallstone. Thoracic empyema denotes an accumulation of pus in the pleural cavity.

Ulcerative Inflammation

Inflammation of body surfaces or the mucosa of hollow organs, like the stomach or intestines, may result in *ulceration,* or a loss of epithelial lining. An *ulcer* is defined as a defect involving the epithelium, but it may extend into the deeper connective tissues as well. A peptic ulcer typically occurs in the stomach or duodenum (Fig. 2-16).

Pseudomembranous Inflammation

Pseudomembranous inflammation is a particular form of ulcerative inflammation that is combined with fibrinopurulent exudation. The exudate of fibrin, pus, cellular debris, and mucus forms a pseudomembrane on the surface of the ulcers. For example, *Clostridium difficile* causes pseudomembranous colitis. This bac-

terial overgrowth, which is secondary to intake of broad-spectrum antibiotics, may affect the entire large intestine. Pseudomembranes can also form in the throat in diphtheria. These pseudomembranes can be scraped away to expose ulcerated defects that bleed profusely.

Chronic Inflammation

Chronic inflammation is best defined by its duration—it lasts a long time. Because of its prolonged duration, such an inflammation produces more extensive tissue destruction, heals less readily, and is associated with more serious functional deficiencies than an acute inflammation.

Chronic infections are marked by an exudate which, on histologic examination, is found to contain lymphocytes, macrophages, and plasma cells. The secretory products of chronic inflammatory cells stimulate proliferation of fibroblasts and also perpetuate the inflammation by constantly recruiting new inflammatory cells. Loss of parenchymal cells is, thus, accompanied by scarring (i.e., the replacement of normal cells with fibroblasts and collagen), which may distort the organs involved. For example, fallopian tubes affected by chronic pelvic inflammatory disease (PID) are twisted and obliterated. Kidneys affected by chronic disease are small and shrunken (so-called end-stage kidneys).

The functional consequences of chronic inflammation cause many clinical symptoms. For example, the fibrosis associated with chronic lung disease causes thickening of the alveolar walls, which impairs the passage of oxygen from the air into the blood and causes dyspnea (shortness of breath). Constrictive pericarditis prevents dilatation of the heart during diastole and adversely affects the pump function of the heart. Chronic myocarditis with scarring may prevent the normal transmission of electric signals from the atrioventricular node to the myocardium and cause cardiac block. Loss of pancreatic

FIGURE 2-16

Peptic ulcer. An ulcer represents a defect of the epithelial lining.

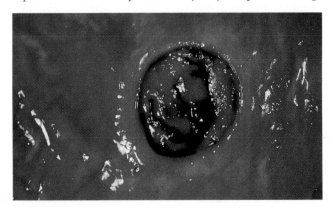

parenchyma causes severe digestive problems owing to the resultant deficiency of pancreatic enzymes.

Granulomatous Inflammation

A **granuloma** is a special form of chronic inflammation that typically is not preceded by an acute, PMN-mediated inflammation. It may be caused by antigens that evoke a cell-mediated hypersensitivity reaction, or by antigens that persist at the site of inflammation. Granulomas are typically formed in tuberculosis, but are also found in tissues infected with fungi, such as *Histoplasma capsulatum.*

Granulomatous reactions are mediated by macrophages and T lymphocytes (Fig. 2-17). These cells accumulate at the site of injury, forming nodules in which the macrophages interconnect with one another and transform into so-called epithelioid cells.

The granulomas of tuberculosis and other infectious granulomas are often associated with central caseous necrosis. In contrast, the immunologically mediated granulomas of *sarcoidosis,* a disease of un-

FIGURE 2-17
Granulomatous reaction. The lesion is composed of epithelioid cells, lymphocytes, and multinucleated giant cells.

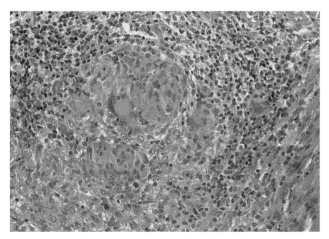

known origin, do not show central caseating necrosis (and are thus termed noncaseating granulomas).

The granuloma typical of syphilis is called a *gumma.* In the central zone of the gumma, there is coagulation necrosis of tissue, in which the cells have retained their normal outlines. The rim of inflammatory cells around the necrotic central zone include epithelioid cells, giant cells, and lymphocytes, as well as plasma cells. This reflects the ability of *Treponema pallidum* to provoke antibody production. As a consequence of this, antitreponemal antibodies appear in the serum. These antibodies can be measured and are useful in the serologic diagnosis of syphilis.

Granulomas destroy tissue and tend to persist for a long time. In the lungs, confluent necrotizing granulomas may cause cavities, erode blood vessels, and ultimately destroy the entire lung. Bleeding from eroded blood vessels into the cavities was a well-known complication of pulmonary tuberculosis. Fibrosis induced by chronic inflammation may destroy the organ and completely incapacitate the patient.

Clinicopathologic Correlations

The classical symptoms of inflammation are still the most important local findings and most useful indicators in the diagnosis of inflammation. For example, acute inflammation of the nail fold (*paronychia*) will present with redness (*rubor*), swelling (*tumor*), warmth (*calor*), and pain (*dolor*). Movement may also be limited by pain (*functio laesa*).

Similar symptoms could characterize an acute attack of appendicitis, but this organ is hidden from sight and so all the symptoms cannot immediately be recognized. The swollen hyperemic appendix may produce pain, or the pain may be elicited by the physician palpating the abdominal wall in the right lower quadrant. Clearly, one cannot see the appendix through the skin; thus, the signs of inflammation do not become evident until the surgeon intervenes and removes the affected organ. At operation, the appendix is typically swollen, red, and warm, and if the patient were not anesthetized, he or she would confirm that it was also painful.

Localized inflammations like appendicitis typically produce two important clinical findings: fever and leukocytosis. *Fever*—an elevation in body temperature that exceeds 37°C—is a typical response to acute inflammation caused by endogenous pyrogens. These substances—primarily IL-1 and tumor necrosis factor (TNF)—act on the thermoregulator centers in the hypothalamus, which serve as a thermostat (Fig. 2-18). If the threshold of the thermostat (like the heating sensor in a house) is raised, the temperature of the body rises.

Fever is mediated by prostaglandins that are re-

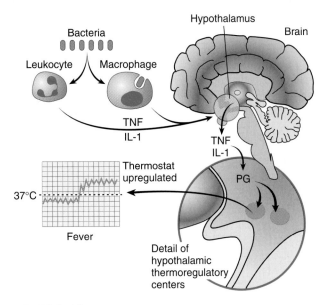

FIGURE 2-18
Pathogenesis of fever. Interleukin-1 (IL-1) and tumor necrosis factor (TNF) are endogenous pyrogens released from leukocytes or macrophages during inflammation. The action of IL-1 and TNF on the thermoregulatory centers in the hypothalamus is mediated by prostaglandins. This can be inhibited by aspirin, which blocks prostaglandin synthesis by inhibiting cyclooxygenase.

leased by pyrogens in the hypothalamic center. Prostaglandin synthesis can be inhibited by antipyretic drugs, such as aspirin. However, in most cases, the fever will abate on its own as soon as the inflammation is eradicated.

Leukocytosis is yet another important sign of inflammation. Normal blood has less than 10,000 white blood cells per mm³. Mediators of inflammation act on the bone marrow, stimulating a rapid release of leukocytes. When their number in the circulation exceeds 12,000 to 15,000, this is called leukocytosis. Leukocytosis is usually transient except in certain forms of chronic inflammation when it may be prolonged. Such chronic leukocytosis is associated with overstimulation of bone marrow by leukocytic growth factors.

Other symptoms of inflammation are mostly nonspecific and are called *constitutional.* These include fatigue, weakness, depression, lack of appetite, generalized pain, and exhaustion. The pathogenesis of these symptoms is not understood, but could be related to the action of mediators of inflammation, like IL-1 or TNF. These cytokines and others, known as acute phase reactants, act adversely on various cells and also stimulate the metabolism in general. This hypermetabolism may then cause fatigue and exhaustion.

Healing and Repair

Acute inflammation may heal without any consequences, or it may progress to chronic inflammation. Mild inflammation usually resolves spontaneously after the inciting stimuli have disappeared and the mediators of inflammation are no longer being secreted. However, if the inflammation was accompanied by considerable destruction of tissue, complete healing may be postponed or never accomplished.

Tissue loss has different consequences in different organs, depending primarily on the nature of the cells forming those tissues. In general, cells can be classified into three groups according to their capacity to proliferate (Fig. 2-19).

1. *Continuously dividing* or *mitotic cells* (also known as labile cells) are cells that divide throughout the entire life span. Such cells are typically known as stem cells and are found in the basal layer of the skin or in the mucosa of internal organs. These cells divide at a regular rate and give rise to more differentiated cells. Their descendants replace the superficial epithelial cells that have been shed after having reached the end of their predetermined life span.
2. *Quiescent, facultative mitotic cells* (also known as stable cells) do not divide regularly, but can be stimulated to divide if necessary. Such cells form the parenchymal organs (e.g., the liver or kidney). Loss of liver parenchyma following partial hepatectomy stimulates the remaining liver cells to enter mitosis and, by dividing, to replace the loss. Once the liver has regenerated, the cells become quiescent again and do not proliferate.
3. *Nondividing, postmitotic cells,* also known as permanent cells, do not have the capacity to proliferate under any circumstances. This category includes neurons and myocardial cells. Loss of postmitotic myocardial cells cannot be compensated; rather, the defect is repaired by fibrous scarring. Loss of brain cells is also irreversible.

Thus, it is clear that continuously dividing cells can easily repair a defect in the epithelial covering. Likewise, skin wounds or mucosal ulcers heal readily under appropriate conditions as the superficial layers are replenished from the descendants of cycling stem cells in the basal layer or the intestinal crypts. Loss of liver or kidney tubular cells may be replenished by regeneration to complete the healing. However, necrosis of heart muscle or brain cells leads to permanent defects that cannot be remedied by the proliferation of equivalent, highly specialized cells.

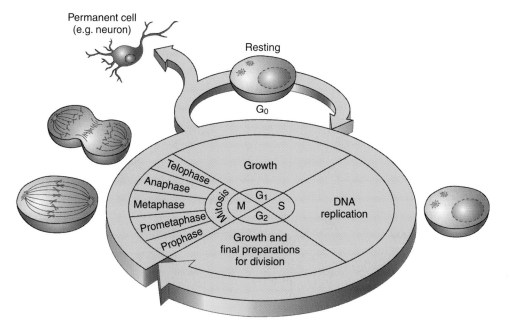

FIGURE 2-19

Three cell types in relation to the mitotic cell cycle. Mitotic cells may be in any of the four phases of the normal mitotic cycle. Facultative mitotic cells are arrested in the G_0 phase, but can enter the cycle if necessary. Postmitotic cells have left the mitotic cycle and cannot reenter it. Mitosis, marked in red, is a relatively short phase of the mitotic cycle. Following mitosis, the mitotic cells enter the G_1 (gap) phase, which is of variable duration. The facultative mitotic cells enter a G_0 phase, during which they perform various specialized functions. The G_1 phase is followed by the DNA synthetic phase (S) and a second gap (G_2).

Wound Healing

Wound healing is an important event that takes place at many anatomic sites. It is perhaps best illustrated by the sequence of events following skin incision. However, before discussing wound healing, it is important first to identify the main cells that participate in healing, as well as their primary secretory products.

Cells Participating in Healing. The most important cells that are involved in wound healing are leukocytes, macrophages, various connective tissue cells, and epithelial cells. PMNs play a brief role in scavenging the initial site of injury. Macrophages are much more important. These cells stay long at the site of healing and produce many cytokines, growth factors, and mediators that act on other connective tissue cells, most notably myofibroblasts, angioblasts, and fibroblasts.

Myofibroblasts, as their name implies, have hybrid properties of smooth muscle cells and fibroblasts. This enables them to contract like muscle cells and secrete matrix substances like fibroblasts. The contraction of myofibroblasts that occurs within the first few days of healing reduces the defect and holds the margins of tissue in close approximation.

This enables the proliferating epithelial cells to cover the surface defect and to restore the integrity of the surface epithelium.

Angioblasts are the precursors of blood vessels. They proliferate like sprouts from the several small blood vessels at the margins of the wound. These appear 2 to 3 days after incision, and by the fifth or sixth day, the entire field is permeated with newly formed blood vessels that serve two functions: (1) to provide a route for the scavenger cells to remove the scab and tissue debris and (2) to allow the influx of blood and its accompanying oxygen and nutrients.

Fibroblasts are the cells that produce most of the extracellular matrix. Of the numerous matrix components, the most important are fibronectin and collagen. *Fibronectin* has numerous functions in wound healing, the most important of which are the formation of scaffold, the provision of tensile strength, and the ability to "glue" other substances and cells together. *Collagens* form fibrils in the interstitial spaces. At least 6 different collagens have been isolated and characterized thus far, and it is likely that several others will be identified in the near future. Initially, fibroblasts synthesize predominantly type III collagen, which is typical of "young" or "immature" connective tissue temporarily formed in the wound. Later, type III collagen is replaced by type I collagen, which is the most common form of collagen in the body, providing tensile strength for all tissues.

The secretion of collagen is rather complex (Fig. 2-20) and requires several essential elements, such as zinc and vitamin C. Furthermore, collagen does not acquire its full strength until it is laid down in the extracellular spaces. This occurs several weeks after injury, when the collagen fibers are cross-linked with each other to form a dense meshwork.

Clinical Wound Healing. Healing of sterile surgical wounds occurs by *first intention* (Fig. 2-21). The incision site initially contains coagulated blood that forms a scab. The scab is invaded by PMNs whose function is to scavenge debris. These are replaced 2 to 4 days later by macrophages. The cytokines and growth factors secreted by macrophages promote the ingrowth of myofibroblasts, angioblasts, and fibroblasts.

The vascularized connective tissue that is rich in macrophages, myofibroblasts, angioblasts, and fibroblasts is called *granulation tissue* (Fig. 2-22). Gran-

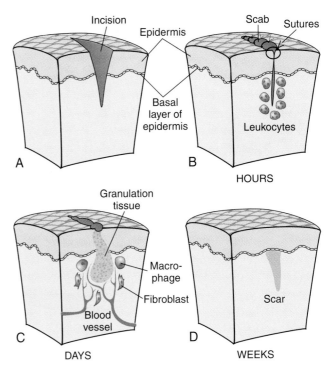

FIGURE 2-21
Wound healing by first intention. The sequence of events includes (A) formation of a scab and scavenger action of polymorphonuclear leukocytes, (B) formation of the granulation tissue, and (C) scarring.

FIGURE 2-20
Schematic representation of the synthesis of collagen. Collagen is synthesized in the rough endoplasmic reticulum and excreted. The collagen fibers in the interstitial spaces are cross-linked to form a firm lattice.

FIGURE 2-22
Diagram of the histologic appearance of granulation tissue. (A) In the early stages, it contains numerous macrophages, myofibroblasts, and blood vessels. (B) In the late stages, the granulation tissue is less vascular. Moreover, it contains more matrix and fibroblasts and only scattered macrophages.

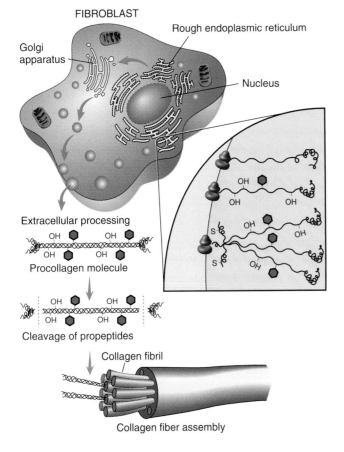

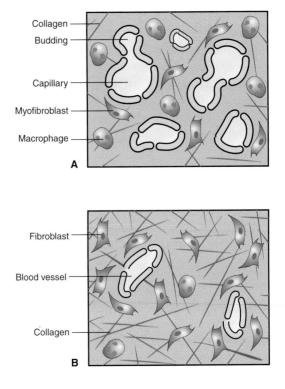

ulation tissue represents a temporary, makeshift structure that changes over time. Initially, it contains many myofibroblasts, which contract the wound and then disappear. Macrophages also become less prominent, and the blood vessels that are initially prominent slowly collapse. As a result, if everything goes well, the wound will become less inflamed and, by the second week, will start blanching. The interstitial spaces that were initially filled with extravasated blood will become edematous and finally will be filled with matrix. With time, the composition of this matrix changes from fibronectin and fibrin to collagen type III and, finally, to predominantly collagen type I. This final collagenous structure is called a *scar*.

Changes in the dermis are accompanied by a proliferation of epithelial cells from the margins of the wound. These cells cover the defect within 3 to 7 days. Under ideal circumstances, the granulation tissue filling the skin defect in the wound is trans-

formed into a scar within 3 to 6 weeks. The scar is then remodeled, and most of the disorderly formed collagen is replaced with collagen that is indistinguishable from that in the normal skin.

In contrast to the orderly sequence of events that characterizes the healing of sharp, sterile, surgical wounds by first intention (primary union), large defects and essentially all infected wounds heal by *secondary intention* (Fig. 2-23). Large defects cannot readily be bridged, and the surgeon cannot juxtapose the gaping tissue margins. Wound contraction cannot be accomplished by myofibroblasts in such cases, and the granulation tissue remains exposed to the external world. Wound healing by secondary intention is usually prolonged, and some wounds never heal completely.

Delayed Wound Healing. Wound healing may be complicated by local or systemic influences. Overall, the most important determinants of wound healing

FIGURE 2-23
Wound healing by secondary intention occurs in wounds that are marked by a large defect of tissue, that contain foreign material, or that are infected. The healing is slower because the epithelial cells proliferating from the wound margin take longer to cover the defect. Granulation tissue is more abundant; consequently, scarring is more prominent.

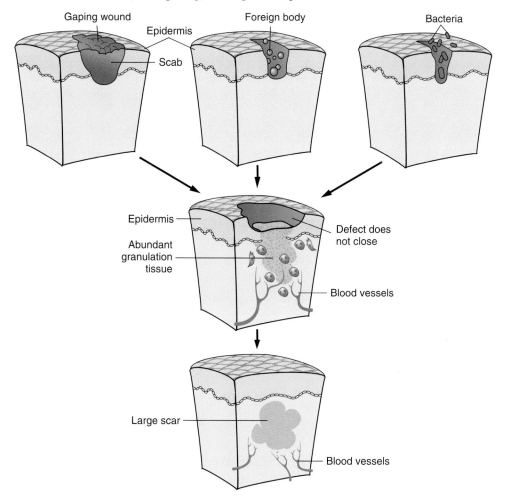

are: (1) site of the wound, (2) mechanical factors, (3) size, (4) presence or absence of infection, (5) circulatory status, (6) nutritional factors, and (7) age.

1. *Site of the wound.* Skin wounds heal well, whereas brain wounds do not heal at all.
2. *Mechanical factors.* Wounds heal faster if the margins can be juxtaposed neatly by a surgeon and the field can be kept immobile. Tension at the wound margins, if the skin had to be stretched to cover the gap, will impede healing. Movement may slow healing, which is why patients often remain confined to bed for some time after an operation. Foreign particles in the wound also retard healing.
3. *Size of the wound.* Small wounds heal faster than large ones.
4. *Infection.* Sterile wounds heal faster than those that are infected. Unfortunately, infections are sometimes inevitable. Indeed, approximately 5 percent of hospitalized patients develop wound infections postoperatively. Antibiotic treatment is, therefore, important for all patients with wounds, especially when the surgeon operates in an infected field.
5. *Circulatory status.* Wounds involving ischemic tissues heal poorly. Diabetes mellitus, a disease marked by chronic ischemia secondary to small blood vessel disease (*diabetic microangiopathy*), is typically associated with poor wound healing.
6. *Nutritional and metabolic factors.* General well-being promotes wound healing. Proteins are essential for wound healing; thus, malnutrition delays wound healing, as does vitamin C deficiency. Metabolic disturbances, such as those caused by diabetes mellitus, also cause delayed wound healing. An excess of endogenous corticosteroids, caused by endocrine oversecretion or exogenous intake for medicinal purposes, adversely affects scar formation.
7. *Age.* Wounds heal faster in children than in the elderly.

Complications of Wound Healing. Wound healing may be less than optimal as a result of the factors just discussed. In general, these complications may lead to:

- *Deficient scar formation.* Sluggish formation or granulation tissue occurs in diabetic patients, partly as a result of the ischemia caused by diabetic microangiopathy and partly as a consequence of the metabolic disturbances of diabetes. Inadequate collagen production has been reported in patients treated with corticosteroid hormones. Scars in such patients may not have sufficient tensile strength, and wound *dehiscence* (separation of tissue margins) may occur.
- *Excess scar formation.* Excessive scarring leads to the formation of *keloids,* which are hypertrophic scars composed predominantly of type III collagen, rather than type I collagen. Keloids result from defective remodeling of scar tissue and the persistence of type III collagen, which is typical of immature scar. Large scars, especially those caused by skin burns, tend to be irregularly shaped, which can give rise to *contractures.* Contractures over the joints may impede movement and, in some cases, may even completely immobilize an extremity.

Review Questions

1. Explain why inflammation cannot occur in an ameba or in a dead body.
2. Does inflammation have beneficial or noxious effects on the human body?
3. What are the cardinal signs of inflammation?
4. Explain the sequence of events that leads to active hyperemia in inflamed tissues.
5. What happens to the leukocytes inside the blood vessels in inflamed tissue?
6. Why does the permeability of blood vessels increase during acute inflammation?
7. Describe the consequences of activation of Hageman factor in acute inflammation.
8. Why are some complement fragments called opsonins, anaphylatoxins, or chemotactic factors?
9. How is membrane attack complex (MAC) formed and how does it damage red blood cells?

10. Explain the formation of leukotrienes and prostaglandins in acute inflammation.

11. How does a transudate differ from an exudate?

12. How do polymorphonuclear neutrophils emigrate from blood vessels toward bacteria in the tissue?

13. What are the most important chemotactic substances and how do they promote inflammation?

14. How do polymorphonuclear neutrophils engulf and kill bacteria?

15. What is pus and how is it formed?

16. Why are polymorphonuclear neutrophils best suited to combat acute bacterial infection?

17. How do eosinophils differ from polymorphonuclear neutrophils?

18. Which inflammatory reactions are mediated by eosinophils and basophils?

19. What are the main functions of macrophages?

20. How do platelets differ from other white blood cells?

21. Compare acute with chronic inflammation.

22. Compare cellular inflammatory response to a typical viral infection with that occurring in bacterial infection.

23. What are the main causes of inflammation?

24. Give an example of both a localized and a systemic inflammation.

25. Give an example of a serous inflammation and describe the pathologic findings.

26. Give an example of fibrinous inflammation and describe the pathologic findings.

27. Give an example of a purulent inflammation and describe the pathologic findings.

28. Give clinical examples of an abscess, sinus, fistula, and empyema.

29. What is the difference between an ulcerative and pseudomembranous inflammation?

30. Describe tissue changes in chronic inflammation, such as pelvic inflammatory disease.

31. Describe possible chemical symptoms of chronic inflammation involving the lungs, heart, and pancreas.

32. What are the main features of a granulomatous inflammation?

33. Compare caseating and noncaseating granulomas with gumma.

34. Correlate the typical clinical features of acute appendicitis with the pathologic changes found at surgery.

35. What are endogenous pyrogens and how do they act on the hypothalamus?

36. Explain the differences between continuously dividing, quiescent, and nondividing cells, and give examples of each.

37. Which cells participate in wound healing?

38. What is granulation tissue and how does it evolve during wound healing?

39. Compare wound healing by primary and secondary intention.

40. Explain why various adverse factors delay wound healing.

41. Compare wound dehiscence with keloid formation.

Learning Objectives

After reading this chapter, the student should be able to:

1. Define and distinguish between natural immunity and acquired immunity.

2. List the main organs and cells that participate in the immune response.

3. Describe the main differences between subsets of lymphocytes: B cells, T cells, and NK cells.

4. Describe the antigen-presenting cells and discuss their functions.

5. Describe the functions of lymphokines.

6. Describe the basic features of immunoglobulins and their reaction with antigen.

7. Describe the role of MHC in antigen presentation.

8. List four mechanisms of hypersensitivity reactions.

9. Describe type I hypersensitivity reaction and how it induces hay fever and asthma.

10. Describe type II hypersensitivity reaction and how it induces hemolytic anemia, myasthenia gravis, and Graves' disease.

11. Describe type III hypersensitivity reaction and how it induces glomerulonephritis.

12. Describe the cell-mediated hypersensitivity reaction and how it induces granuloma formation.

13. Describe the main forms of transplants: homograft, isograft, autograft, and xenograft.

14. Discuss the medical uses of transplantation, and give three examples.

15. Discuss the principles of blood transfusion.

16. Describe Rh incompatibility between the mother and the fetus.

17. Discuss the pathogenesis of autoimmune diseases.

18. List three congenital immunodeficiency diseases and three acquired immunodeficiency states.

19. Explain the pathogenesis of AIDS and list its most important complications.

20. List the three forms of amyloid and relate them to clinical presentations of amyloidosis.

Additional Key Terms and Concepts

Agglutination

Anaphylactic reaction

Contact dermatitis

Glomerulonephritis

Hydrops fetalis

Kaposi's sarcoma

Serum sickness

Chapter Outline

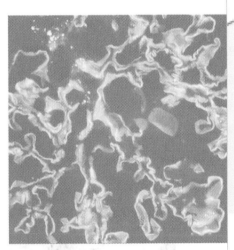

Immunopathology
Chapter 3

Immunity, derived from the Latin term denoting exemption from duty (*munus,* meaning duty or service) was originally defined as resistance to infections. Immune persons would be "exempt from suffering" inflicted by the infectious diseases. Subsequently, it became apparent that immune reactions are not elicited only by bacteria, but also by many other substances, as long as they are perceived as foreign by the immune system. Furthermore, we have learned that these reactions occur in many forms, and that immunity not only provides protection, but also can cause diseases. To appreciate the beneficial and not-so-beneficial consequences of immunity, a review of the *basic mechanisms of immunity* is provided and then discussed in relation to *immunopathology.* The *secondary immune reactions* that accompany most infectious diseases, many systemic diseases, and tumors are not presented here. However, it is worth remembering that there are few human diseases that do not affect the immune system.

Immunologic techniques are useful in research but are also used daily in clinical laboratories. This applied immunology forms the basis for *immunodiagnostics.* Finally, *immunotherapy* should be mentioned, as it provides new modalities for the treatment of diseases. *Immunopreventive* techniques, such as vaccination and active and passive immunization, have contributed enormously to the fight against diseases in humans and animals. It is fair to say that immunization has probably saved more human lives than all other drugs together.

Immune Response

The immune response has two different forms: a relatively primitive, nonspecific set of *natural protective mechanisms* and a complex system of cellular and humoral reactions that evolve in response to repeated exposures to foreign substances, known as *acquired immunity.*

Natural Immunity

Natural protective mechanisms are inherited and do not depend on previous exposure to foreign substances (Fig. 3-1). These defense mechanisms include various mechanical barriers (e.g., the epidermis), physical forces (e.g., the ciliary movement of bronchial epithelium), and secretory substances. For example, *properdin* is a plasma protein that activates the alternative complement pathway, thus generating a set of protective substances. *Lysozyme* is a basic protein of low molecular weight found in tears, and in nasal and intestinal secretions. It is a potent bactericidal agent that nonspecifically kills many bacteria.

Acquired Immunity

Acquired immunity is based on specific responses elicited by substances that act as antigens. An *antigen* is any chemical substance that can induce a specific immune response. The initial antigen-antibody reaction is amplified by a series of events that involve the cells of the immune system and closely related auxiliary (helper) cells, such as macrophages, basophils, and eosinophils. Acquired immunity is based on the ability of the body's immune system to distinguish *self* from *non-self,* to generate an immunologic memory, and to mount an integrated reaction of various cells.

The ability of the body to mount an appropriate immune response is termed *immunocompetence.* Immunocompetence depends on adequate structural and functional development of the immune system, as well as on the coordinated action of its components. A brief description of the organs and cells that constitute the immune system is presented, along with a review of their function. After that, various pathologic changes mediated by immune mechanisms are discussed.

Cells of the Immune System

All cells of the immune system are descendants of primitive hematopoietic stem cells originally found in the bone marrow (Fig. 3-2). The bone marrow stem cells give rise to two major cell lineages: lymphoid cells and all other hematopoietic cells. In this context, note that macrophages are descendants of the nonlymphoid premyeloid stem cells in the bone marrow that give rise to other leukocytes.

Lymphocytes

Lymphocytes are small cells, only slightly larger than erythrocytes. They have a round nucleus and very little cytoplasm. All lymphocytes are derived from bone marrow prelymphoid stem cells, which give rise to two distinct cell lineages. Descendants of one lineage migrate to the thymus and mature into *T lymphocytes. B lymphocytes,* descendants of the other lineage, remain in the bone marrow from which they colonize the peripheral lymphoid tissues. The bone marrow and thymus are called *primary lymphoid organs,* and the differentiation of T and B cells in them is developmentally programmed and unrelated to antigenic stimulation. From the primary lymphoid organs, the T and B lymphocytes enter the blood circulation and colonize various *secondary lymphoid organs.* Among these, the most prominent are the lymph nodes and spleen in which lymphocytes constitute a significant percentage of the total cell popu-

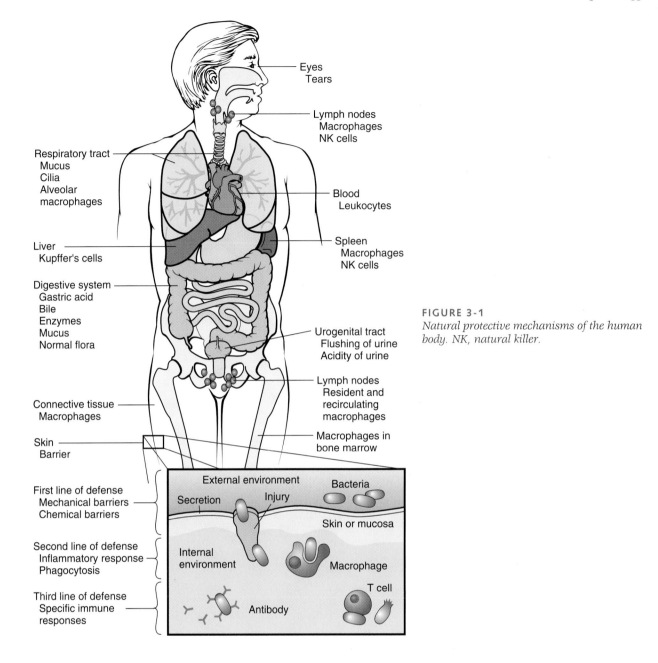

FIGURE 3-1
Natural protective mechanisms of the human body. NK, natural killer.

lation. Lymphocytes are also present in other organs and are most prominent in the gastrointestinal and bronchial mucosa, where they form the so-called mucosa-associated lymphoid tissue (MALT). In contrast to encapsulated lymph nodes and spleen, MALT has no capsule, and its cells are an integral part of the mucosa.

T and B lymphocytes have distinct functions, even though morphologically, they cannot be distinguished by light or electron microscopy. Subtle differences between T and B lymphocytes can be recognized by immunochemical techniques designed to identify unique marker molecules on the cell surface of these cells. In practice, this can be done by immunocytochemical staining of tissue sections or cell smears with specific, color-coded antibodies. Anti-

bodies to so-called cluster differentiation (CD) antigens have been most useful in this regard. CD antigens are selectively expressed during specific stages of lymphocyte development. Some CD antigens are selectively expressed on T cells, whereas others are selectively expressed on B cells. Several subsets of T and B lymphocytes and their immature precursors can be recognized using this approach. Using cell sorters, such as the fluorescence-activated cell sorter (FACS), it is possible to distinguish T from B lymphocytes or to determine their ratio in circulation or in various lymphoid organs. FACS also can be used for separation of subsets of T lymphocytes, which is important for the diagnosis of immunodeficiency diseases, such as acquired immunodeficiency syndrome (AIDS).

Major lymphoid organs

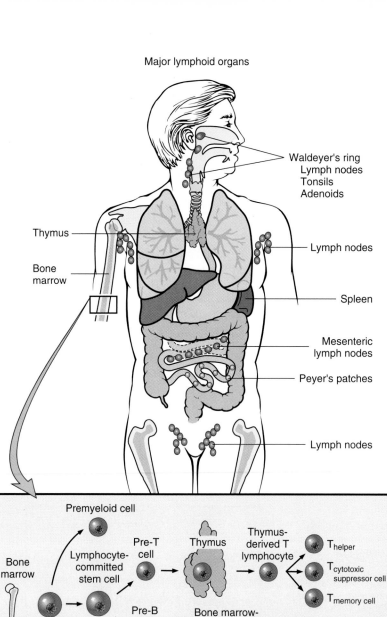

FIGURE 3-2
Immune system. Lymphocytes, like all other hematopoietic cells, are derived from a common pluripotential bone marrow stem cell. These stem cells give rise to myeloid cell precursor and the stem cell committed to lymphocytic lineages. There are three lymphoid cell lineages that lead to mature T and B cells (plasma cells), or natural killer cell formation.

T Lymphocytes. T lymphocytes are lymphocytes that have matured in the thymus. They account for two thirds of all lymphocytes in the blood and also are found in the paracortical zone of the lymph nodes and the periarteriolar sheath of the spleen. There are several subsets of T cells, the most important of which are the *T helper/inducer* and *T suppressor/cytotoxic* cells. T helper/inducer cells, known as T helper cells for short, actively participate in the immune responses to antigens, helping B cells produce antibodies. T suppressor/cytotoxic cells suppress un-

wanted antibody production and mediate killing of virus-infected cells or tumor cells that are recognized by the body as foreign.

Common to all T cells is the surface T-cell receptor (TCR), which is linked to a membrane protein known as CD3. T cells use TCR for recognition of antigens. TCR-CD3 complex is, thus, essential for the activity of T cells. Like all other genes inherited from our parents, the gene for TCR is in all the cells of the body. However, the gene is activated only in T cells. TCR gene activation occurs through rearrangement of parts of the gene. Because TCR rearrangement occurs only in T cells, it is a unique genetic marker for T lymphocytes. This is important to note because 10 percent to 15 percent of peripheral lymphocytes have the same surface markers as T lymphocytes, but do not have TCR gene rearrangement. These cells are known as *natural killer* (NK) *cells.* NK cells are not involved in T- and B-cell–mediated immune reactions. Their function is to react against virus-infected cells and to kill tumor and foreign cells without previous sensitization.

T helper cells carry CD4, whereas the T suppressor/cytotoxic cells carry the CD8 antigen. CD4 and CD8 are used as markers for these lymphocytes and for the counting of T helper and T suppressor/cytotoxic cells in blood. In normal blood, CD4-positive cells predominate, and the cell ratio of CD4:CD8 is approximately 2:1. In individuals with AIDS, CD4 cells are selectively lost, and the cell ratio of CD4:CD8 is less than 1.0.

B Lymphocytes. *B cells* are lymphocytes that are primed to differentiate into immunoglobulin-producing plasma cells. This differentiation occurs in a step-wise manner. Each of these intermediate stages is characterized by distinct cell surface and cytoplasmic changes that can be recognized by immunohistochemical methods. However, some features are shared by all B cells and their mature descendants, the plasma cells. The most important shared feature is the activation of the immunoglobulin gene, which occurs only in the B-cell lineage. The immunoglobulin gene is similar to TCR, and its activation also occurs through a rearrangement of parts of the gene. The immunoglobulin gene rearrangement enables B cells to produce immunoglobulins.

Plasma Cells

Plasma cells are fully differentiated descendants of B lymphocytes. These cells have an oval shape and an eccentrically located round nucleus. The cytoplasm of plasma cells is basophilic because it contains an abundance of ribosomes. On electron microscopy, the cytoplasm of plasma cells contains numerous stacks of rough endoplasmic reticulum (RER) (Fig. 3-3). The RER is the site of synthesis of immunoglobulins, the primary secretory products of plasma cells.

Antibodies

Antibodies are serum proteins of the immunoglobulin class that are secreted by plasma cells. There are five classes or isotypes of immunoglobulins: IgG, IgM, IgA, IgE, and IgD.

These immunoglobulins share some common features:

- All immunoglobulins are composed of light and heavy chains (Fig. 3-4). All immunoglobulins have the same light chains, which are either kappa or lambda. A single molecule contains either two kappa or two lambda chains. Heavy chains are immunoglobulin class–specific. These are called gamma, mu, alpha, epsilon, and delta and correspond to IgG, IgM, IgA, IgE, and IgD, respectively. Heavy chains are the primary determinants of the class of each immunoglobulin, their properties, and their function.

FIGURE 3-3
Electron microscopic photograph of a lymphocyte and a plasma cell. (Left) The cytoplasm of the lymphocyte is scant and contains few organelles. (Right) The cytoplasm of the plasma cell is well developed and contains prominent rough endoplasmic reticulum (RER). The RER serves as the site for production of immunoglobulins.

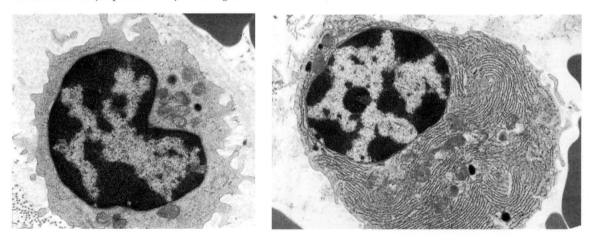

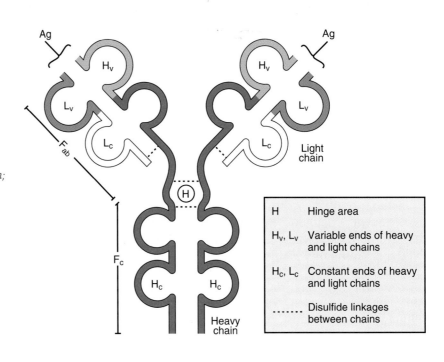

FIGURE 3-4
Diagram of immunoglobulin. L_c, light chain; H_c, heavy chain. The F_{ab} and F_c portions are also indicated.

H	Hinge area
H_v, L_v	Variable ends of heavy and light chains
H_c, L_c	Constant ends of heavy and light chains
......	Disulfide linkages between chains

- Each chain has a constant and a variable part. The *constant* part extends from the C terminal (called so because it ends with a COO⁻ [carboxy] group) across the *hinge* region to the *variable* part, which occupies the N terminal (called so because it ends in an NH_3^+ [amino] group).
- Each antibody is made up of domains of about 110 amino acids that form loops held together by disulfide bonds on cysteine residues.
- Each antibody can be cleaved enzymatically into two fragments: the F_c portion, which contains the constant region, and the F_{ab} fragment, which contains the variable region. F_c binds to specific F_c receptors that are expressed on macrophages and polymorphonuclear leukocytes (PMNs) and some other cells. Fab serves as the antigen-binding site.

IgM is composed of five basic units and is thus the largest immunoglobulin (macroglobulin) held together with a linker-J chain. Its function is to neutralize microorganisms. It is an avid complement activator because it has five complement-binding sites. IgM is the first immunoglobulin to appear after immunization, and it is a natural antibody against blood group antigens ABO.

IgG has the smallest molecular weight of the immunoglobulins but is, nevertheless, the most copious immunoglobulin. It is produced in small amounts upon initial immunization, but its production is boosted by reexposure to the antigen. Fc receptors for IgG exist on macrophages, PMNs, lymphocytes, eosinophils, and platelets, and in the placenta. This allows the passage of IgG across the placenta into the fetus. IgG acts as an opsonin; that is, it coats the bacteria and thus facilitates their phagocytosis.

IgA is predominantly found in mucosal secretions and milk, where it functions as a primary protective immunoglobulin. It is usually joined into a dimer with a J chain. The dimers usually carry a secretory piece that protects the immunoglobulin that is discharged into the intestine from the action of digestive enzymes.

IgE is present in trace amounts in serum. This immunoglobulin is secreted by sensitized plasma cells in tissues and is locally attached to mast cells. IgE mediates allergic reactions in tissues. Systemic release of IgE may lead to anaphylactic shock.

IgD is a cell membrane–bound immunoglobulin found exclusively on B cells. It participates in the antigenic activation of B cells and is not released into serum or body fluids.

Antibody Production

Antibody production begins with contact between an antigen and the cells of the immune system. All substances identified by the body as foreign could serve as antigens and incite an immune response. This activation of B cells culminates in the production of specific antibodies that can react with the antigen. Antigens that can elicit an immune response are called *complete antigens,* in contrast to incomplete antigens, or *haptens.* Haptens are low-molecular-weight substances that are not immunogenic by themselves. However, if attached to a larger carrier molecule, haptens become immunogenic. Once the antibodies have been induced against a hapten, they will react with this hapten, even if the hapten is not linked to the carrier.

In order to elicit antibody production, the antigen must be presented to B lymphocytes (Fig. 3-5).

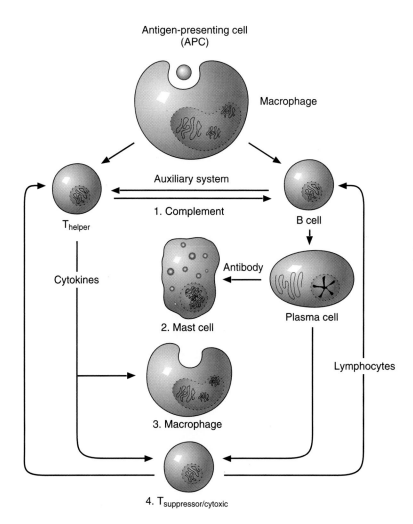

Antigen-presenting cell
(APC)

Macrophage

Auxiliary system

1. Complement

T_{helper}

B cell

Cytokines

Antibody

2. Mast cell

Plasma cell

3. Macrophage

Lymphocytes

4. T_{suppressor/cytoxic}

FIGURE 3-5
Diagram of antigen presentation. The antigen-presenting cell (APC) (macrophage) presents the processed antigen to B or T lymphocytes. Stimulated B cells differentiate into immunoglobulin-secreting plasma cells. The function of helper T and B cells is regulated by suppressor T cells. T and B cells and macrophages act upon one another, stimulating or inhibiting each other.

Only a minority of antigens can directly stimulate B cells, whereas others require the initial involvement of T cells. The *T-cell–independent* antigens are also known as nonspecific B-cell mitogens because they directly stimulate proliferation of previously sensitized B cells. Most antigens must be presented to B cells by antigen-presenting cells (APCs), such as macrophages. The response of B cells depends on the interaction with T helper and T suppressor cells. Thus, most antigens are *T-cell–dependent.*

The interaction of antigens and T and B lymphocytes is mediated by receptors expressed on the surface of these cells. The receptors on B cells are immunoglobulins, whereas those on T lymphocytes are TCR and CD3, differentiation antigens of all T lymphocytes. **Macrophages** and other APCs, such as Langerhans' cells in the skin or the follicular dendritic cells in the lymph nodes, have receptors for the F_c portion of the immunoglobulin, as well as complement C3. These receptors enable macrophages to phagocytize opsonized antigens (e.g., bacteria coated with C3 or IgG). Antigens that are not opsonized can also be processed by APCs, but less efficiently.

Major Histocompatibility Complex

All processed antigens are presented to T cells in the context of the *major histocompatibility complex* (MHC) proteins expressed on the surface of APCs. These MHC proteins, also known as *human leukocyte antigens* (HLAs), are expressed on all nucleated cells in the body. A unique set of MHC antigens determines the individuality of each person. Only identical twins have the same MHC antigens. In immune reactions, the MHC antigens regulate the cell-to-cell contact during antigen presentation (Fig. 3-6).

Human MHC antigens belong to two groups. Type I MHC proteins serve as the receptors for CD8, thus linking macrophages to suppressor and/or cytotoxic T lymphocytes. Type II MHC molecules react with CD4, mediating the attachment of macrophages to helper T lymphocytes. The antigen is passed to B lymphocytes, which become activated and differentiate into memory cells. Simultaneously, both APCs and T lymphocytes produce **lymphokines,** such as interleukins (labeled from IL-1 to IL-12), interferons (alpha, beta, gamma), tumor necrosis factor (TNF), and various colony-stimulating factors. These soluble

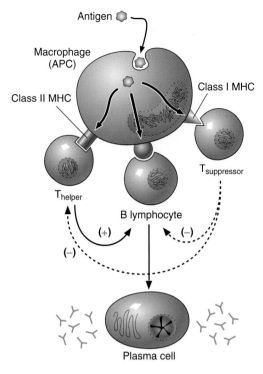

FIGURE 3-6
Major histocompatibility complex (MHC) participates in the antigen presentation. MHC-I links macrophages to suppressor T cells, whereas MHC-II links them to helper T cells. APC, antigen-presenting cell.

factors regulate and promote the interaction of cells of the immune system.

The first response to exposure to an antigen, based on IgM production, is weak and transient (Fig. 3-7). The initial IgG response, which follows IgM, is also temporary. Upon second exposure to the same antigen, a much stronger *anamnestic* (Greek root meaning recall or memory) reaction occurs. This is characterized by IgG production.

Each sensitized B cell gives rise to an antibody-producing cell, a memory daughter cell. The former cell differentiates into plasma cells. Each B cell descendant is clonal and capable of producing only one

FIGURE 3-7
Primary and secondary antibody response. The primary response is marked by IgM, which is followed by IgG. The secondary response involves predominantly IgG secretion.

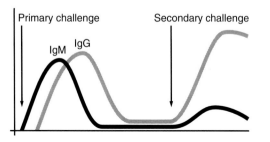

antibody of defined specificity (Fig. 3-8). Clonal expansion, which is mediated by cytokines released from the activated T lymphocytes, amplifies the immune response. The number of memory cells also increases. A switch from IgM to IgG occurs simultaneously in effector cells. Hence, if an anamnestic secondary immune response is induced by reexposure to antigen, it is much stronger and is based on IgG production.

Antigen-Antibody Reaction

Most antigens carry more than one antigenic site, or *epitope,* and are thus able to bind more than one antibody to their surface. Antigens are thus multivalent. Antigens and antibodies are bound to each other by complex physical and chemical bonds, forming *antigen-antibody complexes.* If the antigen is soluble and circulating in the blood, the complexes will also be soluble and will circulate in the plasma, the fluid portion of blood. However, these complexes tend to enlarge as more and more antibodies and antigen molecules are included in the meshwork. Finally, the complexes reach the size of small particles, which are phagocytized in the spleen and the liver by fixed macrophages. The smaller complexes may remain in the circulation, depending on their overall solubility, size, and electrical charge. Depending on these three properties, the immune complexes may remain suspended in circulation for a long time; alternatively, they may be attached to red blood cells (RBCs) or endothelial cells, or filtered through the capillary walls with other proteins.

Antibodies to insoluble antigens, such as cell surface antigens, become fixed to the cell membrane (Fig. 3-9). This is best illustrated by the antibodies to RBCs that typically coat the cell surface. Antibodies bind RBCs to one another, which is recognized as *agglutination*—that is, clumping of RBCs and their separation from serum. If the antigen-antibody complex activates the complement cascade, cell lysis will occur (*hemolysis*). This occurs almost invariably with all IgM- and IgG-containing complexes because these immunoglobulins fix complement.

Complement activation results from circulating, soluble, or cell-surface–fixed immune complexes inside the blood vessels. Antigen-antibody complexes formed outside the vessels, or those that are pathologically deposited in tissues, also activate complement. As previously stated, antigen binds to the F_{ab} region of the antibody. The F_c region that protrudes on the opposite side serves as a binding site for complement. At the same time, F_c can attach to all cells that have F_c receptors. The most important among these are the macrophages and PMNs, which act as scavengers of immunoglobulin-coated (opsonized)

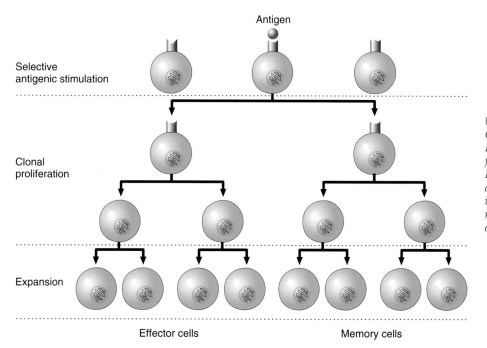

Antigen

Selective
antigenic stimulation

Clonal
proliferation

Expansion

Effector cells

Memory cells

FIGURE 3-8
Clonal selection and expansion of B-lymphocyte populations occurs following antigenic stimulation. Each antigen stimulates a single B cell, which gives rise to clones of identically imprinted effector, immunoglobulin-secreting, and memory cells.

bacteria. RBC membrane fragments that are coated with antibodies and the large soluble immune complexes are taken in the same way by macrophages and removed from circulation.

In summary, the antibody response has many biologically important features. These can be recognized in the living organism and reproduced experimentally in animals, or in vitro in the test tube. Immune reactions primarily have a protective role, which can be fully realized only in the context of the coordinated participation of APCs and T and B lymphocytes, which interact one with another. The critical role of MHC in antigen presentation and the complex regula-

tory role of cytokines produced by T lymphocytes and macrophages should not be forgotten. Finally, the process of antibody production and the nature of antibodies must be fully appreciated to understand the protective, as well as the potentially pathologic, consequences of antigen-antibody reactions.

Hypersensitivity Reactions

An abnormal immune response to exogenous antigens or a reaction to endogenous autoantigens is called a *hypersensitivity* reaction. Hypersensitivity re-

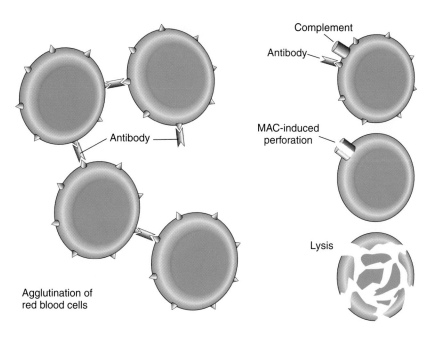

Complement

Antibody

MAC-induced
perforation

Antibody

Lysis

Agglutination of
red blood cells

FIGURE 3-9
Reaction of antibody with antigen on the surface of RBCs (red blood cells). This could lead to agglutination of RBCs or hemolysis mediated by activated complement. MAC (membrane attack complex).

actions are the basis of **hypersensitivity diseases,** which are also known as *allergic disorders.*

Hypersensitivity diseases are pathogenetically classified into four major groups, each of which is mediated by distinct mechanisms:

Type I—anaphylactic-type reaction

Type II—cytotoxic antibody–mediated reaction

Type III—immune complex–mediated reaction

Type IV—cell-mediated, delayed-type reaction

Type I Hypersensitivity

Type I hypersensitivity reaction is mediated by IgE and mast cells or basophils. IgE is produced by plasma cells derived from B lymphocytes that are sensitized to foreign antigens, such as pollen. The antibody, which is produced in tissues exposed to antigens, diffuses locally toward mast cells and is fixed to the Fc receptors on their surface (Fig. 3-10). Reexposure to the antigen leads to the formation of antigen-antibody complexes on the surface of mast cells. This triggers the release of vasoactive substances stored in mast cell granules. The most important among these is histamine, the well-known vasoactive biogenic amine. The release is instantaneous, as any sufferer of hay fever can testify. It is accompanied by increased vascular permeability, edema, and accumulation of inflammatory cells, most notably eosinophils. Eosinophilia—an increased number of eosinophils in the blood—is a common systemic feature of type I hypersensitivity reactions.

Type I hypersensitivity reactions also produce a *late-phase response* that usually occurs 4 to 6 hours after exposure to allergens. Basophils and mast cells play an important role, but are not the only cells involved in this reaction. The late-phase response is mediated by slow-reacting substances of anaphylaxis (SRS-As). SRS-As are arachidonic acid derivatives classified as leukotrienes. Late-phase response is typical of bronchial asthma.

The most important clinical examples of type I

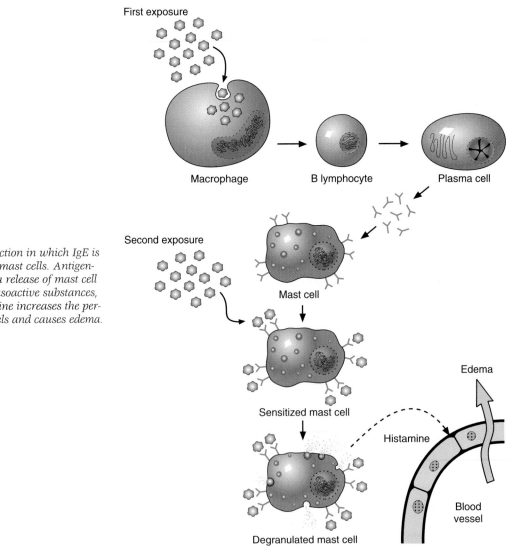

FIGURE 3-10
Type I hypersensitivity reaction in which IgE is bound to the F_c receptor of mast cells. Antigen-antibody reaction triggers a release of mast cell granules, which contain vasoactive substances, such as histamine. Histamine increases the permeability of the blood vessels and causes edema.

First exposure

Macrophage

B lymphocyte

Plasma cell

Second exposure

Mast cell

Sensitized mast cell

Histamine

Edema

Blood vessel

Degranulated mast cell

hypersensitivity are hay fever, bronchial asthma, atopic dermatitis, and anaphylactic shock.

Hay fever, or allergic rhinitis, occurs typically as a seasonal allergy to pollens. It may also be caused by other foreign substances, such as cat dandruff, and it is not always seasonal.

Exposure to inhaled allergen causes nasal itching and sneezing. Swelling of the nasal mucosa is often associated with similar irritation and inflammation of the conjunctiva (*conjunctivitis*). All symptoms can be attributed to the effects of histamine, and can be neutralized by antihistamines. Drugs that stabilize mast cells and prevent the discharge of their granules are also effective. Long-term relief can be achieved by desensitization to specific allergens. This treatment is based on repeated prophylactic injections of antigen, which induce a neutralizing IgG response. When a desensitized patient encounters the allergen again, the IgG that is bound to the antigen will prevent its contact with the IgE in the sensitized tissue. The adverse response of mast cell is thus prevented.

Atopic dermatitis is typically a disease of childhood, presenting as a chronic skin irritation known as *eczema* (derived from the Greek term for "boiling over" or erupting). Eczema affects approximately 10 percent of all children, 50 percent of whom have a family history of similar problems. This genetic predisposition is associated with hyperproduction of IgE in response to potential environmental allergens. However, a nonfamilial form of atopic dermatitis can occur as well.

Exposure to allergen usually occurs through direct skin contact. Other allergens may be inhaled or ingested in food. Atopic dermatitis improves with age, although affected children have a tendency to develop other type I hypersensitivity diseases in adulthood, such as asthma or hay fever.

Asthma is considered to be a type I hypersensitivity reaction affecting the bronchi. However, as will be presented in Chapter 8, there are several forms of asthma, not all of which are immunologically mediated. Asthma caused by hypersensitivity to inhaled antigens is mediated by SRS-As and usually affects children. Attacks of asthma are marked by coughing and wheezing related to the constriction of bronchi and overproduction of mucus by bronchial glands.

Anaphylactic shock is a life-threatening, severe, systemic response to an allergen to which the body was previously sensitized. Anaphylactic shock following a bee sting in a person sensitized to bee venom is a typical example. In the hospital, it is most often encountered following intravenous injection of anesthetics or radiographic contrast media. Shock develops as a result of a massive release of histamine and other vasoactive substances into the circulation. Typical symptoms include *choking* secondary to laryngeal edema; *wheezing* and shortness of breath resulting from bronchial spasm; and *pulmonary edema*

and systemic *circulatory collapse* with fainting, caused by hypotension secondary to vasodilation and increased leakage of fluid from the hyperpermeable blood vessels. Treatment includes the administration of epinephrine (adrenalin) to simulate both contraction of the precapillary arterioles and heart action, thus restoring normal blood pressure. Bronchodilators are used to alleviate bronchospasm and improve respiration.

Type II Hypersensitivity

Type II hypersensitivity is mediated by cytotoxic antibodies that react with antigens in cells or tissue components, such as basement membranes. The antigen may be extrinsic or intrinsic, as is often the case in some autoimmune diseases. Intrinsic antigens include macromolecules, such as proteins, RNA, or DNA. The reasons why these body components become antigenic are not known. Foreign antigens include drugs or simple chemicals that usually act as haptens. These substances bind to soluble plasma proteins or proteins on the surface of RBCs or other cells in the body and immunize the body. Foreign substances released from bacteria, as well as cells infected with viruses, may provoke a similar response. Hypersensitivity reaction occurs upon reexposure to the pathogenic antigen. Persistent antigens, as in chronic infection, and a slow release of endogenous autoantigens provoke deleterious hypersensitivity reactions.

Type II hypersensitivity reaction is mediated by IgG or IgM, which forms antigen-antibody complexes on cell membranes or extracellular matrix, such as basement membranes (Fig. 3-11). These complexes activate *complement*, which is the major effector mechanism accounting for the cell lysis that occurs, for instance, in the acute hemolytic reaction caused by transfusion of mismatched blood. Immunoglobulins attached to the antigen also may evoke an *antibody-dependent, cellular, cytotoxic (ADCC) reaction.* The antibody typically binds to the antigen with the Fab end, whereas the Fc portion is free and serves as the attachment site for various effector cells, such as NK cells, macrophages, and other leukocytes. Finally, some type II hypersensitivity reactions do not require either complement or an ADCC reaction. Such reactions are based on the binding of antibodies to the receptors on cell surfaces. The binding of antibodies to receptors may stimulate or inhibit the function of such cells.

The best examples of type II hypersensitivity reaction are hemolytic anemia, Goodpasture's syndrome, Graves' disease, and myasthenia gravis.

Hemolytic anemia is the prototype of a cytotoxic antibody-mediated reaction. It may occur in several forms. For example, hemolytic anemia may develop in systemic autoimmune disorders, such as systemic

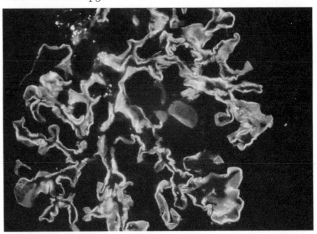

FIGURE 3-11

Pathogenesis of type II hypersensitivity. (A) Binding of the antibody to the antigen on the surface of the cell activates complement, resulting in cell destruction. (B) An antibody-dependent cellular cytotoxic (ADCC) reaction involves effector killer cells, which destroy the target cell coated with the antibody.

lupus erythematosus (SLE). The RBC antigens of these patients become antigenic and are recognized as foreign by the body's own immune system. In some circumstances, foreign chemicals, such as drugs, attach to the surface of the RBCs and act as haptens. The antibodies against haptens on the RBCs cause hemolysis.

Goodpasture's syndrome is marked by renal and pulmonary pathologic changes. These develop because of autoimmunity to a component of collagen type IV which has become autoallergenic. An epitope, which is normally hidden, becomes inappropriately exposed in the glomeruli and the pulmonary blood vessels. Antibodies to collagen IV attach to the basement membrane, damaging the glomeruli and the lungs. These antibodies may be seen in the glomerular basement membrane on immunofluorescence microscopy (Fig. 3-12).

Graves' disease is a form of hyperthyroidism that typically develops in women who have autoantibodies to the thyroid-stimulating hormone (TSH) receptor on the surface of their own follicular cells of the thyroid. The binding of the antibody to the receptor leads to the stimulation of the cells, which is similar to the action of TSH itself. This results in hyperthyroidism, or overproduction of thyroid hormones.

Myasthenia gravis is a muscle disease marked by severe muscle weakness. This autoimmune disease is mediated by antibodies to the receptor for acetylcholine on the surface of striated muscle cells. Acetylcholine is the neurotransmitter released from the nerves at the neuromuscular junction, and it mediates the transmission of signals for muscle contraction. Blockade of acetylcholine receptors prevents the binding of the neurotransmitter, causing progressive muscle weakness and even paralysis.

Type III Hypersensitivity

Type III hypersensitivity is mediated by immune complexes that are formed between antigens and appropriate antibodies. In systemic reactions to soluble antigens, the immune complexes are in the circulation, whereas in localized reactions, the immune complexes are formed in tissues.

Serum sickness, which was common previously when horse serum was used extensively for passive

FIGURE 3-12

Goodpasture's syndrome. Antibodies deposited in the basement membrane of the glomerulus appear as linear, greenish-yellow fluorescent areas when the tissue is processed for immunofluorescence microscopy.

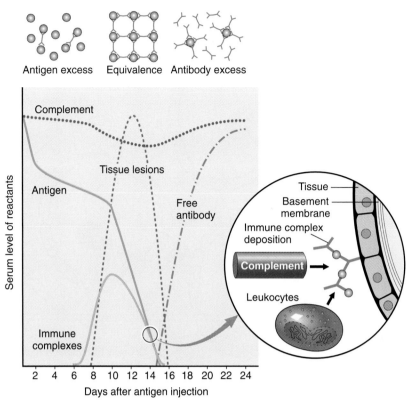

Antigen excess   Equivalence   Antibody excess

Complement

Tissue lesions

Antigen

Free antibody

Immune complexes

Serum level of reactants

2 4 6 8 10 12 14 16 18 20 22 24
Days after antigen injection

Tissue
Basement membrane
Immune complex deposition
Complement
Leukocytes

FIGURE 3-13
Serum sickness. This type III hypersensitivity reaction is mediated by formation of circulating immune complexes. Pathogenic immune complexes are formed only during the phase of antigen excess. The tissue lesions are caused by activated complement and leukocytes attracted to the site of antigen-antibody complex deposition.

immunization against tetanus, is the prototype of type III hypersensitivity (Fig. 3-13). A few days after the injection of the serum, foreign proteins appear in the circulation. As the titer of antibodies rises, the concentration of antigen decreases until all of it is completely complexed with antibodies and eliminated from circulation. Initially, the antigen-antibody complexes are small and sparse, but with time, the antibody excess becomes overwhelming and the antigen is completely bound into large complexes. During the time of equilibrium or mild antibody excess, antigen-antibody complexes form that are rather soluble and not large enough to be phagocytized by macrophages. Such soluble antigens remain in circulation and are filtered through the basement membranes of glomeruli and other sites where the plasma is ultrafiltered to produce body fluids (Fig. 3-14). Such anatomic sites include the anterior chamber of the eye, the choroid plexus of the brain, and the serosal surface covering the pleura, pericardium, and the peritoneal cavity. Immune complexes that are trapped in these semipermeable membranes activate complement which, in turn, forms chemotactic fragments and complexes. PMNs respond to such stimuli and migrate toward the deposited complexes, causing acute inflammation. In acute serum sickness, such a reaction is short-lived and transient. In SLE, another example of type III hypersensitivity reaction, there is a sustained production of immune complexes and the disease is chronic.

Localized immune complex formation occurs typi-

cally in various forms of vasculitis, such as *polyarteritis nodosa*. This disease can be reproduced experimentally in the form of the so-called *Arthus phenomenon*. The antigen is injected subcutaneously to produce sensitization and to stimulate antibody production. Upon rechallenge with the same antigen injected into another site, the antibodies from the circulation diffuse toward the antigen in the tissue and react with it at the site of contact. Antigen-antibody complexes precipitate at the site of equilibrium, and this occurs typically in the vessel wall (Fig. 3-15). Antigen-antibody complexes formed in the vessel wall activate complement, which attracts leukocytes. A localized acute inflammation develops, characterized by fibrinoid necrosis. Fibrinoid necrosis reflects the influx of plasma proteins that permeate the site of injury. Fibrinogen, which is also present, undergoes polymerization into fibrin, leading to localized clotting in the vessel walls.

The most important clinical entities mediated by type III hypersensitivity reactions are SLE, poststreptococcal glomerulonephritis, and polyarteritis nodosa. Rheumatoid arthritis, a very common autoimmune disorder, probably also represents an immune complex disease, although this has not been proven conclusively.

Systemic lupus erythematosus is an autoimmune disease of unknown origin, which will be discussed later in greater detail. Here, it should be mentioned that patients with SLE have circulating immune complexes formed between various autoantigens and

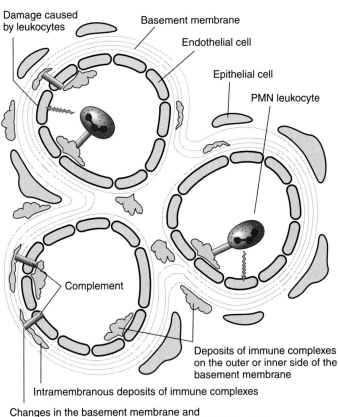

FIGURE 3-14

Diagrammatic depiction of glomerulonephritis. The lesions are produced by activated complement, which acts as a chemotactic stimulus and attracts leukocytes that take part in damaging the tissue. PMN, polymorphonuclear.

FIGURE 3-15

Pathogenesis of the Arthus phenomenon. Localized formation of antigen-antibody complexes results in complement activation and leukocytic inflammation. Necrosis of the vessel wall is accompanied by an influx of plasma proteins. Fibrin formed from insudated fibrinogen is the most prominent feature, accounting for the term fibrinoid necrosis used to describe such lesions.

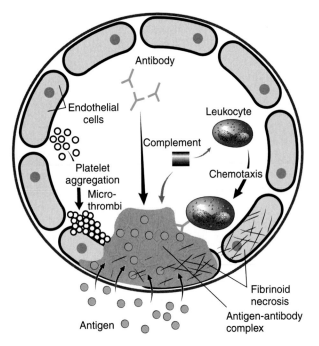

equivalent antibodies. Although it is not clear what elicits the autoimmune reaction, the consequences of immune complex deposition in tissues are well known. These include kidney disease, arthritis, skin disease, and a variety of other diseases. In all these tissues, one can demonstrate the immune complexes by immunofluorescence microscopy.

Poststreptococcal glomerulonephritis is an acute renal disease that typically follows an upper respiratory tract infection caused by certain strains of streptococci that are nephritogenic (i.e., capable of inducing nephritis). Persons sensitized to streptococcal antigens during acute infection produce antibodies that react with the residual bacterial antigen to form circulating complexes. Such antigen-antibody complexes are deposited in the glomerular basement membrane, evoking a complement-mediated inflammatory response.

Glomerulonephritis also may be caused by complexes that are locally formed in the glomeruli. Some soluble streptococcal antigens are "retained" in the glomerular basement membranes during filtration from the plasma. Such hidden foreign antigens may react locally with the circulating antibody. Like in the Arthus phenomenon, antigen-antibody complexes are formed in the vessel wall (i.e., glomerular capillaries) where they activate complement and elicit an inflammatory reaction. This acute glomerulonephritis is usually short-lived and, in most cases, resolves without any serious consequences.

Polyarteritis nodosa, which is the clinical equivalent of the Arthus phenomenon, is a disease that typically involves small to medium-sized arteries. It can affect any organ in the body, and there is nothing typical in the clinical presentation of this disease. The pathologic changes are, however, characteristic. In the early stage, the affected vessels show focal fibrinoid necrosis and acute inflammation. In the chronic stage, the disease is marked by destruction of the vessel wall and formation of microaneurysms (i.e., bulges in the vessel wall) whose elastic and muscle layers have been focally destroyed. The damaged vessels tend to thrombose and become occluded. Occlusion of the arteries causes infarcts and various ischemic symptoms.

The cause of polyarteritis is usually unknown, although in some cases, the disease appears to be linked to chronic hepatitis B viral infection. The treatment includes immunosuppressive drugs, but the results are not always satisfactory, especially if the vessel wall has been damaged and the lumen has been occluded by thrombosis.

Type IV Hypersensitivity

Type IV hypersensitivity is also known as cell-mediated or delayed-type immune reaction. It involves T lymphocytes and macrophages, which typically aggregate at the site of injury to form *granulomas.*

Type IV hypersensitivity reaction is initiated by complex antigens that are taken up by macrophages or equivalent APCs, such as Langerhans' cells of the epidermis. The antigen is processed and presented to T lymphocytes. Helper T lymphocytes that are exposed to the antigen and the cytokines produced by the APCs become primed and activated. This leads, on one hand, to formation of immune memory, which is important for subsequent exposure and the recruitment of other cells, most notably macrophages, and additional helper T and suppressor/cytotoxic T lymphocytes. Under the influence of cytokines, the macrophages transform into epithelioid cells, which produce even more varied mediators of inflammation than their predecessors, further promoting the formation of granulomas. *Interferon gamma,* considered to be the most important cytokine responsible for the formation of granulomas, acts on epithelioid cells by augmenting their phagocytic activity and their ability to kill antigen-bearing cells and bacteria (e.g., *Mycobacterium tuberculosis* or tumor cells). Interferon gamma also promotes the fusion of epithelioid cells into giant cells. Hence, fully formed granulomas consist of epithelioid cells, giant cells, and lymphocytes (Fig. 3-16). Traditionally, the giant cells in tuberculous granulomas have been

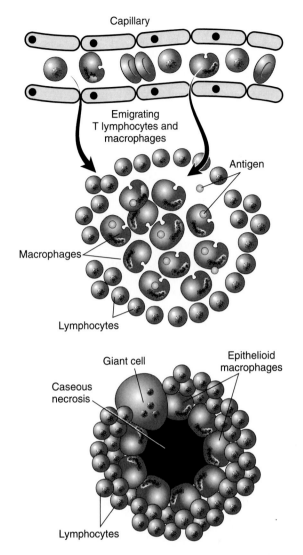

FIGURE 3-16
Granulomas, which are typical of type IV hypersensitivity, consist of epithelioid cells, giant cells, and lymphocytes.

called Langerhans' giant cells, but today we know that these cells are not diagnostic of tuberculosis, but can occur in other granulomas as well.

Type IV hypersensitivity reaction occurs in response to complex antigens of *M. tuberculosis* and *M. leprae,* and various fungi. In addition to infectious granulomas, type IV hypersensitivity reaction accounts for granulomas that develop in response to tumors, as well as idiopathic granulomatous diseases, such as *sarcoidosis.*

Granulomas can be induced by injecting humans or animals with the antigen. For example, tuberculin, prepared from *M. tuberculosis,* may induce delayed hypersensitivity reactions. Thus, it is possible to test whether somebody was exposed to tuberculosis by injecting purified tuberculin into the skin. If the tested person develops localized induration of the skin within 48 hours, the test is considered to be positive and the person is assumed to have been exposed to tuberculosis (or to have persistent disease).

Contact dermatitis, the most common clinical form of type IV hypersensitivity, also does not present with granulomas. In this disease, which may be caused by allergy to a variety of allergens, such as rubber gloves, gold rings, or poison ivy, the skin usually contains infiltrates of T lymphocytes and macrophages, but no granulomas. The inflammatory cells typically show perivascular cuffing, which correlates with altered vascular permeability and wheal formation, as well as edema of the affected skin.

Most of us are sensitized to common childhood viral pathogens, such as mumps, or widespread fungi, such as *Candida albicans.* Antigenic extracts prepared from such microorganisms can be used, therefore, to test the functional capacity of the T cells. If the organism of an adult does not respond to intradermal injection of mumps or Candida antigen, one can conclude that that individual's T cells are unreactive (i.e., that that person has developed *anergy*). This typically occurs in immunosuppressed persons, such as those suffering from AIDS.

Transplantation

Solid tissues can be transplanted successfully from one individual to another, but the graft will be viable only if the donor and the recipient are immunologically similar enough to avoid immunologic rejection. Alternatively, the graft will "take" only if the immune system of the recipient is unable to react against foreign antigens. This is the case in congenitally immunodeficient children born without a thymus, or in nude athymic mice, which represent an animal model of this human immunodeficiency. The immune system can be partially inactivated with various *immunosuppressive* drugs, which are used in clinical medicine to facilitate the acceptance of transplants.

In the clinical setting, there are several forms of **transplantation.** If the patient is serving as both donor and recipient, the transplant is called an *autograft.* Such grafts are typically used for skin grafts, hair transplantation, and replacement of blood vessels of the heart with leg veins.

Tissue transplantation between genetically identical individuals of the same species, as in genetically syngeneic mouse strains or identical twins, is called an *isograft.* Such ideal grafts do not elicit a transplant reaction because the recipient does not recognize the tissue as foreign. Transplants between individuals of the same species who are not genetically identical are called *homografts or allografts.* In clinical practice, homografted tissues are accepted only if the donor and the recipient are matched at several major histocompatibility loci (human leukocyte antigens [HLAs]) and have the same blood group. Best results are obtained with transplantation between relatives or siblings. However, to avoid immune reaction against foreign antigens, the recipients routinely receive immunosuppressive therapy prior to transplantation. *Xenografts*—tissue transplants between animals of different species (as in liver transplantation between monkeys and humans)—are poorly tolerated. However, avascular tissues, such as the cornea or heart valves, can be used for xenografting. Porcine heart valves are used to replace damaged human heart leaflets.

Before transplantation, the donor's tissue must be matched with that of the recipient. This is done by crossmatching the peripheral blood lymphocytes, as the lymphocytes carry the same major histocompatibility antigens as the cells of the solid organs. This test provides basic information on the similarities and disparities of the two individuals and makes it possible to determine to what extent they are *histocompatible.* The **histocompatibility antigens** form four major loci (HLA-A, HLA-B, HLA-C, and HLA-D). Together with a closely related antigen called HLA-DR, these antigens are inherited as a single unit of five loci known as the *haplotype.* Because haplotypes are inherited as single alleles, each of us has a 1 in 4 chance that a brother or sister has a haplotype that is identical to ours. Thus, siblings are ideal tissue donor-recipient pairs. If an ideal match cannot be arranged, however, tissues from the patient's closest relatives or from unrelated donors may be used.

Transplant Rejection

All homografts invariably evoke some transplant rejection, which is mediated by antibodies and a delayed cellular immune reaction. Several clinically distinct forms of transplant rejection are recognized (Fig. 3-17).

Hyperacute reaction typically occurs because the recipient has preformed antibodies to the donor's antigens. Typically, the reactions occur during the operation. When the surgeon connects the donor's and recipient's blood vessels and the recipient's blood enters the graft, the preformed circulating antibodies react with the endothelial cells. Damage to the endothelial cells leads to thrombosis, and the graft cannot perfuse normally. Such transplants must be removed immediately to prevent even more serious and inevitable complications.

Acute rejection occurs most often within the first few weeks of transplantation, but may also evolve later when the immunosuppressive treatment becomes ineffectual. It involves both antibody-mediated and cell-mediated immune reaction. Antibodies tend to damage the blood vessels, which show signs

Clinical Use of Transplantation

Transplants are used extensively in clinical practice. Kidney transplants have been performed with considerable success for more than 30 years. Skin transplants are used for the treatment of burns. Liver, heart, lung, or pancreas that has been terminally damaged also can be replaced successfully with transplants.

Bone marrow transplantation is used to treat aplastic anemia and bone marrow failure. This procedure is also used in the treatment of leukemia, a neoplastic disease of the bone marrow. In such cases, the bone marrow of the leukemic patient is irradiated to kill all the tumor cells and the bone marrow is then replenished with the stem cells removed from the bone marrow of a histocompatible donor.

The best way of preventing transplant rejection is to match the donor and recipient carefully. Because an ideal match is not always possible, recipients must be prepared for transplantation with adequate immunosuppression. This is accomplished by administering drugs, like cyclosporin, which inhibit IL-2 production and thus impair T cell response, or cyclophosphamide, which inhibits proliferation of lymphocytes. Antibodies to T cell antigens are also used to reduce the number of these cells. However, immunosuppression is not an innocuous procedure, and it predisposes the patient to infections. Some drugs, like cyclosporine, may have significant side effects and are nephrotoxic. Immunosuppressed patients are at increased risk for developing infections with ubiquitous bacteria and fungi, which are then difficult to eradicate.

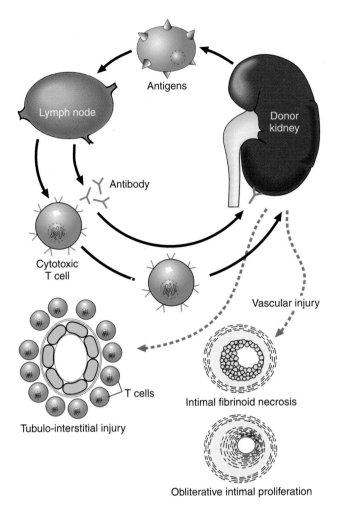

FIGURE 3-17
Transplant rejection is either antibody- or cell-mediated, or both. Antibodies bind to endothelial cells of the transplanted kidney and cause fibrinoid necrosis and thrombosis typical of hyperacute rejection. Chronic vascular rejection is characterized by obliterative endarteritis. Cell-mediated transplant rejection, typical of chronic transplant rejection, is characterized by chronic tubulointerstitial inflammation.

of vasculitis. The inflammatory reaction is most evident in the intima of medium-sized arteries. Cell-mediated immune rejection presents in the form of tissue infiltrates which consist of helper T and suppressor/cytotoxic T lymphocytes and macrophages. B lymphocytes and plasma cells are also present, indicating that this is a mixed reaction.

Chronic transplant rejection evolves slowly over a period of several months or years. It also involves both antibody- and cell-mediated responses. Vascular changes cause obliteration of the arterial lumen (endarteritis), which in turn leads to hypoperfusion of tissues and chronic ischemia. Interstitial tissue inflammation contributes to the destruction of parenchymal cells and the ultimate deterioration of the function of the transplanted organ.

Graft-Versus-Host Reaction

An important complication of transplantation, especially that of bone marrow, is the *graft-versus-host (GVH) reaction* that develops as a result of the transfer of a donor's immunocompetent lymphocytes. In response to antigens on the recipient's tissues, the donor's lymphocytes initiate a cell-mediated type IV immune reaction. Because the host is usually immunosuppressed, the transplanted immunocompetent cells cannot be rejected; as a result, these cells proliferate and overwhelm the donor's body. The donor's lymphocytes attack various tissues in the host, especially the epithelial cells of the gastrointestinal tract, the skin, and the liver. Severe *dermatitis* develops, with scaling of the epidermis. *Diarrhea* and fever are typical signs of gastrointestinal GVH reaction. *Jaundice* is the most prominent sign of liver involvement. GVH reaction may be difficult to treat, and the patient usually dies secondary to overwhelming infection.

Blood Transfusion

Transfusion of blood from one person to another is a form of transplantation. In contrast to solid organs, however, blood is a tissue that is composed of dissociated cells circulating inside the vessels. Because RBCs outnumber white blood cells by an order of magnitude, the success or failure of blood transfusions depends primarily on the compatibility of the donor and the recipient with regard to their RBC blood group antigens.

Every RBC carries a set of surface antigens, which can be divided into three groups: major blood group antigens, minor blood group antigens, and Rh blood antigens.

Major blood group antigens (ABO) are encoded by three genes that can give the following six genotypes: AA, AB, AO, BO, BB, and OO. The A and B gene are dominant over the O gene, so there are only four blood groups: A (AA, AO), B (BB, BO), AB, and O.

ABO antigens have corresponding natural antibodies: A group blood contains anti-B antibodies, B group blood contains anti-A antibodies, and the O group contains both anti-A and anti-B antibodies. Group AB blood does not contain natural antibodies to A or B antigen. Thus, A blood can be given to group A and group AB recipients, whereas AB blood can be given only to AB group recipients. O group blood can be given to recipients of all blood groups. Accordingly, individuals with AB blood are called *universal recipients* and those with O blood are considered to be *universal donors* (Fig. 3-18).

If the blood of an A group donor is infused into a B group recipient, the natural antibodies to A in the recipient hemolyze the donor's RBCs. This will cause a *transfusion reaction* that is clinically manifested by chills, shivering, and even mild fever. If the transfusion is not discontinued, a state of shock, with microthrombi and disseminated intravascular coagulation (DIC) develops, and the patient may even die. Jaundice, from the bilirubin released from hemolyzed RBC, develops in those who survive. Acute renal failure is a common complication.

In order to avoid transfusion reaction, the donor's blood must be crossmatched with the blood of the recipient. This is done before the transfusion by mixing the serum of the donor with the RBCs of the recipient and vice versa. The RBCs are incubated at body temperature in a test tube. The RBCs that are compatible with the serum will remain suspended in the fluid. However, if there are antibodies in the serum, these will attach to the RBCs and agglutinate them. Blood that agglutinates in the crossmatch is not suitable for transfusion.

Crossmatching of donor and recipient blood is essential for avoiding transfusion reactions caused by ABO incompatibility. Additionally, this procedure

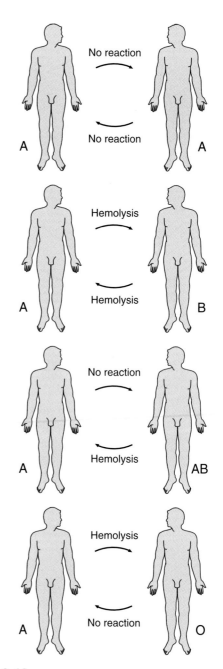

FIGURE 3-18

ABO blood groups. There are three genes—A, B, and O—which can yield six combinations. Because A and B are dominant over O, there are only four blood groups; A, B, AB, and O. Blood transfusion is well accepted between persons of the same group (A to A). The transfusion of A blood to a donor with group B blood causes hemolysis. A person with group AB blood can receive blood of all groups ("universal recipient"). A person with group O blood can give blood to all other groups ("universal donor").

can also detect significant incompatibilities of minor blood group antigens. These blood group antigens are known as Lewis, Kell, and so on. In most instances, incompatibility at these loci has no consequence, but occasionally, it may cause a significant hemolytic reaction.

Rh Factor Incompatibility

The Rh blood group system consists of a group of antigens expressed normally on the surface of human RBCs. Only three antigens, known as cde/CDE are strong antigens, and of these, only the d/D antigen is of practical significance. Persons that have the dominant allele D are called Rh positive (Rh⁺) and those that have two recessive d/d alleles are Rh negative (Rh⁻). Approximately 15 percent of Caucasians and 5 percent of African Americans are Rh⁻, whereas most others, including Native American Indians and Asians, are Rh⁺.

In contrast to the ABO antigens, which are complemented with natural antibodies, Rh antigens do not have natural antibodies. Thus, antibodies to dominant Rh antigens will be formed in Rh⁻ persons who are transfused with Rh⁺ blood. Furthermore, it is important to note that the antibodies to the ABO antigens are of the IgM class, whereas the newly generated anti-Rh antibodies are IgG. As mentioned previously, the IgG antibodies can cross the placenta, which is an important consideration in maternofetal **Rh factor incompatibility.**

Maternofetal incompatibility involving the Rh antigen D has, until recently, been the most important cause of neonatal *hemolytic disease* and several syndromes known as *icterus gravis neonatorum, hydrops fetalis,* and *erythroblastosis fetalis.* These conditions, which involve Rh⁻ women with Rh⁺ mates, are all caused by the same mechanism; the different names for the syndromes merely reflect the extent of

injury and its timing. If the child is Rh⁺ because it has inherited the paternal D allele, its Rh⁺ blood could sensitize the mother. During the first pregnancy, the Rh⁺ child will not be affected because the mother does not have natural antibodies to the Rh antigen D (Fig. 3-19). However, the mixing of fetal and maternal blood at the time of delivery may expose the Rh⁻ mother to the dominant D antigen on fetal RBCs. This will immunize the mother and cause her to produce IgG-type anti-Rh antibodies. If the fetus in the subsequent pregnancy is again Rh⁺ (i.e., d/D), the antibodies to D will cross the placenta and affect the fetal Rh⁺ RBCs. Hemolysis will ensue in the fetal circulation and the fetus may die in utero showing signs of severe *hydrops fetalis* (Fig. 3-20).

Essentially, the hemolysis destroys fetal RBCs. The fetus becomes anemic and develops severe hypoxia and congestive heart failure. The term *erythroblastosis fetalis,* used as a synonym, indicates that the fetal bone marrow is maximally stimulated by the loss of RBCs and is trying to compensate for the loss. There is marked extramedullary hematopoiesis in the liver, spleen, and lymph nodes. The fetus is also jaundiced owing to bilirubin released from the hemolyzed RBCs.

In milder cases, there is comparatively less hemolysis and massive edema does not develop. The newborn child does not show signs of massive edema, and the only external evidence of hemolysis is marked jaundice (*icterus gravis*). The major danger associated with icterus gravis is *kernicterus* (*Kern* meaning nucleus in German) or jaundice of the basal

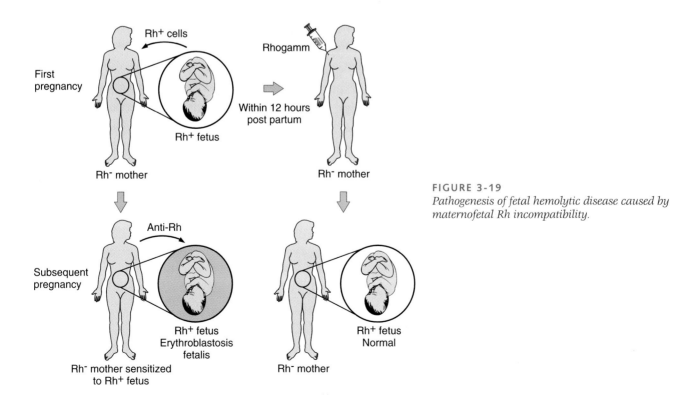

FIGURE 3-19
Pathogenesis of fetal hemolytic disease caused by maternofetal Rh incompatibility.

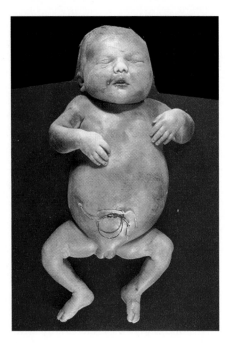

FIGURE 3-20
Hydrops fetalis caused by maternofetal incompatibility.

ganglia (nuclei) of the brain. The massive elevation of serum bilirubin breaches the blood–brain barrier and the bilirubin that normally does not cross into the brain is deposited preferentially in the basal ganglia. This bilirubin is toxic and may cause permanent neural damage.

Clearly, maternofetal Rh incompatibility has serious repercussions, and once the disease develops, it cannot be treated efficiently. Fortunately, this disease can be prevented by immunoprophylaxis. At the time that an Rh⁻ mother first delivers an Rh⁺ fetus, it is possible to prevent Rh immunization of the mother by injecting her with anti-D immunoglobulin (RhoGAM). This procedure, if performed during the first 12 hours postpartum, will prevent maternal immunization and erythroblastosis fetalis in subsequent pregnancies. Unfortunately, if a pregnant Rh⁻ woman becomes immunized to the D antigen during pregnancy or during previous abortions, immunoprophylaxis with RhoGAM is of no avail.

Immunoprophylaxis of Rh maternofetal incompatibility has almost completely eliminated this medical problem in the United States. Hemolytic disease of the neonate still occurs, albeit rarely, as a result of the incompatibility of the fetal and maternal major blood groups or some minor blood group antigens. In practice, this is usually encountered in fetuses of the A_1 subtype born to group O mothers who have acquired IgG antibodies to the A_1 antigen. Fortunately, this incompatibility results only in mild hemolysis and the newborn child usually shows only anemia and jaundice. There is no prophylactic measure that could be applied to prevent the consequences of maternofetal incompatibility in ABO or minor blood group antigens.

Autoimmune Diseases

As stated before, immune response is based on the ability of cells of the immune system to distinguish between self and non-self. The body is generally tolerant to antigens expressed on its own cells. Numerous control mechanisms have been devised in nature to suppress the response against self-antigens. Breakdown of autotolerance results in **autoimmune diseases.**

There are several theories for the development of autoimmunity, but only three are presented here. The *clonal deletion theory* postulates that autoimmunity occurs if the autoreactive T or B clones have not been eliminated. Under normal circumstances, the body does not react to its own fetal and neonatal antigens, recognized because the corresponding T and B cell clones have been eliminated from the immune system during the fetal period or early after birth. If such "forbidden clones" of autoreactive B cells remain active, producing antibodies to self-antigens, an autoimmune disease develops. This frequently involves helper T cells, which lose the ability to regulate B cell function. A second theory proposes that autoimmunity can be triggered by an exogenous antigen, assuming that the antibodies produced to it cross-react with some similar determinant on the body's own cells. Finally, it is also possible that some antigens that are normally nonimmunogenic ("hidden antigens") become autoimmunogenic and stimulate the immune system to react against "self." Normal antigens could also transform into autoimmunogenic "neoantigens" by combining with a foreign hapten.

The diagnosis of autoimmune disorder is made when (1) the existence of autoantibodies can be documented, (2) there is evidence that the immune mechanisms are pathogenetically important and have caused the pathologic lesions, and (3) there is direct or indirect evidence of the immune nature of the disorder. For example, a disease is presumably autoimmune if it shows a favorable response to treatment with immunosuppressive drugs or if it can be diagnosed by immunologic techniques. The existence of autoantibodies cannot always be demonstrated, and their pathogenicity is often even more difficult to prove.

Autoimmune disorders occur with increased frequency in some families, suggesting that genetic factors have an important pathogenetic role. The genetic basis of these disorders has been best documented by studying the linkage of autoimmune disorders and certain HLA haplotypes. For example, HLA-B27 is strongly associated with *ankylosing spondylitis.* More than 90 percent of all patients with this disease of the spine have this particular major histocompatibility antigen.

Most autoimmune diseases are more common in women than in men. The preponderance of women

Table 3-1 Autoimmune Diseases

Systemic Diseases	Organ-Specific Diseases	
Systemic lupus erythematosus	Brain	Multiple sclerosis
Rheumatic fever	Thyroid	Hashimoto's thyroiditis
Rheumatoid arthritis	Blood	Autoimmune hemolytic anemia
Systemic sclerosis	Kidney	Glomerulonephritis
	Liver	Primary biliary cirrhosis
Polyarteritis nodosa	Skin	Pemphigus vulgaris
	Muscle	Myasthenia gravis

among the population affected by SLE, rheumatoid arthritis, or autoimmune thyroiditis suggests that *nongenetic* factors are also important and could influence the predisposition to these diseases.

Autoimmune diseases may present in two forms: a systemic, multiorgan disease or a disease limited to a single organ. Table 3-1 lists some of the more common autoimmune diseases. It is worth mentioning that many of these diseases were previously classified as collagen-vascular disorders or "collagenoses." Although many of these diseases adversely affect collagen and other components of the connective tissue, it would be incorrect to consider them primarily as connective tissue disorders. It has been conclusively shown that the primary defect for almost all of these disorders is the dysregulation of the immune response, and that this, rather than the connective tissue lesions themselves, is the most important unifying aspect for the entire group of diseases.

Systemic Lupus Erythematosus

SLE is a prototype of an autoimmune disorder characterized by multisystemic involvement. It affects 1 in 2500 persons and is 10 times more common in women than in men. It may occur at any age, but most often affects young adults. The disease, which is most severe among African Americans, shows a familial preponderance. There is a 30 percent concordance among identical twins. Collectively, these facts show that both genetic and nongenetic factors play important pathogenetic roles.

Pathogenesis. The etiology and pathogenesis of SLE are poorly understood. Generally, it is believed that the basic defect is a malfunction of suppressor T cells which allows polyclonal activation of B cells. Plasma cells derived from these uncontrolled B cell clones secrete antibodies of variable specificity against both autoantigens and foreign antigens. A variety of antigens can be detected in the serum of pa-

tients with SLE, but it is not known to what extent these antigens elicit noxious antibodies. Some antibodies represent only a secondary response of the body's immune cells to preexisting injury caused by some other mechanism(s). Some authorities even believe it possible that the tissue lesions could be primarily inflicted by a virus, and that antibody production represents only a secondary response. Initially, such a response can be beneficial, but if it persists, it could clearly be deleterious.

The most important antibodies are to nuclear components: DNA, RNA, and nuclear proteins. These are, therefore, called antinuclear antibodies (ANAs) and are best detected by indirect immunofluorescence microscopy. This test is performed routinely on tissue sections. The tissue sections obtained from an unrelated donor are placed on a histology slide and covered with the patient's serum. If the serum contains ANAs, these will bind to the nuclei. The bound antibodies can be detected with a fluoresceinated secondary antibody. The tissue examined by fluorescence microscopy shows fluorescence of the nuclei. Antibodies to DNA and histones show diffuse staining, whereas antibodies to double-stranded DNA (native DNA) show a rimlike staining along the nuclear membrane; antibodies to nuclear proteins show speckled staining. The concentration of antibodies—i.e., their titer—is then determined by serially diluting the serum until no more staining occurs. For example, a titer of 1:256 means that this dilution still yields a positive result, but the next dilution (1:512) produces no staining.

Practically all patients with SLE have ANAs. One half of them have rim staining and one fourth have speckled staining. Diffuse staining is also seen. However, because diffuse staining is also seen in other autoimmune diseases, the rim staining, and especially the speckled staining pattern, have greater diagnostic import. The latter antigens can easily be extracted and are, therefore, called *extractable nuclear antigens* (ENAs). These include the so-called Sm antigen (named so after the patient Smith in whom it was first discovered), which is the most reliable diagnostic indicator of SLE. Unfortunately, Sm is found in only about 20 percent of patients. In practice, then, one must compromise between sensitivity and specificity of the test, and use all laboratory data in the proper clinical context.

Pathology. Antibodies of patients with SLE react with antigens in tissues, but also with those released from cells damaged by other means. Skin exposed to sunlight is often affected. One hypothesis is that the damaged cells release their nuclear content, which then diffuses toward the antibodies, permeating the tissues. Antigen-antibody complexes form in the skin along the epidermodermal junction.

If the antigens reach the circulation, they form

complexes with the antibodies in the serum. Such circulating antigen-antibody complexes are usually deposited in semipermeable membranes, like the glomerular basement membranes. Other sites at which the deposits are seen include the synovial membrane of the joints, the serous membranes of the pleura and peritoneum, the endocardium of the heart valves, the choroid plexus in the ventricles of the brain, and the anterior eye chamber. In all these sites, the plasma is filtered across a membrane into a body cavity (e.g., joint space), or it penetrates into the tissue by diffusion (e.g., endocardium). The immune complexes are relatively large and are retained during this ultrafiltration. At the site of deposition, the immune complexes activate complement; this, in turn, elicits an inflammatory reaction, resulting in a number of organ-specific inflammatory diseases, such as glomerulonephritis, dermatitis, arthritis, and others (Fig. 3-21).

Clinical Features. The symptoms of SLE are highly variable. Inflammation of the joints (arthritis), manifested by swelling, redness, and painful movement, and skin eruptions are found in most patients. There is kidney involvement in 75 percent of affected patients. Kidney symptoms may be mild, with renal involvement sometimes causing only minor urinary abnormalities, such as hematuria or proteinuria. Nevertheless, glomerulonephritis is common, and renal problems are among the most important manifestations of SLE. Kidney disease associated with SLE must be treated vigorously to prevent loss of kidney function.

Circulatory antibodies damage the RBCs and cause anemia, a common sequela of the disease. The polyclonal activation of lymphocytes is usually associated with enlargement of the lymph nodes and spleen. Other organs are less commonly involved.

The course of SLE is highly variable. Immunotherapy has achieved considerable success; indeed, more than 75 percent of treated patients are alive 10 years after the onset of disease. Kidney failure is still the most common serious complication of SLE. It can be treated only by renal transplantation.

Immunodeficiency Diseases

Immunodeficiency diseases may be *congenital* (*primary*), or they may be *secondary*, occurring as a result of infections, metabolic diseases, cancer, or treatment. Secondary immunodeficiency is more common than primary immunodeficiency. AIDS, the most prevalent disease in this group, is one of the most important human diseases today.

Immunodeficiency, be it primary or secondary, may involve primarily B cells or subsets of T cells, or it may be generalized and involve the entire immune

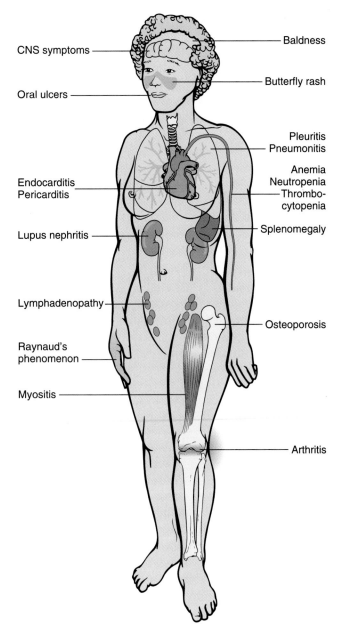

FIGURE 3-21
Clinical and pathologic features of systemic lupus erythematosus.

system. All immunodeficiencies are characterized by *lymphopenia,* a low lymphocyte count in the peripheral blood. B-cell deficiencies are associated with low levels of serum immunoglobulins. Defective or inadequate function of T cells may be detected by immunologic tests for cell-mediated immunity (e.g., a patch test or tuberculin test). All immunodeficiencies cause reduced resistance to infections.

Primary Immunodeficiency Diseases

Primary immunodeficiency diseases are a heterogeneous group of inborn disorders affecting differentiation and maturation of the T and B lymphocytes. The block in differentiation can occur at any step in the developmental sequence that leads from the lymphoid stem cell to T cells on one side and B cells on the other side of the developmental pathway. There are many immunodeficiencies, but only three examples are presented here.

Severe combined immunodeficiency (Swiss type agammaglobulinemia) is related to a defect of lymphoid stem cells, also known as pre-B, pre-T cells. Affected children lack both T and B cells. The thymus is hypoplastic, and the lymph nodes are small and lack germinal centers. Unless placed in strict isolation, these children succumb to infections and die early in infancy.

Isolated deficiency of IgA is the most common congenital immunodeficiency, affecting 1 in 700 persons. The affected person cannot produce IgA, apparently as a result of a block in the terminal differentiation of B cells to IgA-producing plasma cells. Affected persons have a reduced resistance to intestinal infections, but many are otherwise asymptomatic.

DiGeorge syndrome is a deficiency of T cells related to a developmental block in the formation of the thymus. The thymus develops from the branchial clefts, fetal structures that also give rise to the parathyroid glands. Children born without a thymus are unable to mount a cell-mediated immune response and usually die of infection. Owing to congenital hypoparathyroidism, they also develop hypocalcemia and experience severe spastic convulsions.

There are numerous other congenital immunodeficiencies that are beyond the scope of this discussion. Although these are generally not as common as the three described, it is important to keep them in mind. From time to time, an infant or young child will present with a history of recurrent infections and retarded development. In such cases, it is worth remembering that the child may have a congenital defect of the immune system. There are already encouraging experimental data that indicate that some of these children may be saved by genetic engineering. "Bubble children" (so called because they must be placed in strict isolation from all environmental pathogens) have already received transplants of genetically modified lymphoid cells. Transplanted cells have successfully repopulated the bone marrow of these immunodeficient children and colonized the secondary lymph organs. The immune defect has been completely corrected by this procedure in a dozen children.

Acquired Immunodeficiency Syndrome (AIDS)

AIDS, as the name implies, is a syndrome (i.e., a complex of symptoms) that develops as a consequence of a severe acquired immunodepression caused by the human immunodeficiency viruses (HIVs).

Etiology and Epidemiology. HIVs are small RNA viruses that belong to the lentivirus family of viruses. This human virus is related, but distinct from, immunodeficiency viruses that affect monkeys, called simian immunodeficiency virus (SIV), and other lentiviruses that infect horses, sheep, and many other animals. Clinical AIDS is most often caused by HIV-1, although HIV-2 is an important cause of AIDS in Africa.

The medical world became aware of AIDS in the early 1980s, after a series of reports about this "new disease" appeared. Initially, the reports concentrated on homosexual men who developed repeated bouts of pneumonia and various other opportunistic infections and who usually died, completely exhausted by disease and in a state of profound immunosuppression. Subsequently, it became apparent that the disease could occur in other populations as well, and that it could be transmitted in several ways. Ultimately, this led to the discovery of the virus. Serologic tests were developed for the detection of the virus and the antibodies to the virus, which appear in essentially all infected persons. All these scientific advances made it possible not only to diagnose the viral infection, but also to study its spread and define the risk factors that allow the virus to spread from one person to another.

AIDS has a worldwide distribution. In 1994, the World Health Organization (WHO) reported that, for the first time, the number of recorded cases of AIDS had surpassed 1 million. The estimates are that, by the year 2000, there will be at least 40 million people infected with HIV worldwide.

The highest prevalence of AIDS has been reported in Africa, where the disease is still spreading at an alarming pace. In the United States, the number of new cases has leveled off, but more than 100,000 new cases are still reported every year. Reports indicate that 1 percent of all college-aged people (18 to 25 years of age) have serologic evidence of HIV infection.

Pathogenesis. HIV is an RNA retrovirus that cannot survive outside of human cells. Humans are the only source of infection. The virus is transmitted from one person to another by close contact that facilitates the transfer of body fluids. The most common modes of transmission are blood transfusions or contacts that transfer blood from one person to another. Intravenous drug abuse is an important mode of transmission because drug users often share the same blood-contaminated paraphernalia. Hemophiliacs who have received blood products prepared from inadequately tested sources have often been infected. Sexual secretions and sperm also contain HIV, so sexual contact, be it homosexual or heterosexual in nature, is an important mode of transmission of AIDS. In addition to blood-borne and sexually transmitted HIV infections, AIDS can also be acquired by maternofetal, transplacental transmission of the virus. Screening of blood donors has reduced the number of transfusion-related cases of AIDS. The recent emphasis on safe sex—i.e., use of condoms and avoidance of casual sex with unknown persons—has reduced the number of sexually acquired AIDS cases in the Western World. Nevertheless, sexual transmission is still an important mode of infection, especially in Africa. Maternofetal transmission remains an important health problem, especially among HIV-infected drug addicts.

From time to time, there are news reports that AIDS has been acquired by casual contact and without exposure to infected blood or body fluids. There is no scientific evidence that AIDS can be acquired by casual contact. Minor open wounds, an accidental prick with an infected needle, or a minor incision during operation in an HIV-infected person may serve as an entry point for HIV and constitute a risk for health professionals. Nevertheless, with appropriate precautions, the risk is very small. There are only a few health professionals who have died of AIDS acquired in the professional setting.

HIV infection is accompanied by a series of events that can be explained by two factors: selective affinity of HIV for certain human cells and the effects of the virus on the immune system. In the blood, HIV has an affinity for helper T lymphocytes (CD4-positive lymphocytes) and monocytes. Macrophages, which are the tissue-derived descendants of monocytes, can also become infected. Furthermore, fixed tissue phagocytic cells, such as the follicular dendritic cells in the lymph nodes and the microglia of the nervous system (which are also derived from monocytes) are also sites of infection. All of these cells can serve as reservoirs for the virus.

Helper T lymphocytes, macrophages, and their fixed tissue equivalents are essential components of the immune system. HIV is cytotoxic, so a depletion of helper T lymphocytes and other infected cells is typical of AIDS.

Initial infection of an immunologically competent organism stimulates B cells to produce antibodies, which appear in the circulation within weeks of exposure. These antibodies are important for the diagnosis of HIV infection. However, serologic positivity alone, (i.e., the presence of antibodies) does not mean that that person has AIDS. Actually, most infected persons enter a latent phase of infection and are asymptomatic for prolonged periods of time. As the virus replicates and destroys more and more helper T lymphocytes, the symptoms of AIDs begin appearing. Cell-mediated and B-cell–mediated immunity ultimately become depressed and the immunosuppressed organism cannot then defend itself from infection. Death usually occurs because of overwhelming infection. A small number of patients develop tumors that are the cause of death. These tumors can be of any kind, but most commonly are lymphomas or a peculiar tumor of the blood vessels called Kaposi's sarcoma. Lymphomas can arise from B or T cells, the proliferation of which cannot be controlled by the weakened immune system. Many lymphomas originate in the brain, an anatomic site that cannot be "properly policed" by the immune system, even under normal circumstances. The lymphoma cells probably also contain activated cancer genes (oncogenes), and it is also possible that the HIV virus may act as an oncogene itself. Kaposi's sarcoma appears to be caused by an oncogene that is activated selectively in endothelial cells lining the small blood vessels.

Clinical Presentation. According to the Centers for Disease Control (CDC) in Atlanta, Georgia, HIV-infected persons belong to one of four groups; those with acute illness (I); those with asymptomatic infection (II); those with persistent, generalized lymphadenopathy (III); and those with other diseases superimposed on the viral infection (IV). These groups correspond clinically to the early acute, chronic, and crisis phases of the disease (Fig. 3-22).

Acute illness occurs in approximately 50 percent of HIV-infected persons, usually 3 to 6 weeks after exposure. Typical symptoms are nonspecific, and may include fever, night sweats, nausea, myalgia,

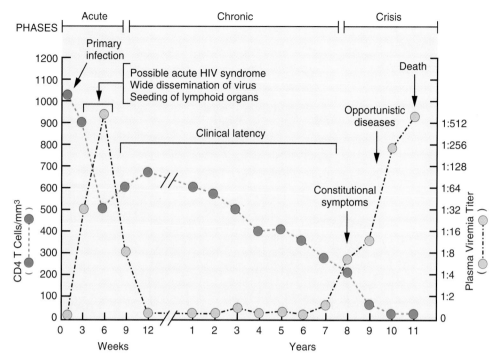

FIGURE 3-22

Typical course of HIV infection. During the early period after primary infection, there is widespread dissemination of virus and a sharp decrease in the number of CD4+ T cells in peripheral blood. An immune response to HIV ensues, with a decrease in detectable viremia followed by a prolonged period of clinical latency. The CD4+ T-cell count continues to decrease during the following years, until it reaches a critical level below which there is substantial risk of opportunistic diseases. (Redrawn and reproduced with permission from Pantaleo, G., Graziosi, C., and Fauci, A.S.: The immunopathogenesis of human immunodeficiency virus infection. The New England Journal of Medicine 328:327, 1993.)

headache, sore throat, skin rash, and mild lymph node enlargement. These symptoms last 2 to 3 weeks and then disappear spontaneously. During this period, some patients develop antibodies to HIV.

The phase of *asymptomatic infection* is of variable duration, lasting from a few months to a few years. The patient is asymptomatic but carries the virus and is infectious. Approximately 50 percent of HIV-infected patients develop AIDS within 10 years of initial diagnosis.

Persistent *generalized lymphadenopathy* may develop in patients who are initially asymptomatic. Alternatively, the lymphadenopathy may develop early in the course of infection and persist for months or years.

Group IV symptoms are categorized, according to CDC recommendations, into several subgroups. These patients show signs of AIDS, the most important of which reflect opportunistic infections, gastrointestinal disorders, central nervous system involvement, and neoplasia.

The diagnosis of HIV infection and AIDS is based on clinical findings and laboratory data. The most important laboratory tests are the test for antibodies to HIV and the lymphocyte count. The antibodies to

HIV appear at a variable rate, 2 to 10 weeks after infection. The presence of the virus in the body can be confirmed by additional tests, which are often used to avoid false-positive results.

The lymphocyte count is very important for the evaluation of immunocompetence. In practice, it is used to determine the ratio of helper T to suppressor/cytotoxic T cells. Normally, this ratio is greater than 2 and reflects an absolute number of helper T (CD4-positive) cells that exceeds 500 per microliter. During the early phases of the disease and during the chronic phase, the CD4-positive cell count exceeds 500. As the disease progresses, helper T cell counts decrease; once the number of CD4-positive cells falls below 200, the crisis phase ensues. In the last stages of disease, almost no CD4 cells are present in the circulation.

Pathologic Findings. The morphologic changes induced in the human organism by HIV are relatively nonspecific (Fig. 3-23). These changes vary with time, the extent of viremia, and the degree of immunosuppression. For example, the lymph nodes initially enlarge and show hyperplasia of the follicles, reflecting the B cell response to viral antigens that

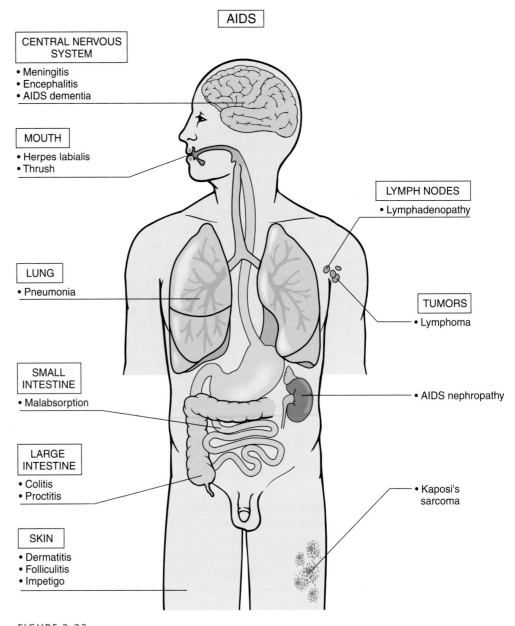

AIDS

CENTRAL NERVOUS
SYSTEM
• Meningitis
• Encephalitis
• AIDS dementia

MOUTH
• Herpes labialis
• Thrush

LYMPH NODES
• Lymphadenopathy

LUNG
• Pneumonia

TUMORS
• Lymphoma

SMALL
INTESTINE
• Malabsorption

• AIDS nephropathy

LARGE
INTESTINE
• Colitis
• Proctitis

• Kaposi's
sarcoma

SKIN
• Dermatitis
• Folliculitis
• Impetigo

FIGURE 3-23
Pathologic changes associated with AIDS.

leads to the appearance of antiviral antibodies. After some time, the lymph nodes involute and become depleted of lymphocytes, especially in the T-cell–dependent parafollicular zones. In the last stages of AIDS, the lymph nodes may be infected with fungi or mycobacteria, which usually do not provoke an inflammatory response, and almost never contain granulomas.

The brain is the only organ that shows HIV-specific changes. In the brain, HIV evokes a microglial response. Microglial nodules with multinucleated giant cells in the gray matter and subcortical gray matter of the cerebrum are typical of AIDS encephalopathy. Overshadowing these changes are le-

sions caused by opportunistic infections, which give rise to meningitis or encephalitis. Of the pathogens affecting the brain, the most important are viruses, such as herpesvirus and cytomegalovirus; fungi, such as Cryptococcus; and protozoa, such as Toxoplasma. These infections may destroy parts of the brain directly, or by occluding blood vessels and causing ischemic infarct.

The respiratory tract is a common site of infection in AIDS patients. In the initial stages of the disease, the infections are typically localized to the upper respiratory tract and present as nasal infection (rhinitis) or throat infection (pharyngitis). Advanced immunosuppression predisposes the individual to pneumonia, which is often caused by fungi, such as *Pneumocystis carinii, Aspergillus fumigatus,* or *Candida albicans.* Mixed bacterial infections are also common. A significant number of patients develop pulmonary tuberculosis.

The gastrointestinal tract is also often infected, usually by the same pathogens that infect the lungs. Furthermore, parasitic infections, with pathogens that are rarely found in otherwise healthy people, are also common. Protozoa, such as Cryptosporidium, worms, such as Strongyloides, and uncommon forms of tuberculosis, such as *Mycobacterium avium intracellulare* (MAI), are not uncommon. Diarrhea and malabsorption of nutrients, caused by such infections, are important cofactors in the pathogenesis of wasting that typically occur in AIDS.

Skin lesions are common in HIV-infected persons. The skin changes may present as mild seborrheic dermatitis (itching skin rash) or persistent infections with various viruses (herpesvirus), fungi (dermatomycoses), and bacteria (streptococcal folliculitis).

Tumors that develop in AIDS are important causes of mortality. Patients with AIDS show an increased incidence of all tumors. The most important among the malignant neoplasms occurring in patients with AIDS are lymphomas and Kaposi's sarcoma. The lymphomas occur in the lymph nodes, spleen, liver, and many extranodal sites. Brain lymphomas are especially common and are associated with a high mortality. Histologically, AIDS-related lymphomas do not differ from other lymphomas. Cytologically, they are often found to be of high grade, which correlates with their rapid proliferation and poor prognosis.

Kaposi's sarcoma is a malignant disease involving endothelial cells. It often occurs in the skin of patients with AIDS, and, for unknown reasons, has an especially high prevalence among male homosexuals. Kaposi's sarcoma is often multifocal and may involve internal organs as well. On gross examination, it presents in the form of bluish red nodules. Histologically, these nodules are composed of anastomosing vascular spaces filled with blood. Kaposi's sarcoma grows slower than lymphoma. Nevertheless, it may cause extensive bleeding, and the mass lesions may compress vital organs and cause death.

Treatment. At the present time, AIDS is an incurable disease. Death can be postponed, however, by vigorous treatment of opportunistic infections and general support of vital functions. New drugs that inhibit replication of viruses have improved the chances for survival of most HIV-infected patients. However, such drugs are expensive and not readily available. Efforts to produce a vaccine against HIV have been unsuccessful so far.

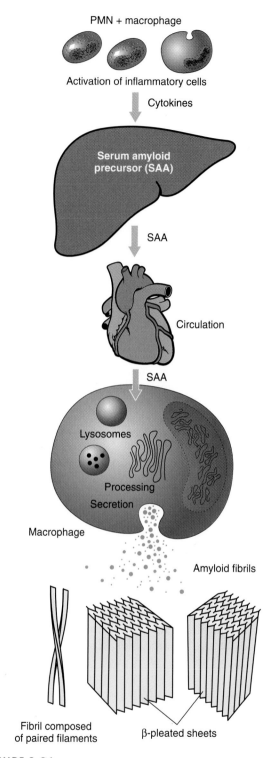

FIGURE 3-24

Pathogens of amyloidosis secondary to inflammation. Cytokines released from inflammatory cells stimulate the liver, which secretes serum amyloid A (SAA). This soluble precursor of amyloid is processed by macrophages and laid down in tissues in the form of fibrils that have a beta-pleated structure.

Amyloidosis

Amyloidosis is caused by deposition of a fibrillar substance called amyloid. As amyloidosis is a multifactorial disease that is often related to abnormalities of the immune system or an abnormal response to chronic infection, it is reviewed in this chapter.

Amyloid, originally named so because it was thought to resemble starch (the meaning of the Greek term *amylon*), is not a chemically distinct entity. Instead, it is defined in terms of its physical properties: fibers that are 7.5 nm thick and arranged into a beta-pleated sheet. Thus, any fibrillar protein that forms a beta-pleated sheet is called amyloid. This conformational state can be recognized by radiographic crystallography. In histologic sections, this would be impractical. Instead, amyloid is detected with Congo red, a dye that has the capacity to intercalate into beta-pleated sheets in a peculiar manner. Congo red, when bound to amyloid, is red. However, when examined under polarizing light, it becomes apple green. Amyloid fibrils also have a distinct appearance on electron microscopy.

Biochemically, there are several forms of amyloids that are all derived from distinct precursors. On the basis of the biochemical structure of the major fibrillar protein, amyloids are divided into several groups, the most important of which are

- *AL amyloid,* derived from the light chain of the immunoglobulins. This is typically formed by neoplastic B cells, as seen in malignant lymphoma and plasmacytoma.
- *AA amyloid,* derived from serum amyloid-associated (SAA) protein. SAA is an acute-phase reactant that is produced by the liver in response to various stimuli, most notably, infection (Fig. 3-24).

As already stated, all amyloids, regardless of their biochemical composition, are deposited in the extracellular spaces as Congo red–positive substances. This material stains pink on slides prepared with hematoxylin and eosin stain. Therefore, the tissue impregnated with amyloid will appear to be hyalinized (i.e., homogeneously eosinophilic and "glassy," without structure).

Amyloid changes the function of tissues and cells. The deposits in the basement membranes of the blood vessels change their permeability. In the glomeruli, amyloid thus leads to proteinuria. The sinusoids of the liver and adrenal gland, which are normally fenestrated, transform into solid, tube-like, impermeable vessels. Furthermore, the deposits of amyloid compress the parenchymal cells, which together with ischemia, causes atrophy and loss of cell function. Hepatic and adrenal insufficiency develop. Deposits of amyloid in the heart weaken myocardial contractions. Deposits of amyloid in the brain, a typical feature of Alzheimer's disease, impair neural cell function and contribute to the dementia ("feeble-mindedness") that is characteristic of this brain disease.

The biochemical properties of amyloids found in various anatomic locations vary. The *AL amyloid* of multiple myeloma, also called *primary amyloidosis,* is deposited in the kidneys, but may be found in the blood vessels of other organs as well. *AA amyloid* is typically found in association with chronic inflammation (e.g., chronic tuberculosis of the lungs, suppurative bronchiectasis, chronic osteomyelitis), but also occurs in association with tumors, most notably, renal cell carcinoma. Deposits of *AA amyloid* cause *secondary amyloidosis,* which typically affects the kidneys, liver, adrenals, and spleen. However, all other organs may show deposits of AA amyloid in their vessels as well.

Clinically, amyloidosis presents in many forms, and the symptoms depend predominantly on the organ system involved. The definitive diagnosis can be made only by demonstrating amyloid in tissue; to this end, a biopsy (e.g., kidney or liver biopsy) must be performed. Kidney and liver tissue that is infiltrated with amyloid is brittle, so the biopsy must be done with extreme care so as not to provoke bleeding. Systemic deposits of AA amyloid can be detected by gingival or rectal biopsies, which are less traumatic. These tissues show deposits of amyloid in the blood vessels. Amyloidosis cannot be treated efficiently.

Review Questions

1. What is the main difference between natural and acquired immunity?
2. What are the functions of properdin and lysozyme?
3. How do you define antigens?
4. What are the main differences between T and B lymphocytes?
5. What is the difference between CD4- and CD8-positive lymphocytes?

6. How are plasma cells related to lymphocytes?

7. What are the most important common features of IgG, IgM, IgA, IgE, and IgD, and what features distinguish one from another?

8. How do antigens induce production of antibodies?

9. How do antibodies react with antigens?

10. What is the role of the major histocompatibility complex and cytokines in the response of the body to foreign antigens?

11. Compare immune-mediated hemolysis with agglutination of red blood cells.

12. What is the mechanism of type I hypersensitivity?

13. Which diseases are caused by type I hypersensitivity reactions?

14. Correlate the pathologic findings and clinical features of respiratory, ocular, and skin manifestations of type I hypersensitivity reactions.

15. What is the pathogenesis of anaphylactic shock?

16. What are the two basic mechanisms of type II hypersensitivity?

17. Which diseases are caused by type II hypersensitivity reaction?

18. Compare the role of type II hypersensitivity in hemolytic anemia, Graves' disease, and myasthenia gravis.

19. Which diseases are caused by type III hypersensitivity reaction?

20. Compare Arthus phenomenon with systemic lupus erythematosus.

21. What is the mechanism of type IV hypersensitivity?

22. Which diseases are caused by type IV hypersensitivity reaction?

23. What is the difference between autografts, isografts, homografts, allografts, and xenografts?

24. What is the significance of haplotypes for transplantation of human organs?

25. What is the difference between hyperacute, acute, and chronic transplant rejection?

26. What is the pathogenesis and what are the clinical features of graft-versus-host reaction?

27. How could one determine whether a unit of donated blood could safely be transfused into a person in need of blood transfusion?

28. What is the cause of transfusion reaction and how does it present clinically?

29. What happens if an Rh⁻ person receives a blood transfusion from an Rh⁺ donor?

30. What is the pathogenesis of erythroblastosis fetalis due to fetomaternal Rh incompatibility?

31. What is kernicterus?

32. What clinicopathologic and laboratory findings must be present to allow the diagnosis of an autoimmune disorder?

33. What are the most common autoimmune diseases?

34. What is the pathogenesis and what are the clinical and pathologic findings in systemic lupus erythematosus?

35. Describe common features of some primary immunodeficiency diseases.

36. How prevalent is HIV infection worldwide?

37. How is HIV transmitted from one person to another?

38. How does HIV spread in the human body and what changes does it induce?

39. What are the clinical phases of HIV infection?

40. What are the pathologic manifestations of AIDS?

41. Which pathogens cause infections at an increased rate in patients with AIDS?

42. Which tumors typically occur in AIDS patients?

43. What is amyloid?

44. What are the most important forms of amyloid and how are the amyloid deposits formed?

45. Which organs are most often involved in amyloidosis?

Learning Objectives

After reading this chapter, the student should be able to:

1. Define neoplasia and its related terms: tumor, cancer, and oncology.
2. Classify tumors on the basis of their clinical behavior and histopathologic features.
3. Describe typical features of benign and malignant tumors.
4. Define metastasis and explain its pathogenesis.
5. List the common forms of carcinoma and sarcoma and their tissues of origin, and describe their benign equivalents.
6. Explain the principles of tumor staging and grading and the TNM system.
7. Describe the various approaches to studying the etiology and pathogenesis of cancer.
8. Discuss environmental carcinogens that could affect humans.
9. Describe the evidence for viral carcinogenesis in humans, with special emphasis on human papillomavirus, Epstein-Barr virus, and hepatitis B virus.
10. Define oncogenes and tumor suppressor genes and explain their clinical significance.
11. Describe host's immune response to neoplasia.
12. Describe the significance and the clinical value of tumor-associated antigens.
13. Describe five local and five systemic adverse effects of tumors on the host.
14. Discuss the changes in cancer incidence that have occurred over the last 100 years, and list the three most common forms of cancer in men and women previously and now.
15. Describe the geographic differences in the incidence of the main forms of cancer.
16. Describe the main contributions of cancer epidemiology to our understanding of neoplasia.

Additional Key Terms and Concepts

Adenoma

Angiogenesis

Cachexia

Carcinogen

Carcinoma

Epstein-Barr virus

Human papillomavirus

Incidence

Prevalence

Sarcoma

Teratoma

Chapter Outline

Neoplasia
Chapter 4

Neoplasia, literally meaning new growth, is a term derived from the Greek words *neos* (new) and *plasia* (growth). It is used to denote uncontrolled growth of cells whose proliferation cannot be adequately controlled by normal regulatory mechanisms operating in normal tissues.

The proliferation of normal cells is regulated internally by (1) the genetic program of each cell, (2) signals transmitted from one cell to another through direct contact, and (3) various soluble substances that have growth-promoting or -inhibiting effects. Once the cells stop proliferating, they assume specialized functions by activating a set of genes specific for each cell type. This selective activation of genes, typically associated with the suppression of other genes, is called *differentiation.* Tumor cells differ from normal cells in that they usually do not achieve the same level of differentiation.

In contrast to the tightly regulated growth of normal cells, the proliferation of neoplastic cells is

- *Autonomous*—independent of growth factors and stimuli that promote the growth of normal cells
- *Excessive*—unceasing in response to normal regulators of cellular proliferation
- *Disorganized*—not given to following the rules governing formation of normal tissues and organs

Terminology

The proliferation of neoplastic cells leads to the formation of masses called **tumors.** This term is derived from the Latin word *tumor,* which means swelling. The Greek term for a swelling, *onkos,* has been used to construct the term oncology, which is the most widely used name for the scientific discipline concerned with cancer. *Clinical oncologists* deal with neoplastic diseases in the clinical setting, primarily from a diagnostic and therapeutic point of view. *Experimental oncologists* work in the laboratory and study the etiology, pathogenesis, and cellular and molecular biology of neoplasms. *Cancer epidemiologists* deal with neoplasia in human populations and also study the environmental causes of tumors.

The terms neoplasm and tumor are used synonymously. However, it is very important to note that not all neoplasms form tumors. For example, leukemia is a malignant disease of the bone marrow, but the malignant cells are in the blood circulation and so do not form distinct masses. Also, not all swellings are neoplasms, as mentioned in the chapter on inflammation in which the Latin term *tumor* was listed as one of the cardinal signs of inflammation. It is also important to note that there are many forms of tumors, and that neoplastic disease is not a single clinical or pathologic entity, but rather a broad spectrum of pathologic processes.

A final note should be added regarding the term *cancer,* which is the most widely used synonym for neoplasms. Cancer is a Latin word, closely related to the Greek term *karkinos,* which means crab. It was introduced into the medical terminology by ancient Latin and Greek physicians who observed that tumors invaded tissues like crawling crabs. The term cancer came to be widely accepted, and even today, is used as a collective designation for all tumors.

Classification of Tumors

Tumors can be classified according to many criteria, none of which are generally valid or universally accepted. The most important classifications are as follows:

- *Clinical classification*—takes into account the clinical presentation and outcome of neoplastic diseases
- *Histologic classification*—based on histologic examination of tumors. On the basis of histologic features, pathologists can determine whether the tumor is composed of epithelial cells, mesenchymal (connective tissue) cells, lymphoid cells, or other cell types. For many years, pathologists have been correlating the clinical course of various neoplastic diseases with the histologic characteristics of tumors. On the basis of this correlation of clinical and pathologic data, criteria for benign and malignant tumors have been established. The histologic classification of tumors thus correlates very well with the clinical classification. In practice, these classifications are used interchangeably and complement one another.

Clinical Classification: Benign and Malignant Tumors

Most tumors can be classified clinically as either benign or malignant. Benign tumors have a limited growth potential and a good outcome, whereas malignant tumors grow uncontrollably and eventually kill the host. As with anything else in nature, though, there are many exceptions to this simple rule.

The clinical behavior of neoplasms—i.e., whether a tumor is benign—can be predicted from a pathologic examination. Typically, such an examination includes naked eye (macroscopic) inspection supplemented by microscopic examination of histologic sections of the tumor. Additional data may be obtained with various ancillary techniques, such as electron microscopy, immunohistochemistry, chromosomal analysis, and molecular biological studies of tumoral DNA.

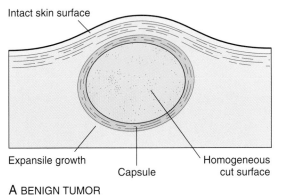

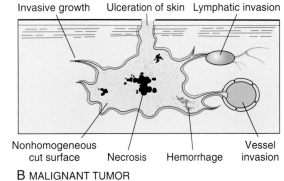

A BENIGN TUMOR

B MALIGNANT TUMOR

FIGURE 4-1
Gross appearance of benign (A) and malignant (B) tumors.

Macroscopic Features. On gross or naked eye examination, benign tumors are sharply demarcated from normal tissue and are often encapsulated (Fig. 4-1). The capsule is usually composed of connective tissue. Benign tumors have an expansive growth and compress the adjacent normal tissue, which undergoes atrophy and fibrosis, often forming a pseudocapsule. The distinction between a capsule and a pseudocapsule is not important, as in both cases, these structures provide a sharp border between the tumor and normal tissue, allowing the surgeon to easily remove ("shell out") the tumor.

Malignant tumors lack a capsule and are not clearly separated from normal tissue as are benign tumors. In contrast to the expansive growth of benign tumors, malignant tumors invade the surrounding tissue by infiltrating normal tissue just as the roots of a tree penetrate the soil. Because of their infiltrative growth and lack of sharp borders, malignant tumors cannot be removed as easily as benign ones.

Microscopic Features. On histologic examination, benign tumors are composed of cells that resemble the tissue from which they have arisen. By contrast, the cells of malignant tumors may differ considerably from cells in normal tissues. It is said that malignant cells show prominent *anaplasia;* that is, they exhibit new features not inherent to the tissue of their origin. In contrast to benign tumors, which show high degrees of differentiation, malignant tumors are *undifferentiated* (Fig. 4-2).

Cellular Features. The differences between benign and malignant tumors also can be appreciated at the level of individual cells. Benign tumors are composed of a uniform cell population in which all cells have approximately the same features. By contrast, malignant tumors consist of heterogeneous cell populations that often show marked pleomorphism (derived from the Greek words *pleo,* meaning variable, and *morpheo,* meaning to shape).

FIGURE 4-2
Comparison of normal glands with carcinoma. (A) Normal glands have smooth contours and uniform nuclei. (B) Adenocarcinoma is composed of irregular glands. (C) Anaplastic or undifferentiated carcinoma forms cell groups that show little resemblance to glands.

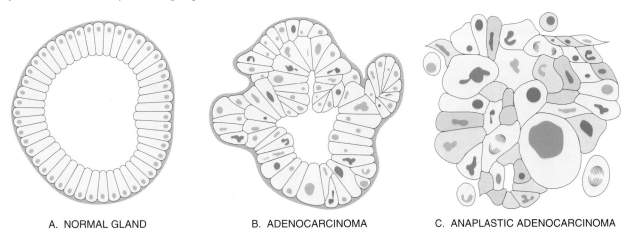

A. NORMAL GLAND

B. ADENOCARCINOMA

C. ANAPLASTIC ADENOCARCINOMA

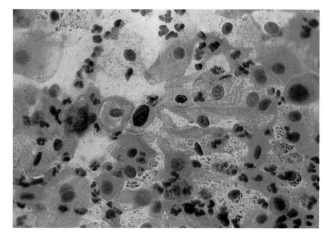

FIGURE 4-3
Cytologic features of malignant disease detected by a vaginal Papanicolaou smear. Malignant cells have enlarged hyperchromatic nuclei in contrast to the small nuclei of normal cells.

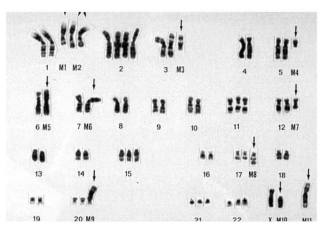

FIGURE 4-4
Abnormal chromosomes in a cancer cell. The cell is polypoid; that is, it contains more than two sets of 23 chromosomes. Many abnormal chromosomes (M1–M5) are marked by arrows.

Benign tumor cells have regularly shaped nuclei that may be round, oval, or elongated, but that are usually of the same size. Malignant cells have nuclei that vary in size and shape. Benign cells have a well-developed cytoplasm, whereas malignant cells have variable amounts of cytoplasm. Like the rapidly proliferating undifferentiated embryonic cells that have no specialized cytoplasmic functions, undifferentiated tumor cells often have very little cytoplasm. In well-differentiated normal and benign tumor cells, the nucleus accounts for a small part of the total cell volume, whereas in malignant cells, the nucleus is relatively larger. Typically, malignant cells have a high nuclear:cytoplasmic ratio. This is best seen in cytologic smears, like the vaginal Papanicolaou smear. In contrast to benign cells, which have a small nucleus and abundant cytoplasm, malignant cells have a larger nucleus surrounded by a narrow rim of cytoplasm (Fig. 4-3).

The nuclei of benign cells exhibit a regular, even distribution of chromatin. The nucleoli are not overly prominent. In comparison with normal cells, the nuclei of most malignant cells are hyperchromatic; that is, they contain more chromatin, and it is distributed unevenly. The nucleoli are often prominent and may be multiple. Malignant tumors contain more cells that are undergoing mitosis (cell division) than do benign tumors.

Chromosomal Studies. Benign tumors usually have a normal number of chromosomes. By contrast, malignant cells are often aneuploid, which means they do not have a normal diploid (46,XX or 46,XY) number of chromosomes. The chromosomes may be structurally abnormal owing to deletions or translocations of chromatics and their fragments caused by

abnormal mitoses that are common in malignant tumors (Fig. 4-4).

Biologic Features. The well-differentiated cells of benign tumors may retain some of the complex functions of the normal cells in the tissue of their origin. Malignant cells, which show no signs of differentiation, have no specialized functions. Their entire metabolism is geared toward supporting rapid growth and replication. To this end, the cells have a modified basic metabolism and function that gives them a growth advantage and allows them to outpace normal cells.

The most important differences between benign and malignant tumors are listed in Table 4-1.

Metastasis

Metastasis (derived from the Greek words *meta*, a prefix for change, and *stasis*, meaning position) denotes a process in which cells move from one site to another in the body. Only malignant tumor cells have the capacity to metastasize. Benign tumors never metastasize and always remain localized.

Metastasis involves a spread of tumor cells from a primary location to some other site in the body. The spread can occur through three main pathways: the lymphatics, the blood, and by seeding of the surface of body cavities. Regardless of the pathway for dissemination of tumor cells, the sequence of events leading to metastasis is essentially the same, and includes several distinct steps, collectively known as the *metastatic cascade* (Fig. 4-5).

Not all malignant cells are capable of metastasis. The first step then, is acquisition of a capacity to metastasize. Cells that have acquired the capacity to

Table 4-1 Comparison of Benign and Malignant Tumors

Feature	Benign	Malignant
Growth	Slow	Fast
	Expansive	Invasive
Metastases	No	Yes
Gross Appearance		
External surface	Smooth	Irregular
Capsule	Yes	No
Necrosis	No	Yes
Hemorrhage	No	Yes
Microscopic Appearance		
Architecture	Resembles that of tissues of origin	Does not resemble that of tissue of origin
Cells	Well differentiated	Poorly differentiated
Nuclei	Normal size and shape	Pleomorphic
Mitoses	Few	Many irregular

metastasize expand clonally, forming a distinct subpopulation. As this clone expands by successive divisions, its cells reach the lymphatics or the blood vessels, or enter a body cavity. The fluid in these spaces (i.e., the lymph in the lymphatics, the blood in the blood vessels, or the pleural and peritoneal fluid)

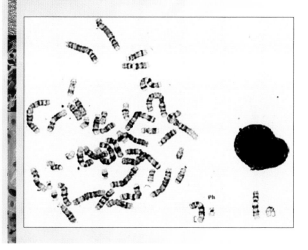

Did You Know?

Chromosomal changes are common in cancer cells. The first chromosomal abnormality linked to a malignant disease in humans was discovered by Nowell and Hungerford in 1960 in Philadelphia. Hence, the abnormal chromosome found in chronic myelogenous leukemia is known as the Philadelphia (Ph) chromosome.

carry the cells from the primary site to distant locations, where the cells attach and begin forming a new tumor mass.

Metastatic cells must escape the deleterious effects of immune cells, such as T lymphocytes, natural killer (NK) cells, and macrophages, which act on circulating tumor cells. In order to survive at the new site, the malignant tumors must elicit *angiogenesis* (new blood vessel formation) (Fig. 4-6). Such new blood vessels are essential for tumor growth because it is through these vessels that the tumor receives blood, with all its nutrients and oxygen. Experimental studies in animals have shown that metastases and tumor growth can be inhibited by strengthening the antineoplastic immune response or by inhibiting angiogenesis.

Histologic Classification of Tumors

The cells of most benign tumors and many malignant ones retain some microscopic features of the tissue of their origin. The tumors are thus named according to the cell type which they resemble the most. The names of benign tumors of mesenchymal cells—i.e., connective tissues, muscles, and bones—are formed by adding the suffix *-oma* to the root of the Latin name for the cell type (Table 4-2). For example, a tumor composed of fibroblasts is called a fibroma; that formed from cartilage cells (chondrocytes) is called a chondroma; that from fat cells (lipocytes) is termed a lipoma (Fig. 4-7); that from bone cells is an osteoma; that made up of smooth muscle cells is termed a leiomyoma; and that composed of striated muscle cells is called a rhabdomyoma.

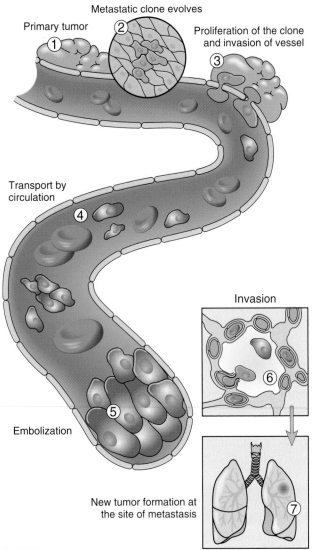

FIGURE 4-5
Metastatic cascade occurs in several steps, marked 1 through 7.

Benign tumors of epithelial cells are called **adenomas** (Fig. 4-8). Without any additional qualifier, the term adenoma refers to a tumor composed of glands or ducts, whereas specific terms, like liver cell adenoma, renal cell adenoma, and salivary gland adenoma, all denote specific tumor types. Adenomas of the gastrointestinal tract carry additional descriptive terms and are known as *tubular* or *villous* adenomas. Because they protrude from the surface of intestinal mucosa, these adenomas are also known as **polyps.** Benign protuberant tumors of the skin, urinary bladder, or mouth and larynx are called **papillomas.** Cystic tumors composed of hollow spaces lined by neoplastic epithelium are called **cystadenomas.**

The names for the malignant tumors of mesenchymal cells are coined from the root of the cell type and a suffix: **sarcoma** (Fig. 4-9). The tumors are thus called fibrosarcoma, chondrosarcoma, liposarcoma, and so on. The malignant tumors of epithelial cells are called **carcinomas** (Fig. 4-10). The tumors of squamous cells are called squamous cell carcinomas and those of transitional cell epithelium, transitional cell carcinomas. All tumors composed of malignant glands or ducts are called **adenocarcinomas.** Tumors composed of unique cell types are named accordingly, such as renal cell carcinoma, liver cell carcinoma, adrenocortical carcinoma, and so on.

There are several important exceptions to these general rules. For example, not all tumors that end in *-oma* are benign, and not all malignant tumors are labeled as carcinoma or sarcoma. The most important examples of such inconsistent nomenclature include

- **lymphomas,** which are malignant tumors of lymphoid cells
- **gliomas,** which are malignant tumors of glial cells
- **seminomas,** which are malignant tumors of the testicular seminiferous epithelium

FIGURE 4-6
Tumor-induced angiogenesis. Malignant tumors, especially those in metastatic sites, induce formation of blood vessels, which serve as routes for the transport of nutrients into the tumor. FGF, fibroblast growth factor.

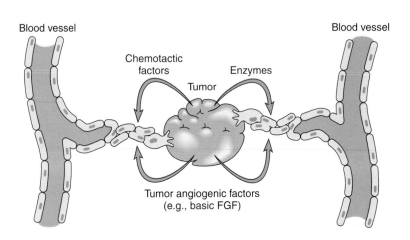

Table 4-2 Classification of Human Tumors

		Examples	
Tumor Type	**Cell/Tissue of Origin**	**Benign Tumors**	**Malignant Tumors**
Mesenchymal tumors	Fibroblast	Fibroma	Fibrosarcoma
	Fat cell	Lipoma	Liposarcoma
	Blood vessels	Hemangioma	Angiosarcoma
	Smooth muscle cell	Leiomyoma	Leiomyosarcoma
	Striated muscle cell	Rhabdomyosarcoma	Rhabdomyosarcoma
	Cartilage	Chondroma	Chondrosarcoma
	Bone cell	Osteoma	Osteosarcoma
Epithelial tumors	Squamous epithelium	Epithelioma (papilloma)	Squamous cell carcinoma
	Transitional epithelium	Transitional cell papilloma	Transitional cell carcinoma
	Glandular/ductal epithelium	Adenoma	Adenocarcinoma
	Neuroendocrine cells	Carcinoid	Oat cell carcinoma
	Internal organ-specific		
	Liver cell	Liver cell adenoma	Liver cell carcinoma
	Kidney cell	Renal cell adenoma	Renal cell carcinoma
Tumors of blood cells and lymphocytes	White blood stem cells	—	Leukemia
	Lymphoid cells	—	Lymphoma
	Plasma cells	—	Multiple myeloma
Tumors of neural cell precursors	Neuroblast	Ganglioneuroma	Neuroblastoma
Tumors of glial cells and neural supporting cells	Glial cells	—	Glioma
	Meningial cells	Meningioma	—
	Schwann cells	Schwannoma	Malignant schwannoma
Germ cell tumors	Embryonic cells	Teratoma	Embryonal carcinoma
			Teratocarcinoma
			Seminoma/dysgerminoma

FIGURE 4-7

Lipoma. (Left) On gross examination, this benign tumor is well circumscribed. It is yellow because it consists of fat cells. (Right) Histologic examination reveals that the tumor is composed of fat cells.

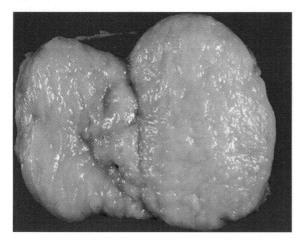
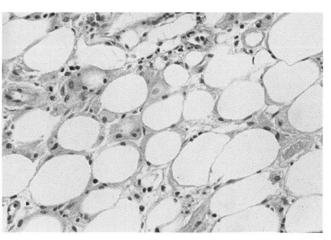

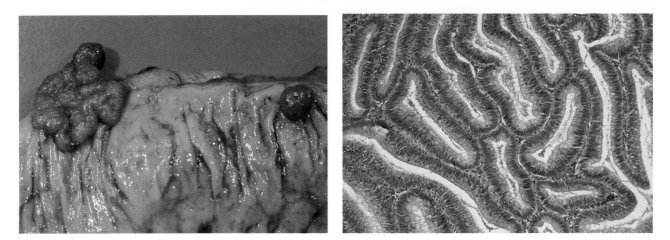

FIGURE 4-8
Adenoma. (Left) Two well-defined polypoid adenomas of the large intestine. (Right) On histologic examination, the tumor is found to be composed of glands that appear uniform.

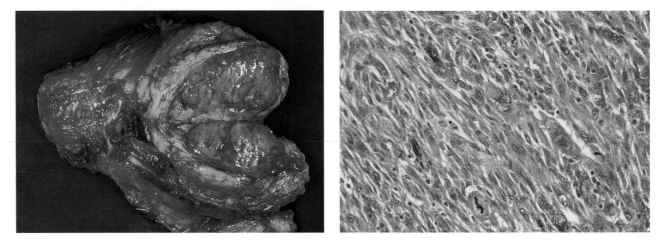

FIGURE 4-9
Sarcoma. On gross examination, the tumor has a fleshlike appearance (left). Histologically, the tumor is composed of elongated cells that resemble fibroblasts (right).

FIGURE 4-10
Carcinoma. (A) Squamous cell carcinoma consists of solid cell nests that show central keratinization. (B) Adenocarcinoma consists of neoplastic glands. In both tumors, the neoplastic cells are surrounded by non-neoplastic stroma.

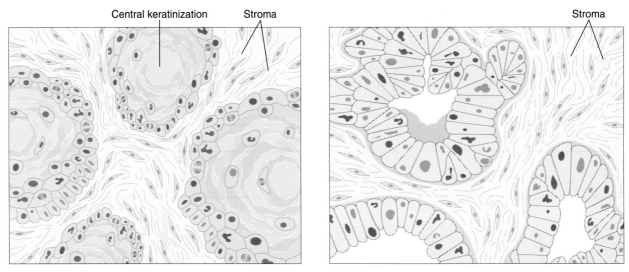

A. SQUAMOUS CELL CARCINOMA

B. ADENOCARCINOMA

Some tumors of the same name can be either benign or malignant, and this must be clearly stated. For example, islet cell tumors of the pancreas can be either benign or malignant. Because the distinction cannot be made clearly on histologic examination, the noncommittal term islet cell tumor is used for most of these tumors. However, if such a tumor is accompanied by metastases, it is clearly malignant and so is designated a malignant islet cell tumor.

Malignant tumors composed of embryonic cells, presumably originating from embryonic primordia (anlage), are often called **blastomas.** Thus, retinal tumors are called retinoblastomas, hepatic tumors hepatoblastomas, and renal tumors nephroblastomas.

Tumors derived from germ cells, mostly in the testis and ovary, contain embryonic cells that differentiate into embryonic germ layers; ectoderm, mesoderm, and endoderm. These germ layers form various tissues, which are intermixed with one another in an irregular manner (Fig. 4-11). Such tumors are called **teratomas** (from the Greek word *teraton,* meaning monster) to indicate their abnormal ("monster-like") histologic structure. Teratomas may be benign or malignant. Malignant teratomas are also called **teratocarcinomas.**

Teratomas must be distinguished from **mixed tumors,** which usually contain only a single epithelial and mesenchymal component. Mixed tumors typically involve the salivary glands, where they are usually benign. Malignant mixed tumors, typically found in the uterus, consist of a malignant epithelial and a malignant mesenchymal component and are also called **carcinosarcomas.**

FIGURE 4-11

Teratoma. The tumor is composed of various tissues intermixed in an irregular manner. Note the variety of tissues in this cystic ovarian tumor. It even contains a tooth.

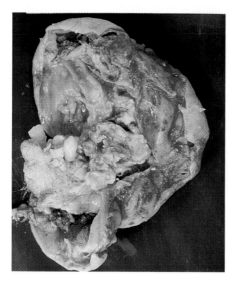

Some tumors cannot be classified according to existing schemes and criteria. Such tumors carry the name of the physician who first described them. Examples of such eponymic tumors are **Hodgkin's disease** of the lymph nodes, **Ewing's sarcoma** of the bones, and **Kaposi's sarcoma** of the skin.

Tumor Staging and Grading

Staging of tumors is done by clinically assessing the extent of tumor spread. This is based on clinical examination, x-ray studies, biopsy, or surgical exploration. Staging takes into account the size of the primary tumor and the presence or absence of lymph node metastases and distant metastases. Tumor stage is expressed on a scale from I to IV or alphabetically (A through D). According to the widely used TNM system of staging, a number is assigned for T (tumor size), N (lymph node involvement), and M (distant metastases). For example, a tumor that is smaller than 2.5 cm and that has spread to a local lymph node but not to distant sites would be staged as T1, N1, M0.

Grading is based on the histologic examination of tumors. Grade I tumors are well differentiated, grade II lesions are moderately well differentiated, and grade III lesions are undifferentiated. Staging and grading are used for prognosis of tumor outcome. Overall, staging has more predictive value than grading.

Biology of Tumor Cells

Most tumor cells differ from the normal cells from which they have arisen. For example, tumor cells may differ biochemically. If explanted into a test tube, tumor cells may behave differently than normal cells. However, these differences are not absolute or constant. Generally, malignant tumor cells differ from normal cells much more than do the cells of benign tumors.

Biochemistry of Cancer Cells

The search for biochemical differences between normal and tumorous cells began in the 19th century and is still in process. Most biochemical differences between normal and neoplastic cells discovered so far are relative and quantitative rather than qualitative. In other words, there are no definitive or absolute biochemical differences between normal and neoplastic cells, and there are no biochemical tests to tell whether a cell is benign or malignant.

As an example of such differences, the metabolism of liver tumor cells is much simpler than the metabolism of adult liver cells. Accordingly, the tumor cells require less oxygen and are better adapted to survive under unfavorable conditions. Most malignant cells contain, therefore, fewer mitochondria than normal cells (Fig. 4-12). Neoplastic liver cells do not contain all the enzymes that are found in the cytoplasm of normal liver cells and often do not synthesize all the proteins normally produced by liver cells. Rough endoplasmic reticulum (RER), the organelle involved in synthesis of proteins for export, is less prominent in malignant cells than in the corresponding normal cells. Tumor cells do not process glucose as efficiently as normal cells and store it in the form of glycogen in their cytoplasm.

Simplified metabolism leads to a loss of highly specialized functions. Malignant tumor cells retain only those functions that are essential for their sustenance and proliferation. Tumor cells require less oxygen and are able to metabolize glucose anaerobically. Lactic acid accumulates in large amounts as the end-product of anaerobic respiration. This anaerobic glycolysis was originally thought to be a common feature of all tumor cells. The German scientist, Otto Warburg, first noticed this in the 1920s and received the Nobel Prize for his discovery. It later became apparent that all hypoxic cells produce lactic acid. In this respect, tumor cells are not appreciably different from normal cells except that they produce lactic acid more readily and are better adapted to survive under suboptimal conditions.

Tumor cells also may acquire some new features and become quite different from normal cells. This acquisition of new, atypical features is called *anaplasia*. Anaplastic cells are larger than normal and often show nuclear irregularity. Tumor cells may also "regress" and assume fetal features. For example, liver cancer cells secrete alpha-fetoprotein (AFP), a major secretory product of fetal liver cells, but one that is not synthesized by normal adult cells. Similar changes occur in intestinal carcinoma cells, which produce carcinoembryonic antigen (CEA), a glycoprotein normally found only on embryonic intestinal cells.

FIGURE 4-12
Comparison of a typical normal (A) and malignant (B) cell. CEA, carcinoembryonic antigen; AFP, alpha-fetoprotein.

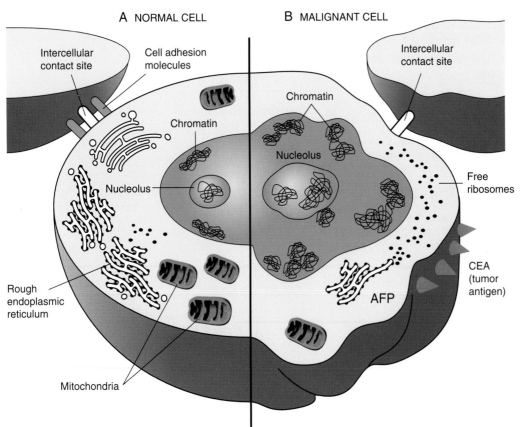

Growth Properties in Cell Culture

Tumor cells have less stringent requirements for nutrients and can survive on their own outside the body. Cell growth in test tubes is called *in vitro* cell culture because the first dishes used for these experiments were made of glass (*vitrum,* meaning glass in Latin). Most differentiated normal cells require complex growth media and survive for only a limited time in vitro. Primitive cells, such as fibroblasts, can survive longer in vitro. Nevertheless, even these cells pass through only a limited number of mitoses and then die. In contrast to normal cells, cancer cells survive much more easily because they require only simple growth media containing carbohydrates, proteins, vitamins, and essential minerals. Many malignant cells are actually "immortal" (i.e., they can be kept in cell culture indefinitely).

Normal cells that are explanted in vitro grow in an orderly manner, and when the bottom of the culture flask is completely covered, the cells stop dividing. This phenomenon is called *contact inhibition.* The malignant cells show no such contact inhibition and tend to pile up, forming aggregates and nodules. Cancer cells lack the adhesiveness of normal cells owing, in part, to a loss of cell surface adhesion molecules. Malignant cells tend to detach from the bottom of the culture flasks and float in the culture medium. All normal cells except the hematopoietic cells require firm support for growth (so-called anchorage-dependent growth). Malignant cells do not require such support and can be grown even in "roller bottles"—vessels that are constantly rotated to prevent cell attachment to the vessel wall. Cancer cells can be explanted into soft agar, in which they float suspended, forming round colonies. By contrast, normal cells, including the relatively sturdy fibroblasts, die if the agar prevents them from attaching to the surface of the dish.

The growth of tumor cells in vitro mimics tumor cell growth in vivo (i.e., in the body). In vitro tumor cell growth is *autonomous* and does not depend on exogenous growth stimuli. Many tumor cells secrete their own growth factors (*autocrine stimulation*) or express growth factor receptors that are amplified and respond to minimal external stimulation. The growth of tumor cells is *excessive* and unregulated because the neoplastic cells do not respond to the normal inhibitory influences of adjacent cells. Inappropriate cell-to-cell adhesion results in a lack of cohesion and detachment of cells, allowing cells to survive in anchorage-independent conditions. The lack of contact inhibition that normally prevents cellular overgrowth results in piling of cells and exuberant proliferation. As in the body, the growth of tumor cells in vitro is irregular and *disorganized.*

Causes of Cancer

The cause of most human cancers is not known. Nevertheless, many potential carcinogens have been identified, and the pathogenesis of many tumors has been elucidated (Fig. 4-13). Because cancer is a multifactorial disease with numerous forms, there are no general rules; for teaching purposes, however, it is convenient to divide the causes of cancer that have been identified thus far into two major groups: exogenous causes and endogenous causes. **Exogenous** causes of cancer include a number of cancerigenic (cancer-forming) factors that can be classified as follows:

* chemicals
* physical agents
* viruses

Endogenous causes of cancer reside in the genome of cells and are, like other genetic traits, heritable. However, as we shall see, exogenous carcinogens cause changes in the genome of the target cells that are similar to those caused by endogenous factors. The distinction of exogenous and endogenous factors has become even more difficult since the discovery that some human cancer genes, so-called **oncogenes,** are identical to exogenous viral genes. Cellular oncogenes can be isolated and used like viruses to infect normal cells. This procedure, called *transfection,* results in malignant transformation of previously normal cells.

Identification of Human Carcinogens

The search for causes of cancer is usually based on a three-pronged approach that includes clinical, epidemiologic, and experimental studies (Fig. 4-14).

Clinical studies include data gathered by practicing physicians treating cancer patients. Some of these clinical observations are reported in the medical literature as *case reports.* Other data are culled retrospectively into a large series that is then analyzed to provide guidance for future medical practice. Still other data are collected prospectively in carefully planned clinical trials. Knowledge about most human cancers is primarily derived from clinical studies.

Epidemiologic studies concentrate on identifying the exogenous causes of cancer in the environment, as well as the endogenous (genetic) factors in the human population. For example, epidemiologic studies have pointed out that lung cancer is caused by tobacco smoking. Asbestos-related lung cancer and pleural mesotheliomas were first identified by epidemiologic studies. Some familial forms of breast

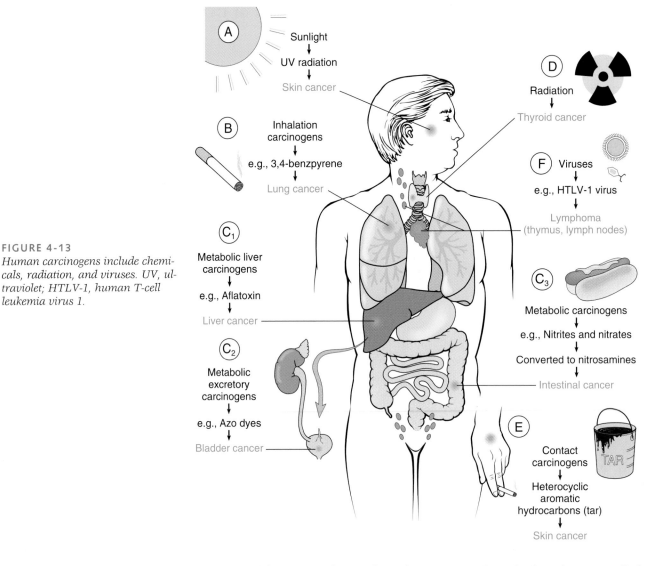

FIGURE 4-13
Human carcinogens include chemicals, radiation, and viruses. UV, ultraviolet; HTLV-1, human T-cell leukemia virus 1.

cancer and colon cancer were also identified by cancer epidemiologists.

Experimental studies can be performed on animals or cells and tissues removed from the clinically identified tumors. Tumors removed by surgeons can

FIGURE 4-14
Study of the etiology of human cancer begins with clinical observations (A), which are amplified by data obtained by epidemiologic study (B), additional clinical studies (C), experimental studies in animals (D), and in vitro studies (E). The final goal is identification and isolation of cancer genes (F).

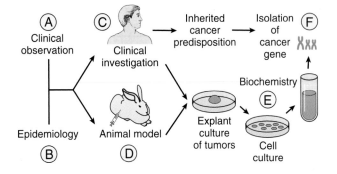

be explanted in vitro and studied under controlled conditions. Many cancer cell lines have been established in such studies. The best known of these tumor cell lines is the HeLa cell line, which was established in 1941 from a cancer patient at Johns Hopkins University in Baltimore, Maryland. To protect the privacy of the patient, she was given the fictitious name Helen Lane and the cell line was identified by the initials HeLa.

Experimental studies of cancer performed on animals may serve as models for human tumors. The presumptive carcinogens in the environment, such as various chemicals and viruses, are given to animals to produce tumors or simply to study the adverse effects of a potential carcinogenic agent. For example, rabbits were taught to smoke, which enabled scientists to study the adverse effects of tobacco smoke on lungs. Human genes isolated from tumors may be inserted into mice and studied further in vivo. Such transgenic animals, called so because they carry genes of another species, are excellent models for the study of human oncogenes.

The search for causes of a particular cancer usually begins with clinical observation. Any clues about the cessation of that cancer based on clinical reasoning must be validated by epidemiologic studies. The suspected causative agent must be identified biochemically. The carcinogenic potential of the putative carcinogen may be tested in vitro and in vivo. The final proof is at hand when the cancer can be reproduced in animals injected with the carcinogen.

The classical story of such a search for causes of common cancer began in 1775 when the British physician Sir Percival Pott reported that the chimney sweeps in England often developed carcinoma of the scrotum. He hypothesized that scrotal cancer developed because of the adverse effects of soot that was rubbed into the scrotal skin when chimney sweeps straddled the chimneys. This observation was received with incredulity and remained forgotten for many years. In 1875, German epidemiologists noted an increased incidence of skin cancer in chemical industry workers who handled tar, which apparently contains the same possible carcinogens as soot. The German study was amplified in 1915 by Yamagiwa and Ishikawa. These Japanese scientists painted tar on the ears of rabbits and induced tumors, thus proving that the tar contained carcinogens. The tumors produced in rabbits were linked to dibenzanthracene, a chemical carcinogen isolated in 1929 from tar. Dibenzanthracene was identified in the soot as well. In the 1960s, it was shown that tobacco smoke also contains dibenzanthracene and related polycyclic hydrocarbons, which are all capable of inducing cancer in animals. These chemicals were applied to normal human cells in culture and were found to interact with DNA and cause genetic mutations which transform normal cells into malignant cells. More than 200 years after the initial observation, the pathogenesis of scrotal cancer in chimney sweeps was explained as a consequence of a chemical injury of the DNA in cells exposed to the adverse effects of polycyclic hydrocarbons.

Industrial Carcinogens. Humans are exposed to chemical carcinogens in many situations. The most important exposure is in the workplace because it can be prevented and the risk of cancer can be minimized by proper industrial hygiene. For example, exposure to asbestos, quite common in the ship-building industry during World War II, has been identified as a cause of lung cancer and is no longer used. Naphthylamine, found in aniline dyes, has been found to cause bladder cancer. Mining of nickel ore has been found to be associated with nasal cancer. Vintners using arsenic as an insecticide have developed skin cancer. All these forms of cancer can be prevented by proper protection and precautionary measures.

Drugs as Carcinogens. Many drugs successfully used in cancer treatment are also carcinogenic. Secondary cancer that develops in patients treated with alkylating agents, such as nitrogen mustard or cyclophosphamide, are unfortunate complications of such treatment. The risk of developing cancer caused by drugs is low, though, so it is still better to try to cure a potentially lethal cancer, even if there is a slight chance that another will develop many years after. For example, Hodgkin's lymphoma has become a treatable disease and most patients are cured by chemotherapy. Nevertheless, a secondary, treatment-related cancer develops in 1 percent to 3 percent of patients so treated.

Chemical Carcinogens

Chemical carcinogens abound in our environment, and it is almost impossible to live without being exposed to some chemical carcinogen. Such carcinogens can be classified according to origin, chemical composition, or their mode of action, as listed in Table 4-3.

Chemical carcinogens can be classified as natural or as man-made. In the most important group of carcinogens, the so-called polycyclic aromatic hydrocarbons, one may find representatives of both (Fig. 4-15). Aflatoxin B_1 is, for example, a very potent natural liver carcinogen produced by the fungus *Aspergillus flavus*. Polycyclic hydrocarbons, like 3,4-benzpyrene, are important components of tobacco smoke. Tar and fossil fuels used in the manufacturing of gasoline contain the same polycyclic hydrocarbons. It should be noted that steroid and sex hormones also have a polycyclic structure. Sex hormones, especially estrogens, may also induce tumors in sensitive tissues. Estrogens produced in excess endogenously by the ovary and adrenals can cause cancer of the breast and uterus. Exogenous estrogens are also manufactured and administered as drugs. Many postmenopausal women who take estrogens must weigh the benefits of these hormones against their possible harmful effects.

Action of Chemical Carcinogens. The chemicals entering the body may act in several ways, as follows:

- *Locally.* Skin carcinogens, for example, act at the site of contact. Pulmonary carcinogens inhaled as smoke act on the bronchial mucosa.
- *At the site of digestion in the intestines.* This type of activation of carcinogens is typically mediated by intestinal bacteria. For example, nitrites and nitrates that are ingested in food are converted into nitrosamines, which may have a carcinogenic effect on the large intestine.

Table 4-3 Examples of Chemical Carcinogens

Category of Chemical	Compound	Source	Mode of Action	Tumor Induced
Polycyclic aromatic hydrocarbons	3,4-benzpyrene	Tobacco tar	Inhalation Skin contact	Carcinoma of lung Skin cancer
	Aflatoxin B_1	Fungi	Metabolic	Liver cancer
Aromatic aminines	β-naphthylamine	Dye and rubber industry	Excretion in urine	Bladder cancer
Nitrosamines	Nitrates	Food additives	Bacterial conversion in the gut	Intestinal cancer
Steroid hormones	Estrogens	Ovary/adrenal or injection	Stimulation of endometrium	Endometrial carcinoma
Metals and inorganic compounds	Arsenic sulfate	Pesticides	Skin contact	Skin cancer
	Nickel sulfate	Ore	Inhalation	Nasal cancer

FIGURE 4-15
Chemical carcinogens. Note the polycyclic structure of all compounds.

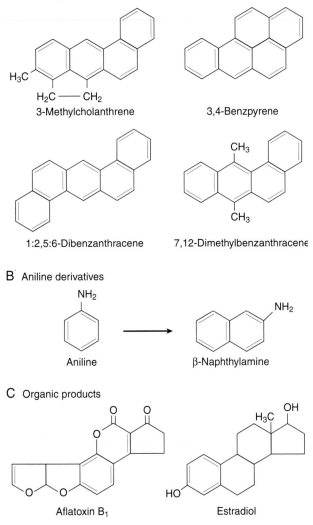

A Carcinogens from tar and cigarette smoke derivatives

3-Methylcholanthrene

3,4-Benzpyrene

1:2,5:6-Dibenzanthracene

7,12-Dimethylbenzanthracene

B Aniline derivatives

Aniline

β-Naphthylamine

C Organic products

Aflatoxin B_1

Estradiol

- *At the site of metabolic activation in the liver.* The liver is the primary organ involved in the degradation or alteration of carcinogens, as well as other chemicals, into other compounds. Aflatoxin is thus activated into a most potent liver carcinogen.
- *At the site of excretion in urine.* Aromatic amines derived from azo-dies are metabolized in the body and converted into potential carcinogens that are excreted in urine. These carcinogens act on the urinary bladder.

Chemical carcinogenesis is a multistep process. The initial step is the conversion of the potentially harmful substance—the procarcinogen—into a carcinogen. This conversion is mediated by enzymes locally active in the exposed cells or in the liver, which acts as the major conversion site for most exogenous chemicals. The carcinogens formed from procarcinogens act on the DNA of the exposed cells. This event, characterized by an induction of irreversible genetic changes in the exposed cells, is called *initiation* (Fig. 4-16). In the second step, called *promotion,* the initiated cells can be stimulated to proliferate. Promotion can be achieved by continuous exposure to the carcinogen or to another substance which is not carcinogenic in itself, but which can promote the growth of initiated cells. These substances are called promoters. The promoters must be applied until the cells acquire an ability to proliferate on their own and convert to a new cell type (*conversion*). *Progression,* the next phase in cancer development, is marked by an acquisition of new genetic features and expansion of cell clones that do not regress after the carcinogen or the promoter has been removed. These cells grow rapidly and give rise to identical daughter cells called clones (*clonal expansion*). Proliferation of divergent clones that arise by mutation of unstable tumor cell

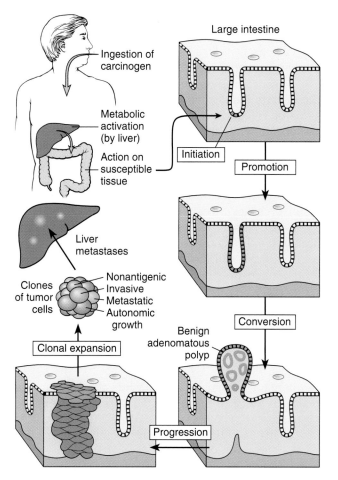

FIGURE 4-16
Carcinogenesis is a multistep process.

genome leads to tumor cell heterogeneity. Some clones are invasive; others are capable of metastasizing, and others become dormant; still others differentiate along the same lines as the normal cells from which they have arisen. Diversification of tumor cell populations is unpredictable. Nevertheless, a *selection* takes place in favor of most vital clones and cells that have adapted best to adverse conditions. Ultimately, these clones outgrow all others.

Physical Carcinogens

The most important among the various physical agents that cause cancer is radiation. Radiation may originate from several sources, such as ultraviolet (UV) light, x-rays, radioactive isotopes, and atomic bombs (see Fig. 4-13).

UV light is a potent skin carcinogen. Long-term exposure to UV light in sunlight causes several forms of skin cancer, such as basal cell carcinoma, squamous cell carcinoma, and melanoma. Persons working in the sun, such as fishermen or farmers, are at increased risk. Skin cancer is most prevalent in the southern United States, and is especially common in

Australia. Light-skinned persons are at increased risk because they lack the protective effects of melanin. Skin cancer is uncommon among blacks.

It is thought that UV light damages the DNA of skin, thus causing mutations that lead to malignant transformation. Incidental UV-induced DNA damage is enzymatically repaired in the damaged cells (Fig. 4-17). Individuals lacking these enzymes, such as those with congenital xeroderma pigmentosum, a genetic defect, are particularly sensitive. Affected persons develop skin lesions early in life and must avoid sun exposure. They tend to develop skin cancer in childhood and puberty.

X-rays have been used extensively in medicine ever since their discovery by Konrad Roentgen in 1895. The pioneers of roentgenology were unaware of the carcinogenic effects of x-rays, and many of them developed cancer. X-rays have been considered a professional risk for radiologists, but with adequate protection, this risk can be reduced to a minimum.

FIGURE 4-17
Repair of DNA damaged by UV light. Patients also have xeroderma pigmentosum and lack DNA repair enzymes. Abnormal DNA repair results in mutations that may lead to cancer.

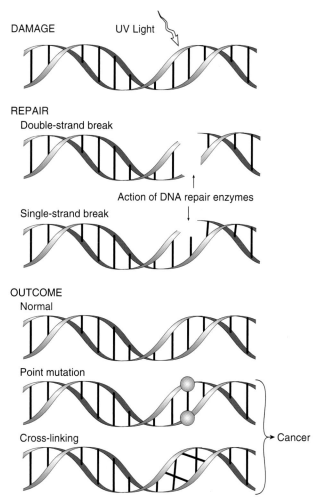

Conventional hospital x-ray instruments pose almost no risk if properly used.

X-rays are also used for treatment of malignant tumors. Such radiation carries a definitive risk. Secondary tumors may develop, but usually after a long latent period, sometimes 20 to 25 years after exposure. The benefits of radiation therapy outweigh the risk of secondary cancer.

Radioactive materials occur in the environment and are also man-made for use in research and for medical purposes. Alpha, beta, and especially gamma rays emitted by these radioactive substances have potential carcinogenic effects. For example, many miners in Joachimsthal, a Polish uranium mine established at the beginning of this century, have developed lung cancer from inhaling the radioactive ore. In those days, the dangers of radioactivity were unknown and workers were not protected adequately. Factory workers who painted early phosphorescent watch dials with radioactive phosphorus in the U.S. plant that was operational after World War I developed bone cancer. Today, we are aware of these risks. The use of radioactive isotopes is tightly regulated and the risk to fully protected laboratory workers is minimal. Similarly, the radioactive material used in atomic power plants poses very little, if any, danger. However, should a mishap occur, as was the case with the Ukrainian power station at Chernobyl in 1986, the emitted radioactive fumes may pose a serious health problem to the exposed populations.

The *atomic bomb* is a powerful source of radioactive material. The first atomic bombs dropped on Hiroshima and Nagasaki in 1945 caused not only immediate massive devastation, but also long-term effects, including an increased occurrence of cancer. The most prominent among these neoplasms were leukemia and carcinoma of the thyroid. The incidence of the more common cancers, such as those of the breast and lung, also increased.

Natural Biologic Carcinogens

Some fungi, such as *Aspergillus flavus,* produce potent carcinogens, such as aflatoxin. *Aflatoxin* was discovered when liver cancer began appearing in flocks of turkeys fed peanuts, imported to England from Brazil, which were contaminated with the fungus.

Various parasites have been associated with an increased incidence of cancer and are thought to be involved in carcinogenesis. For example, infection of the urinary bladder with *Schistosoma haematobium,* a parasitic infection that is quite common in Egypt, is associated with an increased incidence of bladder cancer. Infection with the fluke, *Opistorchis sinensis,* is associated with an increased incidence of liver cancer in China. However, in the Western world, such infections are uncommon, and the most important biologic causes of cancer are thought to be viruses. Most research has concentrated on herpesviruses, human papillomaviruses, and hepatitis viruses. However, data are still inconclusive, and the only proven human oncogenic virus is the human T-cell leukemia virus (HTLV-I), which has been identified as the cause of a rare form of adult T-cell leukemia/lymphoma.

Viral Carcinogens

It has been known for many years that certain animal tumors can be transmitted by cell-free extracts prepared from such tumors and injected into a new host. This was first shown by Whipple Rous, who studied chicken sarcoma and in 1910 induced the same tumor by injecting a cell-free extract of the original tumor into a new host.

Many years later, the cause of these tumors was identified as an RNA virus known today as Rous sarcoma. Numerous other tumor viruses have been isolated from animal tumors since then. Depending on their structure, tumor viruses are classified as DNA or RNA viruses (Fig. 4-18). The oncogenic DNA viruses become directly integrated into the genome of the infected cells. RNA viruses have an enzyme called *reverse transcriptase,* which uses the message encoded in the viral RNA to synthesize fragments of DNA. This DNA is incorporated into the cellular genome.

RNA tumor viruses are of two kinds: acute transforming and slow transforming RNA viruses. *Acute transforming RNA viruses* direct the formation of a cellular oncogene which is the exact copy of the viral oncogene. This process is called *transduction. Slow transforming oncogenic RNA viruses* do not produce a cellular oncogene. Instead, such viruses form a replica of their own RNA, which is inserted into the cellular genome at a point where it activates a latent cellular proto-oncogene into an active oncogene. The transformation of an infected normal cell into a tumor cell occurs only if this insertional mutagenesis occurs at a locus that activates an oncogene capable of transforming the cell. As the insertion is random, numerous insertions must occur before a cell is transformed; therefore, such oncogenic viruses are called slow transforming RNA viruses.

Did You Know?

An increased incidence of thyroid cancer among children was noticed following the meltdown of the Chernobyl atomic power station. Most of the affected children lived many miles away, but all of them were west of the place of the accident. The prevailing east-west winds had obviously carried the radioactive fumes to places initially thought to be safe.

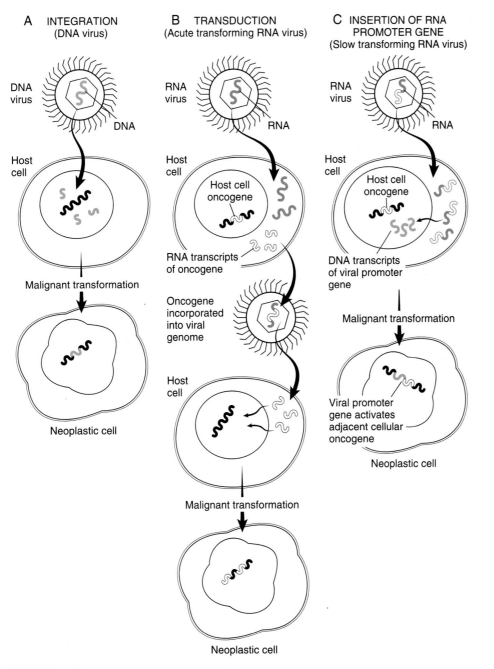

| A INTEGRATION (DNA virus) | B TRANSDUCTION (Acute transforming RNA virus) | C INSERTION OF RNA PROMOTER GENE (Slow transforming RNA virus) |

FIGURE 4-18
Tumor viruses. (A) DNA viruses induce malignant transformation by integration into the genome. (B) Acute transforming RNA viruses produce malignant transformation by transduction. (C) Slow transforming RNA viruses produce malignant transformation by transfection.

Human DNA Viruses. Several human DNA viruses have been linked to cancer, but final proof is still lacking for all of them. The most compelling evidence implicates human papillomaviruses, Epstein-Barr virus, and hepatitis B virus.

Papillomaviruses occur in several animal species. Human papillomavirus (HPV) is classified into more than 70 subtypes, several of which have been linked to human lesions, such as common warts, genital warts, laryngeal papillomas, dysplasia of the cervical epithelium, and cervical carcinoma. Some types of

HPV cause benign lesions, whereas others cause malignant tumors. In the cervix of the human uterus, HPV types 6 and 11 cause lesions that are always benign. However, the lesions caused by HPV types 16, 18, and 33 have a propensity for progressing to cancer. HPV isolated from invasive cervical carcinoma is always of the "unfavorable" type, and such viruses almost invariably belong to groups 16, 18, or 33.

Epstein-Barr virus (EBV) is a human herpesvirus that has a predilection for B lymphocytes. This virus is extremely prevalent. More than 90

percent of adults in the United States have antibodies to it, indicating that they have been infected with it at some point during their life. The infection may pass unnoticed, or it can produce infectious mononucleosis (the so-called "kissing disease"). EBV seems to be related to several forms of cancer, most notably, Burkitt's lymphoma and nasopharyngeal carcinoma. Burkitt's lymphoma is a B-cell neoplasia that occurs most often in Sub-Saharan Africa and typically affects children. Nasopharyngeal carcinoma related to EBV is most prevalent in China, but may occur in other parts of the world as well. As will be shown later, EBV causes chromosomal breaks that result in activation of endogenous cancer genes (oncogenes).

Hepatitis B virus (HBV) is a double-stranded DNA virus that is transmitted from one person to another by blood. Epidemiologists have noted that the high incidence of viral hepatitis in Japan, China, and Southeast Asia is associated with a high incidence of liver cancer. Numerous studies have revealed that the HBV is integrated into the DNA of neoplastic cells. The pathogenesis of HBV-related liver cancer is not understood because the virus does not contain any known oncogenic sequences. Experimentally, HBV cannot transform normal liver cells in culture into malignant cells. However, liver cell tumors develop in transgenic mice that contain human hepatitis B virus.

HTLV-I is an RNA virus that belongs to the same group of retroviruses as the human immunodeficiency virus, HIV, the well known cause of AIDS. Fortunately enough, HTLV-I does not represent such a public health problem as HIV. This virus was originally isolated in southern Japan, where it caused a rare form of adult T-cell leukemia. Subsequently HTLV-I has been identified in Africa, the Caribbean islands, and even in the United States. HTLV-I can infect human T lymphocytes in vitro and transform them into malignant cells, which is definitive proof that the virus is carcinogenic.

Human Oncogenes

Studies of viral carcinogenesis led to the discovery of cellular genes that have the same structure and nucleotide composition as the viral oncogenes. In contrast to viral oncogenes (*v-onc*), these cellular genes were named cellular oncogenes (*c-onc*). It was shown that *c-oncs* are mutated normal cellular genes, called proto-oncogenes. Proto-oncogenes encode for proteins important for basic cell functions. Proto-oncogenes can be transformed into oncogenes by four basic mechanisms: point mutation, gene amplification, chromosomal rearrangement, and insertion of the viral genome (Fig. 4-19).

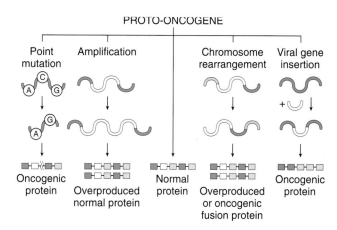

FIGURE 4-19
Activation of cellular oncogenes.

1. *Point mutation.* This event includes a single base substitution in the DNA chain, resulting in a miscoded protein that has an amino acid substituted for another amino acid. Point mutations have been observed in a number of human tumors carrying a mutated *ras* gene.
2. *Gene amplification.* By this mechanism, the cell acquires an increased number of copies of the proto-oncogene. For example, in widespread neuroblastoma of childhood, the tumor cells contain multiple copies of the *N-myc* gene. The more copies of the oncogene the cell contains, the more malignant is the tumor.
3. *Chromosomal rearrangements.* Translocations of one chromosomal fragment onto another, or deletion of a fragment of the chromosome, leads to juxtapositioning of genes that are normally distant one from another. Such gene complexes may result in overactivation of proto-oncogenes, stimulated by an adjacent gene which acts as a promoter. For example, *c-myc,* which is normally located on chromosome 8, is positioned next to the immunoglobulin gene in Burkitt's lymphoma owing to the translocation of chromosome 8 to chromosome 14 (Fig. 4-20). This immunoglobulin gene promotes the activity of *c-myc,* which ultimately results in tumor formation.
4. *Insertion of the viral genome.* This insertional mutagenesis, typical of slow transforming viruses, results in the disruption of normal chromosomal architecture and genetic dysregulation. Hepatitis B virus is found incorporated into the genome of liver cancer cells.

Proto-oncogenes have numerous functions in normal cells. Proto-oncogenes encode proteins that function as growth factors, growth factor receptors, and intracellular signal molecules. All of these proteins are important for cell growth, and their dysregulation can cause neoplastic transformation.

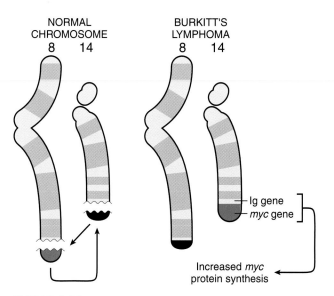

FIGURE 4-20
Chromosomal translocation in Burkitt's lymphoma leads to the activation of myc oncogene. The immunoglobulin (Ig) gene juxtaposed to the oncogene acts as a promoter. Tumors are lymphomas because the immunoglobulin gene is active in lymphocytes. (Adapted from Cotran RS, Kumar V, and Robbins SL: Robbins' Pathologic Basis of Disease, 5th ed., Philadelphia: WB Saunders, 1994:264.)

Tumor Suppressor Genes

Normal cells have regulatory genetic mechanisms that protect them against activated or newly acquired oncogenes. Such genes are called tumor suppressor genes. For example, if a malignant cell is fused with a normal cell, the resultant hybrid cell will be benign because the tumor suppressor genes of the normal cell suppress the oncogenes contributed to the hybrid by the malignant cell.

The two best-known tumor suppressor genes are the retinoblastoma gene (Rb-1) and the p53. However, there are probably many other tumor suppressor genes.

The *retinoblastoma gene* was isolated in studies involving a malignant eye tumor known as retinoblastoma. This tumor occurs in a *hereditary* and *sporadic* form, and becomes clinically evident in early life. The *hereditary form* of retinoblastoma, which is often bilateral, shows a deletion of a segment of the long arm of chromosome 13 that carries the Rb-1 tumor suppressor gene. If the remaining allele of Rb-1 is mutated or lost in any of the retinal cells, such cells will not be able to control the expression of oncogenes. Accordingly, a tumor will develop in the retina. Other malignant tumors may develop in these children, albeit at an older age. Some patients with hereditary retinoblastoma have been cured of eye tumors but have succumbed to osteosarcoma that developed in their bones at puberty. This shows that the Rb-1 gene has a general tumor sup-

pressor function that is not limited to the eye (Fig. 4-21).

In *sporadic retinoblastoma*, the child is born with two normal alleles of the Rb-1 gene. However, if these alleles are mutated owing to some exogenous factor and both Rb-1 genes are inactivated or lost, eye tumors will develop. Such tumors are usually one-sided.

Gene p53, named after the molecular weight of the protein it encodes, is unique in that it acts both as a tumor suppressor gene and an oncogene. It may transform normal cells into neoplastic cells by transfection. A loss of p53 or its mutation leads to tumor formation. It has been implicated in the pathogenesis of numerous human cancers, most importantly, carcinoma of the colon and breast.

Hereditary Cancer

It has been known for many years that certain human cancers occur more often in certain families. These observations have led to an intensive search for possible cancer genes. Rb-1 tumor suppressor gene was identified through such a search, and many

FIGURE 4-21
Retinoblastoma tumor suppressor gene. (A) Patients with hereditary retinoblastoma are born with only one Rb-1 gene; the other one is deleted. Mutation of the remaining Rb-1 gene makes cells of the retina susceptible to cancer because such cells do not have any normally functioning Rb-1. (B) Sporadic retinoblastoma occurs in persons who are born with two Rb-1 alleles. For the tumor to develop, both alleles must be either inactivated or mutated.

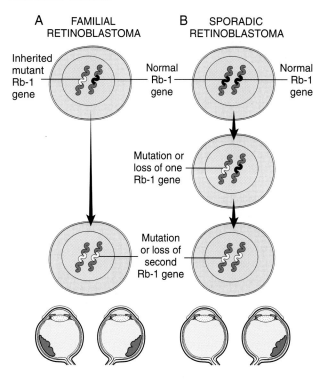

other tumor suppressor genes have been discovered in families with hereditary tumors.

Neurofibromatosis type 1 is the most common autosomal dominant disease in humans. The disease, which affects more than 3 million Americans, presents with numerous subcutaneous neural sheath tumors (neurofibromas). The patients also have pigmented lesions of the skin, called café au lait spots, and often have other tumors, such as intracranial meningiomas and adrenal pheochromocytomas. These lesions have been linked to the NF1 tumor suppressor gene. The NF1 gene product is a protein that inactivates a cytoplasmic signal transduction protein encoded by the *ras* oncogene. If the NF1 gene is defective or missing, the *ras* protein remains active all the time, leading to tumor formation.

There are several other neoplastic syndromes that are inherited as autosomal dominant traits. The most important of these are hereditary polyposis coli and Wilms' tumor.

In *hereditary polyposis coli,* the colon contains numerous polyps, many of which undergo malignant transformation. *Wilms' tumor* (nephroblastoma) is a renal malignant tumor of infancy and childhood. Each of these diseases has been linked to a specific tumor suppressor gene.

The incidence of cancer is increased in families affected by certain inborn errors of metabolism. Among this group of diseases, which are usually inherited as autosomal recessive traits, is xeroderma pigmentosum, which, as already mentioned, is an inborn deficiency of DNA repair enzymes. Affected patients cannot repair the DNA damage induced by UV light and are prone to develop skin cancer. Chromosomal fragility syndromes, such as Bloom's syndrome and Fanconi's syndrome, also show a predisposition to cancer. Inborn immunodeficiency syndromes also predispose individuals to neoplasia, especially malignant lymphomas.

Most common cancers are not inherited as Mendelian traits. Nevertheless, it is known that the incidence of breast cancer and colon cancer is increased in some families. Any woman whose mother or sisters had or have breast cancer has a 5 to 6 times greater risk of developing breast cancer than other women. The tendency for such persons to develop cancer is apparently polygenic and, like other polygenic diseases, is strongly influenced by exogenous factors. Recent discovery of a breast cancer gene is the first step toward elucidating the genetic aspects of this important human disease.

Immune Response to Tumors

Benign tumor cells may resemble the cells in the tissue of their origin, whereas malignant tumor cells differ from their normal ancestors. Malignancy may alter tumor cells so much that they become "foreign" to the body's own immune system. Tumor antigens that are perceived as foreign to the body will induce antibody production and a cell-mediated immune response. Ultimately, this immune response can limit the growth of the tumor. It is believed that many small tumors that form during the human life span are eliminated by the immune system. Many of the tumor cells that have entered into the blood circulation from established tumors are destroyed by the immune system. Some clinically apparent tumors that "heal spontaneously" also are most likely destroyed by the immune system. There is clinical evidence that some tumors may regress if treated by immunotherapy. All these facts point to antitumoral immunity as an important by-product of the *interaction between the tumor and the host.*

Antigenic changes that occur during malignant transformation also have diagnostic value in the clinical laboratory. Among the tumor-associated antigens, the best known is CEA, a glycoprotein normally found on the surface of fetal intestinal cells, but also expressed on adenocarcinoma of the colon. The measurement of CEA in the serum is valuable for monitoring tumor growth in patients with colon carcinoma. AFP, the major product of fetal liver cells, is also produced by liver cell carcinoma and is the most useful marker for this cancer.

The immune response of the host to tumor cells

Did You Know?

Cancer can heal spontaneously. Although this occurs infrequently, the medical literature contains many reports of spontaneous cancer cure. Scientists have been intrigued with such cases. Among these spontaneously healing tumors, the most common are melanoma, a pigmented skin tumor, and neuroblastoma, a tumor of malignant immature neural cells (neuroblasts). The cause of cure in such cases can only be surmised. It seems that the cure of melanoma is related to an immune response of the body. It is known that the immune cells can destroy malignant melanoma cells, and there are documented cases of regression of such tumors. Attacked by immune cells, melanomas lose their pigmentation and ultimately disappear. Neuroblastomas have been shown to undergo a peculiar form of maturation. During this process, the malignant neuroblasts transform into nonproliferating mature neural cells. In other words, in this respect, the malignant cells resemble maturing embryonic neuroblasts. Spontaneous maturation of neuroblastomas has spurred scientists to look for maturation-inducing factors as possible remedies for cancer.

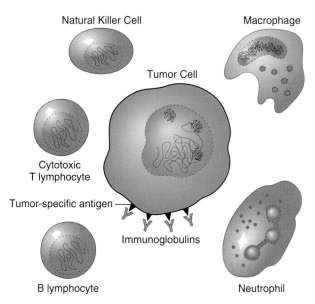

FIGURE 4-22
Host response to tumor cells is mediated by lymphocytes (T, B, and natural killer [NK] cells), macrophages, and neutrophils.

may be augmented for therapeutic purposes. The host response is mounted by NK cells, macrophages, cytoxic lymphocytes, and, to a lesser extent, antibody-producing cells (Fig. 4-22). The tumor cells that are highly immunogenic are the best targets for immunotherapy. Such tumors are typically infiltrated with lymphocytes, many of which belong to the NK cell subset. The lymph nodes draining a tumor-infiltrated area may contain granulomas, which represent a cell-mediated immune response to the tumor.

Immunotherapy of tumors has achieved best results in the treatment of melanomas. These skin tumors evoke a strong lymphocytic response and may even regress spontaneously. Some of the fetal tumors, such as neuroblastoma, also may heal spontaneously. This is probably because such tumors express the fetal antigens that are recognized as foreign by the adult host's immune system. Excellent results have been achieved in bladder cancer treatment by injecting attenuated tuberculosis bacillus, known as bacille Calmette-Guérin (BCG), into the urinary bladder. This nonspecific stimulus evokes an influx of macrophages, which destroy tumor cells. Unfortunately, most human tumors do not respond to any type of immunotherapy.

The important function of the immune system in controlling tumor growth is evident in the frequent occurrence of tumors in immunosuppressed hosts. Patients with acquired immunodeficiency syndrome (AIDS) typically develop rapidly growing lymphomas. Kaposi's sarcoma, a multifocal tumor composed of proliferating blood vessels, is also frequently found in patients with AIDS, especially those who have acquired the infection through homosexual intercourse.

Clinical Manifestations of Neoplasia

Clinical manifestations of neoplasia are highly variable, as cancer is not a single disease. Cancer may present in various forms, and so it is prudent to think of cancer whenever some unusual symptoms of disease occur. The seven warning signals of cancer listed under the mnemonic CAUTION are listed in Table 4-4.

The clinical features of tumors depend on the

- type of tumor
- location of the tumor
- histologic grade of the tumor
- clinical stage of the tumor
- immune status of the host
- sensitivity of the tumor cells to therapy

Overall, these clinical manifestations of neoplasia can be classified as local or systemic.

Local Symptoms

As tumors grow, they compress adjacent normal tissues. The symptoms depend primarily on the location of the tumors (Fig. 4-23). For example, compression of the brain can cause epileptic seizures. Tumor of the lungs may compress the bronchi and cause coughing. Persistent compression of normal tissues may cause atrophy, as is commonly seen in benign tumors adjacent to bones. Malignant tumors invade the tissues and also cause destruction of normal organs. Invasion of blood vessels and erosion of normal tissues by tumors often result in hemorrhage. Hemorrhage is actually the most common presenting sign of tumors of the large intestine, kidneys, and urinary bladder.

Tumors growing into the lumen of hollow organs, such as the intestines, may cause narrowing of the lumen or obstruction. In the large intestine, the stools passing through a narrowed segment appear "pencil-like." Ultimately, the intestinal passage could

Table 4-4 Seven Warning Signals of Cancer*

Change in bowel or bladder habits
A sore that doesn't heal
Unusual bleeding or discharge
Thickening of lump in breast or elsewhere
Indigestion or difficulty in swallowing
Obvious change in wart or mole
Nagging cough or hoarseness

*If you have a warning signal, see your doctor!
These guidelines are currently under revision. Please refer to the American Cancer Society for more information.

SYMPTOMS OF NEOPLASTIC DISEASE

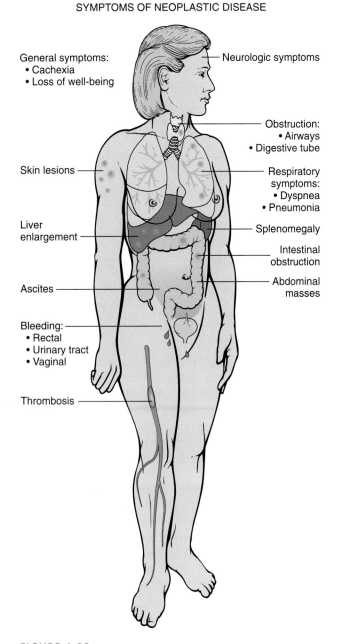

FIGURE 4-23
Symptoms of malignant tumors.

be blocked completely. Bronchial obstruction by lung cancer causes stagnation of mucus in the bronchus and coughing.

Systemic Symptoms

Cancers cause a variety of systemic symptoms. These symptoms include cachexia or generalized weakness, weight loss, loss of appetite (anorexia), and a variety of paraneoplastic syndromes (Table 4-5). Cachexia is caused by wasting secondary to the adverse effects of cancer on the body. Cancer can be considered to be a parasite that drains the energy

from the body and also competes for nutrients. Cancers of the gastrointestinal tract may interfere with nutrition. For example, cancer of the esophagus may impede swallowing. Carcinoma of the pancreas may impede the entry of pancreatic juices into the intestine, which may lead to malabsorption of nutrients, minerals, and vitamins.

Paraneoplastic syndromes are caused by various substances secreted by cancer cells. Paraneoplastic syndromes include various endocrine, hematologic, neuromuscular, cardiovascular, and other changes. For example, carcinoma of the lung may secrete adrenocorticotropic hormone (ACTH) and produce hyperstimulation of the adrenals (Cushing's syndrome). Tumor-derived parathyroid hormone, like polypeptide, may cause demineralization of bone and fractures. Bone demineralization is a common feature of breast cancer and is typically associated with hypercalcemia.

Many patients with cancer have hypercoagulable blood and develop thrombosis. This hypercoagulability results from the entry of tumor degradation products or secretions (e.g., pancreatic enzymes) into the circulation. In pancreatic cancer, thrombosis is often described as migratory; that is, it sequentially affects different veins without apparent order or regularity. Thrombosis is often associated with inflammation of occluded veins (thrombophlebitis). Migratory thrombophlebitis is known as Trousseau's syndrome, named after the doctor who first described it. Although it is most often associated with pancreatic cancer, it may be caused by other cancers as well.

An understanding of clinical symptoms of cancer is most important for the diagnosis and early detection of neoplasia. The most important cancer risk factors and presenting signs are listed in Table 4-6. It should, however, be noted that cancer may present with many other symptoms. There are no symptoms specific to cancer; therefore, the best way to diagnose this disease is to consider it in almost any clinical setting. As most cancers remain incurable if diagnosed in an advanced stage, the best hope of conquering cancer lies in its early detection and regular preventive examinations. Seven safeguards against cancer recommended by the American Cancer Society are listed in Table 4-7.

Cancer Epidemiology

Epidemiology of neoplasia is concerned with the study of cancer in human populations. Epidemiologic studies are based on data gathered from cancer registries and clinical records or by active inquiry. In prospective studies, epidemiologic data are used for vital statistics and for planning of health policies.

Table 4-5 Examples of Paraneoplastic Syndromes

Clinical Symptoms	Cancer Type	Cause
Endocrine Changes		
Cushing's syndrome	Small cell cancer of the lung	ACTH
Hypercalcemia	Squamous cell carcinoma of the lung	PTH-like polypeptide
	Breast carcinoma	TGF-α
Hematologic Changes		
Polycythemia	Renal carcinoma	Erythropoietin
Venous thrombosis	Pancreatic carcinoma	Thromboplastin
Neuromuscular Changes		
Lambert-Eaton syndrome (muscular weakness)	Small cell carcinoma of the lung	Antibodies to NMJ
Myasthenia gravis	Thymoma	Antibodies to NMJ

ACTH, adrenocorticotropic hormone; PTH, parathyroid hormone; TGF, transforming growth factor; NMJ, neuromuscular junction.

The most important epidemiologic data relate to cancer incidence, prevalence, and mortality.

Incidence of cancer is the number of new cases that have been registered over a specific period of time in a defined population. It has been shown that the incidence of cancer varies geographically. For example, gastric cancer is common in Japan and Iceland and is less common in Western Europe and the United States. This discrepancy is thought to be attributable to different dietary habits and the high consumption of raw and smoked fish in the former countries. Indeed, the descendants of Japanese immigrants in the United States have less cancer of the stomach than their relatives who are still living in Japan.

The incidence of cancer in the United States has changed over the last 50 years (Fig. 4-24). Gastric cancer, which was prevalent in earlier years, has become less common than colon cancer. The incidence of lung carcinoma has been rising. This form of cancer was uncommon among women, but today is as common in women as in men. These changes in the incidence of cancer reflect changes in living conditions, habits, and diet. For example, the increased incidence of lung cancer in women is directly related to an increase in smoking that occurred when

Table 4-6 Risk Factors and Presenting Signs of Common Cancers

Cancer Type	Most Important Risk Factors	Most Common Initial Symptoms
Lung	Smoking	Cough
Breast	Family history of cancer	Lump
Colon	Family history of colonic polyps	Blood in stool
Cervix	Promiscuity	Vaginal bleeding ("spotting")
Uterus	Hormonal imbalance and treatment	Vaginal bleeding
Skin	Sun exposure Fair skin	Skin lesion
Prostate	Old age	Dysuria

Table 4-7 Seven Safeguards Against Cancer

Breast: Regular monthly self-examination of breasts for lumps, nodules, or changes in contour; yearly check by physician

Lung: Reduction and ultimate elimination of cigarette smoking; avoidance of smoke-filled environments

Colon-rectum: Rectal examinations as routine part of annual check-ups for those older than 40 years of age; proctosigmoidoscopy or barium enema colon radiographs at age 50 and every 3 to 5 years thereafter

Cervix: Pap test for all adult and high-risk adolescent women

Skin: Avoidance of excessive exposure to sun or tanning lights

Oral: Wider practice of early detection measures; regular dental examinations

Basic: Routine periodic physical examination for all adults

From the American Cancer Society, with permission.

FIGURE 4-24
Death rates for females (A) and males (B), according to site, in the United States arranged by decade from 1930 to 1991. Note the increased rate of lung cancer and decreased rate of stomach cancer. (From Cancer statistics, 1999. CA—A Cancer Journal for Clinicians, 49:18–19, 1999. Published by Lippincott Williams & Wilkins for the American Cancer Society; with permission.)

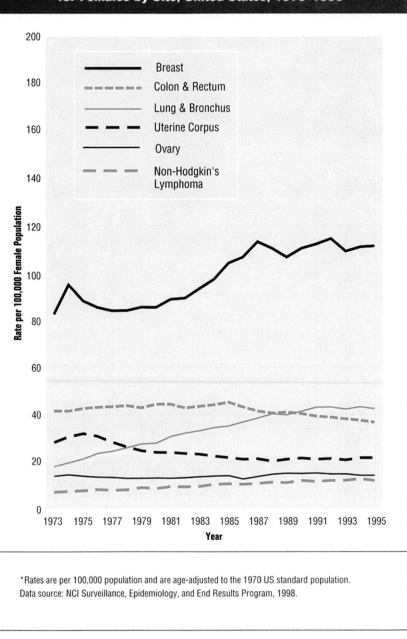

Age-Adjusted Cancer Incidence Rates*
for Females by Site, United States, 1973–1995

— Breast
------ Colon & Rectum
— Lung & Bronchus
– – – Uterine Corpus
— Ovary
– – – Non-Hodgkin's Lymphoma

Rate per 100,000 Female Population

Year

*Rates are per 100,000 population and are age-adjusted to the 1970 US standard population. Data source: NCI Surveillance, Epidemiology, and End Results Program, 1998.

A

women joined the work force during World War II. The most common sites of cancer in males and females and the mortality associated with neoplasms are shown in Fig. 4-25.

Prevalence of cancer is the number of all cases of cancer—new and old—within a defined population at a defined time. The prevalence of cancer has increased over the years. This is, in part, attributable to improved diagnostic methods and life-prolonging treatment, but it may also be the result of increased exposure to environmental carcinogens. Prevalence

of skin cancer is directly correlated with sun exposure. Thus, it is no wonder that skin cancer is more prevalent in the southern United States than in the north. Prostate cancer is more prevalent in the elderly. The increased prevalence of prostate cancer correlates with the generally increased longevity of human populations, especially in the Western world.

Mortality of cancer is the number of deaths attributed to cancer during a specified period in a defined population. For example, the mortality of patients with testicular cancer has decreased dra-

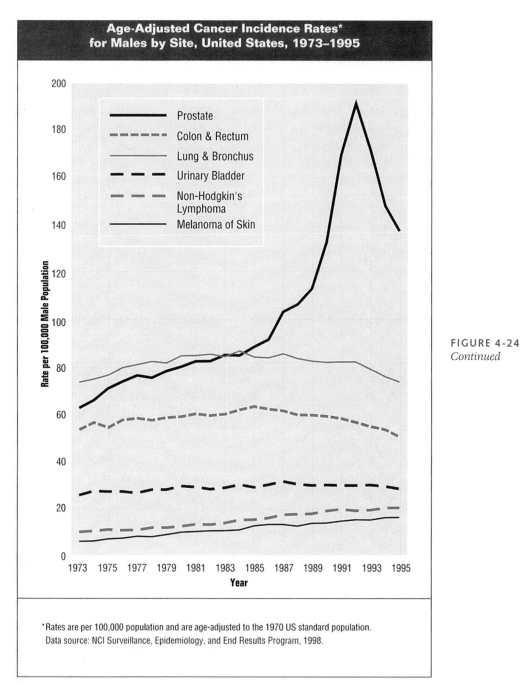

Age-Adjusted Cancer Incidence Rates*
for Males by Site, United States, 1973–1995

Legend:
— Prostate
‑ ‑ ‑ Colon & Rectum
— Lung & Bronchus
– – – Urinary Bladder
– – – Non-Hodgkin's Lymphoma
— Melanoma of Skin

Y-axis: Rate per 100,000 Male Population
X-axis: Year (1973–1995)

*Rates are per 100,000 population and are age-adjusted to the 1970 US standard population.
Data source: NCI Surveillance, Epidemiology, and End Results Program, 1998.

B

FIGURE 4-24
Continued

Did You Know?

The overall incidence of cancer is on the increase. However, cancer is not a new disease. Archeologists have found bone tumors in Egyptian mummies and even in cave men. Because cancer occurs most often in older people, and there are more older men and women than ever before in history, the increased incidence of cancer in our times is not unexpected.

matically since the 1970s. However, the mortality from lung cancer has remained the same over the last 30 years.

The study of epidemiology has provided new insights into the endogenous and exogenous causes of cancer. Among the most important exogenous cancer-provoking agents identified in these studies are

- smoking, as the major cause of lung cancer
- sunlight, as the major cause of skin cancer
- dietary fats, as the possible cause of colon cancer

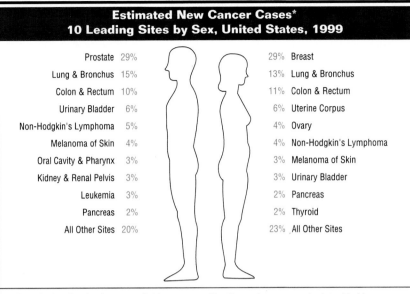

Estimated New Cancer Cases*
10 Leading Sites by Sex, United States, 1999

Male		Female	
Prostate	29%	29%	Breast
Lung & Bronchus	15%	13%	Lung & Bronchus
Colon & Rectum	10%	11%	Colon & Rectum
Urinary Bladder	6%	6%	Uterine Corpus
Non-Hodgkin's Lymphoma	5%	4%	Ovary
Melanoma of Skin	4%	4%	Non-Hodgkin's Lymphoma
Oral Cavity & Pharynx	3%	3%	Melanoma of Skin
Kidney & Renal Pelvis	3%	3%	Urinary Bladder
Leukemia	3%	2%	Pancreas
Pancreas	2%	2%	Thyroid
All Other Sites	20%	23%	All Other Sites

*Excludes basal and squamous cell skin cancers and in situ carcinomas except urinary bladder.

FIGURE 4-25
(Top) Incidence of cancer in various organs. (Bottom) Death rates associated with cancer in various organs. (From Cancer statistics 1999. CA—A Cancer Journal for Clinicians, 49:16, 1999. Published by Lippincott Williams & Wilkins for the American Cancer Society; with permission.)

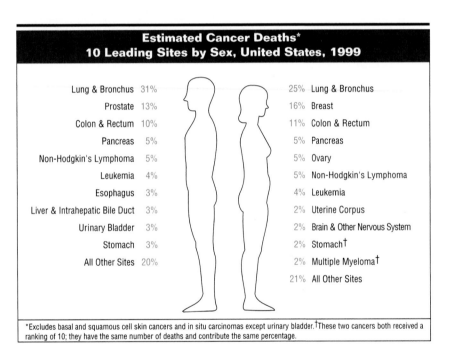

Estimated Cancer Deaths*
10 Leading Sites by Sex, United States, 1999

Male		Female	
Lung & Bronchus	31%	25%	Lung & Bronchus
Prostate	13%	16%	Breast
Colon & Rectum	10%	11%	Colon & Rectum
Pancreas	5%	5%	Pancreas
Non-Hodgkin's Lymphoma	5%	5%	Ovary
Leukemia	4%	5%	Non-Hodgkin's Lymphoma
Esophagus	3%	4%	Leukemia
Liver & Intrahepatic Bile Duct	3%	2%	Uterine Corpus
Urinary Bladder	3%	2%	Brain & Other Nervous System
Stomach	3%	2%	Stomach†
All Other Sites	20%	2%	Multiple Myeloma†
		21%	All Other Sites

*Excludes basal and squamous cell skin cancers and in situ carcinomas except urinary bladder.†These two cancers both received a ranking of 10; they have the same number of deaths and contribute the same percentage.

In the industrial setting, epidemiologic studies have identified such carcinogens as asbestos (as a cause of lung cancer and mesothelioma) and aniline dies (as a cause of bladder cancer). However, the cause of most human cancers remains unknown.

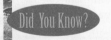

Did You Know?

Cancer is the second most common cause of death in the United States, eclipsed only by cardiovascular disease. More than 500,000 persons die of cancer every year.

Review Questions

1. What are neoplasms?
2. How are human tumors classified?
3. What are the main differences between benign and malignant tumors?
4. How do tumors metastasize?
5. List a few benign mesenchymal tumors and their malignant equivalents.
6. List a few benign epithelial tumors and their malignant equivalents.
7. How do carcinomas differ from sarcomas?
8. Define lymphoma, glioma, seminoma, and teratoma.
9. List three eponymic tumors.
10. What is the difference between tumor staging and grading?
11. Compare normal and malignant cells, taking into account their morphology, some basic biologic functions, and biochemical properties.
12. How do tumor cells grow in vitro?
13. What are the most important exogenous and endogenous causes of cancer?
14. How do scientists identify potential human carcinogens?
15. List some chemical carcinogens and explain how they cause cancer.
16. How does ultraviolet light cause cancer?
17. Compare the carcinogenic action of oncogenic RNA and DNA viruses.
18. Which human DNA viruses have been linked to cancer?
19. How do proto-oncogenes transform into oncogenes?
20. What are tumor suppressor genes and how do they cause cancer?
21. Explain the role of heredity in the pathogenesis of cancer.
22. Describe the immune response to tumors and explain its clinical significance.
23. What are the common warning signs of neoplasia?
24. Explain the pathogenesis of common local symptoms of neoplasia.
25. What is the pathogenesis of tumor-induced cachexia, and hypercoagulability of blood.
26. Define paraneoplastic syndrome and provide specific examples of syndromes dominated by endocrine, hematologic, or neuromuscular changes.
27. List some risk factors for common cancers.
28. What is the difference between incidence and prevalence of cancer?
29. The incidence of which cancers has increased or decreased over the last 40 years?
30. Discuss important safeguards against cancer.

Learning Objectives

After reading this chapter, the student should be able to:

1. Define and describe the following: gamete, zygote, cleavage-stage embryo, blastocyst, germ layers, organ primordia (anlagen), and organogenesis.

2. Define developmental malformations (birth defects).

3. Explain teratogenesis and list the five most common identifiable causes of birth defects in humans.

4. Describe the TORCH syndrome and list the four most common causes of this set of malformations.

5. Define the structural chromosomal abnormalities of deletion and translocation and explain their significance.

6. Define chromosomal monosomy and trisomy and give appropriate examples.

7. Describe three possible functional consequences of single gene mutations.

8. Explain the principles of Mendelian inheritance.

9. List three important autosomal dominant disorders.

10. List three important autosomal recessive disorders.

11. Explain the pathogenesis of lysosomal storage diseases and give three specific examples of prototypic disorders.

12. List three important X-linked recessive disorders.

13. List the cardinal features of multifactorial inheritance and list three important diseases that are inherited in such a way.

14. Describe prenatal diagnosis of genetic and developmental disorders.

15. Define prematurity and list three of its causes.

16. Define fetal pulmonary maturity and describe how immaturity of the lungs causes neonatal respiratory distress syndrome.

17. List three lesions induced by birth injury and explain their pathogenesis.

18. Discuss sudden infant death syndrome.

Additional Key Terms and Concepts

Fetal alcohol syndrome

Fragile X syndrome

Chapter Outline

Genetic and Developmental Diseases

Chapter 5

The beginning of human life cannot be scientifically defined. Without fertilization, there is no human life. For practical purposes, we shall assume that life begins at the moment of fertilization: i.e., the meeting of the female germ cell, or ovum, and the male gamete, or sperm. However, this is an arbitrary definition, as the concepts of life and death are socially determined. These concepts have changed through history and will most likely change in the future as advancing technology inevitably expands our capacity to influence basic events of human life. For the purpose of this discussion, consider the following:

- Human life is just the continuation of the life of two living cells! Both sperm and ovum are living cells. One cannot produce living humans from dead germ cells.
- Germ cells ensure the continuity of life from one generation to another. However, technology has made it possible to modify or temporarily interrupt this sequence. For example, the sperm or ova can be frozen and kept at −70°C indefinitely and then used for in vitro fertilization. Even early embryos can be frozen and stored for indefinite periods of time. Such frozen embryos retain viability and can subsequently be defrosted and implanted into hormonally induced surrogate mothers in whom they develop into normal human beings.
- Human life develops only from cells that carry human genetic material. Human genes can, however, be isolated and transferred to animal germ cells. Such *transgenic animals* may express human genetic trains. In other words, some aspects of human life can be perpetuated outside of the human organism.
- Human life cannot be generated from nonliving material. At this time, we do not know how to produce life from inorganic chemicals. This does not, however, preclude the possibility that one day new life will be generated in the test tube.

Normal Embryonic Development

Following fertilization, the newly formed *zygote* (fertilized ovum) divides into two, and then four and eight cells, reaching the stage of *morula* within 3 to 4 days (Fig. 5-1). A central cavity is formed inside the morula as it transforms into a *blastocyst*. It is important to note that early *cleavage-stage embryos* consist of cells whose developmental potential has not been firmly programmed. Loss of single cells at the 2-, 4-, and 8-cell stages can easily be compensated for without any adverse consequences. However, at the blastocyst stage, the fate of embryonic cells has been determined: cells of the inner cell mass will give rise to the embryo proper, whereas the outer layer, called the trophoblast, will give rise to the placenta. After this stage of development, any cell loss in the inner cell mass will result in embryonic defects because such cell losses cannot be replaced.

The inner cell mass gives rise to the primordial *germ layers:* ectoderm, mesoderm, and endoderm. These germ layers produce the *primordia* of fetal organs (in German, called *anlagen*). For example, the skin and the nervous system develop from the ectoderm, the intestines develop from the endoderm, and the bones and muscle arise from the mesoderm. The development of organs is tightly regulated by special master genes, called "homeobox genes," which regulate and coordinate the expression of other genes in the developing tissues. As the genes are turned on and off, each organ goes through a specific organogenetic period. During the *critical stages* of *organogenesis,* which are those characterized by extensive cell division, migration, and cell-to-cell interaction, the developing organs are very sensitive to adverse external influences. Chemical, physical, and viral agents are most prone to induce developmental defects during these developmental stages. Generally speaking, the critical period for most organs is in the first trimester of pregnancy. However, some organs, like the brain, do not complete development during intrauterine life, and so are susceptible to adverse influences for several months after birth.

In humans, the period of organogenesis that is conventionally called *fetal life* lasts approximately 9 months. During this period, the organs become anatomically recognizable; they assume specific histologic features and become functionally active. Anatomically defined fetal organs can be seen by ultrasonography. For example, by 10 to 12 weeks' gestation, one can recognize the fetal penis and determine the sex of the fetus. One can also see whether the kidneys have been formed, and many other organs can be examined to determine whether they are normal.

Fetal organs have a "fetal histology," being composed of cells that have functions quite different from those of normal adult organs. For example, the red blood cells (RBCs) contain fetal hemoglobin, which, upon birth, is replaced by adult hemoglobin. Likewise, fetal liver cells produce alpha-fetoprotein (AFP) as the major plasma protein in contrast to adult liver cells, which secrete albumin. Fetal lungs are functionally immature because they secrete a different form of surfactant than the adult lung and, therefore, are incompetent for respiration. Functional maturation occurs generally at a slower rate than anatomic maturation. Many organs acquire full functional competence only at puberty, and some need special stimuli to mature. For example, female breast acini develop fully only after pregnancy and during lactation.

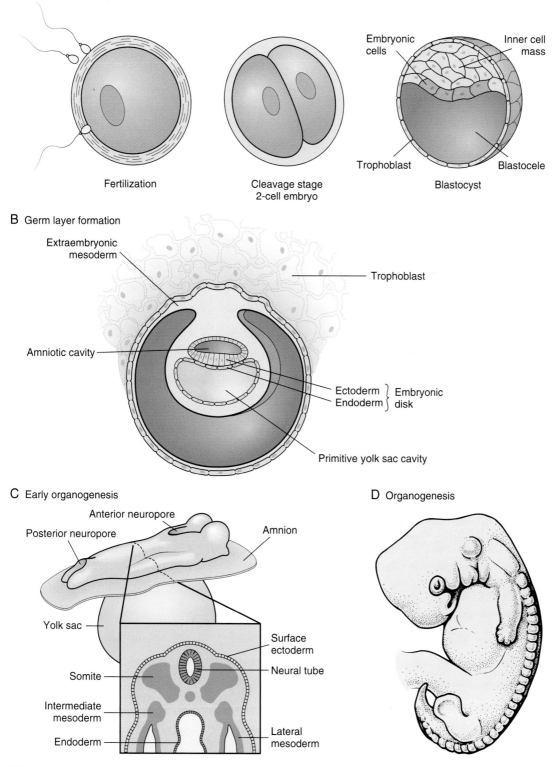

A Preimplantation embryo

Fertilization

Cleavage stage
2-cell embryo

Embryonic cells
Inner cell mass
Trophoblast
Blastocele
Blastocyst

B Germ layer formation

Extraembryonic mesoderm
Trophoblast
Amniotic cavity
Ectoderm
Endoderm } Embryonic disk
Primitive yolk sac cavity

C Early organogenesis

Anterior neuropore
Posterior neuropore
Amnion
Yolk sac
Surface ectoderm
Somite
Neural tube
Intermediate mesoderm
Endoderm
Lateral mesoderm

D Organogenesis

FIGURE 5-1

Normal prenatal development can arbitrarily be divided into several stages. (A) The preimplantation stage, which extends from the first cleavage of the zygote to the formation of the blastocyst. (B) The embryonic stage, which is characterized by germ layer formation during early postimplantation stages of development. (C) Early organogenesis, which is marked by organ primordia formation. (D) Late organogenesis, during which the anatomic and functional maturation of organs occurs.

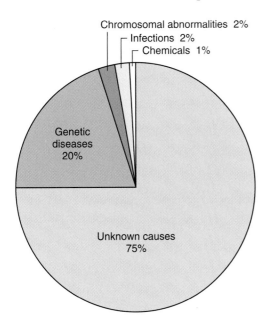

Chromosomal abnormalities 2%
Infections 2%
Chemicals 1%

Genetic
diseases
20%

Unknown causes
75%

FIGURE 5-2
Causes of congenital defects in humans. The etiology of most defects is not known. Among the causes identified, genetic and chromosomal abnormalities are the most common.

Developmental Malformations

Disturbances of development are the subject of a science called *teratology* (from the Greek *teraton*, meaning monster, and *logos*, meaning science). The agents that cause fetal abnormalities (malformations) are thus called **teratogens.** The cause of most malformations (approximately 75 percent) is never established (Fig. 5-2). Among the identifiable causes of developmental malformations, the most prominent are genetic factors (20 percent). Various exogenous teratogens, such as drugs, alcohol, or x-rays, account for a small number of human malformations. Such chemical, physical, and microbial agents are, nevertheless, important to know. By avoiding exposure to potential teratogens, pregnant women can protect their unborn babies and prevent the development of some malformations.

Genetic Factors

Genes inherited from the parents control not only specific traits, such as height or skin color, but also development in utero. The lack of certain essential genes or their mutation (lethal mutations) results in abnormal development. Such embryos and fetuses are not viable beyond a certain stage of development and are usually aborted spontaneously. Numerous studies performed on spontaneously aborted fetuses have shown that most of them had genetic defects, and that many had abnormal chromosomes.

The genetic basis of malformations has been doc-

This child was born with two heads that are incompletely separated from each other. The cause of this congenital malformation, like most others, remains unknown.

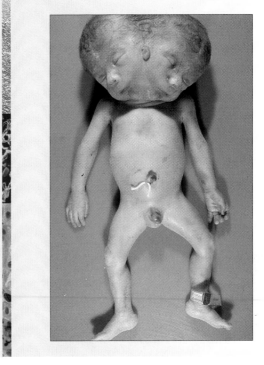

umented for a number of human congenital defects. For example, the incidence of cleft lip (commonly known as "hare lip") is increased in some families and is inherited as a multifactorial trait. Dwarfism, which is characterized by short arms and legs (achondroplastic dwarfism) is inherited as an autosomal dominant Mendelian trait.

Exogenous Teratogens

Exogenous teratogens are classified as physical, chemical, and microbial. Some of the most common of these are presented in the following sections.

Physical Teratogens. The best known physical teratogens are x-rays and other forms of corpuscular radiation (alpha, beta, and gamma rays). Exposure to radioactive radiation during pregnancy thus poses a definite risk. For example, an increased incidence of malformations was noted among Japanese children born to mothers exposed during pregnancy to the atomic bomb explosion in Hiroshima and Nagasaki in 1945. Modern x-ray procedures require small amounts of x-rays and are considered to be safe. Nevertheless, unnecessary exposure to x-rays during pregnancy should be avoided.

The cause of most human birth defects is not known. From time to time, however, we become aware of a substance that can produce birth defects.

The story of thalidomide is a good example. It has taught us an important lesson. This sleeping pill was introduced for medicinal use in the late fifties. Because nobody suspected that it could have any adverse effects, it was given to many sleepless pregnant women. First reports that thalidomide may cause birth defects were ignored. Subsequently, over a period of 5 years, more than 3000 abnormal children were born to women who took thalidomide during pregnancy. The children were born with malformed and shortened limbs resembling the flippers of a seal. (This malformation is called phocomelia, a term derived from the Greek words *phoca*, meaning seal, and *melos*, meaning limb.) Tragedies like this could have been prevented by proper drug testing. U.S. rules and regulations now require that every new drug be tested on pregnant animals to determine whether the drug is safe for use during pregnancy. (Photograph courtesy of Dr. Olav Hilmar Iversen.)

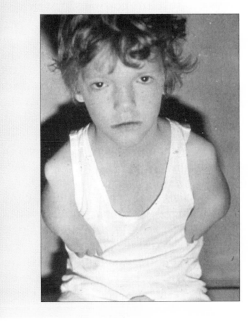

the development of the fetal brain. Children who are born with the full-blown syndrome have typical facial features, such as a small cranium and jaws, a thin upper lip, and palpebral abnormalities (Fig. 5-3). Most importantly, they have reduced mental process and their I.Q. is lower than normal. Other internal organs may be affected as well. Mental retardation can occur, even without these external signs of FAS.

Microbial Teratogens. Various infections during pregnancy may affect the fetus directly or indirectly. Indirect effects, owing to the weakening or physical

FIGURE 5-3

Fetal alcohol syndrome (FAS). Affected children have typical features which, when accompanied by mental retardation, are diagnostic of FAS. The features on the left are those most frequently seen in patients with FAS, whereas those on the right are features that are seen with increased frequency in this population compared to the normal population. (From Drs. Little and Streissguth, Seattle, Washington, 1982.)

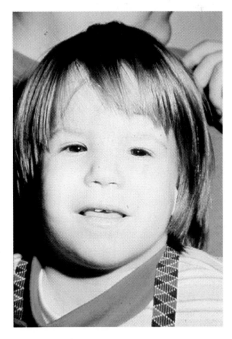

FACIES IN FETAL ALCOHOL SYNDROME

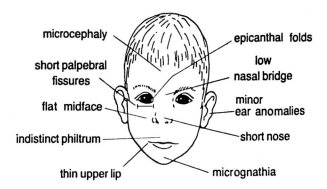

Chemical Teratogens. Many chemical teratogens exist in nature, and even more of them are manmade. These agents are often used in industry or are ingested as drugs. The most important set of preventable fetal malformations related to the maternal ingestion of a chemical is the so-called fetal alcohol syndrome (FAS). Alcohol abuse during pregnancy causes intrauterine growth retardation. It also affects

exhaustion of the mother, typically cause fetal weight reduction, growth retardation, or premature birth. Direct effects, secondary to the transplacental passage of microbes and subsequent infection of fetal organs, are more serious and have more deleterious consequences.

Several human pathogens have been identified as especially noxious to the fetus. These infectious pathogens cause a syndrome of fetal defects known by the acronym *TORCH*. The name is derived from the first letters of the pathogens that cause it: *toxoplasma, rubella, cytomegalovirus (CMV), and herpesvirus.* The letter O stands for *other* less common infectious agents, such as Epstein-Barr virus, varicella virus, *Listeria monocytogenes,* Leptospira, and several other bacteria.

The TORCH syndrome is marked by the involvement of several internal organs. The brain is most often affected, and mental retardation, often combined with neurologic symptoms, dominates the clinical presentation. In congenital rubella, the brain is small (*microcephaly*) and often structurally abnormal. In toxoplasmosis and CMV infection, the brain shows *microcalcifications* of the basal ganglia and dilatation of the lateral ventricles (*hydrocephalus*). Small eyes (*microphthalmia*), inflammation of the inside layers of the eye with calcifications (*chorioretinitis*), and clouding of the lens (*cataract*) are common. Heart defects are most common in congenital rubella infection. Inflammations of the liver and lung, and reactive enlargement of the lymph nodes and the spleen, are common. Skin lesions, such as petechial hemorrhages and vesicles, are also present, especially following herpesvirus infection.

All the symptoms of TORCH can be related to the transplacental passage of infectious agents during the critical stages of organogenesis. For example, the triad of microcephaly, microphthalmia, and congenital heart disease, which is typical of congenital rubella, occurs only if an unimmunized mother is infected with rubella virus during the first trimester (Fig. 5-4). Central nervous system defects, typical of toxoplasma, CMV, or herpes infection, can result even when the infection occurs during the last trimester of pregnancy. Congenital rubella syndrome can be prevented completely by maternal immunization, but there are no vaccines against the other causes of TORCH syndrome.

Chromosomal Abnormalities

Human genes are encoded by triplets of nucleotides. Double-helix DNA is strung into nucleosomes, which, in turn are arranged into larger units called chromatin fibers. During mitosis, the chromatin

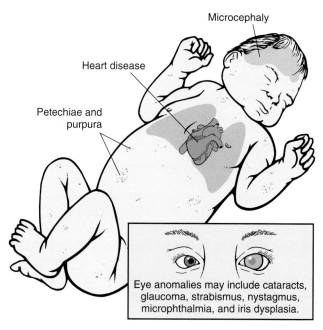

Microcephaly

Heart disease

Petechiae and purpura

Eye anomalies may include cataracts, glaucoma, strabismus, nystagmus, microphthalmia, and iris dysplasia.

FIGURE 5-4
Congenital rubella syndrome is marked by a triad that includes microcephaly, microphthalmia, and congenital heart disease.

fibers condense into **chromosomes,** which can be seen on light microscopy (Fig. 5-5).

Normal human cells contain two sets of 23 chromosomes. Twenty-two of these are in identical pairs, numbered 1 through 22 according to their unique features, and are called *autosomes.* The remaining chromosome, called the sex chromosome, may be either X or Y. Females have two X chromosomes and a 46,XX karyotype, whereas males have an X and a Y chromosome, and a 46,XY karyotype. One set of 23 chromosomes is inherited from the mother and the other from the father. Because all female cells, including the maternal ovum, contain only X chromosomes, it is the paternal sperm (which may carry either the X or Y sex chromosome) that determines the sex of the child.

Chromosomal abnormalities can be classified as either structural or numerical, and can involve either **abnormalities of autosomes** or of the **sex chromosomes.**

Structural Chromosomal Abnormalities

Structural chromosomal abnormalities occur in many forms. The most important of these are *deletion* of a portion of the chromosomal arms and *translocation* of a portion of one chromosome to another chromosome (Fig. 5-6).

Deletions of a portion of a short arm of chromosome 11 is associated with a complex syndrome char-

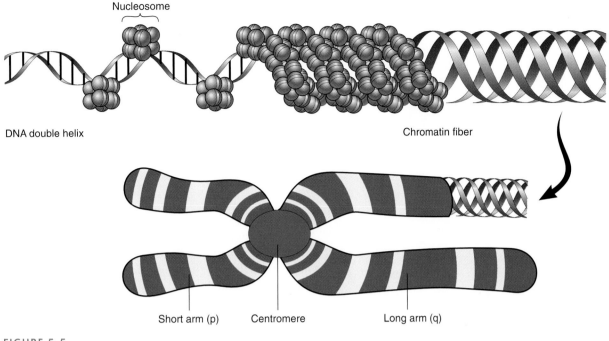

Nucleosome

DNA double helix

Chromatin fiber

Short arm (p) Centromere Long arm (q)

FIGURE 5-5
Human chromosomes are composed of double-stranded DNA that is coiled into nucleosomes which, in turn, are arranged into chromatin fibers. Chromatin fibers are assembled into chromosomes during mitosis.

acterized by congenital Wilms' tumor of the kidney, aniridia (lack of iris), genital malformations, and mental retardation (the so-called WAGR syndrome). Apparently, the lost, deleted part of the chromosome contains several genes that are important for normal development, as well as a tumor suppressor gene (WT, or Wilms' tumor, gene). Children born with deletions of a segment of the long arm of chromosome 13 develop retinoblastomas, which are eye tumors originating in the retina. This segment of the chromosome contains the RB (retinoblastoma) suppressor gene.

Translocations are often associated with infertility, or congenital malformation syndromes. For example, some cases of Down syndrome are associated with translocation of chromosome 21 to chromosome 14.

Numerical Chromosomal Abnormalities

Numerical chromosomal abnormalities involve a loss or a gain of chromosomes, resulting in karyotype known as *aneuploidy*. Instead of the normal diploid number of chromosomes, it may be hyperdiploid (46 + 1, 46 + 2, etc.) or hypodiploid (46–1, 46–2, etc.). The loss of one chromosome is called *monosomy*, whereas the gain of an additional chromosome is called *trisomy*. Autosomal monosomy—loss of an autosome—is not compatible with life. Similarly, the embryo that has only a Y chromosome but no X chro-

mosome usually dies early in pregnancy. On the other hand, embryos with a 45,XO karyotype are viable. Trisomies of sex chromosomes also are compatible with life. Trisomies of autosomes 13, 18, or 21 result in malformations and are often lethal. Most such abnormal fetuses are spontaneously aborted or stillborn. Nevertheless, approximately 1 in 1000 neonates has an autosomal trisomy and is severely malformed.

Trisomy 21 (Down Syndrome). Trisomy 21 is the most common numerical abnormality involving an autosome (Fig. 5-7). It is diagnosed in 1 of 800 neonates. It is clinically recognizable as a constellation of characteristic physical and mental abnormalities known as the Down syndrome.

The pathogenesis of Down syndrome is not fully understood. It is known that trisomy of chromosome 21 is mostly of maternal origin and is a consequence of "nondisjunction" during the meiotic (reduction) division of a maturing oocyte. Abnormal meiosis allocates an extra chromosome 21 to the ovum; if this ovum is fertilized, the zygote and all cells that develop from it in the embryo will have 47 chromosomes. In the notation of cytogenetics, this is registered as 47,XX + 21 or 47,XY + 21, as the baby may be either male or female. The reasons for nondisjunction are not known, but it appears that this mishap occurs more often in older women, suggesting that the final stages of meiotic division are affected by advanced maternal age.

A Deletion

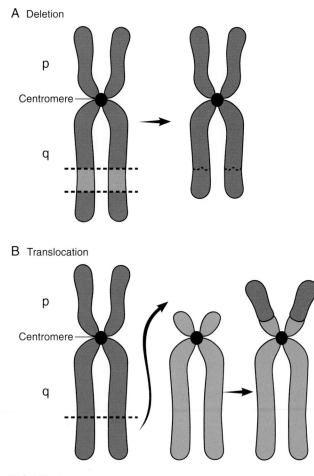

B Translocation

FIGURE 5-6
Structural chromosomal abnormalities. (A) Deletion.
(B) Translocation.

known that Down syndrome predisposes individuals to development of leukemia. Some patients also suffer from immune deficiencies and are susceptible to infections.

Down syndrome represents a severe handicap, primarily because of the incapacitating mental retardation. Furthermore, there is increased mortality related to congenital heart disease and increased susceptibility to infections. With proper care, the life expectancy of affected persons can be prolonged, and the average age at death of these patients is 55 years.

Down syndrome cannot be cured. Nevertheless, the abnormal embryo can be diagnosed cytogenetically by chorionic villus biopsy or amniocentesis, and the abnormal fetus can be aborted. Because the nondisjunction of chromosomes occurs most often in oocytes of older women, who are thus at increased risk of giving birth to children with Down syndrome, prenatal diagnosis should be offered to them on a regular basis.

Abnormalities of Sex Chromosomes

Numerical abnormalities of X and Y chromosomes are more common in clinical practice than those involving the autosomes, and the karyotypic abnormalities of sex chromosomes are less lethal and cause

FIGURE 5-7
The karyotype of Down syndrome consists of 47 chromosomes and shows trisomy 21.

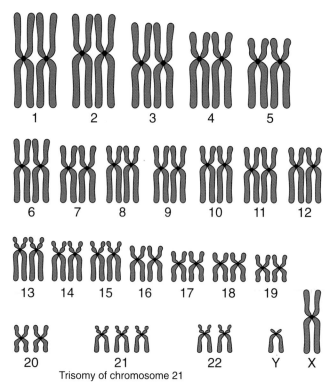

Trisomy of chromosome 21

The symptoms of Down syndrome include the following (Fig. 5-8):

- *Mental retardation*
- *Typical facial features,* including a wide face, a low-bridged nose, and closely set, slanted eyes with epicanthus. *Epicanthus* is a medial fold of the upper lid which gives the eyes an Oriental appearance. There is also *macroglossia* (large tongue), and the tongue often protrudes through the gaping mouth.
- *Abnormal extremities.* The legs and arms of affected individuals are usually short. The hands are wide and show a "simian crease" extending across the entire width of the palms. The fifth finger is shorter than normal and crooked (*clinodactyly*).
- *Congenital defects of internal organs,* which may include heart defects, gastrointestinal atresia or stenosis, and infertility. Men are invariably sterile, but some women with Down syndrome are fertile.
- *Hematologic abnormalities.* These abnormalities may be mild, such as anemia, but it is also

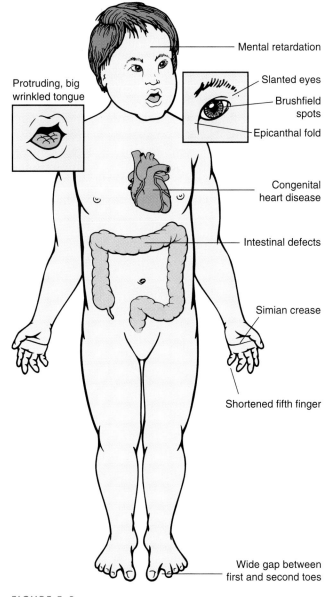

FIGURE 5-8
Typical features of Down syndrome.

Protruding, big wrinkled tongue

Mental retardation

Slanted eyes

Brushfield spots

Epicanthal fold

Congenital heart disease

Intestinal defects

Simian crease

Shortened fifth finger

Wide gap between first and second toes

an X (45,X), a viable child with Turner's syndrome will be born. However, if the fertilizing sperm carries a Y chromosome, a 45,Y zygote will be formed, which is not viable and which will be aborted spontaneously.

Trisomy of sex chromosomes results also from abnormal segregation of chromosomes in meiosis. If the ovum retains both X chromosomes (24,X + X) and is fertilized with a Y sperm, the zygote will have 47,XXY karyotype. The same could result from the fertilization of a normal ovum with a 24,X + Y sperm.

Turner's Syndrome. Turner's syndrome is clinically recognizable by features that include short stature, webbing of the neck, abnormal extremities, a broad chest, and often, congenital heart disease (Fig. 5-10). Patients with Turner's syndrome have normal female genital organs except for the ovaries, which do not develop normally. Ovaries in these patients are unable to nurture germ cells, which disappear early in infancy. They then transform into streak gonads. These women never experience puberty and do not develop secondary sex characteristics. Infertility is the norm. Sex hormone therapy may improve the individual's body image, but it will not cure the infertility.

Klinefelter's Syndrome. Patients with Klinefelter's syndrome are phenotypical males, but are infertile. The testes of 47,XXY men are atrophic and are unable to produce sperm (Fig. 5-11). Secondary sex characteristics in affected males do not develop at

FIGURE 5-9
Pathogenesis of sex chromosome abnormalities. Because of abnormal disjunction during meiotic division, the ovum of the sperm may contain more than one sex chromosome or no sex chromosomes at all. Such gametes, when fertilized with a normal gamete of the opposite sex, will give rise to zygotes that are trisomic or monosomic for sex chromosomes.

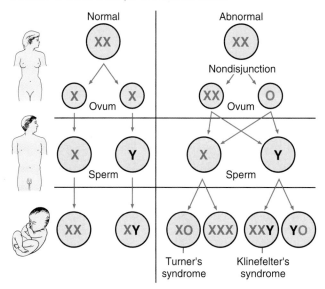

less fetal wastage. The most important of these are monosomy X (45,X or Turner's syndrome), which affects 1 in 3000 neonates, and trisomy of sex chromosomes (47,XXY or Klinefelter's syndrome), which occurs in 1 in 700 newborn infants.

Turner's and Klinefelter's syndromes can be related to abnormal segregation of X or Y chromosomes during meiosis in the female or male gonads (Fig. 5-9). If the sperm does not receive an X or Y, and such a defective sperm fertilizes the normal ovum, the zygote and the embryo that develops from it will lack one sex chromosome. Clearly, this could occur during female meiosis as well, and a zygote resulting from the fertilization of an X chromosome–deficient ovum will also contain only 45 chromosomes. If the sex chromosome in such a zygote is

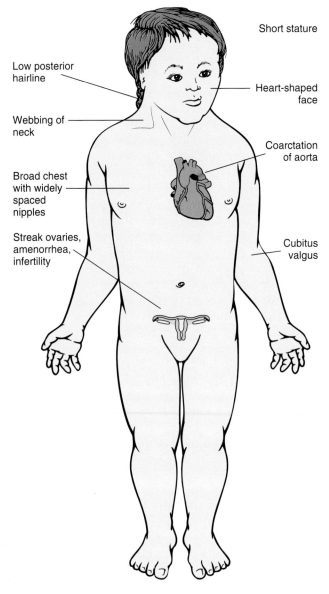

Short stature

Low posterior hairline

Heart-shaped face

Webbing of neck

Coarctation of aorta

Broad chest with widely spaced nipples

Streak ovaries, amenorrhea, infertility

Cubitus valgus

FIGURE 5-10
Typical features of Turner's syndrome.

puberty. The penis is small and the pubic hair is scant. Typically, these patients are tall and effeminate, with eunuchoid proportions and, often, gynecomastia (enlargement of the breasts).

Single Gene Disorders

Single genes are encoded by nucleotide triplets that occupy defined loci on the chromosomes. Genes located on the autosomes are all expressed in duplicate, and are known as *alleles,* each of which is found on the same site of the two homologous chromosomes. In relationship to each other, these genes can be either *dominant* or *recessive.* Dominant genes overshadow the recessive ones. Persons with one dominant and one recessive gene express the trait en-

coded by the dominant gene and are called *heterozygotes.* Recessive genes are expressed only if they are paired with another recessive allele, i.e., in a *homozygous* state. In contrast to autosomes, the sex chromosomes X and Y do not represent identical replicas of one another. In females who have two identical X chromosomes, the rules of gene expression are the same as those for autosomes. However, in males who have an X and a Y chromosome, many recessive genes of the X chromosomes will be expressed as if they were dominant, because the Y chromosome (which is much shorter than the X chromosome) lacks the complementary alleles needed to suppress their expression.

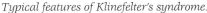

FIGURE 5-11
Typical features of Klinefelter's syndrome.

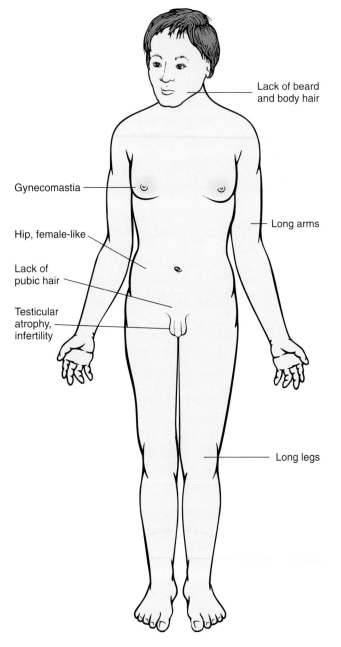

Lack of beard and body hair

Gynecomastia

Long arms

Hip, female-like

Lack of pubic hair

Testicular atrophy, infertility

Long legs

According to the laws of **Mendelian** genetics, human traits can thus be inherited as follows:

- autosomal dominant
- autosomal recessive
- sex-linked recessive
- sex-linked dominant

Only the first three types of inheritance are discussed here, as the sex-linked dominant traits are of limited practical significance.

Autosomal Dominant Disorders

Autosomal dominant traits are encoded by a gene that is located on one of the 22 autosomes and is dominant in relationship to its allele. Thus, it is fully expressed in heterozygotes—that is, even if only one copy of this gene is present. For example, Negroid skin color is dominant over Caucasian skin color; therefore, all children born to racially mixed couples will have dark skin. The basic features of autosomal dominant inheritance are as follows (Fig. 5-12):

- The trait is apparent in heterozygotes.
- The affected heterozygote has a 50 percent chance of transmitting the gene to each offspring.
- The trait is expressed in every generation.
- The unaffected offspring of the symptomatic carrier do not transmit the trait.

These are general rules, and in reality, some additional facts must be taken into consideration. For example, if a dominant trait becomes apparent in a child, one would expect that one of the parents has the trait. Sometimes, a defective gene is, indeed, present in one of the parents, but the expression of the parental gene might have been hindered. This is explained in terms of *low expressivity* of that gene. If neither of the parents has the gene for the abnormal trait, one must assume that the child is affected by a *new mutation*. Finally, some children of affected parents inherit the abnormal gene, but do not express

Table 5-1 Representative Autosomal Dominant Diseases

Affected Organ/Tissue	Disease
Connective tissue	Marfan syndrome
Bones	Achondroplastic dwarfism
	Osteogenesis imperfecta
Cardiovascular system	Familial hypercholesterolemia
Kidney	Adult polycystic kidney disease
	Wilms' tumor
Hematopoietic system	Spherocytosis
Gastrointestinal system	Familial polyposis coli
Nervous system	Huntington's disease
	Neurofibromatosis

the trait. It is assumed that such a gene has low *penetrance*.

For example, neurofibromatosis, a disease characterized by numerous peripheral nerve tumors (*neurofibromas*) and pigmented skin lesions (*café au lait spots*), is inherited as an autosomal dominant trait. However, in more than 50 percent of cases, the parents of the affected person do not have the abnormal gene, and the disease represents a new mutation. The children of some patients have fullblown syndromes associated with numerous tumors, whereas others develop only a few lesions, presumably because of low penetrance of the gene.

There are more than 1000 autosomal disorders; a few of the most important are listed in Table 5-1. From this table, it is clear that any of the major organ systems may be affected, either directly or indirectly. Predisposition to several tumors is inherited as an autosomal dominant trait. The disease is often multisystemic. For example, the defective gene for collagen type I causes *osteogenesis imperfecta,* a disease marked by numerous bone fractures. However, many other organs in the body are also affected because collagen type I is present in almost all tissues. For example, affected children have blue sclerae because of the abnormal refraction of light through the eye, which is composed of abnormal connective tissue.

Marfan Syndrome

Marfan syndrome is an autosomal dominant disease that affects 1 in 10,000 persons. It has been hypothesized that President Lincoln had this disease, as he had a "Marfanoid habitus." This disease is included here to illustrate how a structural protein defect can affect multiple organs.

FIGURE 5-12
Pattern of autosomal dominant inheritance.

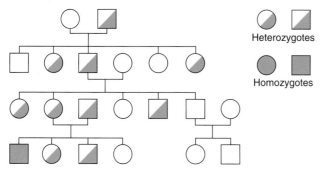

Heterozygotes

Homozygotes

Marfan syndrome is a multisystemic disease (Fig. 5-13). The most important features are as follows:

- *Skeletal changes.* The skeleton is slender and the affected person is tall. The head is elongated (*dolichocephalic*) with prominent frontal bossellation. The joints are loose and the ligaments are weak, resulting in frequent luxations and spinal deformities (*kyphoscoliosis*).
- *Cardiovascular changes.* The connective tissue of the large vessels is weak, resulting in dilatation of the aorta (*aortic aneurysm*), fraying of tissue, and weakening of the vessel wall. The blood sep-

arates the layers of the weakened aorta, ultimately producing *dissecting aneurysms,* which are prone to rupture. The cardiac valves are also loosely structured (so-called *floppy valves*) and tend to malfunction, leading to heart failure.
- *Ocular changes.* The loosening of the ocular connective tissue causes deformities of the eye. The lens may be displaced (*subluxation of lens*), and *cataracts, retinal detachment,* and *blindness* are common.

The pathogenesis of Marfan syndrome is related to the dysfunction of the gene that codes for *fibrillin.* This connective tissue protein is essential for the maintenance of tissue structure of various organs, but most notably, tendons and other connective tissue–rich structures, such as heart valves or blood vessels. Tendons and vessel walls that are devoid of normal fibrillin become loose and cannot support normal body functions. Death is most often caused by heart failure secondary to valvular dysfunction or rupture of aortic aneurysms. Exsanguination from ruptured aortic aneurysms is a well-known complication of Marfan syndrome.

Familial Hypercholesterolemia

Familial hypercholesterolemia is probably the most important autosomal dominant disease. It affects 1 in 500 Americans, and is a common cause of cardiovascular disease in this country.

Familial hypercholesterolemia is caused by a mutation in the gene encoding the receptor for low-density lipoprotein (LDL). LDLs transport approximately 70 percent of the total blood cholesterol and are the principal carriers for the removal of cholesterol from the blood (Fig. 5-14). This occurs through a high-affinity liver receptor that mediates the entry of lipids into the liver cells. In patients with a receptor deficiency, LDL cholesterol is removed from the blood only by a less efficient, receptor-independent mechanism. Inefficient cholesterol removal results in hypercholesterolemia and the deposition of lipids in various tissues, the most important of which are the arteries. This deposition results in accelerated atherosclerosis and an increased incidence of coronary heart disease. Deposition of cholesterol in connective tissue of the skin leads to formation of lipid-rich, yellow nodules called *xanthomas* (*xanthos* meaning yellow in Greek). Xanthomas consist of macrophages that have phagocytized cholesterol.

Familial hypercholesterolemia cannot be cured. However, the progression of the disease can be retarded by dietary measures (low-fat diet). Drugs that block uptake of cholesterol in blood vessels have been introduced recently and show promising results in preventing atherosclerosis in these patients.

FIGURE 5-13
Typical features of Marfan syndrome.

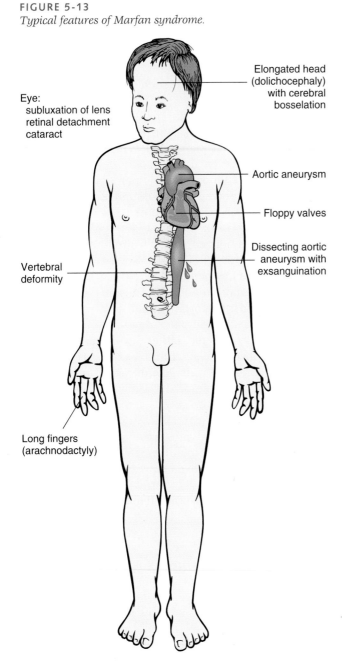

Eye:
subluxation of lens
retinal detachment
cataract

Elongated head
(dolichocephaly)
with cerebral
bosselation

Aortic aneurysm

Floppy valves

Dissecting aortic
aneurysm with
exsanguination

Vertebral
deformity

Long fingers
(arachnodactyly)

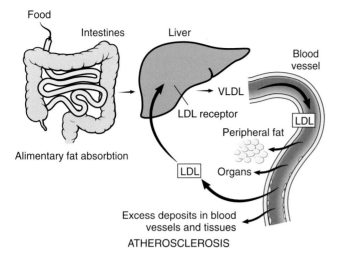

FIGURE 5-14
Familial hypercholesterolemia. The lack of a normal low-density lipoprotein (LDL) receptor results in hyperlipidemia and the deposition of cholesterol in the vessel wall, which leads to accelerated atherosclerosis. VLDL, very low-density lipoprotein.

Autosomal Recessive Disorders

Autosomal recessive traits are encoded by genes located on one of the 22 autosomes. These genes are expressed only under homozygous conditions—that is, only if paired with an identical allele. The basic features of autosomal recessive inheritance are as follows (Fig. 5-15):

- The gene effect is apparent only in homozygotes.
- The parents of the affected homozygote are both asymptomatic carriers of the trait.
- The children of the affected homozygote are not symptomatic, but 50 percent of them carry the gene for the trait.
- Among the siblings of the affected homozygote, 25 percent are symptomatic homozygotes, 50 percent are asymptomatic carriers of the gene

for the trait, and 25 percent are unaffected and do not carry the gene for the trait.

Diseases inherited as autosomal recessive traits are more common than diseases inherited as autosomal dominant traits. Nevertheless, because the symptoms occur only in homozygotes, the overall incidence of such diseases is lower. Still, these autosomal recessive diseases are important causes of morbidity in certain populations. For example, sickle cell anemia affects 1 in 600 newborn blacks, and Tay-Sachs disease affects 1 in 3000 Jews in the United States. Representative autosomal recessive diseases are listed in Table 5-2.

Cystic Fibrosis

Overall, cystic fibrosis is the most common autosomal recessive disease, affecting 1 in 2500 neonates in the United States. It has been estimated that 1 in 25 persons is an asymptomatic carrier of the cystic fibrosis gene. The disease is almost entirely limited to whites, and is extremely rare in other races.

The gene responsible for cystic fibrosis codes for the protein forming the so-called chloride transport channel in the cell membrane. The defect in the transport of chloride across the cell membrane results in a lack of sodium chloride in the glandular secretions of all exocrine glands, most importantly the pancreas, intestine, and the bronchi (Fig. 5-16). Because sodium chloride has an osmotic effect, those secretions contain less water and are viscid. The viscid mucus accounts for the synonym *mucoviscidosis,* another name for cystic fibrosis. Viscid mucus leads to the obstruction of the lumen of these organs (Fig. 5-17). The obstruction of the fetal intestine by dehy-

FIGURE 5-15
Pattern of autosomal recessive inheritance.

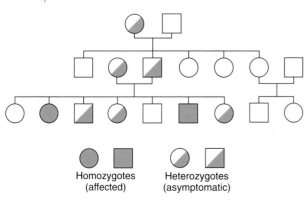

| Homozygotes (affected) | Heterozygotes (asymptomatic) |

Table 5-2 Representative Autosomal Recessive Diseases

Cystic Fibrosis
Anemias
Sickle cell anemia
Thalassemia
Lipidoses
Tay-Sachs disease
Niemann-Pick disease
Mucopolysaccharidoses
Hurler syndrome
Hunter's syndrome
Amino acid disorders
Phenylketonuria
Albinism

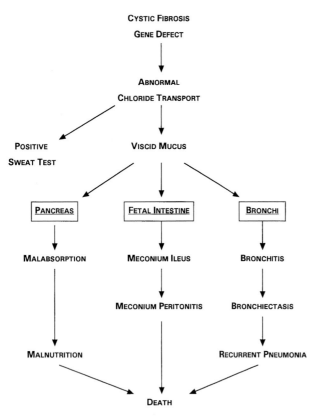

intestine. As the pancreatic enzymes are essential for the digestion of food, malabsorption ensues. The stools contain undigested food and are bulky, greasy, and foul-smelling. Affected children have malnutrition and typically show growth retardation.

The most important complication of cystic fibrosis pertains to the hyperviscosity of bronchial mucus. Bronchial mucus transforms into viscous plugs that prevent normal respiration. At the same time, the mucus provides a fertile ground for bacterial growth, predisposing the individual to recurrent bacterial infections. As a consequence of bacterial infections, patients with cystic fibrosis often have chronic bronchitis and bouts of recurrent pneumonia.

Other exocrine glands are also affected by this disease. From a diagnostic point of view, abnormalities of the sweat glands are the most important. Because the sweat glands cannot reabsorb chloride once it has entered their lumina, the sweat contains increased amounts of salt. This can be measured biochemically by collecting sweat or by stimulating sweating with drugs (the so-called pilocarpine test).

Cystic fibrosis is an incurable disease, and most affected individuals die in their twenties as a result of pulmonary infections. Vigorous treatment of infections and correction of nutritional deficiencies may, however, prolong the life of these patients.

FIGURE 5-16
Pathogenesis of the cardinal symptoms of cystic fibrosis.

Lysosomal Storage Diseases

Autosomal recessive diseases are often related to a deficiency of enzymes involved in intermediary metabolism. The metabolites that cannot be fully degraded, digested, or incorporated into other molecules accumulate inside the affected cells and are

drated meconium (the content of fetal intestines) may cause intestinal rupture and dissipation of intestinal contents throughout the abdominal cavity (*meconium ileus*), as well as **meconium peritonitis.** The obstruction of pancreatic ducts with viscid mucus prevents the flow of pancreatic juices into the

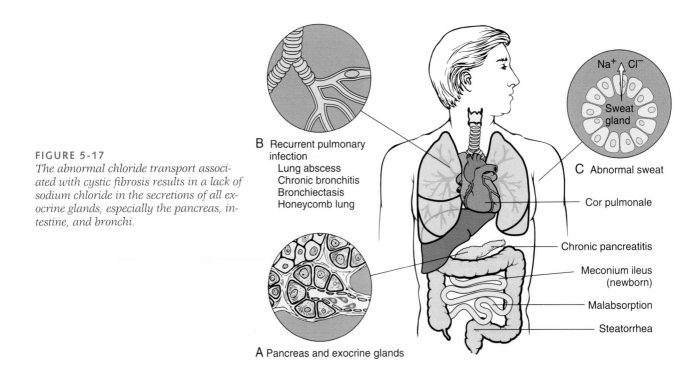

FIGURE 5-17
The abnormal chloride transport associated with cystic fibrosis results in a lack of sodium chloride in the secretions of all exocrine glands, especially the pancreas, intestine, and bronchi.

B Recurrent pulmonary infection
　Lung abscess
　Chronic bronchitis
　Bronchiectasis
　Honeycomb lung

C Abnormal sweat

Cor pulmonale

Chronic pancreatitis

Meconium ileus (newborn)

Malabsorption

Steatorrhea

A Pancreas and exocrine glands

most often stored in lysosomes. These lysosomal storage diseases are classified, depending on the primary metabolic pathway affected, as *lipidoses, glycogenoses, mucopolysaccharidoses,* and so on. Furthermore, they are also known by eponyms relating to the names of the physicians who discovered them, such as Tay-Sachs disease, Niemann-Pick disease, Gaucher's disease, etc. These eponyms are still in clinical use, although many have been renamed according to the basic biochemical defect or the missing enzyme. For example, Tay-Sachs disease is a defect in the function of hexosaminidase A, which leads to the accumulation of GM_2 ganglioside. Thus, it is referred to as hexosaminidase A deficiency or gangliosidosis GM_2.

All lysosomal storage diseases are characterized by the accumulation of metabolites that cannot be processed owing to an inborn enzyme deficiency (Fig. 5-18). These metabolites stored in the lysosomes can be recognized by electron microscopy as amorphous granules or concentric whorls of membranes (myelin figures). By light microscopy, such cells appear to be swollen and granular or vacuolated, especially if the material that fills the lysosomes is lipid (Fig. 5-19). The final diagnosis is usually made on the basis of biochemical tests that demonstrate the specific enzymatic defect.

The symptoms of lysosomal storage diseases are extremely variable. Some of these diseases are lethal in early childhood. Tay-Sachs disease affects the brain and eyes and causes death, usually during the first 3 to 5 years of life. On the other hand, some forms of Gaucher's disease only cause enlargement of the spleen and mild anemia, but do not affect life expectancy. Mucopolysaccharidoses, such as Hunter's or Hurler's syndrome, typically involve the skeletal and the central nervous system and cause gross body deformities ("gargoylism," so called because the body resembles the gargoyle sculptures on Gothic cathedrals), neurologic symptoms, and mental retardation.

At the present time, there is no cure for lysosomal storage diseases. However, most of these diseases can be diagnosed in utero and the affected fetus can be aborted.

Phenylketonuria

Phenylketonuria (PKU), an inborn error of protein metabolism, is included here to show that not only enzyme deficiencies result in lysosomal storage diseases. It is also included to show that the consequences of this enzyme defect can be counterbalanced and its deleterious effects prevented.

Phenylketonuria is a congenital deficiency of phenylalanine hydroxylase (PAH), an enzyme that metabolizes phenylalanine into tyrosine (Fig. 5-20). Phenylalanine is a dietary amino acid, the lack of which leads to accumulation of ingested phenylalanine in blood and tissues. There is also a shifting of its catabolism into another pathway, resulting in the formation of phenylpyruvic acid and related phenylketones, which are excreted in urine. Phenylketones were originally detected in urine, hence the name PKU.

Infants born with PKU are initially normal. Typical features of the disease include a lack of pigmentation secondary to inadequate melanin synthesis, which is inhibited by an excess of phenylalanine in blood. Therefore, the children are fair-haired and fair-skinned and have blue eyes. They also have a mousy odor attributable to the accumulation of intermediary metabolites of phenylalanine.

The diagnosis of PKU is made at the time of birth, usually by routine screening, which is mandatory in the United States. A special phenylalanine-deficient diet is prescribed for affected infants. This ensures normal psychoneural development. However, if the infant receives a normal diet that contains phenylalanine, the resulting hyperphenylalaninemia will adversely affect the developing central nervous system, causing slow, but progressive and irreversible, mental retardation.

FIGURE 5-18
Pathogenesis of lysosomal storage disease. (A) Normal lysosomes digest the material included within the lytic bodies. (B) Lack of degradation enzymes leads to the accumulation of metabolic residues inside the lysosomes.

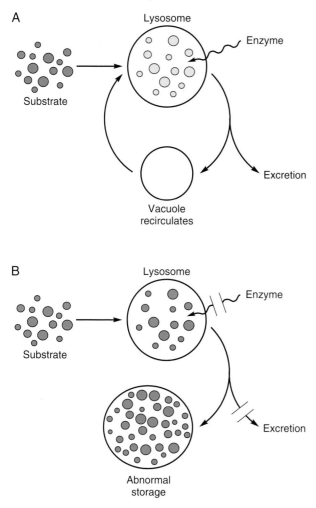

A

Lysosome

Enzyme

Substrate

Excretion

Vacuole
recirculates

B

Lysosome

Enzyme

Substrate

Excretion

Abnormal
storage

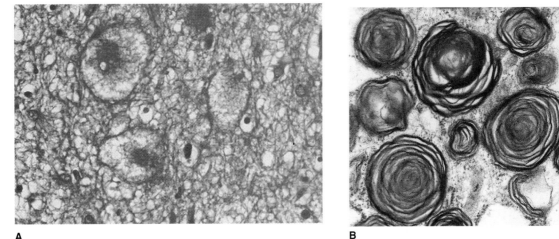

A   **B**

FIGURE 5-19

Tay-Sachs disease. (A) On light microscopy, the neural system cells appear to be swollen and vacuolated because their cytoplasm contains an increased number of lipid-rich lysosomes. (B) On electron microscopy, the cells are seen to contain myelin figures composed of concentric membranes.

X-Linked Recessive Disorders

X-linked recessive traits are encoded by recessive genes that are located on the X chromosome, but that are not found on the Y chromosome. Because they are recessive, these traits are rarely expressed in females, who are usually heterozygous and have a dominant allele for this trait on the other X chromosome. However, males who carry the gene on their X chromosome and are, technically speaking, heterozygous for it, express the gene in a "dominant" manner because the Y chromosome does not have the corresponding alleles to overshadow its expression. Because of their recessive nature, the X-linked genes are not expressed in females unless the person is homozygous, which is extremely rare.

The basic features of X-linked recessive inheritance are as follows (Fig. 5-21):

- The gene effect is usually evident only in males, and only rarely in females.

- The gene is transmitted from an asymptomatic mother.
- Sisters of an affected male are all asymptomatic. They could be carriers of the trait, but may not be. Unaffected brothers do not carry the gene and do not transmit the trait.
- Each son of a carrier female has a 50 percent chance of being affected. Affected males do not transmit the gene to their sons, but all of their daughters are asymptomatic carriers.
- The disease presents rarely in females, who are homozygous. These women have inherited one abnormal allele from the affected father and one from the asymptomatic carrier mother.

More than 100 genes have been identified on the X chromosome, and many of these are linked to important diseases (Fig. 5-22). The most common of these diseases are listed in Table 5-3.

FIGURE 5-20

Phenylketonuria. Lack of phenylalanine hydroxylase blocks the transformation of phenylalanine into tyrosine. Unmetabolized phenylalanine is shunted into the pathway that leads to the formation of phenylketones. Excess phenylalanine also inhibits formation of melanin from tyrosine.

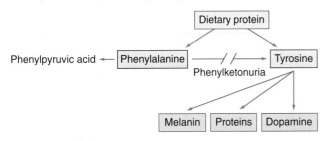

FIGURE 5-21

Pattern of X-linked recessive inheritance.

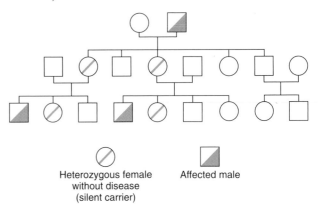

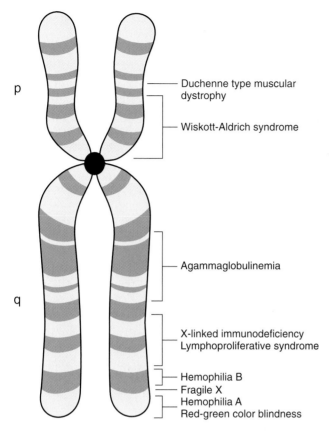

p — Duchenne type muscular dystrophy

— Wiskott-Aldrich syndrome

q

— Agammaglobulinemia

— X-linked immunodeficiency
Lymphoproliferative syndrome

— Hemophilia B
— Fragile X
— Hemophilia A
— Red-green color blindness

FIGURE 5-22
Representative genes encoding clinically important diseases mapped to the short (p) and long (q) arms of the X chromosome.

Hemophilia

Hemophilia, a hereditary bleeding disorder, is linked to mutations of the genes that code for the coagulation factor VIII or IX. Factor VIII deficiency is the underlying cause of the common disorder, hemophilia A, whereas factor IX deficiency accounts for hemophilia B. One in 5000 boys is affected by hemophilia A, whereas 1 in 30,000 is affected by hemophilia B. The gene for factor VIII is located on the terminal portion of the long arm of chromosome X. It is a very

Table 5-3 Representative X-Linked Recessive Diseases

Hemophilia A and B

Muscular dystrophy

   Duchenne type

   Becker type

Congenital immunodeficiencies

   Agammaglobulinemia

   Wiskott-Aldrich syndrome

   X-linked immunodeficiency

   Lymphoproliferative disorders

long gene that accounts for 0.1 percent of the total genome of the X chromosomes. Such a long gene is subject to point mutations, deletions, or insertions that alter its expression. This is reflected in the frequent occurrence of new mutations, evidenced by the fact that 50 percent of all patients have the inherited form of the disease, whereas the others have a new mutation. The gene for factor IX is much shorter and less prone to mutations. Hemophilia B thus is less common.

Hemophilia A can occur in a severe, moderately severe, or mild form. The severity of the disease depends on the extent of the gene defect; more severe defects cause severe bleeding problems, whereas minor defects may prove to be asymptomatic or may cause only minor bleeding episodes. Hemophilia B is, unfortunately, always a severe bleeding disorder. Hemorrhage in the hemophiliac may be spontaneous, or it may follow minor trauma. Internal hemorrhage, especially into the joints (*hemarthrosis*) is common. Deformity of the joints resulting from hemarthrosis remains a common complication. Cerebral hemorrhage, previously a frequent cause of death, is rare today, as the course of the disease can be ameliorated by administration of the deficient clotting factors and by blood transfusions. The genes for factors VIII and IX have been cloned, and the recombinant clotting factors produced in the laboratory are available for treatment of hemophilia.

Muscular Dystrophy

Muscular dystrophies are diseases of unknown etiology marked by progressive wasting of muscles. In this group of diseases, two specific forms—known as *Duchenne type* and *Becker's muscular dystrophy* (DBMD)—are linked to a single gene. This disorder, which affects males and is only rarely found in females on the X chromosome, is inherited as an X-linked recessive trait.

The gene for DBMD, which has been localized to the mid-portion of the short arm of X chromosome, codes for *dystrophin,* a structural cell protein forming a network beneath the plasma membrane that interacts with other cytoskeletal and contractile proteins. Without dystrophin, the cells cannot retain their proper form or adapt to stress and, therefore, tend to disintegrate. Although dystrophin is a widespread protein, the consequences related to its abnormality are most prominent in the skeletal muscles. The dystrophin gene is one of the largest human genes. The size of the gene defect may vary from one patient to another. This may result in either severe muscular disease, which is clinically known as Duchenne type dystrophy, or a less severe disease, known as Becker's dystrophy.

Duchenne type dystrophy affects 1 in 3300 males, most of whom are born to asymptomatic parents. In two thirds of cases, the mother is the carrier of the gene. It has been estimated that the spontaneous mutation rate of the DBMD gene is approximately 1 in 10,000. One third of all affected persons have a nonfamilial disease related to new mutations. Becker's dystrophy is less common, affecting 1 in 20,000 males.

Duchenne type muscular dystrophy is characterized by severe muscle wasting that begins in utero. The symptoms become evident early in infancy. By the time they reach school age, affected children are confined to a wheelchair and show marked deformities of the body owing to muscle weakness. Most affected boys die in their late teens. Becker's dystrophy is less incapacitating. Its symptoms begin in late childhood and the signs of muscle weakness are not clinically significant until midlife. Nevertheless, most patients die in the fourth and fifth decade.

Fragile X Syndrome

Fragile X syndrome is a form of mental retardation linked to increased fragility of the subterminal portion of the long arm of the X chromosome. In affected persons, this chromosomal region, known as Xq27, consists of an amplified number of repeats of three nucleotides: cytosine, guanine, guanine (termed the *CGG triplet repeat*). The chromosomal site occupied by an amplified number of triplet repeats appears to be more fragile than normal, and can be detected by special cytogenetic techniques. It has been shown that 80 percent of males with this chromosomal abnormality have mental deficiency. Mental retardation can also occur in females with fragile X chromosome, but less often than in males.

Children born to mentally normal carriers of the fragile X can be mentally retarded. This underscores the peculiar features of inheritance of trinucleotide repeats. These genetic anomalies seem not to follow all the rules of Mendelian genetics, and the symptoms related to the abnormal gene tend to become more prominent in each subsequent generation. One could predict that the incidence of mental retardation related to fragile X chromosome might increase in the future from the current rate of 1:1250 males and 1:2500 females. Even now, it is already the most common form of hereditary mental deficiency in males.

Multifactorial Inheritance

Familial diseases that are not inherited according to the rules of Mendelian genetics are considered to be the result of **multifactorial inheritance** patterns. Such diseases are the product of several genes that interact with each other and are also influenced by exogenous (*epigenetic*) factors. Most of the human traits and diseases are the end-products of a complex interaction of genes and environment. The risk for developing multifactorial disorders can be estimated only approximately, and it is usually in the range of 5 percent to 10 percent. This risk varies from one trait to another and also can be altered by lifestyle, environmental influences, or other diseases. Representative multifactorial traits and disease are listed in Table 5-4.

Multifactorial inheritance has the following features:

- The trait or the disease is the product of several genes. The inheritance cannot be explained in terms of Mendelian single gene inheritance.
- Exogenous and endogenous factors influence the expression of the trait and determine the severity of the disease.
- The genes encoding the trait or the disease show a dose effect, which determines the severity of the disease. Persons affected by a more severe form of the disease have an increased chance of transmitting it to their offspring.
- The risk of disease in siblings can be estimated on the basis of family data, the severity of the disease, and the sex of the affected individuals.

Anencephaly

Anencephaly is a good example of a multifactorial developmental defect (Fig. 5-23). This disorder occurs because of incomplete fusion of the midline structures covering the brain: the meninges, bones of the calvarium, and the overlying skin of the convexity of the head. This type of midline fusion anomaly is termed *dysraphic* (in Greek, *raphe* is the midline seam). The development of the brain and spinal cord, which depends on the protective covering, is severely disturbed. If the calvarium does not form, the child is born severely malformed, without a brain or with only a rudimentary basal part of the brain. It

Table 5-4 Multifactorial Traits and Diseases

Traits/Process	Diseases
Height	Dwarfism
Intelligence	Mental retardation
Blood pressure	Hypertension
Metabolism	
Carbohydrates	Diabetes mellitus
Uric acid	Gout
Development	Anencephaly
	Cleft lip or palate

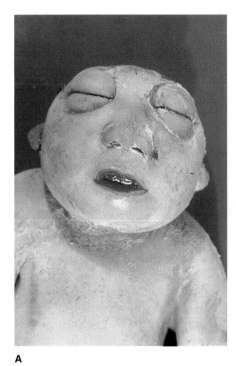 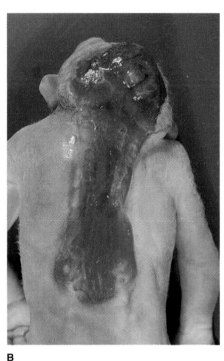

A **B**

FIGURE 5-23
Anencephaly and cranioarchischisis. (A) Frontal view. The entire cranium is missing and the foreshortened face appears frog-like. (B) Posterior view. The brain is missing and the spinal canal is open.

is clear that numerous genes regulate the development of the brain, and that the dysfunction or inappropriate activation of even a single gene can lead to an abnormal developmental cascade. The outcome of altered activity of several genes may result in major defects, such as anencephaly, or a minor defect of the vertebral bones (*spina bifida*). A whole spectrum of pathologic changes has been recorded. For example, if incomplete fusion of the vertebral bodies and the meninges (*meningocele*) is accompanied by a protrusion of the brain, the lesion is called a *meningomyelocele.*

The predilection for developmental gene malfunction is heritable. If one child has anencephaly or related malformations, there is a 5 percent chance that a subsequent sibling will be born with the same defect. If two children are born with these defects, the third child has a 20 percent chance of being born with the defect.

The interplay of genetic and environmental factors in anencephaly is best illustrated by epidemiologic data. The highest occurrence of anencephaly is in Ireland, probably because of the high prevalence of abnormal genes in that population. The risk of anencephaly among Irish living in the United States is five times higher than among blacks. Nevertheless, the risk among the Irish in the United States is only one half of the risk of those living in Ireland. This illustrates further the complex interaction of genetic predisposition and environmental factors. Recent data indicate that folic acid administration during pregnancy may prevent anencephaly in high-risk populations.

Diabetes Mellitus

Diabetes mellitus, a disturbance of intermediate metabolism resulting in hyperglycemia, occurs more often in some families than in others. The adult-onset disease, called noninsulin-dependent diabetes mellitus (NIDDM), is a good example of multifactorial disease with genetic and epigenetic determinants.

The evidence for the genetic basis of this disease includes the following:

- Familial incidence. Almost 50 percent of affected patients have a relative who also has NIDDM.
- High incidence of the disease in some populations with a high rate of intermarriage. A high incidence has been noted, for example, in the Pima Indians in Arizona.
- High concordance of disease among monozygotic (identical) twins. If one twin has NIDDM, the other twin has a near-100 percent chance of developing the disease.

Nevertheless, transmission of the disease from an affected parent occurs only in about 15 percent of offspring. The siblings of affected persons have only a 10 percent to 15 percent chance of becoming diabetic. The development of symptoms also depends on environmental factors. The most important adverse epigenetic factors include diet, obesity, and a sedentary lifestyle (i.e., lack of exercise). However, NIDDM can develop in nonobese persons, and not all obese persons in affected families have the symptoms of diabetes. The interaction in this disease between genetic predisposition and environment is apparently too complex to be explained on the basis of current medical knowledge.

Prenatal Diagnosis

Most genetic and developmental disorders represent complex therapeutic problems, and many are incurable. Such diseases cause considerable human suffering and expenditure of health resources, which can be alleviated in part with adequate prevention and early diagnosis. Gene therapy will likely become available in the not-so-distant future, but for the time being, it is applicable only to a few diseases, and is still considered to be an experimental procedure.

Prevention of genetic and developmental diseases is a complex issue. Common preventive measures, such as rubella immunization, have prevented some forms of prenatally acquired diseases, but many others remain. The best example of the latter is acquired immunodeficiency syndrome (AIDS), which is readily transmitted from infected mothers to their fetus across the placenta in utero. Alcohol is also one of the known causes of human malformations, and thus should be avoided in pregnancy. A healthy lifestyle, safe sex practices, and avoidance of substance abuse should be encouraged. Persons with known hereditary disorders should be counseled, and the risk of congenital malformations in their offspring should be weighed against their wish for parenting children.

Prenatal diagnosis is one of the most important elements of genetic counseling. Many genetic diseases and chromosomal abnormalities can be diagnosed while the fetus is in the early stages of development. Such abnormal fetuses can be aborted early in pregnancy, sparing the parents the suffering and the cost of caring for an incurable child.

Prenatal diagnosis (Fig. 5-24) is based on the following:

- *Ultrasonographic examination* of the fetus and placenta. Ultrasonograms can detect malformations of the head, extremities, and internal organs, as well as abnormal development and positioning of the placenta.
- *Chorionic villus biopsy.* Placental biopsy during early pregnancy is a safe procedure that can provide fetal cells for chromosomal analysis or for biochemical testing for enzyme deficiencies typical of single gene defects. Genetic analysis, using techniques of molecular biology, can also be performed to demonstrate mutant genes.
- *Amniotic fluid analysis.* Fluid aspirated from the amniotic sac during the 12th to 18th week of pregnancy is suitable for biochemical analysis. It also contains fetal cells that can be submitted for chemical, molecular genetic, or chromosomal analysis.
- *Maternal blood analysis.* Certain substances produced by the fetus enter the maternal circulation and can be measured biochemically. For example,

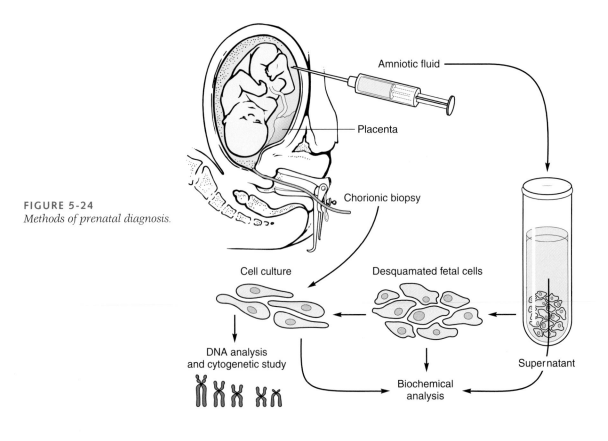

FIGURE 5-24
Methods of prenatal diagnosis.

AFP produced by the fetus is readily detectable in the mother's serum. High levels of AFP are common in pregnancies involving a fetus with anencephaly or congenital kidney malformations.

Prenatal diagnosis is based on rather complex procedures. Because of the high cost, such procedures cannot be performed during every pregnancy, and are presently limited to those considered to have a high-risk pregnancy. Because older women have an increased likelihood of bearing a child with Down syndrome, prenatal chromosomal examination is routinely recommended in women older than 35 years of age. Prenatal diagnosis is also recommended for families known to be affected by Mendelian traits.

Prematurity

The normal pregnancy lasts 40 weeks, by which time the fetus attains viability and an average weight of 3500 g. Children born before the 37th week of pregnancy and those that weigh less than 2500 g are considered to be *premature.* Those weighing less than 1500 g are labeled as *immature.* Such neonates are not only anatomically immature, but also functionally immature, and cannot survive without medical assistance and treatment in special neonatal intensive care units.

Approximately 5 percent to 10 percent of all pregnancies terminate prematurely. There are many causes of **prematurity.** These causes can be categorized into three groups as follows:

- Maternal factors
- Fetal factors
- Placental factors

Unfortunately, in most cases, the cause of premature birth remains unknown. Among the maternal factors, the best known are malnutrition, smoking, and substance abuse. Various infections affecting the mother, or both the mother and the fetus, are also well-known causes of prematurity. Fetal malformations and genetic diseases also predispose the individual to premature birth. Placental insufficiency is often postulated, but it remains poorly documented.

Premature infants show signs of anatomic and functional immaturity of their vital organs, most notably, the lungs and the brain. As a consequence of pulmonary immaturity, these children tend to develop the *neonatal respiratory distress syndrome,* also known as *pulmonary hyaline membrane disease.*

Neonatal Respiratory Distress Syndrome

The maturation of the fetal lungs occurs rapidly during the last 3 months of pregnancy. During this time, the lungs expand and the principal components of the respiratory units of alveoli are formed. In preparation for their respiratory function after birth, the alveolar pneumocytes type II begin secreting a surfactant rich in lecithin. Lecithin is the surface active substance that keeps the pulmonary alveoli open and prevents their collapse. During fetal life, the surfactant is released into the amniotic fluid that fills the fetal lungs. As there is no need for prenatal respiration because of the oxygen being delivered via the placenta from the mother, the surfactant produced by the fetal lungs is not required for pulmonary function in utero. However, if the fetus is born prematurely, the functionally immature lungs cannot sustain normal respiration. The alveoli in such premature infants tend to collapse (Fig. 5-25). The oxygen from the inspired air cannot diffuse into the pulmonary circulation because the respiratory surface has been reduced by the collapse of alveoli (atelectasis). Oxygen can reach the blood only through the wall of the alveolar ducts and terminal bronchioles. Because these anatomic structures are not suitable for oxygen transport, their surface epithelium is easily damaged. The necrotic cells are sloughed off and the epithelial defects of the alveolar ducts and terminal bronchioles are covered with proteinaceous material derived from the plasma. The plasma proteins coagulate and form sheets of fibrin known as hyaline membranes (Fig. 5-26). These impede gas exchange further, and unless the alveolar spaces open up, the infant will die of severe anoxia within the first 48 hours after birth. Those infants that do survive may have respiratory problems for the rest of their lives.

Anoxia caused by the neonatal respiratory distress syndrome affects the entire organism, but most prominently the immature brain, which is prone to *periventricular hemorrhage* (Fig. 5-27). This hemor-

FIGURE 5-25
Pathogenesis of neonatal respiratory distress syndrome.

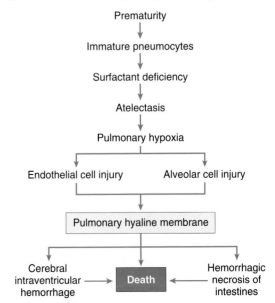

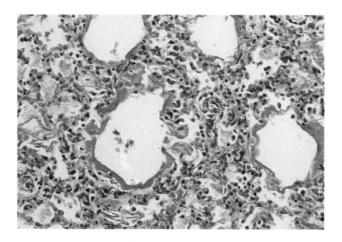

FIGURE 5-26
The appearance of the hyaline membranes in the neonatal respiratory distress syndrome. Pink, fibrin-rich membranes line the respiratory bronchioli and alveolar ducts, whereas the alveoli are atelectatic.

rhage occurs in the so-called periventricular matrix. This part of the brain is occupied by the developing neural cells destined to migrate to the surface of the brain in the last few weeks of intrauterine life. Because these cells are metabolically active, they require a copious supply of blood and oxygen. The blood is supplied by temporary, make-shift vessels that have thin walls. Anoxia at this critical stage of development leads to necrosis of the cerebral germinal matrix and the walled blood vessels. The intracerebral hemorrhage may spill into the ventricles and cause *hematocephalus* (in Greek, meaning "head filled with blood," but a term used only for blood in the cerebral ventricles).

FIGURE 5-27
Intraventricular hemorrhage in a premature neonate affected by respiratory distress syndrome.

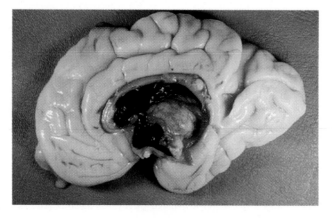

Birth Injury

The term birth trauma is used for various lesions caused by mechanical trauma during delivery. Such lesions occur rarely today and are registered in 1 of 5000 deliveries. Trauma occurs most often during the delivery of very large fetuses or abnormally positioned fetuses, or in cases in which there is a disproportion between the fetus and the birth canal. Most common are lesions of the head and extremities. Rupture of internal organs, such as the liver, spleen, or intestines, has been reported in severe injury.

The minor hemorrhages or edema of the head that normally occur in most children during birth should not be considered to be birth injuries.

Skull fractures may be induced by forcing the infant's head through a narrow pelvis or by applying external pressure with forceps. Minor linear fractures heal without treatment. However, fragmentation of the cranial bones and depressed fractures, which compress the brain and can cause neurologic symptoms, require surgical correction.

Intracranial hemorrhage is caused by the same mechanisms as skull fractures; indeed, skull fracture may be complicated by intracranial hemorrhage. The hemorrhage is typically located between the dura and arachnoid (*subdural hemorrhage*) and is the result of tearing of the major cerebral veins traversing this space. Minor hemorrhages resolve without serious consequences. Massive hemorrhage is usually lethal. Neurologic symptoms are common in children who have survived large intracranial hemorrhages.

Peripheral nerve injury results from severance or avulsion of nerves of the extremities (e.g., *brachial plexus palsy*) or the cranial nerves (e.g., *facial nerve palsy*).

Long bone fractures may occur if the fetus is extracted from the uterus by force, or if the fetal position is unusual and incompatible with spontaneous delivery. The clavicle and humerus are most often affected.

Sudden Infant Death Syndrome

Sudden unexpected death in infants older than 2 months and younger than 9 months of age is called **sudden infant death syndrome** (SIDS) or "crib death." The death of these otherwise healthy infants usually occurs during sleep. No obvious cause of death can be determined by autopsy. SIDS, which is the most common cause of death in infants beyond the immediate neonatal period, has an incidence of 1:500. The cause of SIDS is not known, but it appears to be associated with a set of maternal and fetal risk factors. SIDS is most common in children born to young mothers, women of low socioeconomic status and education, and those who are smokers and substance abusers. SIDS occurs more often in families that have already experienced such an accident. Premature infants and those that have had a previous gastrointestinal disease are at an increased risk. The pathogenesis of SIDS remains unknown. It has been postulated that these children are prone to apnea and stop breathing without any obvious reason. At autopsy, there are signs of anoxia, but otherwise, the morphologic findings are unremarkable.

Review Questions

1. How do germ cells ensure the continuity of life from one generation to another?
2. What is the difference between developmentally pluripotent cells in cleavage stage embryos and those forming the primordial germ layers?
3. How do fetal cells differ from those in the adult organism?
4. What are the main causes of congenital defects in humans?
5. Which physical, chemical, and microbial teratogens have been proven to cause malformations in humans?
6. What is TORCH syndrome?
7. List common structural chromosomal abnormalities and relate them to the congenital defects they cause.
8. List common numerical chromosomal abnormalities and relate them to the clinical syndromes they cause.
9. What are the most common clinical and pathologic findings in Down syndrome?
10. Compare Turner's syndrome with Klinefelter's syndrome.
11. What is the difference between autosomal dominant and autosomal recessive alleles?
12. List the basic features of autosomal dominant inheritance.
13. List the most common autosomal dominant diseases.
14. Describe the pathogenesis and the pathology of Marfan syndrome and familial hypercholesterolemia.
15. List the basic features of autosomal recessive inheritance.
16. List the most common autosomal recessive diseases.
17. Describe the pathogenesis and pathology of cystic fibrosis.
18. Explain the concept of lysosomal storage diseases and give specific examples.
19. Explain the pathogenesis and pathology of phenylketonuria.
20. List the basic features of X-linked recessive inheritance.
21. Describe the pathogenesis and pathology of hemophilia.
22. Describe the pathogenesis and pathology of muscular dystrophy.
23. How is fragile X syndrome related to triple nucleotide repeats?
24. List the main features of multifactorial inheritance and the most common diseases in this category.
25. Explain the pathogenesis of anencephaly and related dysraphic disorders and describe the main pathologic findings in these conditions.
26. What is the evidence that adult-onset diabetes mellitus has a genetic basis?
27. Describe the principles of prenatal diagnosis.
28. Define prematurity and list the most important causes of premature termination of pregnancy.
29. Explain the pathogenesis of neonatal distress syndrome and describe the main pathologic findings in this condition.
30. List the most important pathologic changes related to birth injury.
31. Define sudden infant death syndrome and discuss its possible causes.

Learning Objectives

After reading this chapter, the student should be able to:

1. Describe the distribution of fluid between the intracellular and extracellular compartments, and the basic aspects of normal circulation.

2. Define edema and give five clinical examples.

3. Explain the pathogenesis of edema caused by increased intravascular hydrostatic pressure, a reduction in colloid osmotic pressure of the plasma, and increased retrograde pressure in the veins and lymphatics.

4. Explain active hyperemia and congestion and give clinically important examples of each process.

5. Define hemorrhage and give clinically important examples of this pathologic process.

6. Explain normal hemostasis, and the role of endothelial cells, platelets, and the coagulation proteins in this process.

7. Describe the role of endothelial injury in thrombogenesis.

8. Define and explain hypercoagulability.

9. Describe the morphology of thrombi and explain mural thrombi, occlusive thrombi, and thrombophlebitis.

10. Describe the fate of thrombi with special emphasis on their organization, recanalization, and embolization.

11. Describe the clinical consequences of venous and arterial thrombi.

12. List five conditions that predispose an individual to arterial thrombi.

13. Define emboli and give five clinically important examples.

14. Define infarction and explain its pathogenesis.

15. Define shock and explain its pathogenesis.

Additional Key Terms and Concepts

Adult respiratory distress syndrome

Disseminated intravascular coagulation

Hematoma

Hemostasis

Transudate

Chapter Outline

Fluid and Hemodynamic Disorders

Chapter 6

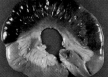

ater accounts for approximately 60 percent of the total body weight. Two thirds of the body fluid water is intracellular, whereas the remaining third occupies the interstitial space in the tissues or circulates in the blood (Fig. 6-1). Plasma—the fluid portion of blood that can be separated from blood cells by centrifugation—accounts for approximately 5 percent of the total body weight in normal adults; for a 70-kg man, this amounts to 3.5 L. Plasma volume can be expanded or reduced, but only within narrow physiological limits and only in counterbalance with other **body fluid compartments.** When these boundaries of normal physiological variation are exceeded, pathologic *overhydration* or *dehydration* ensues. Other derangements include

- redistribution of body fluids
- loss of fluids secondary to bleeding, sweating, or diarrhea
- retention of fluids because of inadequate renal excretion
- disruption of the circulation of fluids in tissues and vessels

Edema

Edema is an excess of fluid in the interstitial spaces and/or the body cavities. It can be localized or generalized. Localized edema may involve any tissue or organ and is then designated descriptively as, for example, *cerebral edema, pulmonary edema,* or *periorbital edema.* Accumulation of edematous fluid in the abdominal cavity is called *ascites* or *hydroperitoneum;* in the pleural cavity, it is termed *hydrothorax* and in the pericardial cavity, *hydropericardium.* Generalized edema is called *anasarca.*

The fluid accumulating in edematous tissues can

be classified as an exudate or a transudate. *Exudate* is rich in protein and blood cells and is typical of inflammation. Indeed, edema is one of the first manifestations of inflammation, and it accounts for one of the cardinal signs of inflammation ("tumor" or tissue swelling). *Inflammatory edema* is primarily related to the increased permeability of the blood vessels, but is also attributable to complex hydrodynamic changes in the peripheral circulation that promote the passage of fluids from the blood vessels into the interstitial spaces.

Transudate contains less protein and fewer cells than exudate. This edema is, in essence, an ultrafiltrate of plasma fluid that may accumulate in tissues as a result of several factors, including

- increased hydrostatic pressure inside the blood vessels
- decreased oncotic pressure of the plasma
- obstruction of the interstitial fluid drainage
- increased tissue hydration because of sodium retention

The fluid in the circulating blood is separated from the interstitial fluid by the vessel wall, which serves as a semipermeable filtration barrier. The movement of fluids across the vessel wall of capillaries is determined by several factors that maintain the typical gradients holding the fluid in circulation or promoting its passage into the extravascular compartment.

Most of the exchange of fluids occurs in the capillaries. As shown in Figure 6-2, the arterial blood enters the capillaries under pressure that is counterbalanced by the oncotic pressure of the plasma. This oncotic pressure is primarily a function of osmotically active proteins, such as albumin. At the arterial end of capillaries, the hydrostatic pressure exceeds the oncotic pressure of plasma, whereas at the ve-

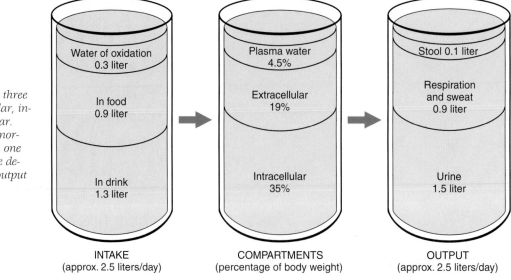

FIGURE 6-1
Body fluid is contained in three compartments: intracellular, interstitial, and intravascular. These compartments are normally in equilibrium with one another, and their volume depends on the intake and output of fluid solutes.

INTAKE
(approx. 2.5 liters/day)

COMPARTMENTS
(percentage of body weight)

OUTPUT
(approx. 2.5 liters/day)

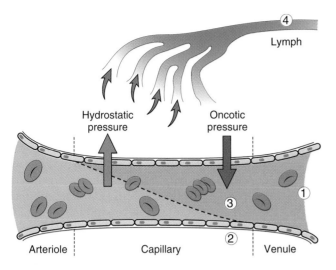

FIGURE 6-2
Pathogenesis of edema. The most important pathogenetic factors are increased venous pressure (1), increased permeability of the vessel wall (2), decreased oncotic pressure of plasma due to low albumin concentration (3), and obstruction of lymphatics (4).

nous end, the oncotic pressure is higher than the hydrostatic pressure, causing the flow of fluids to be redirected from the interstitium into the capillary lumen. The excess of interstitial fluid that is not returned into the capillaries is normally drained from the tissue through the lymphatics.

Edema occurs as a result of an imbalance between the forces that keep the fluid in the vessels and those that promote its exit into the interstitial spaces (Table 6-1). In *inflammatory edema,* the fluid leaks through the vessel wall, which has been made more permeable by the mediators of inflammation and increased blood flow (*hyperemia*). In *hydrostatic edema of hypertension,* the increased arterial blood pressure promotes the transmembranous passage of fluids. The intravascular pressure in the capillaries can be increased in a retrograde fashion by venous pressure. Venous stagnation is actually the most

common cause of hydrostatic edema and is typically found in individuals with congestive heart failure (so-called "backward heart failure").

Oncotic edema is caused by a reduction in colloid osmotic pressure (oncotic pressure) of the plasma. Because albumin is the most active osmotic plasma protein, oncotic edema is, in clinical practice, a consequence of hypoalbuminemia. Hypoalbuminemia may be caused by increased loss of protein in the urine (proteinuria), as seen in nephrotic syndrome, or decreased protein synthesis, as seen in chronic liver disease (cirrhosis).

Oncotic edema is usually generalized, but shows a predilection for loosely textured tissues. Therefore, it is prominent in the area of the face ("puffiness"), especially around the eyes (periorbital edema).

Obstruction of the lymphatics is a rare cause of edema. Because the lymphatics serve as a drainage route for the tissue fluid that has not been resorbed at the venous end of the capillaries, any obstruction of these thin-walled vessels will produce edema. The lymphatics are most often occluded by tumor cells or chronic inflammation. In parts of Africa infested with parasites, lymphatic edema may be caused by worms, such as filaria, which can produce massive swelling of the legs. This is referred to as elephantiasis because the legs resemble those of elephants!

Hypervolemic edema is typically caused by retention of sodium and water. The excretion of sodium and water is controlled by a complex system of regulators and depends on the normal structure and function of the kidneys, as well as on the action of renin, angiotensinogen, and aldosterone. Kidney disease promotes the release of renin, which stimulates the formation of angiotensin. Angiotensin acts on the adrenal cortex, which releases aldosterone. Aldosterone promotes renal sodium retention, which is accompanied by retention of water.

In clinical practice, edema is often multifactorial. For example, edema caused by chronic heart failure is usually a combination of hydrostatic and hyper-

Table 6-1 Forms of Edema

Form of Edema	Mechanism	Example(s)
Inflammatory	Vessel permeability	Acute inflammation
	Hyperemia	
Hydrostatic	Increased arterial pressure	Hypertension
	Increased venous backpressure	Heart failure
Oncotic	Hypoproteinemia	Nephrotic syndrome
	Increased protein loss	
	Decreased protein synthesis	Cirrhosis of the liver
Obstructive	Lymphatic obstruction	Lymphatic blockade (e.g., tumor)
Hypervolemic	Retention of sodium	Hyperaldosteronism

volemic edema (Fig. 6-3). Due to heart failure, the kidney is hypoperfused with blood, which stimulates the release of renin and renal retention of fluid. Increased venous backpressure resulting from pump failure of the heart further promotes edema. Edema of heart failure is most prominent in the lower extremities because it is gravity-dependent. It is also referred to as "pitting edema," because the compressed

subcutaneous tissue rebounds slowly and shows finger marks after compression.

Clinicopathologic Correlations. Edema is a very important clinical symptom that indicates dysfunction of major organs, such as the heart, kidneys, or liver. The distribution of edema depends on its cause. As mentioned earlier, edema of the lower extremities is typical of heart failure. Because edema secondary to heart failure is gravity-dependent, in patients confined to bed, it becomes redistributed and is most prominent on the back. Cardiac edema, caused by left ventricular failure and consequent pulmonary hypertension, is most prominent in the lungs. This pulmonary edema is characterized by an accumulation of proteinaceous fluid in the lungs. By contrast, edema associated with renal failure or with nephrotic syndrome is typically diffuse. Patients with liver cirrhosis accumulate fluid in the abdominal cavity (ascites); this is partially attributable to hypoalbuminemia and partially to hydrostatic pressure because of the increased portal venous pressure caused by the deformed and heavily scarred liver.

Edema is not only a symptom of a major disease, but it may often be, in itself, a cause of clinical problems. For example, pulmonary edema fills the alveolar spaces, thus preventing the normal entry of oxygen from the inhaled air into the blood. Shortness of breath (dyspnea) is, therefore, a typical consequence. Brain edema causes an expansion of the brain. Because the brain is enclosed in a rigid, bony structure—the skull—this causes intracranial hypertension. If the increased pressure is not relieved, the compression of vital centers of the brain will cause death.

FIGURE 6-3

Edema of heart failure. Left heart failure leads to pulmonary congestion, edema, and pleural effusion. Right heart failure leads to chronic congestion of the liver and spleen, formation of ascites, venous congestion of lower extremities, and edema. Hypoperfusion of the kidneys leads to increased secretion of renin, which acts on the adrenals, stimulating the release of aldosterone. These hormonal changes contribute to renal retention of sodium and water, which aggravates heart failure and contributes to generalized edema.

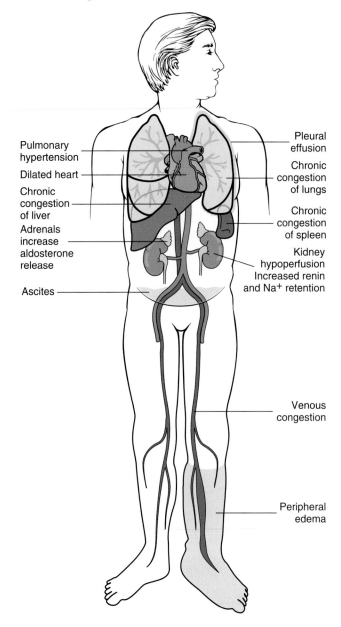

Pulmonary hypertension

Dilated heart

Chronic congestion of liver

Adrenals increase aldosterone release

Ascites

Pleural effusion

Chronic congestion of lungs

Chronic congestion of spleen

Kidney hypoperfusion Increased renin and Na+ retention

Venous congestion

Peripheral edema

Hyperemia

Hyperemia, a Greek term meaning "too much blood," denotes accumulation of blood in the peripheral circulation. Hyperemia can be either active or passive, acute or chronic.

Active hyperemia is a consequence of dilatation of arterioles—i.e., precapillary sphincters—and the resultant influx of blood into the capillaries. This typically occurs during blushing or exercise, and is mediated by neural signals that lead to the relaxation of the arteriolar smooth muscles. Hyperemia is also a feature of acute inflammation.

Passive hyperemia or congestion is caused by increased venous backpressure. Typically, it is a consequence of heart failure and most often occurs in a chronic form. The stagnation of venous deoxygenated blood contributes to a bluish discoloration of the tissue (*cyanosis*) and is often associated with hydrostatic edema. Chronic passive congestion in the

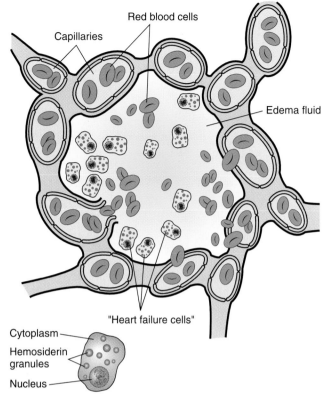

FIGURE 6-4
Chronic passive congestion of the lungs. Increased venous pressure leads to extravasation of red blood cells into the alveoli and alveolar edema. The hemosiderin formed from hemoglobin released from hemolyzed red blood cells is taken up by intra-alveolar macrophages ("heart failure cells").

lungs leads to the formation of edema and also to extravasation of blood into the alveoli (Fig. 6-4). Disintegrated red blood cells (RBCs) are taken up by alveolar macrophages. The hemoglobin of the RBCs is degraded into brown pigment (hemosiderin), which accumulates in the lysosomes of the macrophages. These macrophages, called *heart failure cells,* can be recognized in histologic sections of lung tissue as well as in cytologic smears of expectorated mucus. Chronic passive congestion is accompanied by anoxia and often results in pulmonary fibrosis.

Hemorrhage

Hemorrhage, or extravasation of blood, refers to passage of blood outside of the cardiovascular system (from the Greek *haima,* meaning blood, and *rhegnymi,* meaning bursting forth). Depending on the source, hemorrhage may be classified as cardiac, aortic, arterial, capillary, or venous. Clinically, it may be of sudden onset (acute) or it may be long-standing (chronic), or it may be recurrent and marked by repeated episodes of blood loss (Fig. 6-5).

Cardiac hemorrhage may result from a gunshot or stabbing wound and is often fatal. Additionally, a softening of the heart muscle caused by a myocardial infarct can result in ventricular rupture and lethal cardiac hemorrhage.

Aortic hemorrhage is often caused by trauma, such as that sustained in a car accident. Aortic wall weakening and dilatation (*aortic aneurysm*) also may occur, resulting in aortic rupture and massive hemorrhage and death.

Arterial hemorrhage is most often caused by penetrating wounds inflicted by bullets or a knife. Fractured bone may also tear arteries and cause hemorrhage. All of these mechanisms of hemorrhage involve arterial blood, which is oxygenated and, therefore, bright red. The blood squirts out of the arteries under pressure and its flow is usually pulsating. Unless stopped, these hemorrhages are usually lethal.

Capillary hemorrhage is marked by pinpoint droplets of blood appearing on the surface of the

FIGURE 6-5
Hemorrhage may be cardiac, aortic, arterial, capillary, or venous.

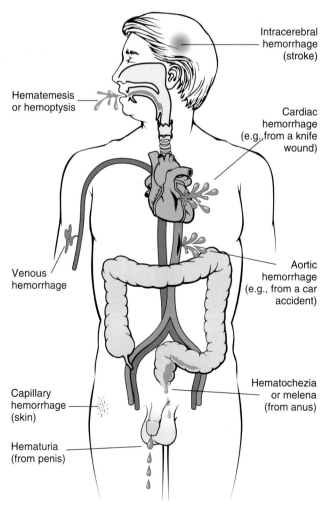

skin, mucosa, or in various tissues. This form of hemorrhage may be related to trauma, increased venous pressure, or weakening of the capillary walls, as may occur in vitamin C deficiency (*scurvy*).

Venous hemorrhage is usually traumatic. Venous blood is deoxygenated and so is dark red or bluish; it does not have the pulsatile flow characteristic of arterial blood.

Hemorrhages can be classified as external or internal. During external hemorrhage, the blood flows out of the body, which may result in exsanguination and death or a marked reduction in blood volume (*hypovolemia*). Blood released by internal hemorrhage may fill various body cavities (causing, for example, *hemothorax, hemoperitoneum,* or *hemopericardium*) and form *hematomas* (literally, a blood-filled swelling or tumor [*-oma*]). Small hemorrhages into the skin and mucosa that are less than 1 mm in diameter are called *petechiae;* those that measure 1 mm to 1 cm in diameter are termed *purpura,* and larger, blotchy bruises are called *ecchymoses.*

Several clinical terms denoting various forms of hemorrhage are worth noting:

hemoptysis—respiratory tract bleeding with expectoration

hematemesis—vomiting of blood

hematochezia—anorectal bleeding

melena—passage of black, discolored blood in the stool. This represents upper gastrointestinal tract bleeding in which the blood is exposed to gastric hydrochloric acid, which produces the color change.

hematuria—blood in urine

metrorrhagia—uterovaginal bleeding. In contrast to profound menstrual bleeding, which is called *menorrhagia,* metrorrhagia is unrelated to the normal monthly bleeding of menstruation.

Both hematomas and small tissue hemorrhages contain RBCs and plasma. The clotting factors of plasma are activated upon contact with tissue, which leads to coagulation of the extravasated blood. The clot or *thrombus* that forms usually occludes the tear in the vessel wall, thus contributing to cessation of the hemorrhage. The clot in the tissue has essentially the same fate as intravascular thrombi, which will be described later.

Clinicopathologic Correlations. The clinical consequences of hemorrhage depend on the amount of blood loss, the site of hemorrhage, its duration, and many other factors. For instance, a healthy young person will tolerate a massive hemorrhage much better than will a chronically ill older person. Moreover, a single episode of hemorrhage has fewer consequences than do repeated hemorrhages.

Massive acute hemorrhage should be treated as a potentially life-endangering event. Most adults can lose 500 mL of blood without any adverse consequences. This is the amount of blood routinely removed from blood donors for transfusion. Loss of 1000 to 1500 mL of blood, however, may result in profound circulatory shock, and loss of blood in excess of 1500 mL is usually lethal.

Chronic hemorrhages, such as those from a bleeding gastric ulcer, usually result in anemia. Anemia can result even from heavy menstruation. Normal menstrual hemorrhage contains about 70 mL of blood; if the lost hemoglobin iron is not replenished in adequate amounts, iron deficiency anemia will ensue.

The extravasated blood may damage tissues. For example, bleeding into the brain ("stroke") is usually associated with loss of neurons and paralysis caused by the destruction of motor centers. Large hematomas are space-occupying lesions in any site, and these may compress normal structures, cause pain, or irritate tissue by the substances released from the disintegrated blood cells. The release of hemoglobin-derived bilirubin in large hematomas may even cause jaundice.

Thrombosis

Thrombosis, or clotting, is transformation of the fluid blood into a solid aggregate encompassing blood cells and fibrin. Fibrin is polymerized fibrinogen; it forms a meshwork of thin filaments that bind together the cellular elements of the blood, forming a *thrombus* (Greek term for clot), or a hemostatic plug.

Pathogenesis of Thrombosis. Thrombi form only in living organisms. This distinguishes thrombi from postmortem clots or coagulated blood in a test tube. Thrombi are the end-products of the coagulation sequence, which is normally activated to prevent blood loss from disrupted vessels. When the same coagulation sequence is activated in intact vessels, pathologic intravascular thrombosis develops.

The normal blood consists of a protein-rich fluid, called plasma, and blood cells. In order to circulate, the blood must be fluid and the blood cells must be freely suspended in the plasma. The fluidity of plasma is the product of interaction between factors that promote coagulation and those that inhibit it. Under normal conditions, the clotting and anticlotting factors are in balance. Plasma clotting factors and platelets promote thrombosis, whereas endothelial cells and plasmin counteract it.

Intravascular coagulation is the result of the interaction of three factors: (1) coagulation proteins, (2) platelets, and (3) endothelial cells (Fig. 6-6). The

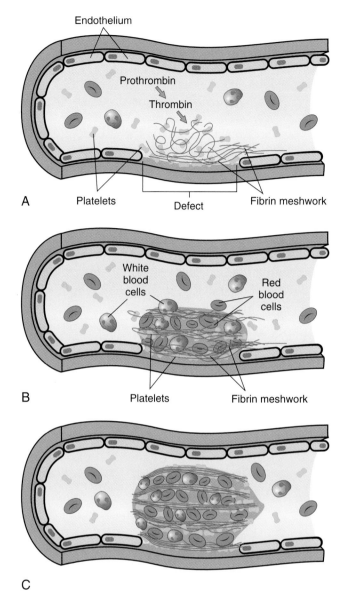

Endothelium

Prothrombin

Thrombin

A

Platelets

Defect

Fibrin meshwork

White blood cells

Red blood cells

B

Platelets

Fibrin meshwork

C

FIGURE 6-6
The formation of thrombi involves platelets, coagulation proteins, and endothelial cells, and occurs in several sequences. (A) An endothelial cell defect is covered with fibrin and platelets. (B) Fibrin forms a meshwork that anchors the blood cells into the nascent thrombus. (C) The fully formed thrombus consists of layers of fibrin and blood cells.

coagulation process may be activated through an endogenous and/or exogenous pathway. In the sequence of events that follows activation, the coagulation factors act on each other and finally form thrombin. Thrombin acts as a catalyst, promoting the polymerization of fibrinogen into fibrin. The meshwork of fibrin represents the framework for the clot, which includes all the blood cells and many plasma proteins.

A thrombus attaches to the vessel wall, reflecting the fact that the coagulation factors of the plasma are actually interacting with the *endothelial cells*. Normal,

resting, endothelial cells have an antithrombotic function. However, if activated, endothelial cells may also initiate coagulation. This usually occurs in inflammation or trauma. Mediators of inflammation, such as interleukin-1 (IL-1) or tumor necrosis factor (TNF), activate the endothelial cells, which then lose their negative charge and antithrombogenic properties; they can then become initiators of thrombosis.

A third component of normal thrombogenesis is the role of *platelets*. Platelets participate in blood clotting in several ways, the most important being their ability to neutralize heparin and other anticoagulation factors and to secrete thromboxane, which directly stimulates the coagulation process. Thrombi formed under normal circumstances are typically small and short-lived. Small thrombi are easily washed away by the circulating blood or degraded by thrombolytic substances, such as plasmin. Pathologic thrombi disrupt the circulation and can have serious functional consequences for the organs in which they have been formed. The formation of pathologic thrombi can be traced to one of three predisposing conditions known as Virchow's triad:

- endothelial cell injury
- hemodynamic changes
- hypercoagulability of the blood

As mentioned earlier, the intact endothelium has distinct anticoagulant properties. Under the influence of mediators of inflammation, however, the endothelium loses its anticoagulant properties and becomes thrombogenic. For example, stimulated endothelial cells release the so-called von Willebrand factor, which is important for the activation of coagulation factor VIII and the adhesion of platelets. More severe injury—e.g., necrosis of endothelial cells and their loss—exposes the blood to connective tissue of the blood vessels and perivascular collagen, which serve as strong activators of the extrinsic coagulation pathway.

Hemodynamic factors that promote coagulation are of two kinds: those that disturb the normal laminar flow of blood, causing turbulence, and those that slow the blood flow. Under both conditions, there is separation of blood elements that allows the platelets to be exposed to the blood vessel wall and to discharge their granules as a result of mechanical stimulation. Slow blood flow promotes sedimentation of blood cells and formation of blood eddies. The resulting turbulence in the blood flow promotes coagulation and also damages the endothelial cells. The slow fluid flow is less efficient in washing away small thrombi than the normal, more vigorous blood flow. Small thrombi that are not dissolved by antithrombolytic substances tend to persist and even grow in the sluggish blood stream.

Hypercoagulability of blood is, to a great extent,

a function of platelets and the soluble coagulation factors of the plasma. Hypercoagulability of blood is usually hard to document, although there is ample evidence that this occurs in pregnancy, in cancer, and even in chronic cardiac failure. The blood is hypercoagulable in severely burned persons, probably because of fluid loss and hemoconcentration. Disseminated intravascular coagulation (DIC), a feature of shock, will be discussed later.

Pathology of Thrombosis. Thrombi are classified on the basis of their location, as follows (Fig. 6-7):

- *Intramural thrombi* are attached to the mural endocardium of the heart chambers and are commonly found overlying a myocardial infarct.
- *Valvular thrombi* appear as small, fibrinous excrescences in debilitated persons and cause

changes that mimic those of endocarditis. Accordingly, these lesions are called *nonbacterial (marantic)* or *sterile thrombotic endocarditis.*

- *Arterial thrombi* are attached to the arterial wall and typically cover ulcerated atheromas in an atherosclerotic aorta or the coronary arteries. Aortic *aneurysms* also contain thrombi.
- *Venous thrombi* are usually found in dilated veins (*varicose veins*). Long-standing venous thrombi are organized by granulation tissue, which may give an impression of inflammation (*thrombophlebitis*).
- *Microvascular thrombi* are found in arterioles, capillaries, and venules, and are typical of DIC.

On the basis of gross features, thrombi are classified as either *red (conglutination) thrombi*, which are composed of tightly intermixed RBCs and fibrin; or

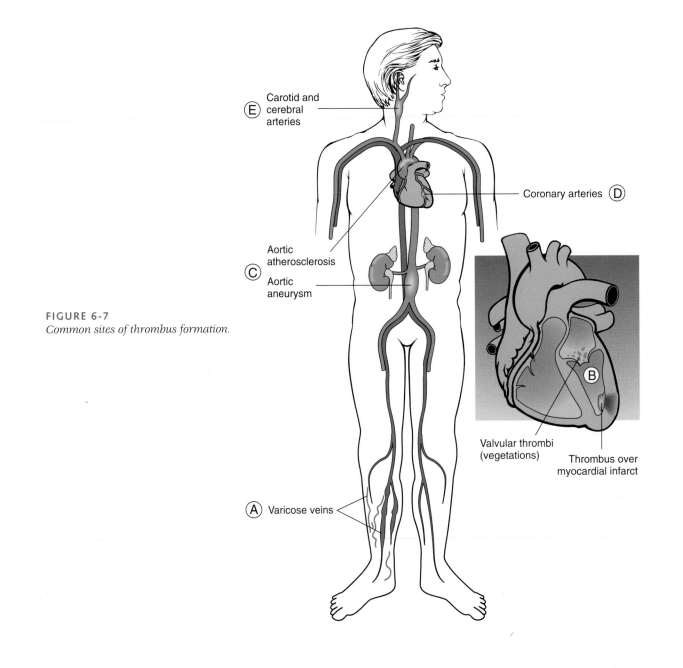

FIGURE 6-7
Common sites of thrombus formation.

E Carotid and cerebral arteries

Coronary arteries D

Aortic atherosclerosis

C Aortic aneurysm

Valvular thrombi (vegetations)

Thrombus over myocardial infarct

B

A Varicose veins

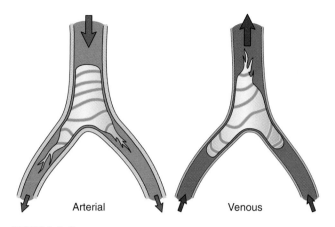

FIGURE 6-8
Diagram showing the gross appearance of a thrombus, depending on its site of origin. Note the lines of Zahn, which are composed of fibrin and platelets.

layered (*sedimentation*) *thrombi*, which show distinct layering of cellular elements and fibrin (Fig. 6-8). The white layers in these thrombi are called the lines of Zahn. Thrombi in small vessels tend to be red. Thrombi in large arteries and veins, as well as mural thrombi, tend to be layered. Histologically, all thrombi consist of RBCs that appear dark red, as well as lighter red strands of fibrin. Nucleated cells and platelets are intermixed with the fibrin and RBCs.

The fate of thrombi depends on their size, location, and the general state of hemodynamics in the vessels. Most small thrombi are *lysed* with no consequences (Fig. 6-9). Larger thrombi remain attached to the surface of the vessel wall or endocardium. Initially, this attachment is mediated by the action of adhesion molecules, such as fibronectin or fibrin. With time, the thrombus stimulates the ingrowth of inflammatory cells and vessels. This granulation tissue provides a much firmer anchorage. This process is called *organization*. The inflammatory cells of the granulation tissue dissolve the thrombus. Ultimately, the thrombus is replaced by collagenous fibrous tissue that develops from granulation tissue. Occlusive thrombi may also be recanalized, and blood could flow again through the previously unpassable lumen with reestablishment of the circulation from the coalescence of anastomosing blood vessels. However, if the thrombus cannot be organized and firmly attached or dissolved, it may break off from the anchoring surface, giving rise to *emboli*. Thromboemboli are carried by the circulating blood to another anatomic site, and if they occlude other blood vessels, they may cause an *ischemic infarction*.

Clinicopathologic Correlations. The clinical significance of thrombi cannot be overemphasized. Thrombotic occlusions of cardiac and cerebral arteries are major causes of death in the United States.

Pulmonary emboli are associated with significant mortality, but the exact prevalence of this complication of thrombosis is not known because pulmonary embolism is often not recognized clinically. The autopsy data indicate that at least one third of all pulmonary embolisms are not diagnosed correctly before death.

The clinical symptoms of thrombosis depend on the site, the extent of thrombi, the rapidity with which they are formed, the duration of thrombosis, and the widespread nature of the disease and its distant complications. Thrombi may

- *occlude the lumen of the blood vessel.* Arterial occlusion typically causes ischemia. Thrombotic occlusion of the coronary arteries is the most common cause of myocardial infarction.
- *narrow the lumen of blood vessels and reduce blood flow.* This results in hypoxia and reduced function of the affected organ. Chronic heart failure is often caused by such narrowing, which is mostly a combination of atherosclerosis and thrombosis.

FIGURE 6-9
The fate of thrombi.

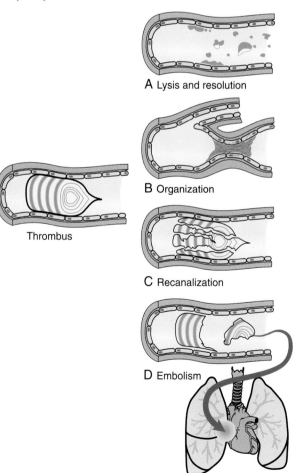

Thrombus

A Lysis and resolution

B Organization

C Recanalization

D Embolism

- *serve as a source of emboli.* Detached thromboemboli carried by blood cause infarcts. Pulmonary emboli stem from venous thrombi in the legs. Cerebral infarct, caused by thromboemboli that become detached from the myocardial chambers overlying the infarct, is one of the most serious late complications of myocardial infarction.

In addition to these three major complications, thrombosis plays a major role in the pathogenesis of atherosclerosis, as discussed in Chapter 7. Thrombi are also fertile grounds for bacterial growth and are prone to infection. These infected thrombi give rise to *septic emboli.*

Embolism

An *embolus* is a freely movable, intravascular mass that is carried from one anatomic site to another by blood. There are several forms of emboli, including the following:

- *Thromboemboli.* These represent fragments of thrombi carried by venous or arterial blood. Infected thrombi give rise to septic emboli.
- *Liquid emboli.* These may include fat emboli that occur after bone fracture, and amniotic fluid emboli caused by the entry of amniotic fluid into uterine veins during delivery.
- *Gaseous emboli.* Air embolism can be produced by injecting air into veins. Air that is liberated under decreased pressure (causing caisson disease or decompression sickness) is another form of embolism.
- *Solid particle emboli.* Cholesterol crystals that detach from atheromatous plaques, tumor cells, or bone marrow emboli (fragments of bone marrow forcibly pressed into the circulation after bone fracture) can also embolize. Cholesterol emboli may cause occlusive symptoms. Bone marrow emboli are usually of no clinical significance and may be found coincidentally at autopsy following rib fractures caused by energetic cardiac resuscitation. Tumor emboli are important for metastasis.

Clinicopathologic Correlations. The clinical significance of emboli lies in the fact that all emboli can occlude blood vessels (**embolism**), thus interrupting the blood supply to an organ. Thromboemboli account for most of the emboli in clinical practice, and thus deserve particular emphasis. All other forms of embolism are rare.

Thromboemboli are classified on the basis of the vessels through which they are carried in the blood (Fig. 6-10). *Venous emboli* originate in veins and are carried by the venous circulation. These typically

> ### Did You Know?
>
> Hospital records show that pulmonary thromboemboli cause more than 50,000 deaths every year in the United States. The number of people dying of pulmonary embolism outside of hospitals is probably even higher.
>
> The symptoms of pulmonary embolism are often nonspecific. Autopsy studies show that 30 percent to 40 percent of all pulmonary emboli discovered postmortem were not even suspected while the patient was alive.

lodge in the pulmonary artery and its branches, causing pulmonary embolism. *Arterial emboli* originate in the left atrium or ventricle, aorta, and major arteries. They are carried by arterial blood and are an important cause of infarction resulting from the occlusion of peripheral arteries. Venous emboli that reach the arterial circulation through the foramen ovale or an interventricular septal defect or some other anastomoses are called *paradoxical emboli.* These emboli are, by origin, venous, but they can travel by both venous and arterial blood and cause symptoms similar to those of arterial emboli.

Pulmonary embolism is the most important complication of venous emboli. These emboli typically originate in the veins of the lower extremities and are carried by venous blood to the vena cava and then through the right atrium and ventricle into the pulmonary artery. A massive thromboembolus may occlude the pulmonary artery or its main branches. Such *saddle emboli* are often lethal (Fig. 6-11) because they prevent the entry of blood into the lung and cause acute anoxia. Smaller emboli lodge in the minor branches of the pulmonary vascular tree and cause pulmonary infarcts. Pulmonary infarcts are triangular, corresponding to the area supplied by the occluded branch, and are often subpleural. These infarcts cause irritation of the pleura, which is associated with typical "pleuritic pain." Pleuritic pain is sharp, its location can be pinpointed by the patient, and it is accentuated by inspiration.

Arterial emboli are important and rather common causes of ischemia in various organs. Most arterial emboli originate from cardiac mural or valvular thrombi. In cases of bacterial endocarditis, the emboli may be infected. Other sources of arterial emboli are the thrombi on ulcerated atherosclerotic plaques of the aorta and its major branches. Moreover, aortic aneurysms often contain thrombi, which may give rise to emboli.

Arterial emboli are mechanically fragmented inside the vessels because arterial blood flows fast and

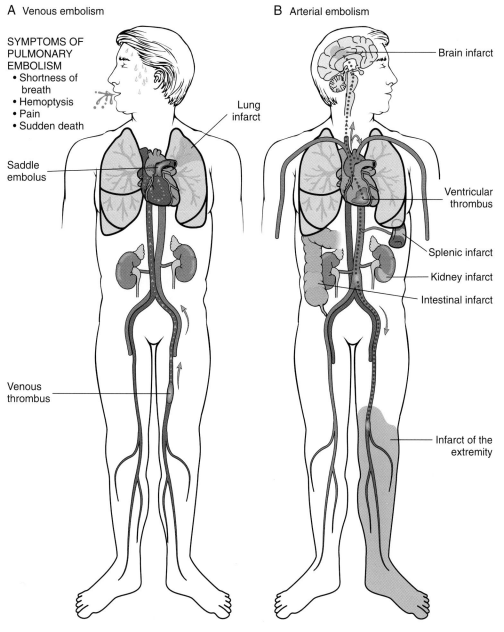

A Venous embolism

SYMPTOMS OF
PULMONARY
EMBOLISM
• Shortness of
  breath
• Hemoptysis
• Pain
• Sudden death

Lung
infarct

Saddle
embolus

Venous
thrombus

B Arterial embolism

Brain infarct

Ventricular
thrombus

Splenic infarct

Kidney infarct

Intestinal infarct

Infarct of the
extremity

FIGURE 6-10
*Venous and arterial emboli. (A) Venous emboli can lodge in the lung, causing a variety of
symptoms and conditions. (B) Arterial emboli may occlude arteries in many organs.*

disrupts them. Thus, they tend to lodge in medium-sized and small arteries. The greatest risk is associated with emboli of the cerebral circulation, which typically lodge in the middle cerebral artery and cause infarcts of the basal ganglia. Cerebral embolization is associated with high mortality, and patients who do survive often have residual neurologic defects.

Other organs commonly affected by arterial emboli are the spleen, kidneys, and intestines. Infarcts that develop from splenic emboli are functionally unimportant. The only symptom is usually a sharp, subcostal pain. Renal infarcts may also be painful, and are often associated with hematuria. Intestinal

infarcts often represent major medical emergencies. If an embolus lodges in one of the major intestinal arteries, and if this happens in an elderly person who already has compromised circulation through the intestinal blood vessels, the embolus may cause gangrene of the large segments of the intestine.

Infarction

Infarction is an insufficiency of blood supply of sudden onset that results in an area of ischemic necrosis. The terms for the process (infarction) and the

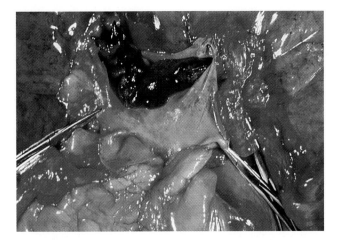

FIGURE 6-11
Saddle embolus of the pulmonary artery.

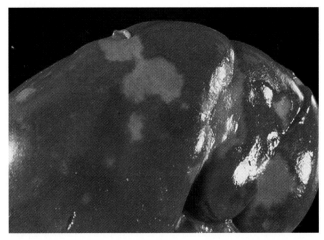

FIGURE 6-12
White infarcts of the kidney.

anatomic lesion (infarct) are often used synonymously. Most infarcts are caused by thrombi or emboli. Depending on the site of vascular occlusion, infarcts may be arterial or venous.

On the basis of their gross appearance, infarcts may be classified as either white or red. *White or pale infarcts* are typical of arterial occlusion in solid organs, such as the heart, kidney, or spleen (Fig. 6-12). The area of ischemic necrosis caused by the obstruction of the arteries is typically paler than the surrounding tissue. It is often rimmed by a thin red zone containing extravasated blood that was destined to reach the ischemic zone from surrounding anastomotic blood vessels. Because the heart and kidney have functionally terminal arteries that do not form large anastomoses among themselves, these abortive attempts to resupply the area with blood from another source are inefficient. If blood from collateral blood vessels ultimately reaches the infarcted area within a few days after the occlusion, the pale infarct will become mottled. In recurrent infarct of the heart, the tissue may exhibit several colors: brown, indicating a normal heart that has survived ischemia; pale brown muscle that is ischemic; yellow necrotic tissue, often infiltrated with polymorphonuclear scavenger leukocytes; RBCs extravasated into the tissue; and white or gray fibrous tissue indicative of connective tissue repair.

Red infarcts are typical of venous obstruction involving the intestines or testis. In these sites, the venous circulation may be interrupted as a result of twisting of the organ around its supporting structure. Twisting of the sigmoid colon (*volvulus*) causes compression of the blood vessels in the mesentery. As the veins have thin walls, they are compressed much more easily than the arteries. This leads to sudden onset of venous congestion, local ischemia, and necrosis—i.e., hemorrhagic infarction (Fig. 6-13). Similar changes result from torsion of the testis, a fairly

common, sport-related lesion in children and adolescents. Thrombosis of the major veins has the same effect. Red infarcts are also typical of organs that have a dual blood supply, such as the lung or liver.

The fate of infarcts depends on many factors, such as their anatomic site, the general circulatory status of the affected person, and the body's capacity to repair the area of infarction. Ischemic necrosis in organs composed of postmitotic cells, like the heart, cannot be repaired except by replacement of damaged cells with fibrous tissue. This results in myocardial fibrosis or scarring. Necrotic brain cells cannot be replaced by regeneration either. Fibrous scars do not form, and the liquefied necrotic brain tissue is ultimately resorbed, leaving behind a cyst filled with clear fluid.

Infarcts involving tissues composed of mitotic or facultative mitotic cells, such as the liver, heal with relatively few residual effects. Small infarcts of the intestine or mucosa also may be repaired by regeneration. However, larger infarcts usually result in defects that cannot be replaced, and this results in scarring.

FIGURE 6-13
Red infarct of the intestine.

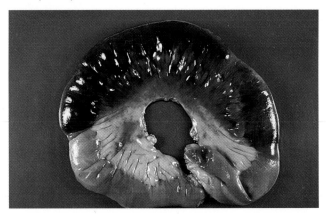

Shock

Shock is a state of hypoperfusion of tissues with blood. It is caused by one of three possible mechanisms:

- pump failure of the heart
- loss of fluid from the circulation
- loss of peripheral vascular tone resulting in overexpansion of the peripheral vascular space and redistribution of fluids

Common to all of these conditions are a collapse of circulation and a disproportion between the circulating blood volume and the vascular space. The resulting hypoperfusion of tissues produces tissue anoxia and multiple organ failure. Anoxia potentiates the loss of vascular tone, which ultimately leads to death in cardiorespiratory failure (Fig. 6-14).

Cardiogenic shock results from pump failure of the heart. Most often, it is secondary to an infarction that destroys a large part of the functioning myocardium. Loss of contractile elements dramatically decreases the ability of the heart to pump blood. Similar consequences may result from myocarditis or valvular heart disease, such as endocarditis. Sudden heart stoppage secondary to cardiac conduction block or arrhythmia also may result in cardiogenic shock.

Hypovolemic shock results from a loss of circulatory volume. This may be attributable to massive hemorrhage or to water loss related to burns, vomiting, or diarrhea. *Hypotonic shock* results from the loss of vascular tonus and the pooling of blood in dilated peripheral blood vessels. This typically occurs in individuals with anaphylactic shock caused by exposure to an allergen (e.g., a bee sting), neurogenic stimuli (e.g., pain caused by trauma; spinal cord injury), or bacterial endotoxins (e.g., sepsis).

Shock represents a series of events, which, if uninterrupted, act synergistically with each other, causing vicious cycles that ultimately result in death. Early stages of shock are reversible and treatable. However, once serious organ failure ensues, the shock becomes irreversible. Cardiac failure and the resultant hypoperfusion are initially compensated for by peripheral vasoconstriction. This redirects blood to vital organs, such as the brain, and preserves their critical function. Central pooling of blood in the abdominal organs and the lungs is accompanied by pallor of skin, which also is clammy and cold. Vasoconstriction of the renal blood vessels results in renal hypoperfusion and a decreased glomerular filtration rate. Low urine output and even anuria are typical of this stage of shock.

Anoxia of tissues and underexcretion of metabolites by the kidneys lead to metabolic acidosis. Acidosis has a depressive effect on the heart and further potentiates pump failure. It also causes vasodilatation and promotes peripheral pooling of blood. Left ventricular insufficiency raises the intrapulmonary

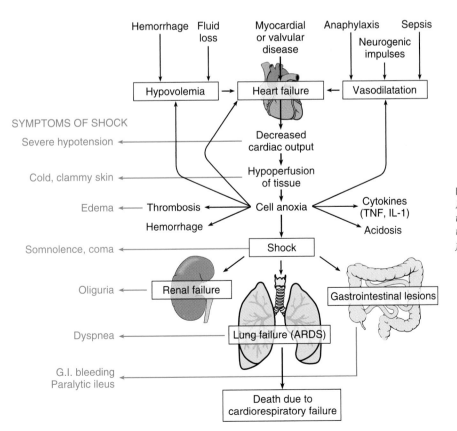

FIGURE 6-14
Pathogenesis of shock. G.I., gastrointestinal; ARDS, adult respiratory distress syndrome; TNF, tumor necrosis factor; IL-1, interleukin-1.

venous pressure, causing stagnation of blood in the pulmonary circulation. Pulmonary venous pressure favors the formation of pulmonary edema. Pulmonary circulatory breakdown affects the alveolocapillary functional units, resulting in a condition known as shock lung, or adult respiratory distress syndrome (ARDS). Lungs that are affected by ARDS cannot function properly, and this further contributes to generalized hypoxia. Respiratory acidosis caused by retention of carbon dioxide further aggravates the patient's already critical condition.

Anoxia of the tissues results in a release of numerous cytokines, the most important of which are TNF and IL-1. These cytokines cause vasodilatation and promote loss of fluids into tissues by increasing the permeability of the peripheral blood vessels. As bacterial endotoxins represent some of the most potent stimulators of cytokine release, they are the primary mediators of septic shock. Antibodies to TNF and IL-1 appear effective in combating shock, at least in experimental animals, and probably could be used one day in human medicine as well.

Anoxic endothelial cells lose their antithrombogenic properties and actually revert into clot-forming cells. Stimulated endothelial cells release clotting factors and, at the same time, serve as anchorage sites for platelets and the plasma clotting factors. The sluggish blood flow that results from circulatory collapse further promotes clotting. All this results in widespread clot formation, known as DIC.

Pathology of Shock. Autopsies performed on patients who have died of shock have revealed numerous pathologic changes. On external inspection, the body is usually edematous (anasarca), and the body cavities contain fluid (ascites, hydrothorax). The internal organs appear to be congested and wet from edema. The most prominent changes are in the lungs, which are heavy, usually exceeding two to three times their normal weight. This reflects the accumulation of fluid in the alveoli (*pulmonary edema*), the most notable feature of ARDS. The liver is congested and enlarged, and blood oozes from its cut surface. The intestines are dark owing to pooling of blood in their vessels, and they are also wet because of the edema of the entire wall. The kidneys are swollen, and on cross-section, will reveal a pale cortex and congested medulla resulting from constriction of the cortical blood vessels and consequent corticotubular necrosis. The brain is almost always edematous and shows flattened gyri and shallow sulci. Because of DIC, hemorrhages are widespread and involve almost all organs. Most prominent are the gastrointestinal mucosal hemorrhages, which usually result in the accumulation of blood in the lumen of the stomach and the intestines.

Clinicopathologic Correlations. In the clinical setting, it is possible to distinguish three stages of shock:

- early or compensated shock
- decompensated but reversible shock
- irreversible shock

Compensated shock is characterized by a set of adaptations that compensate for the circulatory imbalance. Typical of this stage of shock are the following:

- *Tachycardia* (increased heart rate). The heart beats fast in its attempt to pump more blood by increasing the rate of contractions.
- *Vasoconstriction of peripheral arterioles.* This leads to redistribution of the blood and ensures normal perfusion of vital organs, such as the brain and heart. Skin pallor is typical.
- *Reduced urine production.* This represents an attempt of the body to preserve the volume of circulating blood.

During this phase of shock, the blood pressure is normal and there are no serious signs of vital organ ischemia.

Decompensated shock results when the compensatory mechanisms of early shock fail. The following conditions are typical of this stage of shock:

- *Hypotension.* Blood pressure and cardiac output decrease progressively.
- *Tachypnea and shortness of breath.* In response to anoxia, the respiratory rate is increased. Owing to heart failure, pulmonary edema develops, which impedes respiration and ultimately leads to ARDS.
- *Oliguria.* Marked constriction of the renal cortical vessels reduces the glomerular filtration rate, and the renal fluid output decreases precipitously.
- *Acidosis.* This acidosis is partially metabolic, owing to renal excretory failure and the retention of acidic metabolites; partially related to tissue anoxia favoring anaerobic glycolysis and lactic acid production; and partially related to respiratory insufficiency with retention of carbon dioxide.

Irreversible shock is the end result of decompensated shock. It is marked by the following:

- Circulatory collapse
- Marked hypoperfusion of vital organs
- Loss of vital functions

Such patients are typically in great distress and apprehensive of the consequences of their grave condition, or unconscious. There is marked hypotension, respiratory distress, acidosis, and anuria. DIC is common. Despite major therapeutic advances, irreversible shock still is associated with high mortality.

Review Questions

1. What are the main body fluid compartments?
2. What is the pathogenesis of edema?
3. Compare inflammatory and oncotic edema.
4. Explain the pathogenesis of edema in heart failure.
5. Compare active and passive hypermia.
6. List common clinical forms of hemorrhage and explain how they present.
7. Explain the most important clinical terms denoting hemorrhage from various anatomis sites.
8. Compare the clinical findings relating to massive acute hemorrhage with those relating to chronic hemorrhage.
9. Explain the pathogenesis of thrombosis.
10. Which conditions predispose an individual to thrombosis?
11. Classify thrombi according to their anatomic location.
12. Compare arterial with venous thrombi.
13. What is the fate of thrombi?
14. List the most important forms of embolism.
15. Compare venous, arterial, and paradoxical emboli.
16. Compare pale (white) and red infarcts and explain their pathogenesis.
17. What is the fate of infarcts?
18. Compare the pathogenesis of cardiogenic and hypovolemic shock.
19. List the most important pathologic findings associated with shock.
20. Compare the clinical features of compensated and decompensated shock with those of irreversible shock.

Learning Objectives

After reading this chapter, the student should be able to:

1. Describe the normal components of the cardiovascular system and their function.

2. List the five most common forms of heart disease in the United States.

3. List the three most common congenital heart diseases and describe the pathogenesis of each.

4. Discuss the pathogenesis and risk factors of atherosclerosis.

5. Describe the major pathologic lesions of atherosclerosis and list three major complications.

6. Describe the gross and microscopic features and complications of myocardial infarct and correlate these pathologic findings with site and clinical symptoms.

7. Discuss the pathogenesis of hypertension and compare primary and secondary hypertension.

8. Describe the typical gross and microscopic lesions of endocarditis, myocarditis, and pericarditis, and correlate the pathologic findings with the clinical findings.

9. Discuss the pathogenesis of rheumatic heart disease and describe the typical cardiac lesions of rheumatic fever.

10. List three causes of cardiomyopathy and describe the pathologic findings in this disease.

11. Describe two surgical operations performed on the heart and their consequences or complications.

12. Discuss the pathogenesis of arteritis and relate it to its pathologic and clinical features.

13. Describe varicose veins and list the possible causes and consequences of this disease.

14. Describe lymphangitis.

Additional Key Terms and Concepts

Angina pectoris

Aneurysm

Hyperlipidemia

Polyarteritis nodosa

Septal defect

Tetralogy of Fallot

Chapter Outline

The Cardiovascular System

Chapter 7

The cardiovascular system, as the name implies, comprises the heart (the Greek term *cardia* means heart) and vessels. The primary function of this system is circulation of the blood; therefore, it is also called the circulatory system. The **heart** is the centerpiece of the circulatory system which, through its incessant rhythmic action, pumps the blood and keeps it flowing. The vessels represent the venues through which the blood circulates. However, blood vessels also regulate the blood flow and thus actively participate in the circulation.

Heart

The heart weighs approximately 250 to 350 g and is the size of a person's fist. The heart is located in the **pericardial sac.** The inside of the pericardial sac is lined with a smooth surface epithelium that also covers the opposing external surface of the heart, the **epicardium.** When these two surfaces slide over each other during heart movements, they are separated only by a few drops of clear pericardial fluid that keep the surface moist and prevent friction.

The heart consists of four **chambers:** two upper chambers called *atria* and two lower chambers called *ventricles.* The right atrium is separated from the left atrium by an interatrial septum composed of connective tissue. By comparison, the interventricular septum is much thicker and is composed of cardiac muscle cells. The atria are separated from the ventricles by *atrioventricular* **valves** that regulate the proper inflow and outflow of blood from each chamber during heart contractions. The outflow tract of each ventricle also has a valve, known as the semilunar valve, so named because its cusp is half-moon–shaped.

The wall of the ventricles (**myocardium**) is formed by striated muscle cells resembling skeletal muscle. In contrast to skeletal muscles, which contract only when stimulated with nerve impulses, the myocardial fibers contract rhythmically on their own. However, these muscle fibers also respond to the electrophysiologic impulses of the cardiac **conduction system** and can be influenced by various chemicals, transmitters, and drugs. The internal surface of the heart chambers is covered by **endocardium,** whereas on the outside, the heart is covered by epicardium. The epicardium is continuous with the **pericardium.**

Blood is supplied to the heart by two **coronary arteries** (Fig. 7-1). These arteries originate from the proximal **aorta,** just above the aortic semilunar valve. The left coronary artery usually bifurcates into two major branches, the anterior descending and the left circumflex arteries, which provide most of the blood for the anterior and lateral side of the left ventricle and the anterior portion of the interventricular septum. The right coronary artery does not bifurcate, but forms a single major trunk from which several major branches originate. The right coronary artery provides the blood for the right ventricle and the posterior wall of the left ventricle, as well as the posterior portion of the interventricular septum.

Normally, the heart contracts rhythmically at a rate of 60 to 80 times per minute. The contraction of the heart is called *systole,* whereas the relaxation of the myocardium that results in dilatation of the cardiac chambers is called *diastole.*

In diastole, the heart chambers dilate, allowing filling of the right heart with peripheral venous blood while the left heart is filled with oxygenated pulmonary venous blood (Fig. 7-2). During diastole, the ventricles and atria are dilated, and the semilunar pulmonary and aortic valves are closed to prevent regurgitation of blood from the large vessels across these orifices. At the same time, the mitral and tricuspid valves are opened to allow inflow of blood into the dilated ventricles from the atria.

Contraction of the heart and the closing and opening of the valves and heart generate *sounds* and *murmurs* stemming from the flow of blood through the cardiac chambers and across the valves. Various pathologic lesions are associated with distinct auscultatory findings, and an experienced cardiologist can diagnose many important cardiac diseases, especially those involving the valves, by *auscultation.*

Blood Vessels

The blood vessels form the second major compartment of the cardiovascular system (Fig. 7-3). These include arteries, veins, and capillaries, sealed into a closed system through which the blood circulates back and forth from the heart to the peripheral tissues. All blood vessels are lined by endothelial cells, which form the innermost layer of the arteries and veins. The endothelium is the only cell layer of the capillaries. Overall, the arteries are thicker than the veins, and although both consist of several concentric tissue layers, those forming the arteries are generally more cellular and contain more extracellular matrix than those forming the veins. Therefore, the arteries have thicker walls than veins.

The **arteries** are of two types. The larger arteries, including the aorta, are classified as *elastic,* whereas the smaller arteries are called *muscular.* The elastic arteries expand with the internal pressure generated by blood flow during the systole and then

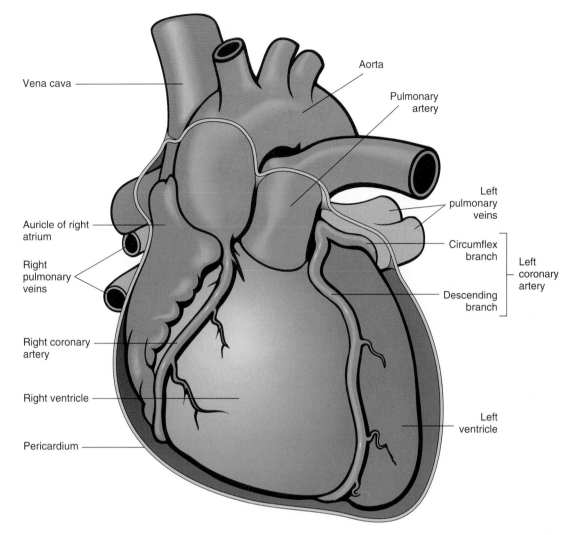

FIGURE 7-1

Normal heart. The heart is located in the mid-portion of the thorax. It is attached to the aorta and the inferior and superior cava. There are two coronary arteries. The left coronary artery branches into a circumflex and a descending branch. It provides the blood to the anterior and lateral part of the left ventricle. The right coronary artery provides blood to the right ventricle and the posterior side of the left ventricle.

recoil during diastole. The muscular arteries contract or dilate to accommodate the blood volume in their lumen, the tissue requirements for blood, and the velocity of circulation.

The **veins** have thinner walls than do the arteries, and generally do not have the elasticity or the contractile capacity of the arteries. These properties are not essential for their function as the venous blood flow is less pulsatile and is under less pressure than flow in the arteries. To prevent backflow of blood, the veins have *valves* that hinder the retrograde blood flow that could easily develop in this low-pressure system.

The **capillaries** are the primary sites at which oxygen is transferred from blood into the tissues and metabolites are exchanged. To this end, the capillar-ies have a thin wall composed of a single endothelial cell layer. Capillaries and venules are also the primary sites at which the blood cells exit into the interstitial spaces, and through which fluids enter the interstitial spaces or reenter the circulation from the peripheral tissues.

Lymphatics

The lymphatic vessels form the third component of the circulatory system. The primary function of the lymphatic system is to facilitate and enable the centripetal flow of lymph from the peripheral tissues toward the heart. Lymph is similar to blood, but differs from it in that it does not contain red blood cells or

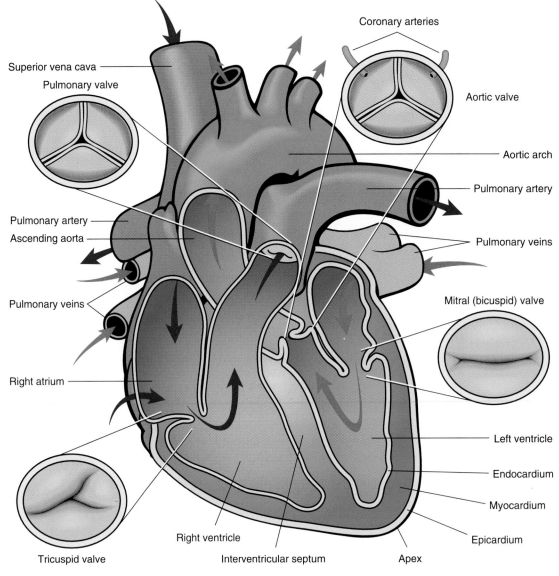

FIGURE 7-2

Chambers of the heart. The right heart pumps the venous blood into the lungs. The oxygenated blood returns from the lungs into the left atrium and is propelled by the left ventricle into the aorta. The insets show closed valves; the tricuspid valve has three leaflets, whereas the mitral valve has two leaflets. The aortic and pulmonary artery valves have three valves and resemble one another except for the fact that the coronary arteries originate from behind the cusps in the aorta.

clotting factors (i.e., it will not coagulate). This fluid is formed in the peripheral tissues and various organs from serum and other extracellular fluids. The lymph enters the open-ended, thin, capillary-like lymphatics and is then transported to the central lymphatic vessels under pressure generated in the peripheral tissues. These vessels converge into the main lymphatic vessels and the thoracic duct, which empty their contents into the large veins in the neck. The lymph that enters the venous circulation does not recirculate like the blood.

In contrast to blood circulation which occurs through continuous channels, flow through the lymphatic channels is interrupted by lymph nodes. These lymph nodes serve as barriers or large filters that clear from the lymph bacteria and other noxious substances. At the same time, lymph nodes contain white blood cells, primarily lymphocytes, which enter the lymph and are transported into the central circulation. Many lymphocytes recirculate, returning to the lymph nodes from which they originated or reaching some other tissue to which they are transported for special functions, as in inflammation.

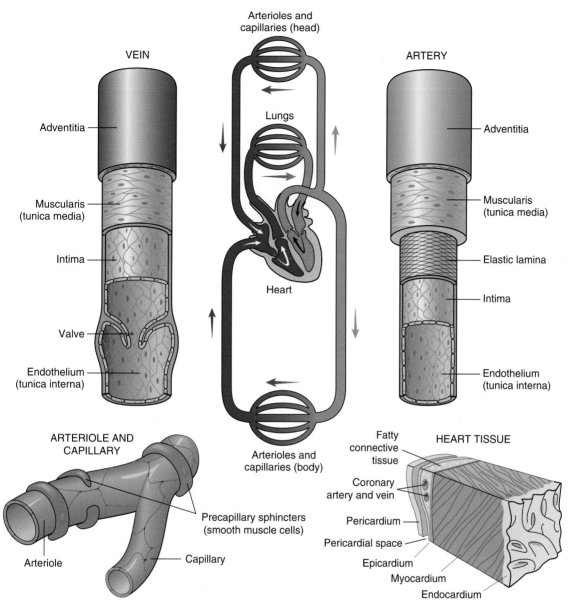

FIGURE 7-3

The peripheral vascular system consists of arteries, which carry oxygenated blood (red), and capillaries and veins, which carry deoxygenated blood (blue). Note the thick wall of the arteries, which is composed of distinct layers of smooth muscle cells and elastic laminae that separate these layers. In comparison, the veins have much thinner walls. The walls of the capillaries consist of a single layer of endothelium. The cross section of the heart is included for comparison.

OVERVIEW OF MAJOR DISEASES

The most important diseases of the cardiovascular system can be classified into the following categories:

- Congenital heart disease
- Ischemic vascular disease
- Hypertension-related disease
- Inflammatory disease (infectious and autoimmune disorders)
- Metabolic disease

Two major arterial diseases are presented: atherosclerosis and arteritis. Among the diseases involving the veins, discussion will be limited to varicose veins and the complications of venous thrombosis. Diseases involving the lymphatics will not be discussed in great detail except for lymphangitis, an acute inflammatory condition involving the small lymph vessels.

Several facts important to an understanding of cardiovascular pathology are presented here, before a discussion of specific pathologic entities.

1. *Cardiovascular diseases account for more than one half of all mortality in industrialized countries.* Atherosclerosis, along with its major manifestations, is the cause of death in more than 50 percent of all adults who die in the United States and the industrialized countries of the West (Fig. 7-4). Atherosclerosis of the coronary arteries, the aorta and its main branches, or the cerebral blood vessels accounts for

FIGURE 7-4
Incidence of cardiovascular diseases. (A) Note that cardiovascular diseases are more common than any other disease. (B) Atherosclerosis accounts for 80 percent of the total mortality from cardiovascular diseases.

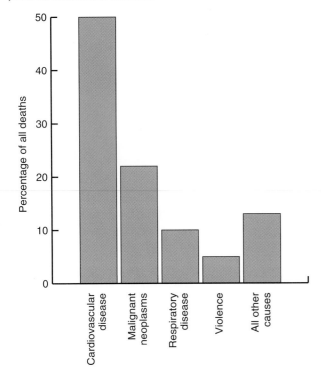

A Mortality due to all causes

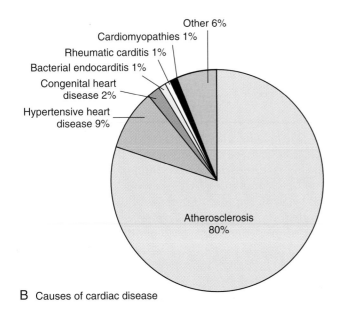

B Causes of cardiac disease

most of the related morbidity. *Hypertension* is an important complication of atherosclerosis. It contributes to the severity of the disease and aggravates its symptoms. Hypertension can, however, occur independent of atherosclerosis and it may even precede it. Hypertension accounts for approximately 10 percent of all heart diseases. *Clotting disturbances* often complicate atherosclerosis. Thrombosis of atherosclerotic coronary arteries is the main cause of cardiac infarction. Thrombi may also occur without preexisting atherosclerosis and are especially common in the venous part of the cardiovascular system. Other cardiovascular diseases are not as common and are less important from the perspective of public health.

2. *Abnormal development of the heart during fetal life is a significant cause of heart disease.* The development of the heart, most of which is completed during the first 2 months of fetal intrauterine life, involves complex embryologic processes (i.e., induction, resorption, inversion, rotation, and so on). These processes are more complicated than their names suggest, and are not yet fully understood. It is important to recognize that, with such a complex morphogenesis, much can go wrong. Congenital heart disease, resulting from abnormal fetal heart development, is, therefore, very common. At least 1 in 100 of all neonates has a minor cardiac abnormality. Luckily, most such defects produce no symptoms or heal on their own.

3. *Heart action is critically dependent on a constant supply of nutrients and oxygen.* Occlusion of the arteries or reduction of the lumen secondary to narrowing impedes blood supply and causes ischemia. Sudden occlusion of the arterial blood flow causes an *infarct*, whereas chronic ischemia leads to pump failure of the heart, which is typical of *chronic coronary heart disease*. This may be associated with bouts of chest pain known as *angina pectoris*.

4. *Arterial blood pressure, which primarily depends on heart action and the elastic and contractile properties of arteries and arterioles, is regulated by hormones and biogenic amines.* Blood flow depends on pressure gradients generated by the action of the heart and the peripheral resistance of arteries and arterioles. The smooth muscle cells in the muscular arteries and arterioles contract under the influence of adrenergic nerves, which release the *catecholamines* epinephrine and norepinephrine. These biogenic amines are also produced by adrenal medullary cells and released into the circulation. Hence, catecholamines also have a systemic effect and act both on blood vessels and the heart. Other humoral regulators of blood pressure include *renin, angiotensin,* and *aldosterone.* Abnormalities in the regulation of blood pressure result in hypotension or hypertension. Hypotension was previously discussed in Chapter 6. Hypertension is an important disease, and it is discussed in greater detail later in this chapter.

5. *The large volume of blood that passes through the heart makes this organ susceptible to blood-borne infections.* Bacteria and other pathogens found in infected blood during *bacteremia (septicemia)* may invade the endothelium of blood vessels and the endocardium of the heart. The endocardium, because it is in direct contact with blood, is involved most often. *Bacterial endocarditis* is, therefore, the most common infectious lesion of the heart. Intramural bacterial abscesses of the myocardium and bacterial pericarditis are less common today, except in immunosuppressed persons.

Preexisting lesions, such as congenital heart defects, deformities of the valves, or mural thrombi, predispose individuals to cardiac infections. Such lesions facilitate the penetration of bacteria into the tissues and their local growth. Clotted blood seems to be the most suitable growth medium for bacteria; therefore, clots in the ventricles (mural thrombi) or those attached to the valves (endocardial vegetations) often become infected. Infected thrombi may give rise to emboli (*septic emboli*). Embolization of the peripheral arteries may cause *infectious arteritis.* Destruction of the vessel wall leads to the formation of *mycotic aneurysms,* suppurative areas of inflammation causing eccentric dilatation of the arteries. Infection of the veins is usually related to preexistent thrombosis (*thrombophlebitis*).

6. *Immunoglobulins in the blood and circulating immune complexes may be deposited in the heart and blood vessels and may cause inflammatory and destructive lesions.* Normal blood contains immunoglobulins, which are normal components of the serum. These immunoglobulins have no adverse influences on the heart and blood vessels. When circulating immunoglobulins are complexed with antigen into immune complexes (as in systemic lupus erythematosus), they may become pathogenic and cause *vasculitis* or *endocarditis.* Immune complexes may also form locally in the vessel wall, as in *polyarteritis nodosa.* Hypersensitivity reactions that elicit formation of autoantibodies—that is, antibodies to the body's own tissues—can damage the heart and blood vessels, as in *rheumatic fever.*

7. *Systemic metabolic diseases often affect the heart and the blood vessels.* The most important metabolic disease affecting the cardiovascular system is diabetes mellitus. This systemic disorder of intermediary metabolism, caused by a relative or absolute deficiency of insulin, or a resistance of tissues to insulin, primarily affects small blood vessels (*microangiopathy*). It also represents an important risk factor for atherosclerosis. Diabetes is discussed in greater detail in Chapter 12.

8. *The cardiovascular system rarely gives rise to malignant tumors.* Malignant tumors of the heart, which by their mesenchymal origin are classified as sarcomas, are extremely rare. Hemangiosarcomas, the malignant tumors of blood vessels, are somewhat more common but still rare overall. On the other hand, *hemangiomas,* which are small benign tumors, are very common but of limited clinical significance. Benign tumors of the heart (rhabdomyomas) and atrial myxomas are also rare.

Congenital Heart Disease

Any defect involving the heart and/or the large arteries and veins that is present at birth is considered to be a **congenital heart disease.** Approximately 25,000 babies with a heart defect are born annually in the United States.

The symptoms of congenital heart disease may be evident at birth or during early infancy, or they may become evident only later in life. These defects may be classified as either *minor* (those that are either asymptomatic or produce only negligent symptoms) or *major* (those that cause serious problems and may be lethal, if not treated adequately).

Etiology and Pathogenesis. The causes and the pathogenesis of most congenital heart defects are not known. Because the heart develops early in embryonic life and is completely formed and functioning by 10 weeks, all congenital heart defects develop before the tenth week of pregnancy. This is important to know because some of these defects can be prevented by avoiding toxic substances, viral infections, and x-ray exposure during the early critical stages of pregnancy.

The fetal heart develops like a tube, being subdivided by a septum that grows from one end while the tube undergoes twisting and segmentation by the primordia of the future valves (Fig. 7-5). If the left side of the heart is not completely separated from the right side, various *septal defects* develop. If the twisting of the heart and its subdivision into the four chambers does not occur normally, complex anomalies form such as *tetralogy of Fallot.* In that anomaly, the base of the heart seems to be twisted too much to the right, causing the aorta to be displaced to the right (*dextroposition of the aorta*). The malpositioned aorta causes narrowing of the adjacent pulmonary artery, which results in *pulmonary stenosis.* There are many other examples of abnormal positioning of the large vessels, but these are relatively uncommon.

The causes of congenital heart diseases can theoretically be classified as either exogenous or endogenous. Among the former, the most important are viruses and alcohol, whereas chromosomal abnormalities are among the most important endogenous causes.

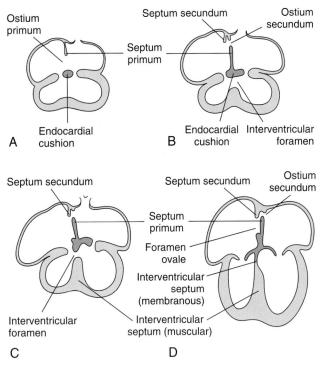

FIGURE 7-5
Schematic drawing of the development of the heart 4 to 8 weeks after conception. Note that the left and right heart are not completely separated during fetal life. Some of these communications between the right and left heart may persist after birth. These are the causes of most congenital heart defects.

- *Viruses.* The best known cause of a congenital heart defect is the *rubella virus,* the cause of German measles. Infection of the mother during the first 3 months of pregnancy is associated with a high incidence of congenital heart disease in offspring. Apparently, the virus crosses the placenta, enters the fetal circulation, and damages the developing heart. Rubella can be prevented by immunization. Widespread immunization against rubella in the United States has decreased the incidence of heart defects caused by this virus.

- *Alcohol.* The complex syndrome of fetal anomalies called *fetal alcohol syndrome* is often associated with heart defects. Alcohol affects the fetal heart directly and interferes with its development. It has been proposed that alcohol is toxic to fetal heart cells and destroys them, but the exact teratogenic mechanism of alcohol remains unknown.

- *Chromosomal abnormalities.* Chromosomal abnormalities are associated with several developmental syndromes, many of which include congenital heart disease. The best known example is the Down syndrome or trisomy 21, which often is associated with heart defects.

Pathology. Pediatric cardiologists have recognized more than 50 congenital heart defects, the diagnosis

and treatment of which are usually coordinated by highly specialized teams that include a pediatric cardiologist, radiologist, and cardiac surgeon. Two examples are presented: one of an isolated, simple defect (septal defects) and one of a complex congenital heart defect (tetralogy of Fallot).

Septal Defects

The left heart is separated from the right heart by a septum. This septum may be defective—that is, it may have a hole in it which, according to its location, may be called either *atrial* or *ventricular.* Septal defects represent the most common form of congenital heart disease, accounting for 30 percent to 40 percent of all clinically recognized cases.

The entire interatrial portion of the septum and the uppermost part of the ventricular septum are made up of connective tissue, whereas the interventricular septum is composed of muscle. During fetal life and until birth, the venous blood enters the left atrium from the right atrium through an opening called the *foramen ovale.* Closure of interatrial communications occurs in several stages, the last of which (closure of the foramen ovale) occurs only after birth. *Atrial septal defects* result from incomplete formation of the septum or incomplete closure of the foramen ovale.

The uppermost part of the interventricular septum is composed of the same connective tissue as the interatrial septum. The lower part of the interventricular septum is composed of muscle. Because the thin fibrous portion of the septum is formed in a complex manner, it is more often affected than the thicker muscular part. Furthermore, because development of the connective tissue septum is intricately connected with the development of the great vessels at the base of the heart and the atrioventricular valves, it is likely that the defects of this part of the septum may occur in concert with other cardiovascular complex malformations.

Atrial and ventricular septal defects may occur as *isolated defects,* which is most often the case, or they may be part of *complex malformation syndromes.* Of the two, interventricular septal defect is the more serious condition.

Ventricular septal defect is the most common congenital heart defect recognized in clinical practice. The symptoms of this condition result from the mixing of blood in the left and right heart chambers as a consequence of the septal defect (Fig. 7-6). Because pressure within the left heart generally exceeds the pressure in the right heart, the arterial blood from the left ventricle or atrium will flow to the right heart. This is called *left-to-right shunt.* Owing to the increased backflow of blood, this left-to-right shunt overburdens the right ventricle, causing it to work twice as hard as normal and resulting in right ven-

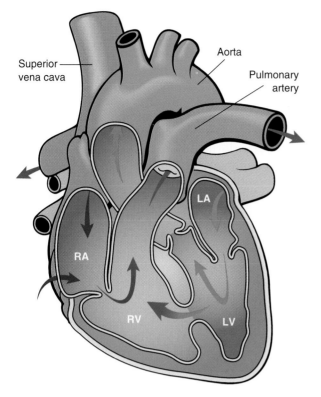

FIGURE 7-6
Ventricular septal defect. In the early stages of this disease, the blood flows from left to right. Once pulmonary hypertension develops, the direction of the blood flow through the shunt reverses, and the venous blood from the right ventricle (RV) enters into the left ventricle (LV) where it mixes with the arterial blood. This dilution of arterial blood with unoxygenated venous blood leads to cyanosis ("late cyanosis"). RA, right atrium; LA, left atrium.

tricular *hypertrophy*. The increased flow of blood through the pulmonary arteries leads to pulmonary hypertension, which is usually accompanied by anatomic changes in the pulmonary artery and its branches. The rising pulmonary hypertension and the narrowing of pulmonary artery branches finally reaches a point at which the pressure in the right ventricle exceeds the pressure in the left ventricle. This reverses the blood flow. A *right-to-left shunt* ensues, at which point the unoxygenated venous blood from the right ventricle and atrium enters the systemic circulation. The venous blood dilutes the arterial blood and reduces its oxygen content, resulting in *cyanosis,* or a bluish discoloration of the skin (in Greek, *kyanos* means blue color).

Septal defects are easily detected by experienced pediatricians because they produce distinct heart murmurs. Most patients have no symptoms. Some of the small defects close spontaneously. However, the larger ones require surgical intervention, whereby a patch of Dacron or some similar artificial material is sutured over the defect. A patient's own connective tissue, removed from other parts of the body, may

also be used to patch the septal defect. The results usually are excellent.

Tetralogy of Fallot

This complex congenital defect of the heart and the major vessels is the most common cause of cardiac cyanosis in newborn children, and it accounts for 10 percent of all congenital heart defects. The pathologic changes associated with this condition, first described by the French physician Fallot, include four typical lesions (Fig. 7-7):

- Valvular stenosis (narrowing) of the pulmonary artery
- Ventricular septal defect involving the uppermost membranous part of the septum
- Dextroposition of the aorta whereby the aorta is moved to the right of its normal position and overrides the septum, thus receiving blood from both the left and the right ventricle
- Hypertrophy of the right ventricle, which is adaptive in nature and develops as a result of the increased workload of the right ventricle

Infants affected by this defect develop cyanosis early after birth and present as "blue babies." The skin turns bluish, most notably over the fingers and toes, lips, cheeks, and earlobes.

The reason for the cyanosis can be deduced from Figure 7-7. Note that the pulmonary artery is narrowed, which limits the amount of blood that can enter the lungs to become oxygenated. The right ventricle attempts to overcome this obstacle at its own outflow tract by pumping more blood. This additional effort causes hypertrophy of the right ventricle. The venous blood in the right ventricle that cannot enter into the narrowed pulmonary artery is shunted through the septal defect into the aorta. The mixing of blood from the right and left ventricle is facilitated by the abnormal position of the aorta, which overrides the septum. Thus, the aorta can be filled with blood from both ventricles, and will contain both venous and arterial blood.

Without surgical repair, most children born with this defect die before puberty. Surgical correction of the defect provides some hope, but the outcome depends on the severity of the defect and other extenuating circumstances.

Atherosclerosis

Atherosclerosis is a systemic disease affecting the arteries. The term—derived from the Greek word *athere,* meaning gruel or porridge, and *scleros,* meaning hard—describes the simultaneous hardening and softening of the arteries that occur in this disease.

Although atherosclerosis may affect all arteries

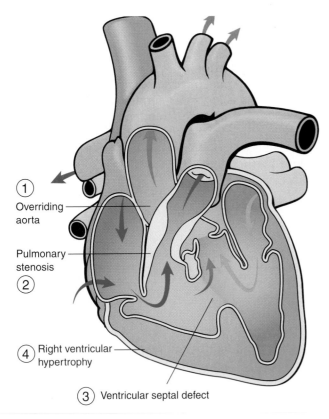

FIGURE 7-7
Tetralogy of Fallot. The heart shows dextroposition of the aorta, which is overriding a ventricular septal defect and is associated with pulmonary stenosis. As a result of the congenital stenosis of the pulmonary artery, which prevents the outflow of blood from the right ventricle, there is right-to-left shunting of the blood and early cyanosis.

in the body, in clinical practice, it is common to encounter patients in whom the symptoms of a single organ predominate. Thus, in addition to the *generalized form,* it is customary to recognize four major *localized* forms of atherosclerosis (Fig. 7-8):

- Atherosclerosis of the coronary arteries, known as *coronary heart disease*
- Atherosclerosis of the brain arteries, known as *cerebrovascular disease* or, more commonly, as a cause of cerebrovascular accidents (CVAs)
- *Atherosclerosis of the aorta,* which usually presents in the form of aortic calcifications and aortic aneurysms
- Atherosclerosis of the arteries in the extremities, known as *peripheral vascular disease*

Etiology and Pathogenesis. Atherosclerosis is, in general, a disease of old age. However, the earliest arterial lesions usually develop long before they become symptomatic and clinically apparent. It is believed that the first damage occurs at the interface between the blood and the arterial wall. This endothelial cell injury, which may be a consequence of metabolic derangements or physical force (e.g., hy-

pertension) is accompanied by the deposition of blood platelets and serum lipoproteins. Growth factors released from platelets stimulate the proliferation of smooth muscle cells in the wall of the artery (Fig. 7-9). The altered environment and the changes in the internal metabolism of smooth muscle cells promote the accumulation of cholesterol and other lipids in their cytoplasm. Typically, the smooth muscle cells transform into foam cells. Some of the lipid-laden smooth muscle cells die, releasing lipid into the interstitial spaces; this is either oxidized, degraded, or deposited in the form of cholesterol crystals. These lesions then attract macrophages, which act as scavengers. Macrophages take up cell remnants and the lipid released from dying or injured

FIGURE 7-8
The four major forms of atherosclerosis are classified as coronary (A), cerebral (B), aortic (C), and peripheral vascular (D).

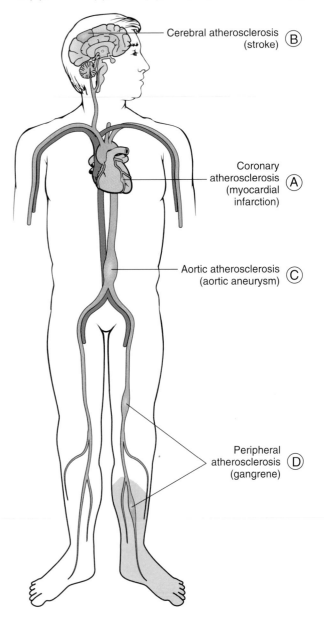

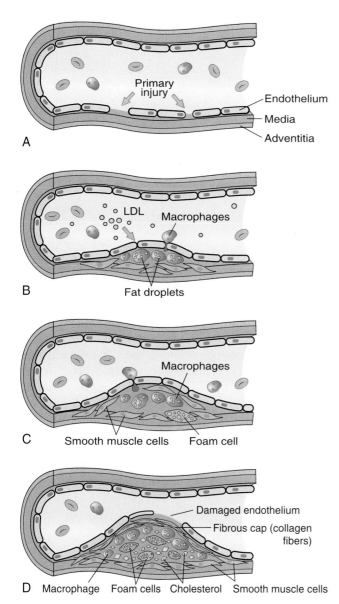

A

B

LDL   Macrophages

Fat droplets

C   Smooth muscle cells   Foam cell

Macrophages

Endothelium
Media
Adventitia

Primary
injury

D   Macrophage   Foam cells   Cholesterol   Smooth muscle cells

Damaged endothelium
Fibrous cap (collagen
fibers)

FIGURE 7-9
Pathogenesis of atherosclerosis. (A) Endothelial injury. (B) Influx of lipids. (C) Accumulation of lipids in the vessel wall, proliferation of smooth muscle cells, and accumulation of macrophages. (D) Atheromas consist of a lipid-rich soft part and a firm fibrous cap. LDL, low-density lipoprotein.

smooth muscle cells, and also transform into foam cells. Macrophages secrete cytokines and biologically active substances, such as tumor necrosis factor (TNF), transforming growth factor beta (TGFβ), and others, which affect other cells in the atheroma, causing more damage.

The repair of the initial arterial wall lesion involves scarring. Collagen deposition leads to hardening of the arteries (*sclerosis*), which surrounds the porridge-like, lipid-rich soft parts (*atheroma*). Typical lesions of atherosclerosis are, therefore, partially soft and partially hard.

Atheromas are the prototypical lesions of atherosclerosis. As shown in Figure 7-9, atheromas bulge

into the lumen of the artery. The central part of the atheroma is soft and consists of lipids and cellular debris. This soft core is covered on the surface by fibrous tissue that forms a *surface cap* on such lesions. However, even this reinforcement is not adequate to preserve the integrity of the vessel wall. The pressure of the liquefied porridge-like material may cause rupture of the surface cap, transforming the atheroma into an intimal *ulceration*. The content of the atheroma is highly thrombogenic, and it initiates formation of a blood clot that typically covers the rough base of this ulcer (Fig. 7-10). In large arteries like the aorta, these *thrombi* do not cause immediate symptoms, but eventually become organized, ultimately transforming into fibrous scars. In smaller arteries, like the coronary or cerebral arteries, formation of the thrombus is usually accompanied by complete occlusion of the lumen of the vessel with subsequent infarction.

The major complication of atherosclerosis is *hardening* of vessels, primarily a consequence of calcification. In pathogenetic terms, this calcification is dystrophic—i.e., precipitated by local tissue degeneration. Lipids released from dead cells and abnormal extracellular matrix extract calcium salts. Calcium salts are thus deposited both in atheromas and in the fibrous tissue. Calcified arteries can be seen on radiographic studies because calcium salts are radiodense.

The atherosclerotic aorta tends to dilate and form *aneurysms* (from the Greek *aneurysma*, meaning dilatation). Blood flow in the aneurysms is irregular. Eddies and whorls inside the aneurysm predispose the individual to thrombosis. Such thrombi can have a beneficial effect because they prevent further widening of the aneurysm. Nevertheless, most aneurysms dilate progressively owing to internal pressure.

Risk Factors. Atherosclerosis is considered to be a multifactorial disease with many risk factors (Table 7-1). The exact role of these risk factors is not known, but it is important to remember that the risks can be diminished by changing one's lifestyle. The beneficial effects of an atherosclerosis prevention program are evident from a review of public health records, which show a significant reduction in atherosclerotic heart disease and other forms of atherosclerosis in the United States. This reduced incidence of atherosclerosis is probably related to changes in the American diet, increased emphasis on exercise and physical fitness, and reduced smoking.

The following risk factors are clinically important:

• *Age.* Atherosclerosis is a disease of older age.
• *Sex.* Atherosclerosis affects more males than fe-

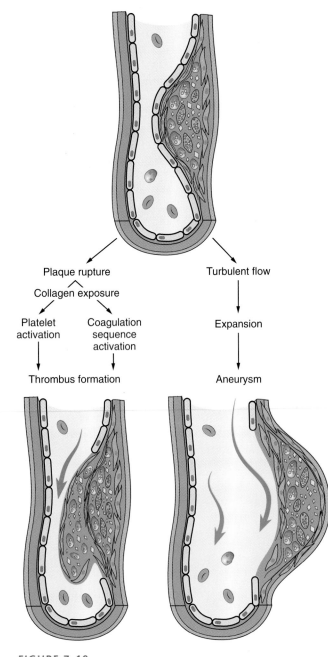

Plaque rupture   Turbulent flow

Collagen exposure

Platelet activation   Coagulation sequence activation   Expansion

Thrombus formation   Aneurysm

FIGURE 7-10
Complications of atheroma. Ulcerated atheromatous lesions are frequently sites of thrombosis. The weakened arterial wall may bulge outward, giving rise to an aneurysm.

males. After menopause, the sex difference becomes less prominent. Apparently, the female sex hormones have a beneficial effect. In postmenopausal women, regular intake of estrogens may reduce the progression and extent of atherosclerosis.

- *Heredity.* It has been known for many years that atherosclerosis affects some families and spares others. However, even the hereditary forms of atherosclerosis have many causes, and the inheritance is considered to be *polygenic.*

Table 7-1 Cardiovascular Risk Factors

Risk Factors That Cannot Be Changed	Risk Factors That Can Be Changed	Protective Factors
Age	Lipid metabolism–related factors	Exercise
Gender	Diet	Estrogen
Heredity	Hyperlipidemia	
	Obesity	
	Diabetes mellitus	
	Hypertension	
	Clotting factors	
	Cigarette smoking	
	Behavior	

- *Lipid metabolism–related factors.* Lipid accumulates in atheromas and is, unquestionably, one of the major pathogenetic factors in the formation of atherosclerotic lesions (Fig. 7-11). Elevated serum levels of lipids—cholesterol, lipoproteins, and triglycerides—directly correlate with the extent and severity of atherosclerosis and, most importantly, with the early onset of clinical symptoms.

  Hyperlipidemia can occur as a primary, familial, or secondary (externally induced) disease. *Familial hyperlipidemias* occur in several forms. In most instances, these polygenic diseases may

FIGURE 7-11
Endothelial cell injury plays a crucial role in atherosclerosis. Hyperlipidemia and thrombosis are major contributing factors. PDGF, platelet-derived growth factor.

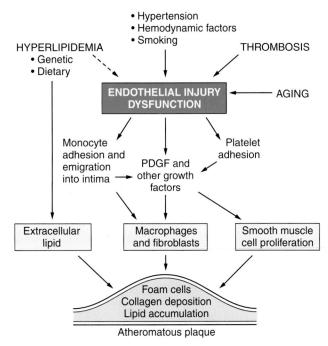

Atheromatous plaque

be significantly modified by exogenous factors, most notably by the diet. Hyperlipidemias are aggravated by overeating, and especially by a diet rich in polyunsaturated fats, such as animal fats or coconut oil. A high-fiber diet that is low in fat, and the intake of vegetable oils, such as olive oil, have a favorable effect.

Secondary hyperlipidemia is most often encountered in obese people. Some of these persons have an underlying genetic predisposition which, combined with overeating, results in an overall increased deposition of fat in the body. Because the tissue fat is in equilibrium with the circulating lipids, the increased total body fat leads to hyperlipidemia. Overall, obese people develop atherosclerosis at an earlier age and have more pronounced atherosclerotic lesions than do age-matched controls of normal habitus. Several disturbances of intermediate metabolism affect the metabolism of fats, but the most important disease in this category is *diabetes mellitus*. Diabetes predisposes individuals to atherosclerosis and also aggravates the course of the disease. Thus, most diabetics whose disease is *inadequately controlled* develop arterial lesions early in life and have more prominent atherosclerosis than those whose diabetes is controlled with a strict diet or insulin.

- *Hypertension.* Clinical studies have shown that hypertension correlates with atherosclerosis. If the hypertension develops at an early age and is not properly controlled, it will accelerate the development of atherosclerosis. Medical control of hypertension has greatly contributed to the reduced incidence of atherosclerosis in the United States that has been observed during the last two decades. The exact role of hypertension in the development of atheromas is not fully understood. Hypothetically, it is possible that the elevated pressure of the blood compresses the intimal cells, making them ischemic or stimulating them to release some cytokines that promote atherosclerosis or initiate proliferation of smooth muscle cells. The jet stream of blood could also contribute to the *insudation* of lipids into the vessel wall, a process likened to forceful filtration of plasma across the intimal layer. Finally, hypertension may cause changes in the clotting system by damaging the *platelets,* causing their aggregation and the release of bioactive substances from their cytoplasm.

- *Clotting factors.* Soluble clotting factors, such as fibrin, thrombin, and platelets, play an important role in the initiation of atherosclerotic lesions. The exact mechanism of action of the clot on the endothelium and the underlying smooth muscle cells is poorly understood. However, it has been shown that aspirin, which prevents clotting, may reduce the incidence of atherosclerotic complications, if given prophylactically.

- *Cigarette smoking.* Epidemiologic studies have implicated cigarette smoking as one of the most important risk factors of atherosclerosis. The adverse effects of cigarette smoke on blood vessels are not fully understood, but they are partially related to nicotine and partially related to tar and other harmful components of smoke. It is hoped that the campaign against smoking will contribute further to the decreased mortality from atherosclerosis. In Eastern European countries and the Far East, where smoking is still highly prevalent, the incidence of atherosclerosis is still on the rise.

- *Behavior.* Clinical studies indicate that constant stress may accelerate or aggravate atherosclerosis, but such claims are not fully documented and therefore not generally accepted. It appears that individuals who are under constant pressure to perform develop atherosclerosis more often than relaxed phlegmatics. However, the lifestyle of the overachievers is so much different from those who "take it easy" that it is not possible to separate the consequences of "endogeneous personality trait" from the influences of the environment in which they live. It is widely accepted, however, that a healthy lifestyle—work and relaxation practiced in moderation, and a healthy dose of exercise interjected on a regular basis—can reduce the risks of atherosclerosis.

Did You Know?

Hyperlipidemia, one of the most important risk factors for atherosclerosis, can be treated medically with drugs that inhibit endogenous cholesterol formation or promote cholesterol excretion in the bile. However, the best way to prevent hyperlipidemia is to eat a low-fat diet, to exercise, and to try not to gain too much weight. Persons who have a genetic form of hyperlipidemia should be placed on a low-fat diet as soon as the genetic disease is diagnosed, and that sometimes means even in childhood.

Atherosclerosis of the Aorta

Atherosclerosis of the aorta is a very common finding in older men. Almost all persons older than 50 years of age have atherosclerosis of the aorta of some degree. The lesions vary from mild to severe and may be focal to diffuse. Clinically, such lesions may be symptomatic, but most often, they are asymptomatic.

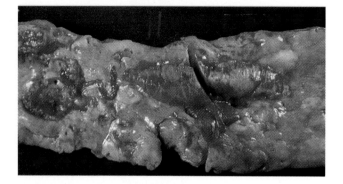

FIGURE 7-12
Gross appearance of an atherosclerotic aorta. The surface of the aorta is rugged and irregular.

The mildest forms of atherosclerosis are found in young or middle-aged persons. Such individuals have fatty streaks, slightly raised fibrotic plaques, and only occasionally, atheromas. As the disease progresses, the atheromas become more numerous and coalesce, occupying large surface areas. Atheromas may rupture, at which time they are covered with thrombi that narrow the lumen of the aorta or distort the blood flow. Calcifications of the atheromas and the fibrous tissues surrounding them reduce the elasticity of the blood vessel. In the final stages of the disease, the aorta transforms into a rigid, calcified tube that has a rugged, partially ulcerated, internal surface covered focally with thrombi (Fig. 7-12).

The atherosclerotic aorta cannot adapt to the changes of blood pressure that occur during the normal cardiac contraction cycle. Because the aorta cannot expand during systole, *hypertension* develops as the same amount of blood now passes through a narrower blood vessel. The pressure from inside causes dilatation of the inelastic aorta, which leads to the formation of an *aneurysm.*

Aneurysms are dilatations of the aortic lumen that may occur in several forms. Most often, they are spindle-shaped (*fusiform*) or appear as eccentric dilatations (*saccular*) (Fig. 7-13). Aneurysms can occur in any part of the aorta. Atherosclerotic aneurysms are most often located in the abdominal aorta.

Aneurysms are often clinically silent, and many are discovered accidentally during a detailed medical examination. The major danger is that the aneurysm may rupture and cause death by exsanguination. In such cases, the jet of blood may also dissect through the wall of the aorta and form a periarterial second lumen. Such bulging lesions are called *dissecting aneurysms.*

Aneurysms can be resected surgically and replaced by an artificial vessel made of Dacron or some similar plastic material. Rupture of aneurysms is associated with high mortality.

Peripheral Vascular Disease

Peripheral vascular disease refers to atherosclerosis involving the arteries that supply the blood to the extremities and the major abdominal organs, such as the intestines and kidney. Atherosclerosis of the peripheral arteries is common in elderly people, diabetics, and in those who have hyperlipidemia and hypertension. It is often part of a generalized atherosclerosis and is associated with atherosclerosis of the aorta and coronary and cerebral arteries. From a

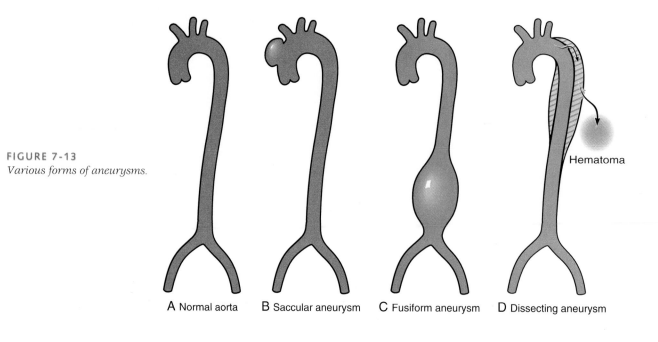

FIGURE 7-13
Various forms of aneurysms.

A Normal aorta   B Saccular aneurysm   C Fusiform aneurysm   D Dissecting aneurysm

Hematoma

clinical point of view, it is customary to distinguish between symptoms caused by ischemia of the major organs and those caused by ischemic changes in the extremities.

Atherosclerosis of the renal arteries is common in persons with atherosclerosis of the aorta. The renal arteries originate from the aorta and are relatively short. Thus, aortic atherosclerosis easily spreads into the renal arteries. Because the renal arteries are much narrower than the aorta, symptoms caused by their occlusion are often more prominent. Reduced flow of blood through the renal arteries causes hypoperfusion of the kidneys, which results in reduced renal functional capacity. This renal dysfunction, combined with an increased release of *renin* (a hormone produced by the kidney in response to ischemia), leads to hypertension. Reduced excretion of urine and urinary sodium further aggravates hypertension which, in turn, damages the kidneys. Atherosclerosis may thus cause irreversible (end-stage) kidney failure.

Atherosclerosis of the intestinal arteries causes ischemia in the small and large intestines. Such ischemia may be chronic or acute. Chronic ischemia caused by narrowing of the arteries and partial occlusion of their lumina is the most common form. Chronic ischemia usually has a gradual onset and causes nonspecific gastrointestinal problems: constipation, poor digestion, intolerance of certain foods, and malabsorption. These symptoms may fluctuate, but generally they are progressive. Many older persons have chronic constipation and a variety of other intestinal ailments.

Acute occlusion of the intestinal arteries causes massive intestinal infarction. Usually, it is a consequence of thrombotic or embolic occlusion of a major intestinal artery. Intestinal infarction is associated with a high mortality.

Atherosclerosis of the extremities typically affects the legs more often than the arms. It may present as *chronic ischemia* or as *acute occlusion* of the blood flow.

Chronic ischemia of the lower limbs secondary to the progressive narrowing of the femoral artery or popliteal artery results in underperfusion of the leg muscles. When a person is at rest or moves around slowly, the blood supply is adequate and no symptoms are present. However, if the same person walks a long distance or tries to run, the blood supply becomes inadequate and the leg muscles develop cramps. This is called *intermittent claudication* (from the Latin term *claudicatio,* meaning limping). Surgical cleansing of the vessels (*endarterectomy*) or removal of the atheromas with catheters may improve the clinical picture.

Sudden occlusion of the arteries, usually at the level of one of the smaller branches, results in gangrene. The necrotic tissue, which is typically black and mummified (*dry gangrene*), may become infected and diffluent (*wet gangrene*). Both forms of gangrene require surgical treatment, which usually entails resection of the extremity.

Coronary Heart Disease

Atherosclerosis of the coronary arteries may present in several clinical forms, all of which have the same underlying pathogenetic mechanism: myocardial ischemia. The clinical presentation depends on several factors:

- Extent of the occlusion (Fig. 7-14)
- Rapidity with which the ischemia develops
- Extent of atherosclerosis in other branches of the coronary system
- Anatomic location of the occluding lesion
- Presence or absence of other changes, and of diseases, such as hypertension or hyperthyroidism, which may complicate the course of ischemia

Myocardial ischemia may develop owing to a slowly progressive narrowing of the coronary arteries or a sudden occlusion. Chronic progressive ischemia results in hypoperfusion of the myocardium

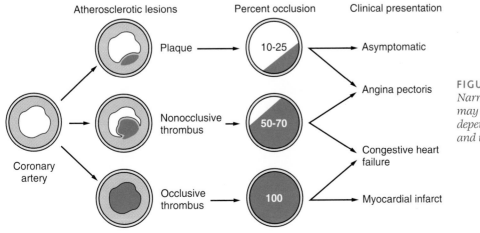

FIGURE 7-14
Narrowing of the coronary artery may cause different clinical symptoms depending on the extent of occlusion and the speed at which it develops.

Atherosclerotic lesions — Plaque → Percent occlusion 10-25 → Clinical presentation: Asymptomatic

Coronary artery — Nonocclusive thrombus → 50-70 → Angina pectoris

Occlusive thrombus → 100 → Congestive heart failure / Myocardial infarct

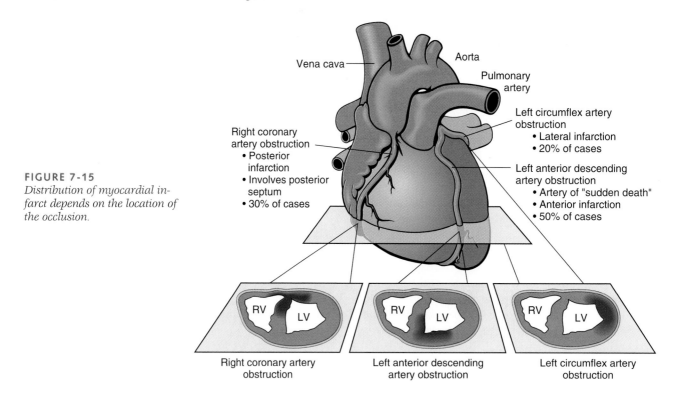

FIGURE 7-15
Distribution of myocardial infarct depends on the location of the occlusion.

Vena cava

Aorta

Pulmonary artery

Left circumflex artery obstruction
- Lateral infarction
- 20% of cases

Right coronary artery obstruction
- Posterior infarction
- Involves posterior septum
- 30% of cases

Left anterior descending artery obstruction
- Artery of "sudden death"
- Anterior infarction
- 50% of cases

RV   LV
RV   LV
RV   LV

Right coronary artery obstruction

Left anterior descending artery obstruction

Left circumflex artery obstruction

and slowly evolving pump failure. The patient may be asymptomatic or have precordial pain, known as angina pectoris. Ultimately, progressive ischemia leads to congestive heart failure. Coronary thrombosis is common in arteries narrowed by atherosclerosis.

Sudden occlusion of a major coronary artery results in an infarct in an anatomically defined area. Thus, an anterior wall infarct is typically caused by occlusion of the descending branch of the left coronary artery, an infarct of the lateral wall of the left ventricle is usually the result of occlusion of the circumflex branch of the left coronary artery, and an infarct of the right ventricle and the posterior wall of the left ventricle is usually caused by occlusion of the right coronary artery (Fig. 7-15). Occlusion of the anterior descending branch of the left coronary artery accounts for approximately 50 percent of all cases, whereas the right coronary artery is occluded in 30 percent to 40 percent of cases, and the remaining 15 percent to 20 percent of cases involve occlusion of the left circumflex artery.

Pathology. The coronary arteries affected by atherosclerosis are typically transformed into rigid, heavily calcified cylinders that can be palpated beneath the epicardium as thick nodular sinews. On cross-sectioning, their lumina are narrowed owing to prominent fibrotic plaques and atheromas (Fig. 7-16). The wall of the coronary arteries contains deposits of calcium salts. In acute occlusion, the plaques may be covered with fibrinous clots occluding the narrowed

lumen. In older lesions, such thrombi are partially organized by granulation tissue that has grown into them from the vessel wall. Some thrombi appear to be recanalized—that is, traversed by numerous small blood vessels that have reestablished blood flow across the occluded segment of the artery.

Sudden occlusion of a coronary artery leads to *myocardial infarction.* An infarct is characterized by ischemic cell death, which can be recognized morphologically first by typical microscopic changes and then by macroscopic changes in the heart (Fig. 7-17).

The first light microscopic changes occur approx-

FIGURE 7-16
Coronary atherosclerosis accompanied by marked narrowing of the lumen of the coronary artery and an intraluminal thrombus.

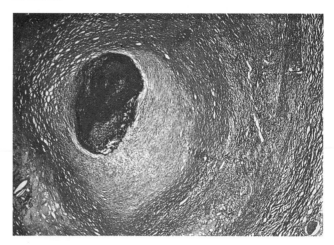

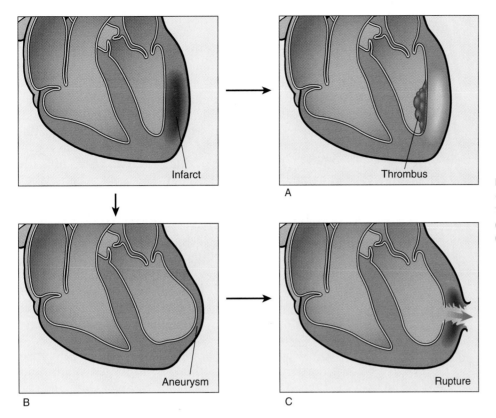

imately 24 hours after the onset of occlusion. These include nuclear signs of cell death, such as pyknosis, karyorrhexis, and karyolysis; cytoplasmic signs of coagulation necrosis; and the appearance of the first inflammatory cells, polymorphonuclear neutrophils (PMNs). PMNs predominate during the next 2 days, and then on day 3 to 4, the infarcted area becomes infiltrated with macrophages. Macrophages persist in the lesion from approximately a week after occlusion, during which time they phagocytize and remove the necrotic myocardial cells. Toward the end of the first week, the infarct is invaded by granulation tissue composed of small blood vessels, myofibroblasts, and fibroblasts depositing extracellular matrix. In older infarcts, fibroblasts predominate and the collagenous matrix is more prominent. Ultimately, the necrotic myocardium is replaced by a fibrous scar.

These histologic changes correlate with the macroscopic findings. On gross examination, the infarcted area cannot be definitively identified during the first 1 to 2 days. There may be some pallor of the infarcted area, but this is not prominent. Approximately 3 to 5 days after the occlusion, the infarct becomes yellow and is surrounded by a hemorrhagic rim. The yellow infarcted myocardium is softened as a result of the action of hydrolytic enzymes released from the leukocytes. This softening is most prominent toward the end of the first week after occlusion. Softened myocardium may rupture, causing sudden death secondary to bleeding into the pericardial sac (*hematopericardium*).

The ingrowth of granulation tissue, which brings into the infarcted area new blood and connective tissue, imparts to the infarct a grayish red and mottled appearance that persists for 1 to 2 weeks. Thereafter, cross-sections of the heart show that fibrosis predominates; old infarcts appear as whitish gray, firm, and irregularly shaped scars that are slightly depressed and easily distinguishable from the brown color of normal myocardium.

Complications. *Complications* of myocardial infarction may include the following:

- *Myocardial rupture.* Softened necrotic myocardium may rupture as a result of the increased pressure of the blood within the ventricle. The blood that penetrates through the ruptured left ventricle fills the pericardial sac, compressing the heart (hematopericardium). *Cardiac tamponade*—compression of the heart by blood in the pericardial cavity—typically occurs 5 to 7 days after infarction and usually is lethal (Fig. 7-18).
- *Cardiac aneurysm.* Massive myocardial infarcts of the left ventricle, which are replaced by fibrous scars, bulge under the pressure of blood in the left ventricle, forming a ventricular aneurysm. The heart is dilated and contracts irregularly because the fibrous scar forming the wall of the aneurysm does not contain contractile elements.
- *Mural thrombus.* The endocardium overlying the infarcted myocardium is often damaged and dis-

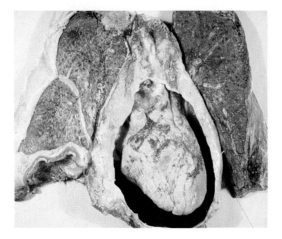

FIGURE 7-18
Hematopericardium caused by rupture of an infarct.

rupted. The blood within the ventricle coagulates in contact with the necrotic endocardium or the exposed myocardium and forms a thrombus attached to the wall of the ventricle (the Latin term *mural* means pertaining to the wall). Such thrombi impede the blood flow and weaken the contraction of the ventricular myocardium, which may contribute to heart failure. Furthermore, fragments of the thrombus may detach, giving rise to *emboli,* which can cause infarcts in distant organs. Cerebral infarcts caused by such emboli are an important complication of myocardial infarcts.

Clinical Features. Coronary heart disease may present clinically as

- congestive heart failure
- angina pectoris
- myocardial infarct (Fig. 7-19)

Congestive Heart Failure. Most of the symptoms of coronary heart disease are a consequence of hypoxia of the myocardium, which results in pump failure.

Because the heart does not pump blood efficiently, back pressure from stagnant blood impedes the venous blood return to the heart. Right ventricular failure causes congestion of the peripheral organs and extremities. Typically, the legs become swollen, especially toward the end of the day. The chronic passive congestion also causes enlargement of the liver. The enlarged liver stretches the capsule, and this stimulates the nerves in the capsule, causing pain below the right costal margin. In addition, pressure in the abdominal veins may lead to the accumulation of fluid in the abdominal cavity (i.e., formation of *ascites*). These changes are schematically shown in Figure 7-20. Failure of the left ventricle leads to pulmonary congestion and *pulmonary edema* secondary to transudation of fluids into the alveoli. *Pleural effusions* also develop, and patients become short of breath (i.e., develop *dyspnea*). In severe heart failure, dyspnea is present at all times. In milder cases, dyspnea develops only when the patient exercises or works strenuously.

Hypoperfusion of the major organs impairs their functions. Owing to the lack of oxygen, brain functions are slowed, and patients become somnolent, cannot concentrate, and easily develop mental fatigue. Hypoperfusion of the kidneys results in a reduction in urine formation (*oliguria*). Renal failure causes retention of sodium and water, which results in generalized edema, called *anasarca.* Affected patients die of progressive heart failure and multiple organ failure.

Angina Pectoris. The myocardium that is inadequately perfused may function normally until additional demands are made by exercise, climbing of stairs, or running. This additional effort cannot be sustained because the narrowed blood vessels do not allow influx of blood into the myocardium. The resulting ischemia causes pain, which is called *angina pectoris,* the Latin term for chest pain. Attacks of angina pectoris are typically precipitated by exercise or strain and can be alleviated by nitroglycerin, a

FIGURE 7-19
Coronary heart disease may present as angina pectoris, congestive heart failure, or myocardial infarct.

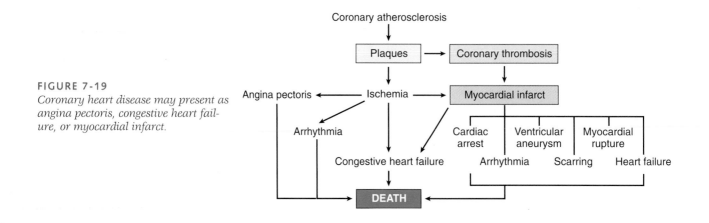

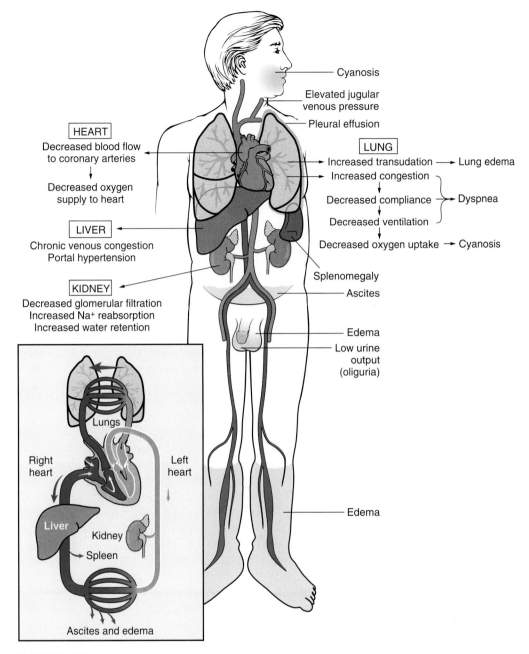

Cyanosis

Elevated jugular venous pressure

Pleural effusion

HEART
Decreased blood flow to coronary arteries

Decreased oxygen supply to heart

LUNG
Increased transudation → Lung edema

Increased congestion

Decreased compliance → Dyspnea

Decreased ventilation

Decreased oxygen uptake → Cyanosis

LIVER
Chronic venous congestion
Portal hypertension

Splenomegaly

Ascites

KIDNEY
Decreased glomerular filtration
Increased Na⁺ reabsorption
Increased water retention

Edema
Low urine output (oliguria)

Edema

Lungs

Right heart

Left heart

Liver

Kidney

Spleen

Ascites and edema

FIGURE 7-20
Chronic passive congestion. Left heart failure leads to pulmonary edema. Right ventricular failure causes peripheral edema that is most prominent in the lower extremities.

drug that dilates the vessels. However, as the atherosclerosis progresses, nitroglycerin becomes less and less efficient.

Myocardial Infarct. Rapid, sudden occlusion of a coronary artery causes an infarct. Myocardial infarct is a serious condition. Sudden death occurs in approximately 25 percent of cases. In most cases, this is a consequence of major arrhythmia (*ventricular fibrillation*), *heart block,* and subsequent pump failure, or *asystole* (cardiac arrest). Patients typically experience crushing precordial pain, often followed by loss of consciousness or fainting. By the time the infarct is recognized, the patient is prostrate, without a pulse, and in severe distress. Unless cardiothoracic resuscitation is initiated immediately, death occurs within minutes. Even with closed chest cardiac massage, mouth-to-mouth resuscitation, and electric shock treatment to restart the heart, the results are poor if the asystole has lasted a few minutes.

Among the 75 percent of patients who survive the onset of an acute myocardial infarct, most develop signs of heart failure and cardiogenic shock (Fig. 7-21). As a result of inadequate perfusion of

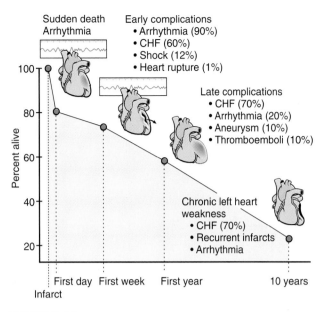

FIGURE 7-21

Outcome of myocardial infarct. Immediate death, early complications (first week), and later complications account for the 40 percent mortality during the first year after the infarct. The 10-year survival rate is approximately 25 percent. CHF, congestive heart failure.

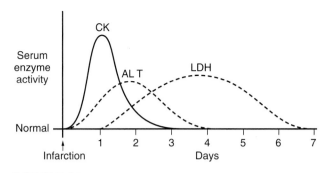

FIGURE 7-22

Enzymatic diagnosis of myocardial infarcts is based on the measurement of creatine kinase (CK), alanine aminotransferase (ALT), and lactic dehydrogenase (LD).

tissues by blood from the failing heart, multisystemic major organ failure develops. Most dangerous are the consequences of cerebral ischemia, which may lead to permanent mental injury and loss of central nervous system functions. Any cerebral ischemia that lasts longer than a few minutes irreversibly damages the brain; the patient becomes *decerebrated* (i.e., without higher nerve functions, like a vegetable). Minor ischemic damages of the brain may cause paralysis or impair motor or mental functions.

Many other organs may be affected, but the *kidneys* are the organs most often damaged. Typical signs of renal failure, such as oliguria, and anuria, are common. Therefore, it is important to monitor urine output in these patients. To this end, most patients in coronary intensive care units have an indwelling urinary catheter.

Diagnosis. The diagnosis of myocardial infarction is made on the basis of typical complaints (e.g., chest pain, shortness of breath, fainting, etc.), as well as clinical and laboratory findings. Electrocardiography and the measurement of enzymes released from the damaged myocardium into the serum are most useful in this respect. The electrocardiogram (EKG), the precardial recording of heart action currents, shows typical changes, and these can be corroborated by other findings. Myocardial infarction is most notably associated with an elevation in creatine kinase (CK), alanine aminotransferase (ALT), and lactate dehydrogenase (LDH) levels. These enzymes rise in

serum in a predictable manner: first CK, then ALT, and finally, LDH. Elevated LDH levels persist the longest (Fig. 7-22).

Newer laboratory tests are based on the fact that myocardial structural proteins, such as myosin, are also released into the blood from damaged heart cells. Troponin elevation in serum has proven to be a most useful laboratory sign of myocardial infarction. This test yields positive results 4 to 6 hours after occlusion of a coronary artery.

Treatment. With modern therapy, the survival of patients with myocardial infarction has improved considerably. Nevertheless, 30 percent to 40 percent of all patients die during the first year. These statistics include acute mortality and death from various complications, or the recurrence of infarcts. The remaining patients recover to a variable extent and lead a normal life. Most require periodic medical control and medication for the rest of their lives. Many undergo a coronary artery bypass to repair the sites of arterial occlusion. Unfortunately, the damaged heart cannot be repaired, but in severe cases, the damaged heart can be replaced with a newly transplanted heart. Cardiac transplantation is currently reserved for younger persons.

Hypertension and Hypertensive Heart Disease

The pressure generated by the left ventricle for the ejection of blood into the aorta is called arterial pressure. It is measured by a sphygmomanometer on the cubital artery. Normal blood pressure is usually in the range of 120 mm Hg during systole and 80 mm Hg during diastole. During exercise, running, vigorous work, or excitement, the blood pressure rises, but subsequently returns to normal values. Individuals with systolic pressures exceeding 160 mm Hg or diastolic pressures greater than 90 mm Hg have **hy-**

Table 7-2 Hypertension

Form of Hypertension	Cause	Treatment
Essential	Unknown	Drugs
Secondary		
Renal	Kidney disease	Treatment of underlying kidney disease
Endocrine	Adrenocortical tumor	Surgery
	Adrenomedullary tumor (pheochromocytoma)	Surgery
Neurogenic	Complex/psychological	Sedatives
Drugs	Examples: oral contraceptives, nasal decongestants, pain-killers	Discontinuing drug intake

pertension. Clinically, hypertension is classified as mild, moderate, or severe.

Etiology and Pathogenesis. In most hypertensive patients (>90 percent), no specific cause(s) for the elevated blood pressure can be found. These people have **primary** or **essential hypertension**. Although the pathogenesis of essential hypertension remains unknown, many contributing factors have been identified, including genetic determinants, occupation, lifestyle, and diet. Even though the causes and mechanisms of essential hypertension are unknown, this disease can be treated successfully with modern drugs and appropriate changes in lifestyle and eating habits.

In approximately 10 percent of patients, the cause of hypertension is an underlying disease or a medication, or it is related to a physiological event, such as pregnancy. These forms of hypertension are called **secondary**. Treatment of the underlying causative disease typically cures the hypertension. The most common causes of secondary hypertension are listed in Table 7-2.

The primary determinants of blood pressure are the *volume of circulating blood,* the *cardiac output,* and the *void space volume* of the cardiovascular system that has to be filled with the circulating blood (Fig. 7-23). Each of these determinants can be modified upward or downward. Therefore, normal blood pres-

sure can be either decreased (*hypotension*) or increased (*hypertension*). A *normotensive* state results from a balanced interaction of the physiologic determinants of blood pressure and their regulators.

Blood Volume. The blood volume is determined by many factors, such as age, body size, and, gender. Seventy percent of the human body is made up of water, and the fluids in circulation are in balance with those in the interstitial spaces in tissues, as well as the intracellular fluids. Various physiologic factors regulate the passage of fluids from one body compartment to another and the accumulation of fluids in these compartments. The intake of fluids and the elimination of surplus fluids through the kidneys, intestines, sweat and excrement, and body secretions are all tightly regulated.

Two examples of the importance of blood volume are presented here. A person with exsanguination secondary to a stab wound will become hypotensive. During such hypotensive shock, the kidneys stop producing urine in order to prevent fluid loss so that the perfusion of the vital organs can be maintained. Diametrically opposing events occur in kidney failure, when pathologically altered kidneys cannot eliminate fluid by excreting it in urine. In such instances, fluids overwhelm the body and overburden the circulation. To pump the extra fluid, the heart must generate increased systolic pressure. When an overburdened heart fails, the diastolic pressure also rises because some blood that cannot be ejected remains in the cardiac chambers. This process causes hypertension, which can usually be treated successfully with diuretics (drugs that increase excretion of urine).

Cardiac Output. Cardiac output can be calculated according to a formula that takes into account the capacity of the heart to pump blood, the amount of blood filling the chambers (*volume load*), and the resistance that it has to overcome in the aorta (*pressure*

Did You Know?

CABAGE is used for treatment of coronary atherosclerosis. This term does not refer to the leafy vegetable; it is the acronym for the surgical procedure used to revascularize the heart: coronary artery *b*ypass grafting. More than 100,000 CABAGE procedures are performed every year in the United States.

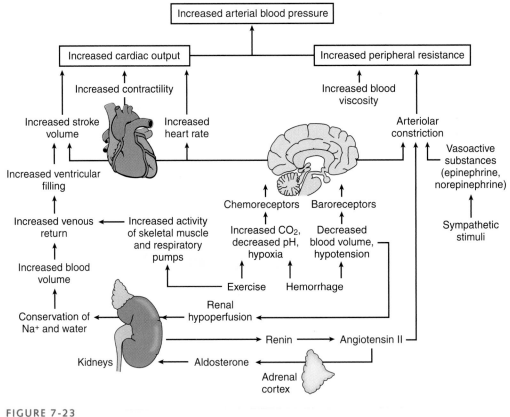

FIGURE 7-23
Regulation of arterial pressure. Increased blood pressure (hypertension) could result from increased cardiac output or increased peripheral resistance.

load). Any stimulus that increases the contractility of the heart, such as adrenaline (secreted from the adrenals in stress) or thyroid hormones (which increase the heart rate), can cause hypertension. Exercise or excitement, both of which are associated with the release of numerous vasoactive and cardiostimulatory substances, has a similar effect.

Peripheral Resistance. Peripheral resistance is regulated at many sites, but most importantly, at the level of the arterioles. The walls of these precapillary vessels are composed of smooth muscle cells that can contract, thereby reducing the capillary blood flow. At the same time, the constricted arterioles increase resistance to the blood entering them from larger arteries, and this is transmitted backward to the aorta and the left ventricle. The left ventricle, confronted with increased resistance in the arterial system, must increase pressure, which leads to hypertension.

The arterioles are critical for regulating blood pressure. The arterioles react to a number of humoral substances that cause their constriction or relaxation and dilatation. Many neurotransmitters bind to the alpha- and beta-adrenergic receptors on the cell membrane of smooth muscle cells in arterioles. Thus, hormonal and neural factors may directly af-

fect this most important regulator of blood pressure in the arterial system.

The most important regulator of arteriolar tonus is the *renin-angiotensin system*. *Renin* is a hormone secreted by the juxtaglomerular apparatus in the kidney. Renin acts on a liver-derived polypeptide called *angiotensin I* and transforms it into *angiotensin II*, which produces vasoconstriction of the arterioles and directly increases blood pressure. Angiotensin II also stimulates the adrenal cortex to release aldosterone. *Aldosterone* is a hormone that acts on the renal tubules to increase resorption of sodium. Sodium retention in the kidney is accompanied by retention of fluid, which also contributes to the elevation of blood pressure. Drugs, such as angiotensin-converting enzyme (ACE) inhibitors, or antagonists of aldosterone, are used effectively in the treatment of hypertension. Diuretics that increase the excretion of sodium and water in urine are also widely used. Atrial natriuretic factor is a natural antagonist of renin and angiotensin, and it also lowers the blood pressure.

Pathology. The morphologic consequences of hypertension are seen in the heart and the peripheral vessels, especially in the kidney, brain, and eye. The heart becomes enlarged (*cardiomegaly*), primarily as a consequence of the concentric hypertrophy of the left ventricle, which increases in thickness from a normal 1.2 cm to 2.5 cm. Histologic examination reveals all muscle fibers to be thickened. Because the enlarged muscle cells need more blood than do normal cells, single cells often die owing to ischemia and are replaced with fibrous tissue. Myocardial fibrosis is, thus, a common histologic finding in cardiomegaly.

Inefficient pumping of the blood from the left ventricle leads to back pressure, which increases pulmonary artery pressure. This, in turn, causes more work for the right ventricle and will eventually cause hypertrophy of the right ventricle. The hypertrophy of the left ventricle is the most common cause of right ventricular hypertrophy. Clinically, the functional consequences of right ventricular hypertrophy and failure are called *cor pulmonale.*

Vascular pathology is an important complication of hypertension. Hypertension accelerates the development of atherosclerosis. In the heart, it is one of the major risk factors for ischemic heart disease. In the peripheral vascular system, hypertension-related changes are most prominent in the arterioles and small arteries. Long-standing hypertension, also known as *benign hypertension,* causes hyalinization of the arterioles and fibrosis of the small arteries. *Malignant hypertension,* which is of sudden onset, may cause fibrinoid necrosis of these vessels. Concentric hyperplasia of the smooth muscle cells in arterioles (which produces so-called onion bulb–like rings) usually accompanies sustained hypertension. Renal ischemia caused by the narrowing of arterioles triggers the release of renin from the juxtaglomerular cells, aggravating the hypertension even more.

Hypertensive encephalopathy is an important complication of hypertension. This term refers to vascular changes in the brain that usually cause acute or chronic cerebral ischemia. Microscopic signs of ischemia, such as focal cell death and microinfarcts, can be detected on histologic examination of the brain. Such patients may have only minor mental problems (e.g., forgetfulness), but often they are rather incapacitated. Hypertensive strokes, caused by sudden rupture of damaged brain arteries, present as intracerebral hemorrhages that can be recognized on gross examination of the brain. Hypertensive strokes produce major neurologic symptoms (e.g., paralysis) and are often lethal. Because of more efficient means of treating hypertension, hypertensive strokes are less common today than 50 years ago.

Retinal changes are an important complication of hypertension because they may impair vision and can eventually cause blindness. Retinal arteries are easily seen with the ophthalmoscope, and retinal changes are among the first signs of hypertension that can be clinically documented. The eye examination is, therefore, an important part of the physical work-up of any patient with hypertension.

Rheumatic Heart Disease

Rheumatic heart disease (RHD) is a major feature of rheumatic fever. **Rheumatic fever** is a systemic, immunologically mediated disease related to streptococcal infections. In addition to the heart, RHD involves the joints, the subcutaneous connective tissue of the skin, and occasionally, the brain. Previously, RHD was an important cause of morbidity and mortality. Although worldwide, there are more than 15 million new cases diagnosed every year, in the United States, the incidence of this disease has decreased dramatically. This is primarily the result of the widespread use of antibiotics and more efficient treatment of the bacterial infections that invariably precede RHD.

Etiology and Pathogenesis. The causes of RHD are not known, although all the scientific evidence collected so far indicates that streptococcal infections of the throat and the upper respiratory tract play a crucial role (Fig. 7-24). Rheumatic fever typically occurs 2 weeks after an episode of "strep throat." The immune response of the body elicited by the streptococcal antigens provides the body with a defense mechanism against the infection, which clearly is beneficial. However, at the same time, the immune reaction damages the connective tissue of the heart and several other organs. It has been postulated that the antibodies against the streptococcal antigens cross-react with similar antigens found in the human heart. In addition to antibodies, the immune response includes a cell-mediated immune reaction which involves lymphocytes and macrophages. Although it is not known whether the initial tissue injury is mediated by antibodies or a cellular immune reaction, it seems that cellular and humoral immune reactions take place.

Antibodies to the streptococcal antigen O, called antistreptolysin-O (ASO), develop in essentially all patients with rheumatic fever. Such antibodies are clinically important because their appearance in the blood of a patient indicates a recent infection. It is, however, worth noting that not all patients with elevated ASO titers develop rheumatic fever. This shows that the streptococcal antibodies, by themselves, are not dangerous, and that some other conditions must be met before rheumatic fever develops. Activation of a T-cell–mediated cellular reaction, which accounts for the pathologic changes in the heart, apparently occurs only in susceptible persons.

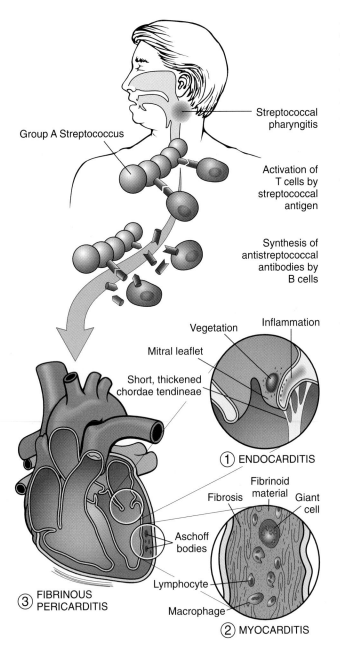

to an ulceration. Surface defects are covered with fibrin thrombi, which progressively grow and assume the form of larger *vegetations* or *excrescences.* Ongoing inflammation inside the valves leads to destruction of the valves, followed by fibrous scarring that causes valve deformities (Fig. 7-25). The chordae tendineae inserting into the mitral valve are typically shortened and thickened, and become fused to one another.

RHD affects the left heart more than the right heart. Owing to the deformity of the leaflets and the changes in the chordae, the valves become incompetent and do not close completely during systole; alternatively, the orifice may become stenotic (from the Greek *stenosis,* meaning narrowing), preventing normal flow of blood from one chamber into another. Mitral *valvular insufficiency* causes reflux of blood across the mitral valve from the ventricle into the atrium during systole. In *aortic insufficiency,* the blood flows back from the aorta into the left ventricle during the diastole. The ventricles of such hearts are dilated and hypertrophic.

Mitral stenosis causes stagnation of blood in the left atrium, which is transmitted into the pulmonary circulation and into the right ventricle. The typical consequences of mitral stenosis are, therefore, left atrial, pulmonary, and right ventricular hypertension, all of which contribute to the clinical entity known as cor pulmonale.

Aortic stenosis impedes the blood flow from the left ventricle into the aorta. To overcome the increased resistance at its outflow tract, the left ventricle increases the ejection pressure, causing left ventricular hypertrophy. As long as the left ventricle is compensated, there are no major clinical symptoms. However, when the hypertrophic heart fails, the back pressure of the blood is transmitted from the left ventricle into the left atrium and into the pulmonary circulation, again resulting in cor pulmonale.

Myocarditis is common in RHD. The histologic hallmark of RHD is the presence of *Aschoff bodies,* which consist of aggregates of lymphocytes and macrophages around a central zone of fibrinoid necrosis. Aschoff bodies destroy the myocardium. Such lesions are relatively small and rarely cause massive myocardial dysfunction. However, if the Aschoff bodies are in the area of the conduction system, they may cause dysrhythmias or cardiac conduction problems.

Pericarditis is found only in severe cases of RHD. Typically, it causes friction between the roughened epicardium and pericardium and is associated with pain. The pericardial sac typically contains fibrin-rich fluid. Pericardial fibrosis and adhesions develop in chronic cases.

FIGURE 7-24
Pathogenesis of rheumatic fever. Following infection ("strep throat"), an immune response elicited by the streptococci acts on the heart and several other organs, most notably the joints, skin, and central nervous system. In the heart, it causes endocarditis, myocarditis, and pericarditis.

Pathology. RHD is a pancarditis; that is, it involves all the layers of the heart, and thus may present as endocarditis, myocarditis, pericarditis, or all of these conditions combined.

Endocarditis is an inflammation of the internal surface lining of the heart chambers. The most prominent changes are seen on the endocardium covering the valves of the left heart. This valvulitis begins with inflammation of valvular surface, leading

AORTIC VALVE

MITRAL VALVE

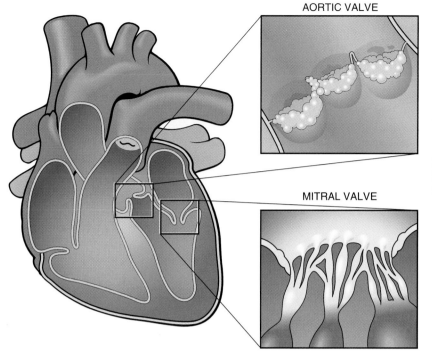

FIGURE 7-25
Chronic rheumatic endocarditis. Mitral and aortic valves are most often involved.

Clinical Features. Rheumatic fever affects children and young adults. The disease is multisystemic and, therefore, cardiac involvement is just one of its symptoms. The diagnosis of rheumatic fever is based on Jones' criteria, which are subclassified as major and minor. Jones' major criteria are (1) polyarthritis (i.e., joint inflammation), (2) carditis (i.e., inflammation of the heart); (3) chorea, a neurologic disorder characterized by involuntary movements caused by brain lesions; (4) subcutaneous nodules; and (5) erythema marginatum, a peculiar skin disease that reflects the changes in the subcutaneous connective tissue. Jones' minor criteria include joint pain (arthralgia), fever, evidence of a group A streptococcal infection preceding the disease, a previous bout of rheumatic fever, an elevated erythrocyte sedimentation rate, and EKG signs of heart damage. Rheumatic fever is diagnosed if two major criteria or one major and two minor criteria are fulfilled.

Complications of RHD are common. Bacterial endocarditis is the most prevalent complication because the thrombotic vegetations on the valves are readily infected. Valvular vegetations also give rise to emboli, which cause infarcts of the brain, kidney, or the extremities.

Rheumatic carditis cannot be cured. Accordingly, most of the lesions that develop are irreversible and can be treated only by surgery. Calcified, deformed valves can be excised and replaced with artificial valves—made of metal and plastic or derived from animal (e.g., pig) valves—that are surgically implanted into the heart. Such interventions prolong the life of these patients who otherwise would die from heart failure.

Infectious Diseases of the Heart

The heart is prone to infections, most of which originate from microbes carried by the blood. As a rule, bacterial and fungal infections affect the endocardium, causing **endocarditis.** Viral and parasitic infections affect the myocardium and cause **myocarditis. Pericarditis** may be caused by viruses or bacteria.

Endocarditis

Bacterial infections of the cardiac valves cause an erosion of the surface layers, allowing entry of the bacteria into the valves. Destruction of the connective tissue ensues because of the action of the bacterial lytic enzymes. The defect of the surface endocardium is soon covered with fibrin and platelet thrombi that serve as nidi to attract even more thrombogenic material. These small bumps on the valves grow rapidly and enlarge into wart-like structures—hence, the term *verrucous endocarditis* (Fig. 7-26). These vegetations or excrescences are more abundant than in rheumatic endocarditis. In contrast to the valvular vegetations of rheumatic endocarditis, which represent sterile thrombi, the verrucae of infectious endocarditis are also composed of thrombi, but they contain bacteria. Bacteria invade the valves,

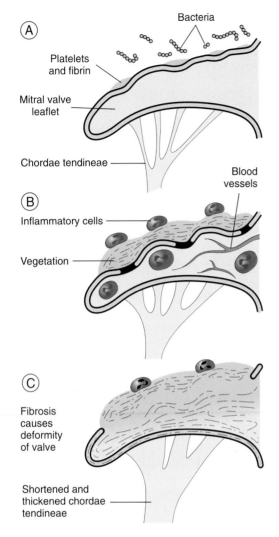

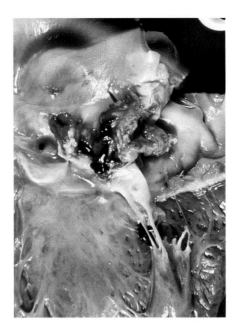

FIGURE 7-27
Bacterial endocarditis. The valves are covered with extensive vegetations.

FIGURE 7-26
Bacterial endocarditis. (A) The initial site of endothelial injury is covered with a fibrin clot, which is infected with bacteria. (B) Inflammatory cells from the blood invade the thrombus. The valve is infiltrated with inflammatory cells and contains blood vessels. (C) The inflammation heals by fibrosis, which causes deformity of the valve.

causing intravalvular inflammation, which, in turn, destroys portions of the valves, thereby causing deformities (Fig. 7-27). Surface defects (ulcers) are common. Severely inflamed valves may rupture.

Infected valvular vegetations may break off and give rise to *septic emboli,* most often involving the brain and kidneys, and the tips of the extremities (Fig. 7-28). Because these thromboemboli contain bacteria, they cause not only ischemic infarcts, like the sterile vegetations of the rheumatic endocarditis, but also form new foci of infection. These *septic infarcts* transform into *microabscesses.*

Bacterial endocarditis may involve normal valves, but most often affects valves that have been altered by some other pathologic process. Individuals with

valves previously destroyed by rheumatic endocarditis and those with congenital valvular defects are especially prone to infection. Cardiac surgery, and even cardiac catheterization, also may damage the valves and predispose them to infection.

Endocarditis is most often caused by pyogenic bacteria, such as staphylococcus and streptococcus. Gram-negative bacteria and even fungi may be isolated from some patients, especially those who have been receiving anticancer therapy and are immunosuppressed and weakened by the disease and the chemotherapy. Mixed infections are a cause of endocarditis in drug addicts who inject themselves intravenously using nonsterile instruments.

Clinical Features. The clinical features of bacterial endocarditis are variable. The disease may present as a febrile illness of sudden onset (*acute bacterial endocarditis*) or as a lingering weakness accompanied by mild temperature elevations that wax and wane over a prolonged period of time (*subacute bacterial endocarditis*). The most characteristic findings are the numerous murmurs produced by the blood flowing over the deformed valves. Because the valves cannot close completely, valvular insufficiency develops, and the blood regurgitates from the aorta into the left ventricle or from the left ventricle into the left atrium. All of these abnormalities impose an increased workload on the heart, ultimately leading to heart failure.

Bacterial endocarditis is more common in the left than in the right heart. Detached vegetations give

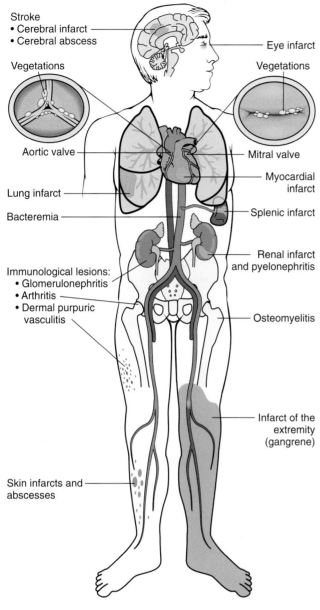

FIGURE 7-28
Septic emboli from endocarditis are carried by the arterial circulation and may lodge in major organs, causing infarcts and new sites of bacterial infection.

Labels on figure:
Stroke
• Cerebral infarct
• Cerebral abscess
Vegetations
Aortic valve
Lung infarct
Bacteremia
Immunological lesions:
• Glomerulonephritis
• Arthritis
• Dermal purpuric vasculitis
Skin infarcts and abscesses
Eye infarct
Vegetations
Mitral valve
Myocardial infarct
Splenic infarct
Renal infarct and pyelonephritis
Osteomyelitis
Infarct of the extremity (gangrene)

rise to arterial emboli. Symptoms of peripheral embolization and dissemination of infection through the septic thromboemboli produced "in showers" contribute further to the progression of the disease. The most dangerous are emboli of the central nervous system. Bacteremia with shaking chills is very common because bacteria are constantly released into the circulation from the infected valves. This may occur even without evidence of embolic phenomena. Endocarditis in drug addicts typically affects the tricuspid valve and causes pulmonary emboli and abscesses.

Bacterial endocarditis can be treated with antibiotics. Treatment may be prolonged until all the bacteria are eradicated. Dysfunctional, deformed, and defective valves remaining after the infection must be surgically replaced with artificial valves.

Myocarditis

Infections affecting the myocardium are typically caused by viruses, such as Coxsackie B virus, or parasites, like Toxoplasma or Trypanosoma. These intracellular microorganisms cannot survive outside the cells, so they must invade the myocardium to survive. In the myocardial cells, they damage the vital organelles and cause cell death. This weakens the myocardium and contributes to heart failure. In addition, the myocardium is invaded by T lymphocytes that are attracted there by the virus. T lymphocytes secrete various biologically active substances (cytokines), such as TNF and interleukins, which are supposed to kill the virus. However, cytokines also kill virus-infected myocardial cells and may have other untoward effects on the heart.

The symptoms of myocarditis are vague and the diagnosis of this disease cannot be made easily. Affected patients usually present with mild fever, shortness of breath, and other signs of heart failure, such as tachycardia, peripheral cyanosis, pulmonary edema, and precardial pressure pain. Severe myocarditis may be indistinguishable from acute myocardial infarction. Viral myocarditis may cause widespread interstitial fibrosis, which clinically presents as dilated cardiomyopathy and progressive heart failure that is resistant to conventional therapy.

Pericarditis

Pericarditis is a term used to describe inflammation of the pericardium as well as of the epicardium, as the inflammation of one of the layers lining the pericardial sac invariably causes changes in the other. Pericarditis may be isolated, but it is most often associated with other infections of the heart, such as myocarditis. Additionally, infections involving the adjacent thoracic structures may spread to the pericardium. Tuberculous pericarditis secondary to lung tuberculosis was common previously, but is rare today.

Pericarditis may be caused by bacteria, viruses, and rarely, by fungi. Rheumatic pericarditis is a form of pancarditis that is typical of severe RHD. Several autoimmune disorders, such as systemic lupus erythematosus, may also affect the pericardium. Finally, inflammation of the pericardium and epicardium can be caused by metabolic waste products that accumulate in the blood in uremia. Trauma and radiation in-

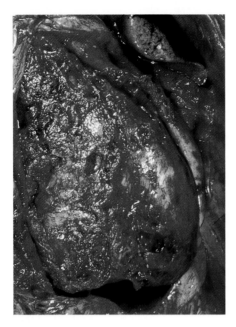

FIGURE 7-29
Pericarditis. The surface of the heart is covered with fibrin and blood, and appears "shaggy."

jury also may cause sterile inflammation. Open heart surgery usually causes sterile pericarditis.

Pathology. Pericarditis is always associated with exudation of fluid into the pericardial sac. The fluid is clear yellow in *serous pericarditis,* and such fluid usually accompanies viral infections. *Serofibrinous* exudate is associated with more severe damage, and is typically found in those with rheumatic fever or early bacterial infection. Fibrin-rich exudates give the heart a "bread-and-butter" appearance, as when one takes apart two slices of bread covered with butter (Fig. 7-29). *Purulent exudate* is a hallmark of bacterial infections and is caused by pus-forming bacteria, such as staphylococci and streptococci.

Cardiomyopathy

Cardiomyopathy, a relatively noncommittal term (literally meaning an ailment of the heart), is used to describe a group of diseases affecting the myocardium. In response to injury, the heart may undergo dilatation or hypertrophy. Cardiomyopathy is divided into three forms:

- Dilated cardiomyopathy
- Hypertrophic cardiomyopathy
- Restrictive cardiomyopathy

In *dilated cardiomyopathy,* the ventricles are markedly dilated and the heart appears to have a myocardium that is either flabby or thinned and that has partially been replaced by fibrous tissue. Among the identifiable causes of this heart disease, alcohol figures highly. Some cases of dilated cardiomyopathy are precipitated by viral myocarditis, but in most instances, the disease has no obvious causes. Anticancer drugs, such as doxorubicin (Adriamycin), may cause similar changes owing to their cumulative cardiotoxicity.

Hypertrophic cardiomyopathy is marked by extensive thickening of the left ventricular myocardium. The cause for this hypertrophy is unknown. The disease typically affects young males, but it can also occur in a familial form that affects males and females equally and is inherited as an autosomal dominant trait. The gene for this familial form of hypertrophic cardiomyopathy has recently been isolated.

The third form of cardiomyopathy is called *restrictive* because the heart cannot expand adequately to receive the inflowing blood. In most cases, this occurs because the myocardium is infiltrated with some abnormal material, such as amyloid. In *endocardial fibroelastosis,* a disease of unknown origin characterized by thickened endocardium, the ventricles cannot dilate.

Cardiomyopathies are incurable diseases and the only hope is heart transplantation.

Cardiac Tumors

Primary tumors of the heart are extremely rare. The only benign tumor worth mentioning is atrial myxoma. This tumor, which is typically polypoid, attaches to the mitral valve and protrudes into the left atrium. It may occlude the mitral orifice.

Secondary tumors may involve the heart; most often, these are spread to the pericardium and surface of the heart from the lung. Myocardial metastases are rare. Apparently, the constantly contracting heart does not provide a fertile environment for growing tumor cells.

Iatrogenic Heart Lesions

Iatrogenic (meaning "doctor-induced" in Greek) lesions of the heart are becoming increasingly prevalent. These include drug- and radiation-induced diseases and surgery-related cardiac changes. Drugs may affect the heart directly and/or indirectly. Many cardiac drugs used to enhance heart function, such as digitalis, are toxic in large doses. Several anticancer drugs, such as doxorubicin, are cardiotoxic.

Radiation therapy delivered to the chest area for the treatment of breast or lung cancer may damage the heart. This occurs only after long-term therapy and high-dose irradiation. The most prominent changes are seen in the epicardium and pericardium; these lead to obliterative fibrous changes (constrictive pericarditis) and may impair the function of the heart.

Surgery is performed often, mostly to repair occluded coronary arteries. Other operations—such as artificial valve insertion and, most recently, heart transplants—are also performed in considerable numbers. In most instances, these operations have few serious complications. Pericarditis caused by blood in the operating field on the surface of the heart may cause adhesions between the epicardium and pericardium, some postoperative pain, and minor discomfort. Functional consequences are rare. The intraoperative death rate is currently in the range of 1 percent to 2 percent.

Cardiac transplants are performed to replace hearts terminally damaged by myocarditis, cardiopathy of unknown origin, and genetic diseases. Younger persons are the prime candidates for such transplantations, which can prolong life considerably. As hearts are transplanted from unrelated donors, the foreign heart almost invariably elicits an immune response in the host. Immunosuppressive drugs are given routinely during the postoperative period and, sometimes, for the rest of the patient's life. Cardiac biopsies are used to monitor the immune reaction against the grafted heart and to determine the appropriate dosage of immunosuppressive drugs. Overall, the results of cardiac transplantation have been most encouraging. The only reasons that more cardiac transplantations are not performed are

the high costs and the insufficient supply of hearts for transplantation.

Arterial Diseases

Atherosclerosis is the most important disease affecting the blood vessels. All other diseases account for less than 1 percent of clinically recognized arterial lesions. Among these are various forms of autoimmune **arteritis,** such as *polyarteritis nodosa;* diseases of unknown origin, such as *giant cell arteritis;* a functional disturbance of arterial contractility called *Raynaud's disease;* and *Buerger's disease,* which affects both arteries and veins of the extremities.

Polyarteritis nodosa is an autoimmune disorder affecting medium-sized and small muscular arteries. As the name implies, it is an inflammation (hence the suffix *itis*) that involves many vessels (*poly* meaning many in Greek). The disease is thought to result from immune complexes formed between antibodies and an antigen, which may be either endogenous (autoantigen) or exogenous (e.g., a virus). The immune complexes are deposited in the wall of the arteries. In the vessel wall, the immune complexes activate complement, which attracts neutrophils. These neutrophils then invade the artery, causing destruction of the vessel wall and fibrinoid necrosis. Damaged arteries often become completely occluded by thrombi that form at the site of injury. Local destruction of the vessel wall results in the formation of microaneurysms.

Polyarteritis nodosa is a multisystemic disease. Symptoms affecting the heart, brain, and kidney predominate in severe cases, whereas nonspecific symptoms involving minor organs abound in other patients. Overall, the clinical picture, the course of the disease, and its outcome are variable and unpredictable. The treatment of choice is the administration of immunosuppressive drugs, but this is often ineffectual.

Giant cell arteritis is a disease of unknown etiology. On histologic examination, this disease is characterized by infiltrates of macrophages and giant cells in the media of medium-sized arteries, causing obliteration of their lumina. Temporary arteries on the lateral side of the head are most often involved, and these arteries resemble tortuous wires coursing beneath the skin. This is typically a disease of the elderly, affecting an estimated 1 percent of all people older than 80 years of age. Usually, giant cell arteritis produces no serious complications, but some patients have visual problems that result from ischemic changes in the eyes.

Raynaud's disease is a functional disturbance affecting the muscular arteries and arterioles. These vessels contract in a disorderly manner, especially in cold weather. This causes ischemia of the distant parts of the body—typically, the tips of the fingers and toes. Upon reheating, the spasm of the arteries subsides, and the blood returns to the extremities.

Diseases of the Veins

In considering the importance of diseases affecting the veins, it is worthwhile to reiterate the following basic facts:

- Veins have thinner and structurally different walls than arteries and do not have the capacity to contract to adjust to the blood flow or to regulate it like the arteries. Moreover, the veins do not respond to adrenergic stimuli the same way as do arteries and arterioles. Thus, veins are not directly affected by the diseases that damage arteries, such as atherosclerosis and hypertension.
- Blood flow in the veins occurs at a lower pressure than in the arteries. However, veins can more easily accommodate an increased amount of blood in their lumina. Thus, back pressure from the failing heart may easily increase the pooling of blood in the veins.
- Back pressure causes retrograde flow and stagnation of blood in the veins. Veins have valves that oppose backflow of blood, but these venous valves easily become incompetent when the veins dilate.
- Once the veins have become dilated, they tend to remain so. Tortuous, dilated veins are called *varicosities* or **varicose veins** (the Latin *varix* meaning dilated vein).
- The slow flow of blood in the veins predisposes an individual to clotting. Clotting is even more likely in dilated varicose veins and those in which the back pressure from the failing heart causes stagnation of the blood. This most often occurs in the leg veins.

Varicose veins develop most often in the lower extremities (Fig. 7-30). Varicose veins are a multifactorial disease with a genetic and environmental component. They are most likely to occur in individuals from families known to have a hypothetical "connective tissue weakness." People in professions that require long hours of standing, like hairdressing or sales, develop such changes more often than those whose jobs do not require long periods of standing. Many women develop varicose veins during pregnancy, in part as a result of the increased blood pressure in the pelvic veins compressed by the pregnant uterus and the subsequent stagnation of blood in the leg veins. Thrombotic occlusion of the veins (**throm-**

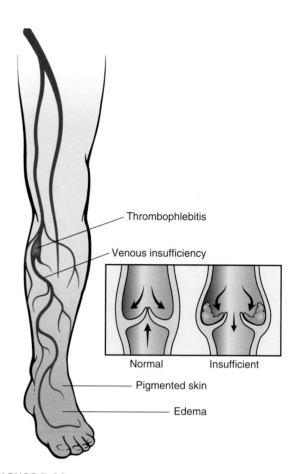

FIGURE 7-30
Varicose veins of the calf. The inset shows venous valvular insufficiency, which accounts for the reflux of blood.

bophlebitis), which prevents the outflow of venous blood, also predisposes individuals to varicosities.

The blood flow in the varicose veins is turbulent and slow. This favors clotting, and thrombi frequently form. Such thrombi are organized by granulation tissue, and the lumen of the vein may become recanalized. However, some thrombi may become loosened and may be embolized to the lungs.

Varicose veins do not drain the blood adequately from the leg, causing pooling of the blood in the lower parts of the leg. Blood leaks from the distended small capillaries and veins into the tissue. The brownish discoloration of the skin in such cases is attributable to the accumulation of blood pigment in the subcutaneous connective tissue. The skin is dry and scaly and shows small, pinpoint hemorrhages from ruptured capillaries. This is called *stasis dermatitis*. Owing to ischemia, the skin may necrotize and a stasis ulcer may form. This is also called *trophic ulcer* (in Greek, *trophein* means feeding) because it evolves in inadequately nourished (ischemic) skin. Stasis ulcers do not heal easily, and if all treatment fails, the affected limb must be amputated.

Lymphatic Diseases

As mentioned previously, the lymphatics are minute channels permeating almost all soft tissue and many internal organs. As a result, they are involved in all inflammatory and circulatory disorders, and many neoplastic disorders, affecting various tissues and organs. Diseases limited to the lymphatics are rare in clinical practice.

Lymphangitis refers to an acute inflammation confined mostly to the lymphatics of an extremity. Typically, such infections are caused by pyogenic bacteria that enter into a skin defect and penetrate to the local lymphatics. The subcutaneous lymphatics can be viewed as extending from the site of entry to the local lymph nodes (typically, from a finger along the forearm to the cubitus or even the axilla). Enlargement of local lymph nodes is common. Lymphangitis can be readily cured by aggressive antibiotic therapy.

Review Questions

1. Compare the anatomy and function of the right and left heart.
2. Compare myocardium with endocardium and pericardium.
3. Compare systole and diastole.
4. Compare arteries and veins.
5. What is the function of lymphatics?
6. How common are cardiovascular diseases?
7. What is the most common cause of heart failure?
8. How common are congenital heart diseases?
9. What is the most common cause of congenital heart disease?
10. List three well-documented causes of congenital heart disease.
11. Compare the blood flow in the early stages of ventricular septal defect with that in the cyanotic stage.
12. Relate the pathology of tetralogy of Fallot to the clinical findings in this condition.
13. What is atherosclerosis and how does it present clinically?
14. What are atheromas and how are they formed?
15. Explain the role of lipids and thrombi in the pathogenesis of atherosclerosis.
16. What are the main risk factors for atherosclerosis?
17. Compare familiar (primary) and secondary hyperlipidemia.
18. What is the evidence that cigarette smoking is a risk factor for atherosclerosis?
19. What are the complications of atherosclerosis?
20. Describe various forms of aneurysms.
21. What clinical symptoms could be caused by atherosclerosis of renal or intestinal arteries?
22. Explain how atherosclerosis can cause intermittent claudication or gangrene of the extremities.
23. What are the principal determinants of the clinical presentation of coronary heart disease?
24. What is the location of myocardial infarctions caused by an occlusion of the left or right coronary artery?
25. Compare the consequences of sudden occlusion of a coronary artery with those of gradual occlusion.
26. List the most important complications of myocardial infarction.
27. Compare the pathogenesis of postinfarction rupture of the myocardium and ventricular aneurysm.
28. What are the pathologic findings in congestive heart failure?
29. Explain the pathogenesis of angina pectoris.
30. How is myocardial infarct diagnosed?
31. What are the causes of primary and secondary hypertension?
32. Explain the pathogenesis of hypertension.
33. What are the main pathologic changes caused by hypertension?

34. How is rheumatic fever related to streptococcal throat infection?

35. Describe the cardiac pathology caused by rheumatic fever.

36. What are Jones' criteria for diagnosing rheumatic fever?

37. Explain the pathogenesis of infectious endocarditis.

38. List the most common complications of infectious endocarditis and relate them to typical clinical symptoms caused by these lesions.

39. Describe the pathology and list the common causes of myocarditis.

40. Describe the pathology and list the common causes of pericarditis.

41. Describe the pathology and list the common causes of cardiomyopathy.

42. Which iatrogenic heart lesions are considered to be related to treatment?

43. What is the main cause of arteritis?

44. What are the main clinicopathologic forms of arteritis?

45. What are the main diseases affecting veins?

46. What is the cause of lymphangitis and how does this disease present clinically?

Learning Objectives

After reading this chapter, the student should be able to:

1. Describe the normal respiratory system and its main functions.

2. List common causes and symptoms of upper respiratory infection.

3. Discuss the pathogenesis, etiology, and symptoms of epiglottitis and laryngitis.

4. Compare acute tracheobronchitis and bronchopneumonia.

5. List the common causes and discuss the pathogenesis of pneumonia.

6. Compare bacterial and viral pneumonia.

7. Describe the pathogenesis and typical lesions of pulmonary tuberculosis.

8. Define chronic bronchitis and describe typical lesions and complications of this disease.

9. Define emphysema, its pathologic changes and clinical symptoms.

10. Discuss the pathogenesis, pathologic changes, and symptoms of bronchial asthma.

11. Discuss sarcoidosis and chronic immune-mediated lung diseases.

12. Define pneumoconiosis and list three common causes of this pulmonary disease.

13. Discuss the pathogenesis of adult respiratory distress syndrome.

14. Discuss the possible causes and the public health significance of respiratory tract cancer.

15. Describe the typical location, gross appearance, and histologic findings associated with various forms of lung cancer.

16. Discuss the pathogenesis of pleurisy and the differential diagnosis of pleural effusions.

Additional Key Terms and Concepts

Bronchiectasis

Bronchitis

Emphysema

Pleuritis

Pneumonia

Tuberculosis

Chapter Outline

The Respiratory System
Chapter 8

The respiratory system can be divided into three parts. The upper and middle respiratory system have traditionally been the domain of *otorhinolaryngologists,* or ear-nose-throat (ENT) specialists. The lower respiratory tract is considered to be the domain of thoracic surgeons and respiratory disease specialists, also known as *pulmonologists.*

NORMAL ANATOMY AND PHYSIOLOGY

The upper respiratory tract comprises the *nose,* the paranasal sinuses, the pharynx, and the larynx (Fig. 8-1). The primary function of these structures is to provide entry for inhaled air, thus enabling respiration. The mucus covering the nasal mucosa serves as a trap for bacteria and foreign particles. Air passing

through the upper respiratory tract is warmed up and moistened.

The air may be inhaled not only through the nose, but also through the mouth. From either entry site, it then reaches the *pharynx,* a structure included in the respiratory and digestive systems. From the pharynx, the air passes through the *larynx,* a highly specialized neck structure that also serves as a speech organ. The larynx is contiguous with the trachea, a long tube located in the midline of the thorax. The *trachea* bifurcates, giving rise to the right and left main bronchi, which enter the lung parenchyma and branch into numerous smaller bronchi. The *bronchi* extend into bronchioli, which terminate blindly in respiratory bronchioli, alveolar ducts, and *alveoli.* The alveoli and the corresponding terminal bronchiole form a functional unit called an acinus.

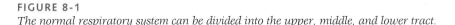

FIGURE 8-1
The normal respiratory system can be divided into the upper, middle, and lower tract.

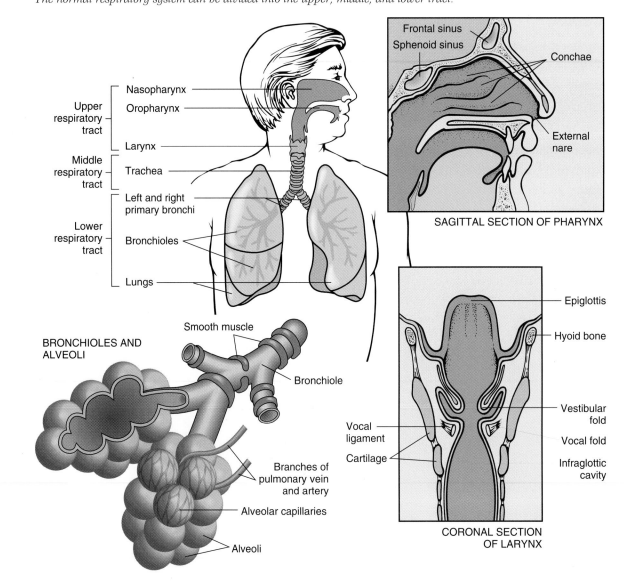

Approximately 5 to 7 acini are arranged into a pulmonary lobule, each of which is surrounded by a connective tissue septum. Pulmonary lobules are arranged into large units that form the pulmonary lobes. The right lung has three main lobes, whereas the left lung has two lobes.

The outer surface of the lungs is called the pleura. The pleura covering the lungs—visceral pleura—is continuous with the parietal pleura that covers the inside of the thoracic cage. These two layers of pleura delimit the pleural cavity. Pleural surfaces are moist, as the pleural cavity contains a few droplets of fluid that allow the pleural surfaces to slide over one another.

Histologically, the nasal cavity and the paranasal sinuses are lined by cuboidal epithelium composed of ciliated and mucus-producing cells. The function of these cells is to keep the air passages moist and to filter the air by retaining large particles and bacteria. The mucus contains bactericidal substances and provides protection against infection. The movement of the cilia helps to remove mucus from the air passages. This usually results in a nasal discharge which, as we all know, is a common feature of upper respiratory tract infections.

The pharynx and larynx are lined by squamous epithelium that is identical to the epithelium of the mouth. This epithelium is sturdy and provides protection against mechanical injury. This is most important in the pharynx, which serves as a passage for air as well as for the food and drinks ingested through the mouth. The mucosa of the pharynx is rich in lymphoid tissue, which is part of the immune system and serves as the source of antibodies and other protective substances. Lymphoid tissue undergoes hyperplasia during infection, which contributes to swelling of the throat.

The larynx is lined by squamous epithelium, which is essential for voicing. It is enclosed in a cartilaginous box that provides support and protection. Similar cartilaginous rings provide mechanical support to the trachea, keeping it patent for the passage of air. Below the larynx, the trachea and the bronchi are lined again with cuboidal epithelium (Fig. 8-2). This epithelium contains four cell types: ciliated cells, mucus-producing cells, neuroendocrine cells, and basal cells. The basal cells or reserve cells are the progenitors of all other more specialized cell forms and are thus considered to be developmentally pluripotent. Under pathologic conditions (e.g., with chronic cigarette smoke irritation), basal cells may proliferate and can give rise to squamous cells (squamous metaplasia). Most lung cancers originate from the bronchial epithelium. Histologically, these tumors may be composed of cell types normally found in the bronchial epithelium or cells formed by metaplasia. This explains why there are several histologic types of lung cancer.

The mucosa of the branches of the bronchial tree all the way to the respiratory bronchioli are lined by the same cells as the main bronchi. All of these anatomic structures also have a connective tissue–rich

FIGURE 8-2

Histology of bronchi and alveoli. Bronchi are lined by cylindrical epithelium that contains ciliated, mucus-secreting, and neuroendocrine cells, all of which originate from basal cells. The wall of the bronchi also contains smooth muscle cells and cartilage. Bronchioli do not contain cartilage. The alveoli are lined by flattened type I pneumocytes and surfactant-secreting type II pneumocytes. The alveolar walls contain centrally located capillaries that are separated from the alveolar lining cells by a thin space.

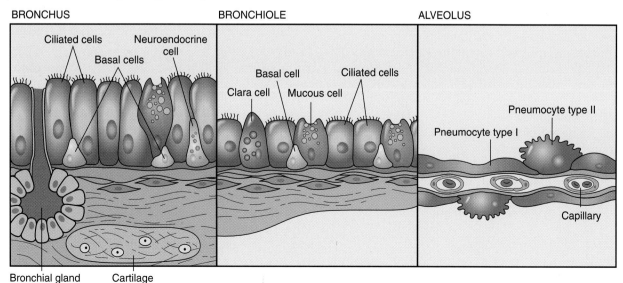

submucosa that contains contractile smooth muscle cells, bronchial glands, and also mucosal lymphoid tissue. The outer third of the bronchial wall, like the wall of the trachea, contains cartilage. As the caliber of bronchi diminishes upon their branching, their wall becomes thinner and finally, as the bronchi transform into bronchioli, the cartilage disappears from their wall.

The transition of bronchi into *alveoli* is abrupt and involves changes in the structure of the epithelium and the support structures. The alveoli are lined by *pneumocytes*. *Type I pneumocytes*, which account for 90 percent of the alveolar surface, are very thin cells designed to allow the passage of air from the alveoli into the blood. *Type II pneumocytes*, which are cuboidal cells, specialize in the production of pulmonary surfactant. **Pulmonary surfactant** is a mixture of lipids, proteins, and carbohydrates. It coats the alveoli with a very thin film which, because of its surface tension, keeps the alveoli open and prevents them from collapsing. The alveolar septa also contain thin capillaries sandwiched between two type I pneumocytes. There is almost no connective tissue between the capillaries and the pneumocytes, an essential factor in the normal passage of air across this respiratory surface. Connective tissue is found only around the acini—in the form of septa. Because the alveoli are so thin, they can be easily ruptured and destroyed, as often occurs in chronic lung disease.

The external surface of the lungs is covered with mesothelium and underlying connective tissue, similar to that forming the interlobular septa. The mesothelium is an epithelial layer that lines both the visceral and parietal pleura.

The lungs have a dual blood supply. The pulmonary artery brings venous blood from the right ventricle into the lungs to be oxygenated in the alveolar septa. The oxygenated blood leaves the lungs through the pulmonary veins, which drain into the left atrium. This functional **pulmonary circulation** provides no nutrients to the lung parenchyma. Oxygen and nutrients are brought into the lungs through the bronchial arteries, which originate in the thoracic aorta. The branches of the pulmonary and bronchial arteries are interconnected by anastomoses, but these are of limited functional significance under normal circumstances.

The primary function of the *lungs* is **respiration,** which includes the transfer of oxygen across the alveolar respiratory membrane into the blood, and the release of carbon dioxide and other gases generated inside the body into the air (Fig. 8-3). The preconditions for normal respiration are as follows:

- The airways must be patent.
- The lungs must be able to expand rhythmically during each respiratory movement.

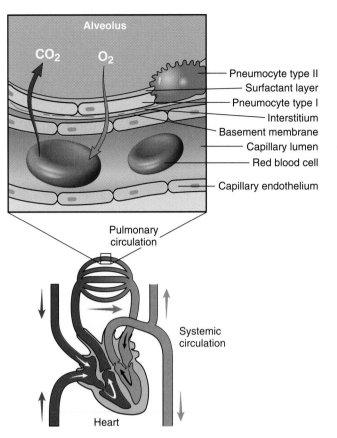

FIGURE 8-3
The primary function of the lung is gas exchange, which takes place in the alveoli. Oxygen enters the blood and is bound to red blood cells; this releases CO_2, which is then released into the alveolar air destined for expiration.

- The alveolar respiratory membrane must be intact.
- The action of the control centers of respiration in the central nervous system (CNS), as well as of the thoracic muscles and the diaphragm, must be properly coordinated.

Any interference with these normal physiologic conditions results in impeded respiration, which is called *dyspnea.*

In addition to respiration, the respiratory system has other functions as well. The larynx produces the voice. Laryngeal pathology may result in *aphonia,* or the inability to produce voice (derived from the Greek a, meaning without, and *phonos,* meaning voice). The mucosa of the respiratory system provides protection against infections. This is a function of the mucosa-associated lymphoid tissue (MALT). MALT forms tonsils in the nasopharynx and pharynx, and lymphoid follicles in the wall of the bronchi. Alveolar macrophages are yet another important component of the **respiratory defense system.** These phagocytic cells are expectorated from the lungs and can also be seen in the sputum. Pulmonary capillaries serve as the peripheral circulatory pool for leukocytes, and these cells can be mobilized from the lungs to the site of infection within a very short time.

The major metabolic function of the lungs is the maintenance of acid–base balance. Failure of this function may result in respiratory acidosis or alkalosis. The lungs also provide compensatory mechanisms for the metabolic acidosis or alkalosis caused by pathologic changes in the kidneys or gastrointestinal tract, or systemic metabolic disorders, such as lactic acidosis secondary to diabetes mellitus.

OVERVIEW OF MAJOR DISEASES

The respiratory tract may be affected by numerous diseases, the most important of which are

- infectious diseases
- immune diseases
- environmentally induced diseases
- circulatory diseases
- tumors

Several facts important to an understanding of respiratory pathology are presented here, before a discussion of specific pathologic entities.

1. *The respiratory system is open-ended and in direct contact with the environment.* As a result, *upper respiratory tract infections* (URIs) are extremely common and occur from infancy to old age. URIs may become so widespread that they are considered to be airborne epidemics, and even world-wide pandemics, as is often the case with influenza. Downward extension of infection into the bronchi or lungs leads to *bronchitis* or *pneumonia.* Pneumonia is still one of the most common causes of death in old people, and in patients with cancer or various forms of immunodeficiency, including acquired immunodeficiency syndrome (AIDS). Indeed, one sixth of all deaths in the United States are attributable to pneumonia.

2. *The respiratory system is exposed to many allergens inhaled in air.* Immunologic diseases of the respiratory tract are very common. The most prevalent of these diseases is *allergic rhinitis* or hay fever. *Bronchial asthma* is also common, especially among children and young adults. It should be noted that many chronic lung diseases have an immune component, and that the immune mechanisms help to eradicate infections, but also may contribute to their perpetuation or progression.

3. *Inhaled air contains pollutants, airborne particles, and gases, which may cause diseases.* Many environmentally induced lung diseases are considered to be occupation-related or related to air pollution. For example, coal-workers' lung disease is caused by particles inhaled in mines. Considerable progress has

been made to reduce air pollution and the dangers of occupational diseases. Nevertheless, cigarette smoking, an avoidable yet major cause of pulmonary diseases, still accounts for most chronic bronchitis, emphysema, and lung cancer. Pulmonary morbidity could be significantly reduced by eliminating cigarette smoking and further improving the quality of air in the human habitat.

4. *The heart and the lungs form a functional unit.* Cardiorespiratory dysfunction is common, especially in the elderly and in many patients with chronic disease. One could almost say that all those who have not suffered from brain death ultimately die of cardiorespiratory failure. Just as lung pathology has a profound effect on the heart, cardiac pathology almost invariably produces changes in the lungs.

The blood flow through the lungs depends on the propulsive forces of the right and left ventricle. Failure of the left ventricle results in the build-up of blood pressure within the left atrium, which is transmitted backward into the pulmonary veins, and then through the entire pulmonary vascular system into the right ventricle. This clinical condition, in which the right ventricle is working against increased pulmonary resistance, is called *chronic cor pulmonale.* Chronic cor pulmonale can also develop owing to vascular changes that develop secondary to chronic pulmonary disease. Other pathologic processes associated with narrowing, such as intrapulmonary thromboemboli, may have the same results.

Massive pulmonary thromboembolism, such as saddle emboli, may block the outflow tract of the right ventricle and cause *acute cor pulmonale.* Inability of the overburdened right ventricle to overcome the block in the pulmonary artery may cause death within minutes of the occlusion.

5. *Inhaled air contains many potential carcinogens.* Malignant tumors of the respiratory system are common. The most important of these tumors is *lung carcinoma,* which usually originates from the intrapulmonary bronchi.

All the currently available evidence indicates that lung cancer is, to a large extent, related to cigarette smoking. However, not all smokers develop cancer and not all lung cancers are caused by cigarettes. The role of individual susceptibility factors, genetic changes, oncogenes, and other carcinogens is being studied intensively.

Congenital Diseases

Developmental malformations of the respiratory system are of limited clinical significance. The only developmental anomaly worth mentioning is *tracheoesophageal fistula.* The trachea develops as an outpouching of the fetal foregut, which also gives rise to the pharynx and esophagus. Incomplete separation of the foregut results in a congenital fistula, a channel linking the esophagus and the trachea. It may be associated with esophageal atresia and other anomalies. It is usually diagnosed shortly after birth when it becomes evident that milk that is swallowed into the esophagus enters the trachea and is aspirated into the lungs. The defect can be surgically repaired, but such delicate operations are associated with considerable mortality.

Infectious Diseases

Infectious diseases of the respiratory tract are traditionally divided into two groups: diseases of the nose and upper respiratory tract (URIs), which are the most common; and *diseases of the lower respiratory tract* (e.g., pneumonia), which are the least common. Pediatricians also recognize the so-called *middle respiratory syndrome,* which includes childhood diseases involving the anatomic structures between the larynx on one side and the bronchioles on the other.

Respiratory tract infections account for 75 percent of all human infections diagnosed clinically, at least after minor skin infections and irritations have been eliminated from consideration. Most infections are limited to the upper respiratory tract; less than 5 percent involve the lungs. Lung infections are most prevalent in hospitalized patients, the elderly, drug addicts, alcoholics, and patients with AIDS. Even if one excludes patients with AIDS, most of whom die of lung infection, pneumonia is listed as the cause of death of 20,000 to 30,000 persons per year in the United States.

Upper Respiratory Infections

Clinically, URIs are most often recognized as common colds. They are characterized by acute inflammation involving either the nose, paranasal sinuses, throat, or larynx, or all of these structures together. These infections have a tendency to extend into the trachea and bronchi, and in a small number of patients, they may be complicated by pneumonia. In children, the infection often extends into the middle ear, causing otitis media (Fig. 8-4).

Etiology and Pathogenesis. Most URIs are caused by viruses. Because it is impractical to isolate viruses in every case, the presumptive diagnosis of a viral etiology is rarely confirmed. Nevertheless, like all other acute viral diseases, URIs are short-lived, heal spontaneously, and do not benefit from treatment with antibiotics. Epidemiologic studies show that the "flu" or common cold is most often caused by influenza virus, parainfluenza virus, and rhinovirus. These pathogens are airborne and tend to cause seasonal epidemics. Epidemics of influenza virus typically occur during the winter, whereas rhinovirus infections are usually the causes of spring and fall mini-epidemics.

URIs are popularly thought to be facilitated by exposure to cold, damp weather, or draft, but there is no scientific evidence to support this premise. On the other hand, it has been documented that physical exhaustion, old age, and general poor health predispose individuals to viral infections by lowering the body's defense mechanisms.

Viral URIs are self-limited diseases that heal spontaneously without any specific treatment. Nevertheless, viral URIs may predispose individuals to

FIGURE 8-4

Acute upper respiratory infection typically affects the nose and the nasopharynx, but it may spread into the middle ear, paranasal sinuses, or tracheobronchial tree.

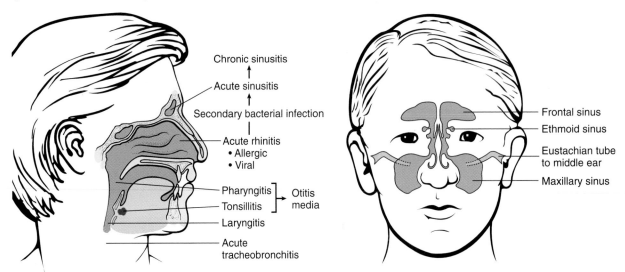

bacterial superinfections, the best known of which is streptococcal nasopharyngitis. Bacteria may spread into the adjacent anatomic structures and cause bacterial sinusitis, otis media, or mucopurulent bronchitis.

Pathology. The pathologic findings in URI are nonspecific. The mucosa of the nose and upper respiratory tract are congested, edematous, and infiltrated with inflammatory cells. In viral infections, the cell infiltrates consist of lymphocytes, macrophages, and plasma cells. Severe infections may cause ulceration of the mucosal epithelial lining, which allows the entry of bacteria. Bacterial infections elicit a reaction of polymorphonuclear neutrophils (PMNs), and many present with a fibrinopurulent exudate. This exudate may form whitish-yellow membranes on the mucosa of the throat, or purulent "plugs" in the crypts and mucosal lacunae of the tonsils. Pseudomembranes— i.e., necrotizing mucosal lesions covered with fibrin, pus, and cell detritus—are typical of diphtheria. Diphtheria is uncommon today because of widespread immunization that effectively prevents the infection.

Clinical Features. URI typically presents with nasal congestion and *rhinorrhea* ("runny nose"). Throat pain or discomfort on swallowing, sneezing, and a hacking cough are common symptoms. General malaise and mild fever are typical systemic manifestations. The disease lasts from a few days to 1 to 2 weeks and abates spontaneously. The appearance of a purulent nasal discharge, sinus or ear pain, and deep throat expectoration are usually signs of bacterial superinfection. In contrast to viral infections, bacterial superinfections do not resolve without antibiotics. "Strep-throat," documented by bacteriologic cultures of material obtained by throat swabs, requires a 7- to 10-day treatment course with antibiotics. If not eradicated, streptococcal infections may be complicated by rheumatic fever or acute glomerulonephritis.

Middle Respiratory Syndromes

The term middle respiratory syndrome (MRS) is used to denote infections of the larynx, trachea, and the major extrapulmonary bronchi. These diseases are most prevalent among children and include isolated laryngitis presenting as "croup," acute epiglottitis, and viral tracheobronchitis. Most often, MRS results from extension of a URI into the lower parts of the respiratory system, and it is commonly associated with pneumonia.

Clinically, it is often impossible to determine whether the infection is limited to the trachea and major bronchi or if it has spread into the smaller pulmonary airways as well. *Whooping cough*, or *pertussis*,

was previously the most important disease in this category. This disease is caused by *Bordetella pertussis* and presents with an unremitting cough. Today, most children are immunized against pertussis and the disease is rare in the Western world.

Croup. *Croup* is an acute, possibly life-threatening infection that involves the larynx (Fig. 8-5). This acute laryngotracheobronchitis is most common in children younger than 3 years of age. Clinically, it is marked by spasm of the vocal cords, which results in inspiratory stridor described as a "barking" or "brass cough." Croup is typically caused by parainfluenza virus, but may be attributable to other viral infections as well. There is no specific treatment for such viral infections. Nevertheless, the child must receive intensive care; in some cases, the larynx must even be intubated to prevent suffocation.

FIGURE 8-5
Acute inflammation of the larynx. (A) Inflammation localized to the epiglottis (so-called acute epiglottitis). (B) Inflammation of the entire larynx causing diffuse laryngeal swelling and laryngospasm (croup).

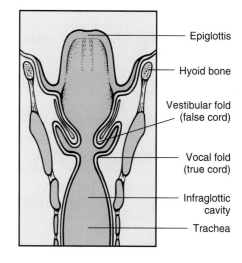

Epiglottis

Hyoid bone

Vestibular fold (false cord)

Vocal fold (true cord)

Infraglottic cavity

Trachea

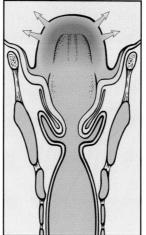

A   ACUTE EPIGLOTTITIS

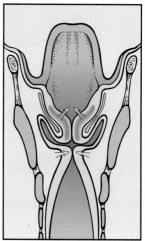

B   CROUP

Epiglottitis. *Epiglottitis* that is caused by *Haemophilus influenzae* has a peak incidence in school-aged children and adolescents. Clinically, it is characterized by a sudden loss of voice and hoarseness, and throat pain on swallowing (see Fig. 8-5). Edema and redness of the epiglottis and the surrounding inflamed pharyngeal mucosa cause narrowing of the air passage. This diagnosis is best confirmed by laryngoscopy, which usually reveals a "cherry-red epiglottis." Antibiotic treatment and supportive therapy with humidified oxygen mask are usually adequate. Occasionally, patients must be intubated to enable air passage so that they do not suffocate.

Bronchiolitis. Bronchiolitis is a term used for the acute childhood disease involving the bronchi and bronchioles but not extending into the alveolar spaces of the lungs. Pediatricians usually lump bronchiolitis together with other middle respiratory syndromes.

Bronchiolitis is a viral infection, and in more than 80 percent of cases, it is caused by the *respiratory syncytial virus*. Other viruses, such as parainfluenza and rhinovirus, can cause the same symptoms. The virus invades the epithelial cells of the bronchi and bronchioli, causing cell death and desquamation. It also incites an inflammatory infiltrate, which consists of lymphocytes, plasma cells, and macrophages. The edema of the small airways and the desquamation of dead cells causes obstruction of the bronchi and bronchioli.

The disease affects infants and small children and occurs in epidemics from fall until spring. Approximately 1 percent of all urban infants and even more of those in nurseries develop signs of bronchiolitis in the course of their first year of life. The clinical picture is dominated by wheezing respiration, low-grade fever, and shortness of breath. Unless pneumonia secondary to bacterial superinfection supervenes, spontaneous recovery occurs within 7 to 10 days.

Pneumonia

Pneumonia is an inflammation of the lung that occurs in two major forms: alveolar pneumonia, which is marked by intra-alveolar inflammation, and interstitial pneumonia, which primarily involves the alveolar septa (Fig. 8-6).

Alveolar pneumonia may be focal or diffuse (Fig. 8-7). Focal pneumonia may be limited to the alveoli, or it may involve both alveoli and bronchi. Focal intra-alveolar inflammation is typical of *hypostatic pneumonia*. It represents bacterial infection superimposed on the pulmonary edema of chronic heart failure, and it is most prevalent in debilitated elderly patients who are confined to bed. Pneumonia that is

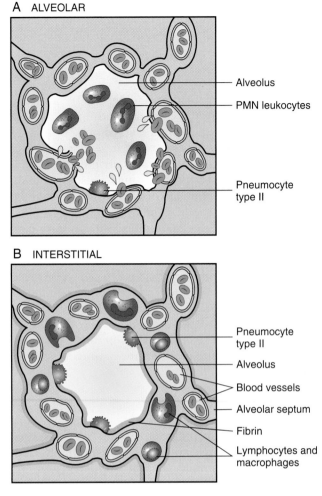

FIGURE 8-6
Diagrammatic representation of pneumonia. (A) Alveolar bacterial pneumonia. (B) Interstitial viral pneumonia. PMN, polymorphonuclear.

limited to the segmental bronchi and surrounding lung parenchyma is called *bronchopneumonia*. Widespread or diffuse alveolar pneumonia is called *lobar pneumonia*. Lobar pneumonia is often the end result of confluent bronchopneumonia in which the infection spreads from one lobule to another until the entire lung is involved.

Interstitial pneumonia is usually diffuse and often bilateral. In contrast to alveolar pneumonia, which is usually caused by bacteria, intestitial pneumonias are viral in origin.

Most bacterial and viral pneumonias are acute. Untreated or incompletely cured, acute pneumonia may become chronic. Recurrent pneumonias, as may occur in children affected by cystic fibrosis, are also classified as "chronic." Chronic pneumonia is typical of tuberculosis and certain fungal infections.

Etiology. Pneumonia may be caused by bacteria, viruses, or less commonly, by fungi, protozoa, or par-

A Bronchopneumonia

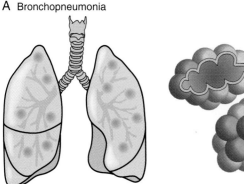

B Lobar pneumonia

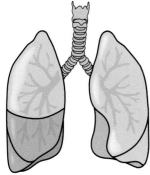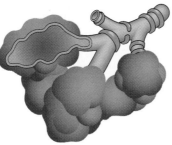

FIGURE 8-7
Clinically and pathologically, the lung infection may be localized (lobular pneumonia or bronchopneumonia) (A) or diffuse (lobar pneumonia) (B). Interstitial viral pneumonia is often bilateral and diffuse (C).

C Interstitial pneumonia

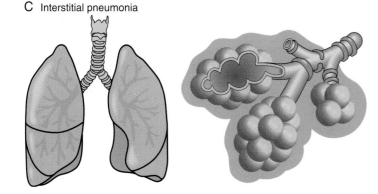

asites (Table 8-1). Bacteria are the most important pathogens and account for 75 percent of the cases of clinically diagnosed pneumonia.

Pneumonias may be classified etiologically as being caused by the following:

• Upper respiratory flora
• Enteric saprophytes
• Extraneous pathogens that are not normally associated with the human body

The normal flora of the upper respiratory tract is a mixture of bacteria. These bacteria, many of which are potential pathogens, normally exist in equilibrium within the human body and cause no disease. Nevertheless, if aspirated into the lower respiratory tract, they will cause pneumonia. The most important among these bacteria are Streptococcus, *H. influenzae,* and Staphylococcus.

The normal upper respiratory tract does not harbor anaerobic gram-negative bacteria, such as *Escherichia coli* or *Pseudomonas aeruginosa.* These bacteria are, however, part of enteric flora. Pulmonary infection may occur if enteric bacteria contaminate the airways or reach the lungs by blood circulation. Bacteria, such as *Legionella pneumophila* or *Mycobacterium tuberculosis,* as well as various fungi and viruses that are not normally present in the nasopharyngeal flora nor on other body surfaces may cause pneumonia if inhaled accidentally. For example, Legionella infection can occur following inhalation of bacteria from humidifiers. The first epidemic caused by this pathogen was isolated from infected members of the American Legion in 1977 and was actually traced to the contaminated air conditioning system of a Philadelphia hotel. Acute viral pneumonias are acquired by close contact with an infected person.

Table 8-1 Common Causes of Pneumonia

Causative Agents	Percentage of All Diagnosed Cases
Bacteria	
Streptococcus pneumoniae	50
Haemophilus influenzae	10
Staphylococcus aureus	5
Mycobacterium tuberculosis	5
Viruses	10
Influenza virus	
Fungi*	
Aspergillus fumigatus	—
Candida albicans	—
Pneumocystis carinii	—
Bacteria-like organisms	
Mycoplasma pneumoniae	10

*Opportunistic infection; rare except in immunosuppressed, debilitated, or terminally ill patients

Some viruses, like herpesvirus or cytomegalovirus (CMV), may be latent in the human body and may cause pneumonia by reactivation in immunosuppressed persons.

Pathogenesis. The pathogens responsible for pneumonia can reach the lung parenchyma through several routes, including the following:

- *Inhalation of pathogens in air droplets.* This is the typical means by which viral infections are spread. *M. tuberculosis* is also acquired by this mode.
- *Aspiration of infected secretions from the upper respiratory tract.* This is typical for streptococcal and staphylococcal infections.
- *Aspiration of infected particles in gastric contents, food, or drinks.* Such aspiration pneumonia is often caused by anaerobic bacteria and is common in people who are unconscious, those who have vomited, and those who have lost control of their body functions (e.g., alcoholics, drug addicts).
- *Hematogenous spread.* Bacteria may be transported to the lungs by the blood. Pneumonia is common in bacteremia (sepsis) and may develop secondary to urinary or alimentary tract infections. Contaminated foreign material introduced by intravenous self-injection is a common cause of pneumonia in drug addicts.

Pathology. Alveolar pneumonia presents in several forms. *Bronchopneumonia* typically begins with bacterial invasion of the bronchial or bronchiolar mucosa. This is typically followed by exudation of PMNs into the lumen of the airways (Fig. 8-8). The inflammation spreads from the bronchi into the adjacent alveoli. In *hypostatic pneumonia,* the infection is preceded by pulmonary edema. In either case, the inflammation may be limited to a small number of single lobules (*lobular pneumonia*), or it may be spread through large portions of the pulmonary parenchyma (*lobar pneumonia*).

As the intra-alveolar exudate accumulates, it replaces the air, and the lung parenchyma becomes consolidated. On gross examination at autopsy, affected lungs resemble the liver; therefore, this process is called hepatization. As consolidated lung parenchyma is denser than normal lung, pneumonia can be recognized on x-ray studies as "infiltrates" or "consolidation of parenchyma." With appropriate treatment, the pulmonary infection can be brought under control and the pneumonia cured. The exudate is resorbed or coughed out with complete restitution of the normal alveolar spaces.

Interstitial pneumonias, which are usually diffuse and often bilateral, differ from alveolar pneumonias in that the inflammation primarily affects the alveolar septa and does not result in exudation of PMNs into the alveolar lumen. In contrast to alveolar pneumonia, which is usually caused by bacteria, interstitial pneumonias are caused by viruses that invade the alveolar lining cells. *Mycoplasma pneumoniae,* another cause of interstitial pneumonia, is a bacteria-like microorganism, but it also resides within cells. These pathogens cause cell necrosis and induce an infiltrate predominantly restricted to the alveolar septa. This accounts for the so-called "reticular pattern," with no major consolidations typically seen on radiographic examination. Fortunately, most viral pneumonias cause only minor alveolar damage and resolve without consequences. However, some viral

FIGURE 8-8

Histologic appearance of bronchopneumonia. The bronchus and the surrounding alveoli contain polymorphonuclear leukocytes.

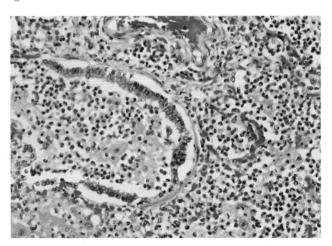

pneumonias may progress to a chronic stage that is characterized by interstitial fibrosis and a honeycomb appearance of lungs. Because viral pneumonias often have an "atypical" course and may pass undiagnosed, it is possible that some cases of "pulmonary fibrosis of unknown origin" are late complications of viral pneumonia.

Complications. Complications of bacterial pneumonia may occur in rapidly progressing cases caused by virulent pathogens, in debilitated patients, or in cases in which treatment is delayed or ineffective (Fig. 8-9). The most important complications of pneumonia are pleuritis, abscess formation, and chronic lung disease.

- *Pleuritis.* Extension of inflammation to the pleural surface commonly leads to pleural effusion. Sometimes, especially with purulent bacteria, pus fills the entire pleural cavity (*pyothorax*); more often,

it is encapsulated by fibrous tissue into pockets called *empyema.* Suppurative pleuritis heals slowly and usually results in pleural fibrosis encasing the entire lung. Pleural fibrosis obliterates the pleural cavity. As the lungs cannot expand during inspiration, restrictive lung disease results.
- *Abscess.* Abscesses are usually associated with highly virulent bacteria, such as staphylococcus, which cause destruction of the lung parenchyma and suppuration. Pus inside the bronchi causes destruction of their walls and bronchial dilatation (*bronchiectasis*).
- *Chronic lung disease* is an important complication of pneumonia that is unresponsive to treatment. Destruction of the lung parenchyma and concomitant fibrosis transform the lung into a honeycomb-like structure ("honeycomb lungs").

Complications of viral pneumonias are rare because most of these infections heal spontaneously. Some viral pneumonias may not resolve and, in such cases, chronic pulmonary interstitial fibrosis will develop.

Clinical Features. Pneumonia is a serious infection that requires prompt and aggressive treatment. It may occur in any age group, but most often affects children younger than 5 years of age or elderly persons older than 70 years of age.

The first prerequisite for diagnosing pneumonia is to suspect that it has developed. In this context, it is worth mentioning that clinicians divide pneumonias into two groups: (1) *primary or community-acquired pneumonias,* which affect previously healthy people, and (2) *secondary pneumonias,* which are hospital-acquired (*nosocomial*) or which arise in persons with preexisting illnesses. The elderly, and debilitated or sick people are at greater risk for developing pneumonia than are healthy persons. Other risk factors are smoking, alcoholism, and immunosuppression caused by diseases or treatment. Pneumonia is a common feature of AIDS.

The symptoms of pneumonia may be classified as follows:

- *Systemic signs of infection.* These include high fever, chills, and prostration.
- *Local signs of irritation.* These are related to bronchial inflammation and the secretion of mucus and include coughing and expectoration. Pleural inflammation causes chest pain.
- *Airway obstruction.* Impaired gas exchange in the damaged alveoli results in shortness of breath (*dyspnea*) and rapid breathing (*tachypnea*).
- *Inflammation and tissue destruction.* Inflammatory exudate causes tissue destruction and bleeding. Consequences include mucopurulent, blood-tinged "rusty sputum," or even frank hemoptysis.

FIGURE 8-9
Pneumonia may extend to the pleura and cause pleuritis, which may heal in the form of pleural fibrosis. Persistence of pus in the pleural cavity is called empyema. Suppurative pneumonia results in abscess formation. Bronchiectasis is a consequence of chronic lung infection. Interstitial fibrosis with cysts accounts for the honeycomb appearance of lungs in chronic lung disease.

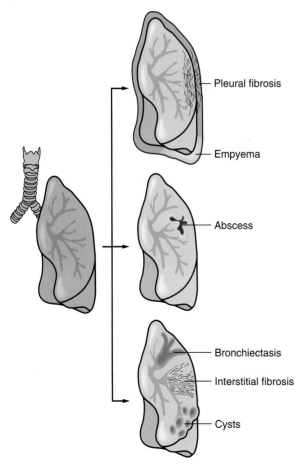

Pleural fibrosis

Empyema

Abscess

Bronchiectasis

Interstitial fibrosis

Cysts

On physical examination, affected patients usually appear in great distress and short of breath. Relentless coughing is a common symptom. Auscultation usually reveals rales, bronchi, and other signs of pulmonary consolidation. A presumptive diagnosis of pneumonia, made on the basis of clinical findings, must be confirmed by additional studies, such as the following:

- *Chest radiography.* Radiologic findings are essential for localizing the pulmonary infiltrates and for assessing the extent of pulmonary consolidation.
- *Bacteriologic studies of the sputum.* Sometimes, the pathogens can be identified in smears of sputum examined under the microscope, but in most cases, bacteriologic cultures of sputum are more reliable and yield more conclusive proof of infection. Bacteriologic data also provide the best guidance for treatment.
- *Peripheral blood studies.* Bacterial pneumonias are accompanied by leukocytosis. Viral pneumonia does not cause leukocytosis, but may be associated with an elevated number of lymphocytes in blood. Hypoxia, and even respiratory acidosis, may be detected by blood gas analysis and pH measurement. Blood gas analysis is performed only in severe cases of pneumonia.

The treatment of pneumonia is based on eradication of the bacterial infection with antibiotics and support of vital functions until the lung function has recovered.

Special Forms of Pneumonia

Infection with *Streptococcus pneumoniae* accounts for more than 50 percent of all bacterial pneumonias. Other forms of pneumonia that have unique features are also recognized. For example, *staphylococcal pneumonia* tends to produce multiple abscesses. *Pseudomonas pneumonial* is the most common gram-negative bacterium causing hospital-acquired pneumonia. It is characterized by vascular lesions that typically cause infarcts and necrosis of the lung parenchyma. *Pseudomonas aeruginosa* is also the most common cause of lung infection in cystic fibrosis.

Atypical Pneumonia

Pneumonias that do not present with classical symptoms are called atypical. This clinical term is used for a variety of conditions and usually implies that a bacterial pathogen cannot be identified. The best examples of atypical pneumonia are diffuse lung diseases caused by viruses or *M. pneumoniae.* In immunosuppressed persons, and especially those who have AIDS, atypical pneumonia is often caused by a fungus, *Pneumocystis carinii.*

Clinical symptoms of atypical pneumonia are milder than in classical pneumonia. The fever is less pronounced, and usually there are no chills. The cough is mild and does not produce mucopurulent or blood-stained sputum. The x-ray findings may be minimal and no distinct condensations are seen. Bacteria cannot be cultured from the sputum. There are usually no signs of septicemia. Purulent pleuritis and abscess formation are not among the complications of atypical pneumonia. There is also no leukocytosis.

Legionnaires' Disease

Legionnaires' disease, a bacterial pneumonia caused by *Legionella pneumophila,* was initially classified as atypical pneumonia because the causative microbes could not be identified by standard bacteriologic techniques. Legionella tends to reside within the cytoplasm of pulmonary macrophages, and it grows only in special bacteriologic culture media. Nevertheless, it is a bacterium and it can be treated efficiently with antibiotics. If not recognized and treated, Legionella causes massive consolidation and necrosis of lung parenchyma associated with high mortality.

Pulmonary Tuberculosis

Tuberculosis is a chronic bacterial infectious disease caused by *M. tuberculosis.* It was widespread in industrialized societies of the 19th century, but its incidence has decreased steadily since the 1950s, when the first tuberculosis drugs were introduced. Nevertheless, tuberculosis infection still affects 25,000 Americans every year, most of whom have lung disease. Because primary pulmonary tuberculosis is clinically unrecognized in most instances, the true incidence of tuberculosis is probably much higher.

The emergence of strains of Mycobacterium that are resistant to drugs has, during the last few years, refocused the attention of the public on this problem.

Etiology and Pathogenesis. Pulmonary tuberculosis is caused by *M. tuberculosis,* a rod-shaped bacterium with a waxy capsule. Because of this capsule, *M. tuberculosis* can effectively be stained only with a special Ziehl-Neelson technique, which renders it red. It is, therefore, called "acid-fast bacillus."

M. tuberculosis does not attract PMNs, and the infection is not marked by acute purulent lesions. Instead, the encapsulated bacteria elicit formation of granulomas. These granulomas are composed of lymphocytes and macrophages. Stimulated macrophages transform into epithelioid cells and often fuse to form multinucleated Langerhans giant cells. The necrotic central portion of the granulomas resembles cottage cheese on gross examination and is, therefore, called caseous necrosis.

Primary infection in a person who has not previously been exposed to *M. tuberculosis* results in a localized lung inflammation. This lesion, known as *Ghon complex,* consists of granulomas in the lung parenchyma and the enlarged regional lymph nodes (Fig. 8-10). In 95 percent of cases, Ghon complex heals spontaneously, usually by undergoing calcification, which can be recognized by x-ray studies. Nevertheless, calcified primary complex may contain *M. tuberculosis,* which can be reactivated, producing secondary tuberculosis. Progressive primary tuberculosis is a rare event that occurs mostly in children and immunosuppressed persons.

Secondary tuberculosis can develop as a result of reactivation of the dormant primary infection or a new reinfection. Most cases represent reactivation of a previous infection. The bacteria typically spread to the apex of the lungs, causing a granulomatous lobular pneumonia. Confluent granulomas tend to produce cavities (*cavernous tuberculosis*). Pulmonary cavities are common sources of hemoptysis.

Tissue destruction facilitates additional intrapulmonary and extrapulmonary spread of infection. Bacillary dissemination in such cases occurs through the lymphatics, the pulmonary blood vessels, or the airspaces (Fig. 8-11). Typical complications resulting from dissemination of tuberculosis include the following:

- *Miliary tuberculosis.* Widespread seeding of bacteria in the lungs or in other organs results in the formation of small granulomas that resemble millet seeds (the Latin *milium* means millet seed).
- *Tuberculous pneumonia.* Fulminant spread of bacteria through the airspaces produces a massive lobular or lobar pneumonia. It may involve the same lung as the primary infection or the contralateral lung.
- *Pleuritis.* Extension of infection to the pleura is accompanied by pleural effusion and the formation of granulomas on visceral and parietal pleura. Thick adhesions regularly form in protracted disease, resulting in obliterative pleural fibrosis.
- *Extrapulmonary tuberculosis.* Expectorated bacilli may infect the larynx and, if swallowed, may cause gastrointestinal tuberculosis, usually in the small intestine. Hematogenous spread may cause tuberculosis of essentially any organ in the body. Extrapulmonary tuberculosis is rarely seen today in Western countries.

FIGURE 8-10
The Ghon complex, typical of pulmonary tuberculosis, consists of a parenchymal focus and hilar lymph node lesions. The detailed section of the diagram shows the typical features of tuberculous granuloma: central caseous necrosis surrounded by epithelioid cells, multinucleated giant cells, and lymphocytes.

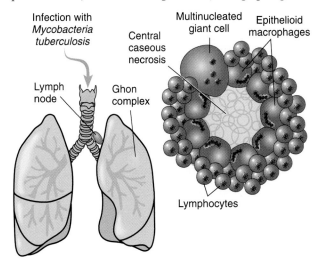

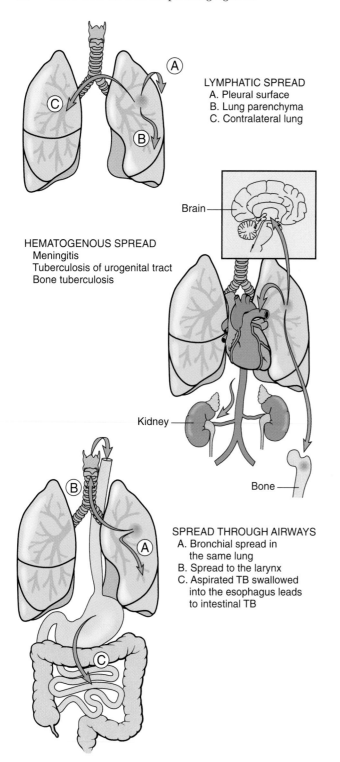

LYMPHATIC SPREAD
A. Pleural surface
B. Lung parenchyma
C. Contralateral lung

HEMATOGENOUS SPREAD
Meningitis
Tuberculosis of urogenital tract
Bone tuberculosis

Brain

Kidney

Bone

SPREAD THROUGH AIRWAYS
A. Bronchial spread in
   the same lung
B. Spread to the larynx
C. Aspirated TB swallowed
   into the esophagus leads
   to intestinal TB

FIGURE 8-11
Spread of tuberculosis (TB). Reactivated bacilli can spread through the lymphatics, blood vessels, or bronchi. Hematogenous spread usually accounts for tuberculosis in distal sites, such as the urogenital tract or the brain. Expectorated bacilli may be swallowed and cause intestinal tuberculosis.

Clinical Features. Tuberculosis may present with a variety of symptoms, most of which are nonspecific. *Primary tuberculosis* is associated with mild pulmonary disease and low-grade fever. It remains clinically unrecognized in more than 95 percent of the cases. The symptoms of *secondary tuberculosis* include a nonproductive (dry) cough, low-grade fever, loss of appetite, malaise, night sweats, and weight loss. Minor hemoptysis from destructive cavitary lesions usually occurs later. Dyspnea may indicate the spread of infection through the parenchyma of the lungs, pulmonary destructive lesions, and pleural effusions.

Chest x-ray studies are essential for the diagnosis, which is definitively established by identifying acid-fast bacilli in sputum stained with the Ziehl-Neelsen technique or in bacteriologic cultures. The *tuberculin test,* performed by injecting 0.1 mL of diluted bacterial extract (called tuberculin), into the skin, is typically positive. However, this test is not absolute proof of tuberculosis. Positive as well as negative tuberculin test data must be interpreted in the context of other clinical and laboratory findings. For example, persons who have developed immunity because of a previous resolved infection or those who have been immunized with attenuated *M. tuberculosis* (called bacille Calmette-Guérin, or BCG) also react positively to injected tuberculin. Anergic patients, as in those with terminal AIDS, have a negative response to tuberculin.

Pulmonary tuberculosis is a treatable disease unless it is caused by drug-resistant strains of *M. tuberculosis.* Tuberculosis in immunosuppressed persons, such as those with AIDS, does not respond to treatment.

Fungal Diseases

Among the causes of primary, community-acquired pulmonary infections, two fungal diseases deserve mention: histoplasmosis and coccidioidomycosis. Histoplasmosis is widespread in the midwestern United States, and coccidioidomycosis is endemic in the Southwest deserts. Both diseases are acquired by inhaling dried out fungi and their spores with the dust. Clinically, these infections resemble tuberculosis. The infection may be asymptomatic, as is usually the case, or it may present as solitary pulmonary lesions, or even in the form of miliary nodules. Fungal infections induce the formation of granulomas, which heal by calcification.

Hospital-acquired fungal infections are common among patients who are terminally ill and those with cancer or AIDS. The most common pathogens are *Candida albicans* and *Aspergillus fumigatus.*

Lung Abscess

Lung abscess is a localized, destructive, suppurative lesion. It is most often caused by staphylococci and less often by other bacteria, such as Klebsiella and Pseudomonas.

Lung abscesses develop under the following conditions:

- As a typical complication of necrotizing staphylococcal pneumonia
- Following aspiration of infected material from the alimentary or upper respiratory tract
- Distal to bronchial obstruction by tumors
- As a result of septic lung emboli

Abscesses may be solitary or multiple. Like abscesses in other sites, lung abscesses are also cavitary lesions filled with pus. In early stages, the central pus is surrounded by granulation tissue, whereas in late stages, it is surrounded by a capsule composed of hyalinized collagen. In contrast to abscesses of other internal organs, which usually remain encapsulated, pulmonary abscesses tend to connect with the airways. The expanding abscesses erode the bronchial wall and extrude their purulent content into the airways. Putrid malodorous expectoration is thus typical of lung abscesses.

Chronic Obstructive Pulmonary Disease

The term **chronic obstructive pulmonary disease** (COPD) is a catch-all clinical term used for lung diseases characterized by chronic airway obstruction. For the sake of simplicity, we shall consider COPD as a spectrum of diseases extending from *chronic bronchitis* on one end to *emphysema* on the other. Although chronic bronchitis and emphysema may occur in "pure" forms, in most cases, these two diseases coexist. Patients can be classified into two groups: those who have predominantly chronic bronchitis and those who have predominantly emphysema.

Chronic Bronchitis

Chronic bronchitis is defined clinically as excessive production of tracheobronchial mucus causing cough and expectoration for at least 3 months during 2 consecutive years. Smoking is the cause of chronic bronchitis in more than 90 percent of the cases. The extent of disease correlates with the number of cigarettes smoked, and cessation of smoking is associated with improvement of clinical symptoms. Other contributory factors include air pollution, oc-

cupational exposure to toxic fumes, and various respiratory infections, especially if recurrent. It has been shown that a single bout of viral pneumonia, especially in childhood, may predispose that individual to COPD in later life.

The pathology of chronic bronchitis is relatively nonspecific. The walls of the bronchi and bronchioli are thickened and their lumen contains thick mucus. Histologically, the mucosa is infiltrated with lymphocytes, macrophages, and plasma cells. The surface epithelium is usually preserved, but it may show focal ulcerations or metaplasia of columnar into squamous epithelium. The most prominent changes involve the submucosa, which shows marked mucous gland hyperplasia, chronic inflammation, and fibrosis.

Bronchiectasis

Bronchiectasis, a permanent dilatation of the bronchi, is the most common complication of chronic bronchitis. It is often associated with bronchiolectasis, a dilatation of the bronchioli. Such dilatation occurs as a result of persistent inflammation inside the airways. Enzymes released from bacteria and leukocytes; mechanical pressure from the inside, exerted by the bronchial contents; and traction of the fibrous scars from the outside all contribute to the formation of bronchiectases.

The larger bronchi usually show *saccular* or *cystic dilatation,* whereas the smaller bronchi and bronchioli show *cylindrical dilatation* (Fig. 8-12). The dilated bronchi and bronchioli are filled with mucopurulent material. This material stagnates and cannot be cleared by coughing. Infection spreads into the adjacent alveoli and recurrent pneumonias are common. Hematogenous spread of the infection into other organs and the systemic consequences of protracted suppuration cause low-grade fever, generalized malaise, and fatigue. These patients often develop clubbing of the fingers. Amyloidosis is a well-known complication and may lead to renal or hepatic failure.

Emphysema

Emphysema is defined, in pathologic terms, as enlargement of the airspaces distal to the terminal bronchioles with destruction of the alveolar walls. Emphysema is a disease affecting chronic cigarette smokers and is, like chronic bronchitis, pathogenetically related to the chemicals contained in smoke. Emphysema is rare in nonsmokers, and most of these patients have a genetic deficiency of α_1-antitrypsin (α_1-AT).

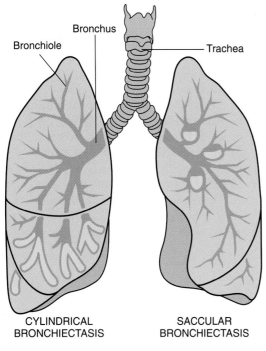

CYLINDRICAL
BRONCHIECTASIS

SACCULAR
BRONCHIECTASIS

FIGURE 8-12
Bronchiectasis. The dilatation may be saccular or cylindrical. The lumina of the dilated bronchi contain pus and mucus.

Pathogenesis. The exact mechanism of tobacco-induced emphysema is not known. It has been hypothesized that the irritants in the smoke provoke an influx of inflammatory cells into the alveoli. Proteolytic enzymes released from the leukocytes presumably destroy the alveolar walls. Oxygen radicals generated by the burning cigarette kill alveolar cells and leukocytes, which release even more degradative enzymes. Increased activity of leukocyte-derived elastase in these lungs probably accounts for the loss of elastin fibers from the alveolar walls. Furthermore, it has been hypothesized that the oxygen radicals inactivate the endogenous antiproteolytic enzymes. Uninhibited by natural inhibitors, the leukocytic proteases act on normal tissues and destroy alveoli.

This hypothesis, which implicates proteolytic enzymes, is supported by observations of congenital *alpha$_1$-antitrypsin* (α_1-AT) *deficiency.* α_1-AT is a serum protein produced by the liver. It circulates in serum and permeates tissues, where its primary function is to neutralize proteases. α_1-AT protects tissues from the adverse effects of proteases released from leukocytes. α_1-AT deficiency results in emphysema, indicating that α_1-AT has a crucial role in counteracting the potentially damaging effects of leukocytes exudated in the pulmonary alveoli. α_1-AT deficiency is uncommon, and it accounts for less than 1 percent of all patients with emphysema. Nevertheless, it is an important "experiment of nature." Extrapolating from observations of this "experiment,"

one could assume that the inhibition of endogenous antiproteases by smoke could result in uncontrollable destruction of the alveolar walls by elastase and other proteases released from leukocytes.

Pathology. Pathologic findings in emphysema are classified according to the pattern of alveolar wall destruction. The most important forms are *centrilobular* (centriacinar) and *panacinar* emphysema (Fig. 8-13).

Centrilobular emphysema is marked by widening of the airspace in the center of a lobule and involves predominantly the respiratory bronchioles. This is the most common form of emphysema. It is typically found in cigarette smokers. The remaining respiratory bronchioles are characteristically infiltrated with

FIGURE 8-13
Emphysema involves the respiratory system distal to the terminal bronchiole. (A) Normal lung. (B) Centrilobular emphysema. (C) Panacinar emphysema.

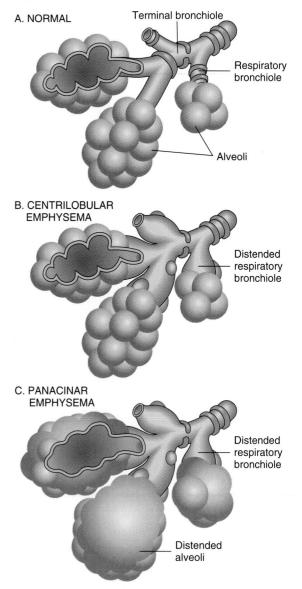

A. NORMAL

Terminal bronchiole

Respiratory bronchiole

Alveoli

B. CENTRILOBULAR EMPHYSEMA

Distended respiratory bronchiole

C. PANACINAR EMPHYSEMA

Distended respiratory bronchiole

Distended alveoli

anthracotic macrophages and chronic inflammatory cells. *Panacinar emphysema* involves all the airspaces distal to the terminal bronchioles. This form of emphysema typically occurs in α_1-AT deficiency, but may also be caused by smoking.

Clinical Features. Clinical symptoms of COPD vary depending on the extent and duration of the disease. Patients are customarily divided into two prototypic groups: those with predominant bronchitis ("blue bloaters") and those with predominant emphysema ("pink puffers") (Fig. 8-14). Table 8-2 compares the clinical features of these two conditions.

Chronic bronchitis results in prolonged bouts of coughing, expectoration of tenacious or purulent mucus, and dyspnea. Hypoxia may be so pronounced during the coughing episodes that it causes cyanosis ("blue bloating"). The pulmonary vasculature is affected by the peribronchial fibrosis, and this results in pulmonary hypertension and chronic cor pulmonale. Right ventricular failure is marked by peripheral venous stagnation, which contributes to cyanosis. Chest x-ray studies show increased bronchiovascular markings and an enlarged heart.

Patients with predominant emphysema have no bronchial obstructions and no irritation that would force them to cough and expectorate. Because of the reduced respiratory surface, they have compensatory tachypnea. The chest is overexpanded ("barrel-chest") and they often must hunch forward while holding onto a table or a window frame to engage the auxiliary respiratory muscles. These patients hyperventilate and thus manage to oxygenate the blood adequately so as not to develop cyanosis or anoxia. Chest radiographs show clear lung fields and "overinflation" with a small heart.

The treatment of COPD is symptomatic and based on supportive measures. The advanced pulmonary lesions are irreversible. Even if patients stop smoking, the symptoms often persist.

Immune Diseases

Among the numerous immune disorders affecting the respiratory tract, the most important are allergic rhinitis (hay fever), bronchial asthma, sarcoidosis, and hypersensitivity pneumonitis.

FIGURE 8-14
Clinically, patients with chronic obstructive pulmonary disease (COPD) can be classified as (A) pink puffers or (B) blue bloaters.

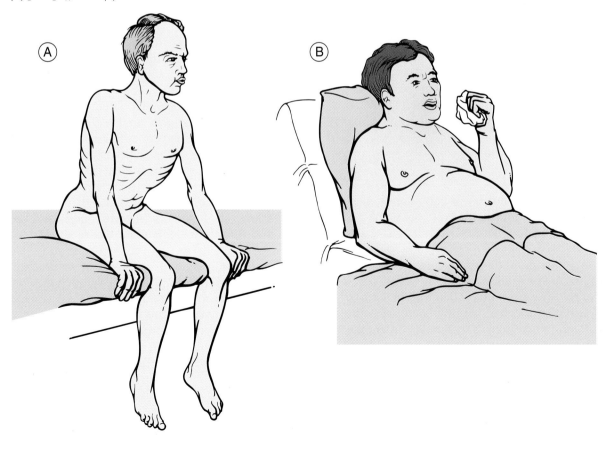

Table 8-2 Chronic Obstructive Lung Disease

	Predominantly Bronchitis ("Blue Bloaters")	Predominantly Emphysema ("Pink Puffers")
Chest	Normal	Barrel chest
Dyspnea	+	+ +
Cough	+ +	+
Sputum	+ +	+ / –
	Mucopurulent	Mucoid
Cyanosis	+ +	–
Pulmonary hypertension	+ +	–
Peripheral edema	+ +	–
Radiographic findings	Densities	Overinflation

Allergic Rhinitis

Hay fever, or **allergic rhinitis,** is a very common disease affecting millions of people. It represents a typical type I hypersensitivity reaction of the nasal mucosa to exogenous allergens. Among these allergens, the most common are pollens—hence, the popular name "hay fever." However, the list of potential allergens is much longer than that and includes such mundane, ubiquitous particles as animal dandruff and various industrial chemicals.

Allergic rhinitis is an acute vasomotor response mediated by histamine and related vasoactive substances released locally in the nose from mast cells coated with immunoglobulin E (IgE). The attack of sneezing may be short-lived or prolonged, but usually stops when the histamine has been depleted. Sneezing can be stopped with antihistaminic drugs and nasal sprays.

Asthma

Asthma is a disease characterized by increased responsiveness of the bronchial tree to a variety of stimuli. Typical "asthmatic attacks" are marked by wheezing during expiration, cough, and dyspnea. Asthma is a common disease, affecting approximately 10 percent of children and 5 percent of adults in the United States. In more than 50 percent of cases, the disease begins in childhood, affecting males two times more often than females. In another 30 percent of cases, signs of asthma develop by the age of 40 years, whereas the remaining 20 percent have so-called "old-age asthma."

Etiology and Pathogenesis. Asthma is a heterogeneous, multifactorial disease. In many instances, the disease has more than one cause and is mediated by more than one pathogenetic mechanism. For the sake of simplicity, two major forms of disease are recognized: extrinsic and intrinsic asthma.

Extrinsic asthma is mediated by exposure to exogenous allergens and represents a type I hypersensitivity reaction. Extrinsic asthma typically affects children and is often associated with other allergies, such as atopic dermatitis or hay fever.

Intrinsic asthma is precipitated by nonimmune mechanisms, most of which are nonspecific and would not produce symptoms were it not for the hyperreactivity of the bronchial tissues. These include

- physical factors, such as heat or cold
- exercise
- psychological stress
- chemical irritants and air pollution
- bronchial infection
- aspirin

The reasons for increased reactivity of the bronchi to various stimuli remain unknown. Current evidence indicates that it is most likely caused by persistent inflammation of the bronchial mucosa. The inflammatory cells, such as lymphocytes, macrophages, eosinophils, basophils, and plasma cells, produce a variety of mediators that act on the blood vessels, increasing their permeability. These substances also act on smooth muscle cells, stimulating their contraction (Fig. 8-15).

The mediators of inflammation in asthma can be divided into two groups: those involved in a rapid, immediate response, and those that have a delayed but prolonged effect. In the first group, the best known are vasoactive substances, such as histamine, bradykinin, prostaglandins, and other derivatives of arachidonic acid. Leukotrienes, which are also derived from arachidonic acid, and platelet-activating factor (PAF) produce delayed and protracted smooth muscle cell contraction. In addition, the inflammatory cells in the mucosa generate chemotactic factors that continuously recruit more inflammatory cells into the bronchial mucosa. Mucous cells stimulated by a variety of mediators secrete and discharge mucus into the bronchial lumen, where the mucus forms viscous plugs. Some of the mediators stimulate nerves that trigger smooth muscle cell contraction and secretion of mucus. Neural dysfunction may play an important role in altering the responsiveness of the bronchial mucosal cells and smooth muscles to cholinergic and beta-adrenergic stimuli.

Pathology. The pathologic changes in the lungs are similar in all forms of asthma, regardless of the etiology of the disease. Histologically, the bronchi show chronic inflammation and overabundance of mucus in the lumen. The mucosal infiltrates consist of non-

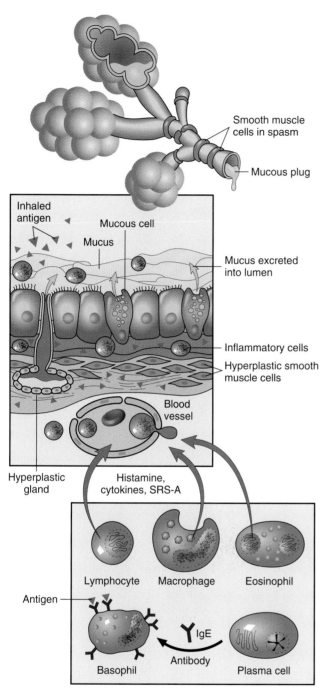

pear to be enlarged, reflecting frequent bronchial spasms.

Autopsy examination of patients who die in status asthmaticus shows overinflation of the alveoli and mucus plugging of the bronchi. The lungs of asthmatic patients who die of other causes usually do not show grossly visible changes at autopsy.

Clinical Features. Extrinsic asthma typically begins before the age of 10 years and lasts for several years. Many children improve spontaneously, but in about 50 percent of those affected in childhood, recurrent attacks persist throughout their life span. The disease is characterized by attacks of wheezing, dyspnea, and cough. These attacks are often precipitated by exposure to specific allergens. Most of these young patients often have a family history of asthma and other allergic diseases, such as atopic dermatitis ("eczema"). Skin testing may be useful for identifying the allergen, and an inhalation test may be used to provoke the attack and thus confirm the diagnosis. The serum of these patients contains elevated concentrations of IgE and often shows eosinophilia.

Intrinsic asthma begins in adulthood, usually before the age of 40 years. The asthmatic attacks, which are similar to those in extrinsic asthma, do not appear to be precipitated by exposure to identifiable

FIGURE 8-15
Pathogenesis of asthma. Allergens can trigger the release of mediators from mast cells which act on the blood vessels and smooth muscle cells. The mediators released from chronic inflammatory cells in the wall of the bronchus also stimulate mucous secretion and contraction of the smooth muscle cells. SRS-A, slow-reacting substance of anaphylaxis; IgE, immunoglobulin E.

FIGURE 8-16
Histopathology of asthma. The lumen of the bronchus contains mucus. The wall is thickened and inflamed and contains hyperplastic smooth muscle cells and bronchial glands.

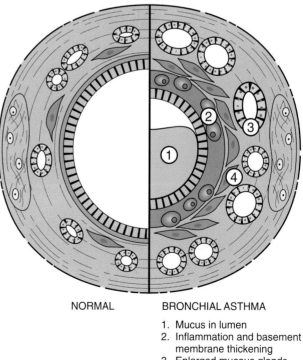

NORMAL   BRONCHIAL ASTHMA

1. Mucus in lumen
2. Inflammation and basement membrane thickening
3. Enlarged mucous glands
4. Smooth muscle hyperplasia

specific chronic inflammatory cells, but often also contain prominent eosinophils (Fig. 8-16). The bronchial walls also show bronchial gland hyperplasia, which correlates with overproduction of mucus. Smooth muscle cells are increased in number and ap-

allergens. Most attacks occur at random, but they may also be related to exposure to cold, environmental pollutants, and toxic gases. Aspirin is a well-known precipitating factor of asthmatic attacks in some people. Emotional stress and exercise can cause asthmatic attacks in others. Respiratory infections—especially chronic sinusitis—are the cause of asthmatic attacks in still others.

The treatment of asthma is symptomatic and is generally directed at preventing or reducing bronchospasm and bronchial inflammation. Drugs that prevent the degranulation of mast cells are especially beneficial. Bronchodilatation with sympathomimetics is an efficient way of stopping the attacks. The prognosis is generally good, and most patients have a normal life span. Death secondary to status asthmaticus occurs only rarely.

Sarcoidosis

Sarcoidosis is a multisystemic granulomatous disease of unknown etiology, presumably mediated by cell-mediated immunity. It has an incidence of approximately 50 per 100,000 and affects blacks 10 times more often than other races. It is twice as common in black women than men.

The cause and pathogenesis of sarcoidosis are not known. For unknown reasons, the disease has a predilection for the lungs and mediastinal lymph nodes. The lungs are infiltrated with T lymphocytes; CD4-positive T-helper cells outnumber the CD8-positive T-suppressor cells by a ratio of 10:1. The number of CD4-positive cells in the circulation is reduced, indicating that these cells have been attracted to the lungs and lymph nodes, where they contribute to the formation of granulomas. It was proposed that granulomas represent a response to putative antigens inhaled into the lungs, but the nature of these antigens has not been elucidated.

Clinical Features. Granulomas of sarcoidosis may involve any organ in the body (Fig. 8-17). The lungs, the lymph nodes of the thorax and the neck, and the liver are most often involved. Granulomas of the lacrimal and salivary glands are found in one third of patients.

Pathology. The clinical symptoms of sarcoidosis vary. Approximately 50 percent of patients are asymptomatic and are diagnosed during routine examination. Most symptomatic patients have a low-grade fever and feel tired and anorexic. Symptoms pertaining to lung involvement are among the most common complaints and include dyspnea, cough, or wheezing respiration. In such patients, x-ray studies show pulmonary nodules and hilar lymph node enlargement. Peripheral lymphadenopathy, hepato-

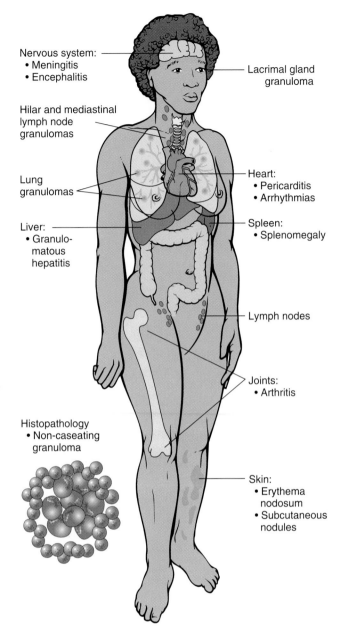

Nervous system:
• Meningitis
• Encephalitis

Hilar and mediastinal lymph node granulomas

Lung granulomas

Liver:
• Granulomatous hepatitis

Lacrimal gland granuloma

Heart:
• Pericarditis
• Arrhythmias

Spleen:
• Splenomegaly

Lymph nodes

Joints:
• Arthritis

Skin:
• Erythema nodosum
• Subcutaneous nodules

Histopathology
• Non-caseating granuloma

FIGURE 8-17
Sarcoidosis. The most common sites of granulomas are the lungs and the thoracic lymph nodes. Other extrathoracic sites are less commonly involved. The inset shows a granuloma composed predominantly of epithelioid cells, macrophages, and lymphocytes. In contrast to tuberculosis, there is no central necrosis.

splenomegaly, and skin nodules are occasionally found. Enlargement of the salivary and lacrimal glands is a useful diagnostic finding which, unfortunately, is seen only in a minority of patients.

The definitive diagnosis of sarcoidosis is made on the basis of biopsy of the lymph nodes, bronchi, liver, or skin. Typical sarcoid granulomas are composed of epithelioid and giant cells surrounded, at the periphery, by a narrow rim of lymphocytes. In contrast to infectious granulomas, such as those caused by *M. tuberculosis* or fungi, granulomas of sarcoidosis do not show central necrosis ("noncaseating granulomas").

The laboratory data are not pathognomonic but can, nevertheless, support the diagnosis. For example, 60 percent of patients have elevated serum levels of angiotensin-converting enzyme (ACE), which is released from macrophages in granulomas. Approximately 10 percent of patients develop hypercalcemia related to elevated serum levels of vitamin D_3. Unfortunately, these findings are not diagnostic, as similar biochemical changes can occur in other granulomatous diseases as well.

There is no specific therapy for sarcoidosis, but more than 70 percent of patients recover spontaneously. When of short duration, the disease has a good prognosis, but if the symptoms last more than 2 years, the prognosis is less favorable.

Hypersensitivity Pneumonitis

Hypersensitivity pneumonitis, or *extrinsic allergic alveolitis,* is an immune disorder caused by repeated inhalation of foreign antigens. Most of these allergens are derived from molds and fungi growing on organic material, such as hay or tree bark, or in contaminated fluid or air conditioning equipment. Bird droppings, animal fur dust, and wood dust are also known to induce hypersensitivity pneumonitis. A short list of such diseases caused in various settings is given in Table 8-3.

Hypersensitivity pneumonitis may occur in an *acute* and a *chronic* form. *Acute pneumonitis* is mediated by antibodies that react with the inhaled antigen in the alveoli. The formation of antigen-antibody complexes activates complement which, in turn, provides chemotactic signals and stimulates an influx of leukocytes. An acute pneumonitis evolves over a period of several hours after the exposure (Fig. 8-18). *Chronic hypersensitivity pneumonitis* is mediated by T lymphocytes and is characterized by a typical cell-mediated reaction. Granulomas, found in most pa-

Table 8–3 Examples of Hypersensitivity Pneumonitis

Disease	Source of Antigen
Farmer's lung	Moldy hay or grain silage
Bagassosis	Sugar cane
Maple bark disease	Maple bark
Mushroom worker's lung	Mushrooms
Humidifier lung	Contaminated fluid
Pigeon-breeder's lung	Pigeon droppings
Furrier's lung	Animal pelts

tients with chronic disease, are primarily located in the alveolar septa, causing their thickening or focal destruction. Damaged tissue cannot be repaired but is replaced by granulation tissue and fibrosis. Loss of parenchyma, scarring, and cystic dilatation of the remaining airspaces is recognized on gross inspection of honeycomb lungs. Such end-stage lung disease of immune origin cannot be distinguished from other chronic lung diseases known under various names, such as fibrosing alveolitis, usual interstitial pneumonitis, idiopathic interstitial pneumonitis, Hamann-Rich syndrome, and others. It is quite possible that some of these diseases are the consequences of an initial immune injury, but in most instances, an immune pathogenesis cannot be proven.

Clinical Features. Acute hypersensitivity pneumonitis presents with dyspnea of sudden onset. Removal of the antigen usually improves the clinical picture. For example, a farmer who has hypersensitivity to silo grain contaminants should be told to avoid close exposure to the silo. Chronic hypersensitivity pneumonitis has a more ominous prognosis. Avoidance of the inciting antigen may provide some relief, but often, the disease has a tendency to progress to end-stage lung disease. In most of these chronic cases, the antigen that has caused the disease is unknown. Destructive lung lesions cause chronic dyspnea and hyperventilation, and ultimately cause respiratory failure. Such end-stage lung disease can be treated only by lung transplantation.

Pneumoconioses

Pneumoconioses are lung diseases caused by inhalation of mineral dusts, fumes, and various organic or inorganic particulate matter. Most of these diseases are classified as occupational and are a consequence of long-term exposure in the workplace. Mineral dust pneumoconioses (most notably, coal-workers' lung disease), silicosis, and asbestosis are the most important diseases in this group. Other air pollutants are listed in Table 8-4.

The lung injury caused by mineral particles is complex, and although the exact mechanisms are not known, it has been shown that the extent of injury depends on

- duration of exposure
- concentration of particles
- the size of the particles, their shape, and solubility
- the biochemical composition of the inhaled dust

Inert material, like coal particles, is less reactive; therefore, coal-miners' pneumoconiosis develops only after very long exposure to high levels of pol-

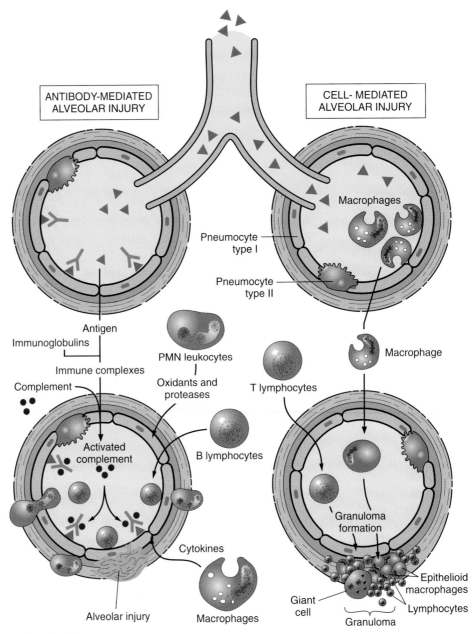

FIGURE 8-18
Pathogenesis of hypersensitivity pneumonitis. The disease may be antibody- or cell-mediated. PMN, polymorphonuclear.

luted air. Silica particles are more reactive and apparently produce more prominent tissue injury. Asbestos particles are insoluble and tend to remain lodged inside the lungs permanently.

The size of the particles is very important. Large dust particles—that is, those measuring more than 10 μm—are retained in the nasal mucus and do not reach the lower respiratory tract. However, particles smaller than 5 μm can enter the alveoli, where they are taken up by macrophages. Such particles, depending on their chemical composition, may produce lung injury.

The response of inflammatory cells to the inhaled particles is also important. Macrophages stimu-

lated by the ingested particles release various cytokines, such as interleukin-1 (IL-1) or tumor necrosis factor (TNF), which promote inflammation and also stimulate the proliferation of fibroblasts and the formation of collagen. Destruction of tissue, the ensuing repair, and fibrosis contribute to a restructuring of the lung parenchyma, and these changes are typically associated with a loss of respiratory surfaces.

The clinical symptoms of pneumoconiosis are variable. Usually, the symptoms are nonspecific and resemble those caused by other restrictive lung diseases. Progressive dyspnea ultimately leads to respiratory failure.

Table 8-4 Examples of Air Pollutants

Pollutant	Source(s)	Consequences
Gases		
Carbon mon-oxide (CO)	Car exhaust Gas stove	Anoxia (Death)
Sulfur dioxide (SO$_2$)	Coal smoke Tobacco	Mucosal irritation
Polychlorinated biphenyls (PCBs)	Air spray Refrigerators	Undefined
Formaldehyde	Laboratory fumes House insulation	Mucosal irritation
Particles		
Carbon	Coal smoke Smog Mining	Anthracosis
Quartz (silica)	Stone cutting	Silicosis
Asbestos	Insulation Shipbuilding	Asbestosis

Coal-Workers' Lung Disease

Coal-workers' lung disease is also known as *black lung disease* because, at autopsy, the lungs of these patients appear black (*anthracotic*). Coal miners working in heavily polluted air suffer from pulmonary ailments. Anthracosis (derived from the Greek *anthrakos,* meaning black), or blackening of the lungs by inhaled carbon particles, is not the only cause of lung injury in such cases, however. Other mineral particles, such as silica, are considered to be pathogenetically important as well.

Amorphous carbon particles are innocuous; indeed, most of them never reach the lungs but instead are retained in the nasal or bronchial mucus. Those that do reach the alveoli are taken up by alveolar macrophages and, in most cases, expectorated. Most urban dwellers have minor anthracosis of the lungs but do not have any clinical symptoms of lung disease. If the burden of coal particles in the dust is overwhelming, as regularly occurs in underground coal mines, the macrophages cannot eliminate it through the bronchi and the anthracotic pigment accumulates in the interstitial spaces of the lung.

It has been hypothesized that the retained mineral particles incite fibrosis. The pathogenesis of pulmonary fibrosis is not understood. It is possible that the lesions occur only after a critical threshold of exposure has been surpassed. Furthermore, some persons might be more susceptible than others. This view is supported by observations that some coal miners tend to develop rheumatoid lung disease (so-called Caplan's syndrome), which is rare in the general population. Finally, it appears that persons who develop coal-workers' lung disease have a predisposition to pulmonary tuberculosis, which was previously prevalent among coal miners.

Pathology. Coal-workers' lung disease is caused by prolonged inhalation of dust that is rich in carbon particles and other earth minerals. These particles are deposited in the centrolobular zones of the lung and may be associated with fibrosis or centroacinar emphysema. Fibrosis may become progressive, replacing broad fields of lung parenchyma (Fig. 8-19).

Clinical Features. The symptoms of coal-workers' lung disease vary in clinical severity from mild to severe. There is no effective treatment, and the disease usually has a slow but unrelenting course. The only good news about this disease is that it apparently does not predispose the individual to cancer. Improved conditions in the coal mines and the protective masks that are currently used have reduced the incidence of this lung disease.

Silicosis

Silicosis is a lung disease caused by inhalation of small (1 to 3-μm) silica crystals, inhaled in dust generated during stone cutting, mining, and sand blasting. The disease typically develops only in persons exposed to silica dust for 10 to 20 years. Silicosis is a relatively mild disease, and only a minority of exposed persons develop progressive massive fibrosis.

Pathology. Silicosis is characterized by fibronodular lesions in the lung parenchyma. Silica particles are initially taken up by macrophages, which are dam-

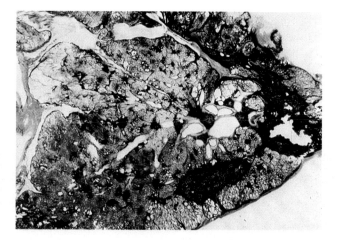

FIGURE 8-19
Coal-workers' lung disease. The lungs appear black owing to massive deposits of carbon particles. (Courtesy of Dr. W. Thurlback, Vancouver, B.C., Canada.)

aged in this process and often killed. Dead macrophages release silica crystals and various biologically active substances that stimulate fibroblasts to produce collagen. This results in the formation of collagenous nodules, which are most prominent along the lymphatics draining toward the hilar lymph nodes. Because silicosis occurs only rarely in an isolated form, but usually presents as anthracosilicosis, these nodules are often black. Confluent silicotic nodules destroy lung parenchyma and cause massive pulmonary fibrosis, which is indistinguishable from other forms of fibrotic lung disease. Tuberculosis is a common complication, probably because silica-laden macrophages cannot effectively combat mycobacterial infections.

Clinical Features. The clinical symptoms of silicosis are generally mild unless a progressive bilateral fibrosis or tuberculosis supervenes. Once the lesions develop, they are irreversible and do not regress upon treatment. Silicosis may be an incapacitating disease, but it is worth noting that it does not predispose individuals to cancer.

Asbestosis

Four lung lesions have been linked to asbestos exposure:

- pulmonary fibrosis
- pleural fibrosis and pleural plaques
- lung cancer
- mesothelioma

Asbestos is a generic name for several fibrous silicates that form natural minerals, such as chrysotile, amosite, or crocidolite. Asbestos fibers have been used in manufacturing and industry for many years. However, only recently—several years after World War II—were the health hazards of asbestos exposure recognized. During the war and thereafter, some 10 million American workers were exposed to asbestos in the workplace, such as those involved in shipbuilding, the construction industry, and the manufacture of car brakes and house insulation. Only a small percentage of these workers developed lung diseases, but, nevertheless, the actual numbers are staggering. Estimates are that approximately 10,000 deaths per year are still directly or indirectly attributable to asbestos exposure during the 1940s and 1950s.

Asbestos fibers vary in size, shape, and biochemical composition. Large and long asbestos particles are innocuous because they do not reach the lungs. Such fibers are retained in nasal and bronchial mucus. Most asbestos fibers presently used in industry, such as chrysotile, are classified as serpentines, which are curly and elongated and produce no harm. On the other hand, amphibole asbestos, the brittle, short, straight fibers of crocidolite and amosite, are potentially more dangerous. These amphiboles are not used today.

The pathogenesis of asbestos lung disease is not known. It is known that short (straight) fibers enter the alveoli and are taken up by macrophages. In contrast to silica, which is toxic to macrophages, asbestos does not kill these cells. Rather, asbestos activates the macrophages and stimulates them to release various fibrogenic cytokines and growth factors. This ultimately results in extensive pulmonary fibrosis.

Pathology. Lungs affected by asbestos show fibrosis that contains beaded bodies with knobbed ends called *"asbestos bodies."* These bodies are coated with hemosiderin pigment and thus appear brown, so they are also called *"ferruginous bodies."* Ferruginous bodies can be found in lungs not affected by asbestosis, but in asbestosis, such bodies are extremely abundant. It has been estimated that, for every iron-coated asbestos body, there are at least 10 that are not coated and therefore cannot be seen by light microscopy. These can best be demonstrated by chemical analysis following microincineration (i.e., burning of the lung tissue sample), with subsequent analysis of the ashes. The asbestos fibers are fire-resistant and will remain in the ashes.

Clinical Features. Asbestosis presents as restrictive lung disease and dyspnea. The dyspnea persists for years, but respiratory failure occurs only rarely. Pulmonary fibrosis is often associated with foci of pleural fibrosis ("pleural plaques"). Solitary or small pleural plaques are usually asymptomatic. Diffuse pleural fibrosis may cause restrictive lung disease.

Lung cancer is an important complication of exposure to asbestos. Malignant tumors develop in fibrotic lungs five to six times more often than in the control population. However, when asbestos exposure is combined with cigarette smoking, the risk of lung cancer is more than 50 times higher. Mesotheliomas are yet another complication of asbestos exposure and will be discussed in the section on lung tumors. These pleural tumors occur almost exclusively in persons exposed to asbestos.

Ventilatory Disturbances, Adult Respiratory Distress Syndrome, and Atelectasis

Respiratory functions of the lung depend critically on the normal inhalation of air, passage of oxygen across the alveolar membrane, and normal blood flow through the lungs. Pathologic changes involving the alveolar septa—i.e., the interface between the air and the blood—have been described in the previous sections on pneumonia and interstitial pulmonary fibrosis. Pulmonary emboli and other circulatory disturbances have previously been presented in Chapter 6. Here, only processes that affect ventilation shall be described. Two complex multifactorial lesions—the adult respiratory distress syndrome (ARDS) and atelectasis—are also included in this discussion.

Disturbances of Ventilation

Normal **ventilation** depends on the unimpeded influx of air into the lungs through the upper and middle respiratory tract. This is effectively achieved through the action of respiratory muscles. It depends on the ability of the thorax to expand and retract with each respiratory movement. Finally, the expansion of the lungs depends on the pressure gradients: the positive pressure inside the airspaces that inflates the alveoli and the negative pressure within the pleural cavity that keeps the lungs from collapsing.

Respiratory difficulties present typically as shortness of breath, which is called **dyspnea.** Various causes of dyspnea are listed in Table 8-5.

Obstruction of the upper respiratory tract can occur under a variety of conditions. **Suffocation** can be caused by occlusion of the larynx with food. For example, a big bite of steak may enter the respiratory system; indeed, steaks kill approximately 30 Americans this way every month! Homicide by suffocation is a common finding in the daily practice of forensic pathology. Small children may suffocate accidentally by pulling plastic bags over their heads. *Small foreign bodies,* such as cherry pits or candy, when aspirated into the larynx and trachea, may completely block the air passage and cause death, especially in children.

Drowning is another example of obstruction of the respiratory tract. It is the third leading cause of accidental death in the United States, and current estimates indicate that more than 5000 people drown every year. The number of near-drowning victims is approximately 10 times that number, which indicates that 9 of every 10 persons thought to have drowned can be saved. Children and adolescents, mostly males, are the most common victims.

During an autopsy examination of a drowned person, one may encounter two sets of changes: a more common form, known as *wet drowning* (90 percent of cases) and a less common form, known as *dry drowning.* In wet drowning, the aspirated water enters the respiratory tract, filling the airways and thus preventing the entry of air. Anoxia results, and if the person is not resuscitated, death occurs within minutes. Dry drowning occurs as a result of reflex laryngospasm and closure of the glottis, which prevents fluid, as well as air, from entering the lower respiratory tract. These patients are more easily resuscitated and many can be saved. It is believed that most persons who experience near-drowning survive because of such laryngospasm.

Aspiration of sea water, which is hypertonic in respect to the blood, causes more pronounced pulmonary edema than does aspiration of fresh water. Whereas hypertonic sea water promotes the entry of water from the circulation into the alveoli, hypotonic fresh water is absorbed into the circulation. In patients who survive near-drowning, these distinctions are of limited clinical significance, as most clinical symptoms stem from hypoxia.

Ischemic brain injury is the most common cause of death. If the patient survives, pulmonary acidosis is the most common short-term consequence of anoxia. Long-term consequences depend on the duration of oxygen deprivation. Neurologic symptoms that develop as a result of brain ischemia and focal necrosis of neurons predominate. The extent of brain injury will ultimately determine the extent to which the patient will recover.

Ventilatory Failure

Respiratory (ventilatory) failure *secondary to alveolar hypoventilation* occurs in several conditions that may affect the following:

- Neural control of respiration
- Respiratory muscles
- Chest wall
- Airways

Neural control of respiration resides in the respiratory centers in the brain stem. It depends critically on peripheral input from chemoreceptors and the content of carbon dioxide in the blood. Brain stem le-

Table 8-5 Causes of Dyspnea

Causes	Examples
Large airway obstruction	Laryngospasm, foreign body
Small airway obstruction	Bronchiolitis, asthma
Intra-alveolar obstruction	Pneumonia, edema
Alveolar septal lesions	
Destruction	Emphysema
Increase in thickness	Interstitial fibrosis
Collapse	Atelectasis
Central nervous causes	Apoplexy of respiratory centers

sions, such as apoplexy, may depress spontaneous breathing. Retention of CO_2 (i.e., prolonged hypercapnia and the resulting acidosis) has the same effect.

The *respiratory muscles*—i.e., the diaphragm and the intercostal and other thoracic chest wall muscles—are striated muscles that are innervated by cranial or spinal nerves. These muscles may become dysfunctional under several conditions. Lesions affecting the nerves, the neuromuscular junction, or the muscles can impair ventilation. *Poliomyelitis,* a disease that affects the spinal cord, was previously known as the most dreaded cause of respiratory paralysis. Similar paralysis can occur following spinal cord trauma. *Tetanus* toxin causes muscle spasm. With tetanus, death is often secondary to respiratory failure because the muscles cannot move. *Myasthenia gravis* affects the neuromuscular junctions and will also depress breathing. *Muscular dystrophy,* especially in its most severe form (known as Duchenne-type dystrophy), is also marked by respiratory muscle failure.

Chest wall lesions that restrict the expansion of the chest wall during inspiration can also cause alveolar hypoxia. Respiratory movement is impaired in persons who have deformities of the chest cage (*kyphoscoliosis*) or pleural fibrosis and pleural tumors that encase the lungs. Extreme obesity can also depress respiration. Impeded respiration secondary to extreme obesity is called *pickwickian syndrome,* named so after the obese boy, Joe, described by Charles Dickens in *The Pickwick Papers.* Joe was so obese that he could not move. He was constantly somnolent, presumably from hypoxia and hypercapnia, related to his shallow and depressed breathing.

Airway pathology causing alveolar hypoxia has been described previously and is mentioned here only as a reminder and for the sake of completeness. The best examples are laryngospasm (croup), the bronchial mucous plugs associated with cystic fibrosis, and the alveolar lesions typical of interstitial pulmonary fibrosis, which may be caused by a variety of factors.

Adult Respiratory Distress Syndrome

Adult respiratory distress syndrome (ARDS) is a clinical term used to describe changes that occur in the lungs under a variety of conditions, all of which cause acute respiratory failure. The most important causes of ARDS are listed in Table 8-6.

Etiology and Pathogenesis. ARDS may develop through several pathways, usually beginning either as an injury of endothelial cells in pulmonary capillaries or an injury of alveolar lining cells (Fig. 8-20). The terminal airways (i.e., the alveolar walls), are in-

Table 8-6 Common Causes of Adult Respiratory Distress Syndrome (ARDS)

Shock
Trauma
Burns
Acute cardiac failure
Pneumonia
Bacterial
Viral
Toxic lung injury
Toxic fumes
Cytotoxic drugs
Bacterial endotoxins
Aspiration of fluids
Near-drowning

variably affected in either case, and their function is severely impaired. The consequences of initial injury are increased permeability of the alveolar blood vessels, loss of alveolar lining cells, and accumulation of fluid in the alveolar spaces. All of these events impair oxygenation of blood, resulting in anoxia. The disrupted pulmonary blood circulation strains the heart and patients die of severe cardiopulmonary failure.

Injury of the *alveolar lining cells* is the initiating event in viral pneumonia or following inhalation of toxic fumes. Leukocytes forming an intra-alveolar exudate in bacterial pneumonia also can damage alveolar cells. *Endothelial cell* injury is the initiating event in patients who are septic. Cytotoxic drugs or anoxia caused by cardiogenic shock can also damage endothelial cells. In many instances, ARDS is attributable to injury of both the alveolar lining cells and the endothelial cells. Inhalation of hot air, for example, may cause pulmonary burns which can destroy the entire alveolar wall (i.e., both the endothelial cells and the capillaries).

Pathology. Regardless of the etiology of ARDS, the lungs show the typical features of diffuse alveolar damage (DAD). On gross examination at autopsy, the lungs are heavy, filled with edema fluid, and are, therefore, airless. Histologically, the alveolar spaces are dilated and filled with proteinaceous edema fluid. The plasma extravasated into the alveoli clots, forming fibrin-rich hyaline membranes (Fig. 8-21). The alveolar capillaries are engorged with blood, which escapes focally into the alveoli. In disseminated intravascular coagulation (DIC), which is caused by shock, intra-alveolar hemorrhages are often associated with microthrombi in small pulmonary vessels.

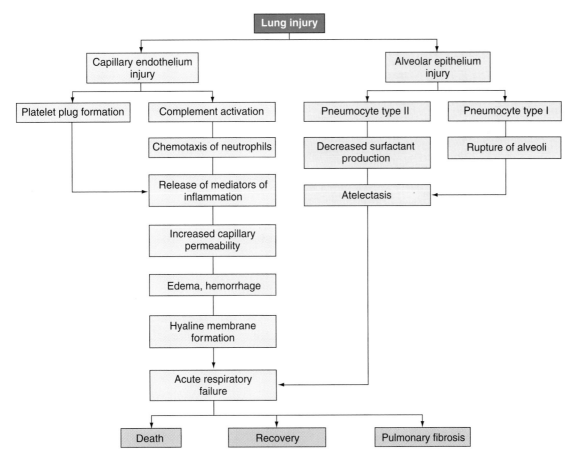

FIGURE 8-20
Adult respiratory distress syndrome (ARDS). The sequence of events may begin with an endothelial cell or an alveolar cell injury. Regardless of the initial injury, progression of the disease leads to a common pathway and respiratory failure.

Clinical Features. The symptoms of ARDS reflect the acute onset of respiratory failure. Initial symptoms usually occur within 24 hours of the inciting event. The patient is in severe distress, short of breath, and gasping for air. Laboratory findings confirm hypoxemia and hypercapnia. Chest x-ray studies show diffuse condensation of the lungs, which appear to be airless. Most patients must receive ventilator (respirator) therapy, and even in those who survive the initial lung injury, there is still a very high mortality. These patients are prone to infections and often die of pneumonia. Those who recover completely tend to have chronic respiratory problems related to the fibrosis of damaged alveolar septa. One third of patients die within days, one third die of pneumonia and heart failure within weeks of ARDS onset, and one third recover. Of those that recover, approximately 40 percent have permanent residual respiratory problems.

Atelectasis

Atelectasis (derived from the Greek *ateles*, meaning incomplete, and *ectasis*, meaning expansion) is a term used to denote incomplete expansion or, more often, collapse of alveoli. Minor focal atelectases are very common and accompany many pulmonary diseases. Massive atelectasis of the entire lungs is less common but is associated with more significant symptoms.

The most important causes of atelectasis, as shown in Fig. 8-22, are

- deficiency of surfactant
- compression of the lungs from outside
- resorption of air distal to bronchial obstruction

Atelectasis secondary to a deficiency of surfactant occurs in premature neonates who are born before their lungs have achieved functional maturity. Alveolar type II pneumocytes of immature lungs do not produce the surfactant. Because the alveoli cannot remain open, the lungs collapse. Because the infant cannot breathe, a respiratory distress syndrome develops that is associated with high mortality.

Compression atelectasis is usually caused by fluid in the pleural cavity. It may represent transudate formed as a result of heart failure, or an exudate caused by inflammation (*pleuritis*). Tumors of the pleura, especially those that are associated with

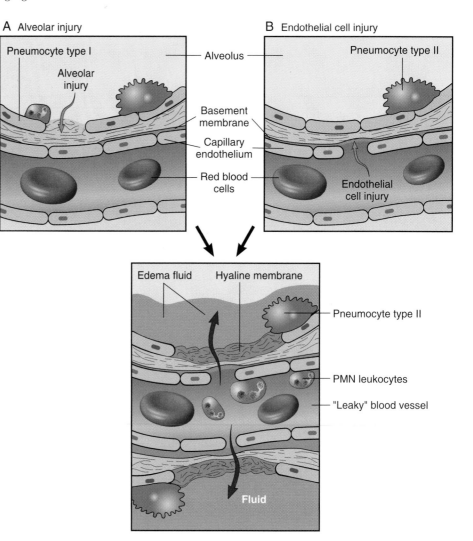

FIGURE 8-21

Pathogenesis of adult respiratory distress syndrome. (A) Alveolar cell injury. (B) Endothelial cell injury. Regardless of the initial injury, the established lesions appear identical and comprise hyaline membranes, ruptured alveolar walls, and intra-alveolar edema fluid. PMN, polymorphonuclear.

FIGURE 8-22

Mechanism of atelectasis. (A) Collapse of the lung in pneumothorax. (B) Compression of the lung by pleural fluid. (C) Resorption of the air from alveoli distal to an obstructed bronchus. Obstructive atelectasis is usually focal. Atelectasis of premature infants, which is caused by a deficiency of pulmonary surfactant, is not shown.

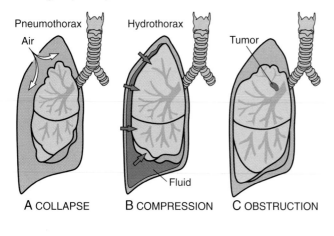

pleural effusion, also can compress the lungs. The fluid compressing the lungs prevents their expansion. Entry of air into the pleural cavity (*pneumothorax*) also causes massive pulmonary atelectasis.

Resorption atelectasis typically develops within a single pulmonary anatomic unit distal to an obstructed bronchus. The obstruction may be caused by a mucous plug, tumor, or foreign material that is aspirated into the bronchial tree. The air from alveoli distal to the obstructed bronchus is resorbed, and the alveolar walls collapse.

Atelectasis is usually reversible. After the causative defect has been corrected, the alveoli expand and resume their normal function.

Neoplasms of the Respiratory Tract

The most important **neoplasms of the respiratory tract** are *lung cancer* and *carcinoma of the larynx*. In comparison with these two neoplasms, all the others

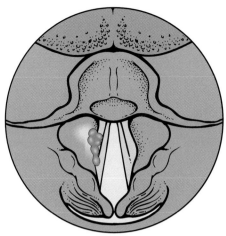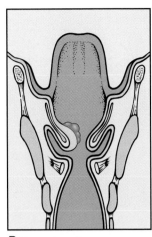

A Mirror view of carcinoma of the larynx. The vocal cord is infiltrated with the tumor.

B Coronal section

FIGURE 8-23
Carcinoma of the larynx. The tumor resembles an ulcerated nodule.

are of minor significance and do not warrant discussion.

Carcinoma of the Larynx

Carcinoma of the larynx accounts for less than 2 percent of all human cancers. The most important facts about carcinomas of the larynx are as follows:

- It has been pathogenetically linked to smoking and chronic alcohol intake. This accounts in part for the high prevalence of laryngeal cancer in males, who are affected seven times more frequently than females.
- Laryngeal cancer is rare in people younger than 40 years of age, and its incidence increases with advancing age.
- Carcinoma may originate from any part of the larynx. Tumors originating above the glottis are called supraglottic, whereas those arising below this demarcation line are termed infraglottic.
- Laryngeal tumors present as nodules or ulcerations of the mucosa (Fig. 8-23). If not resected, these tumors invade locally and tend to metastasize to local neck lymph nodes. Distant metastases are a late event.
- Histologic examination reveals that essentially all laryngeal cancers are squamous cell carcinoma.

Patients with carcinoma of the larynx present relatively early in the course of the disease with symptoms such as hoarseness, loss of voice, or stridorous respiration. Because the tumors are discovered early and are mostly localized at the time of diagnosis, the overall prognosis is very good. The 5-year survival rate of patients who have been treated surgically or by radiation therapy is 75 percent.

Lung Carcinoma

Lung carcinoma is the leading cause of cancer death in the United States and most other Western industrialized countries. Until a few years ago, affected males outnumbered females by a large margin. However, changing work habits and increased smoking among women in the post-World War II era have contributed to an increased incidence of lung cancer among women. The campaign against smoking has only slightly reduced the incidence of lung cancer in the United States, but very little elsewhere. In this context, it is worth remembering the following:

- Lung cancer is the most common malignant disease of internal organs in the United States. It has been predicted that during the 1990s, approximately 150,000 people will die of lung cancer every year.
- Lung cancer is, in most cases, caused by cigarette smoking. Although there is no definitive proof to support this statement, the epidemiologic evidence linking lung cancer to smoking is very persuasive. Approximately 90 percent of patients with lung cancer are smokers!
- Lung cancer is rare before the age of 40 years, but thereafter, its incidence rises in direct proportion with age.
- Lung cancer still has a very poor prognosis. The overall 5-year survival rate is 10 percent to 15 percent, and in most instances, the disease is incurable.

Etiology and Pathogenesis. The events leading to the formation of lung carcinoma are not fully understood. Various chemicals in tobacco smoke probably act as the primary carcinogens. The tobacco smoke contains many potentially harmful substances, the most important of which are chemically classified as polycyclic hydrocarbons. Like the polycyclic hydrocarbons derived from tar, those in cigarette smoke are also mutagenic to bacteria in vitro in the Ames test. In tissue culture, these chemicals can initiate and promote malignant transformation of normal mammalian cells. It is assumed that the exposure to carcinogens in smoke initiates malignant transformation of bronchial cells and promotes their progression into invasive cancer. This probably involves the direct action of carcinogens on cellular DNA, the activation of oncogenes, or mutation and inhibition of tumor suppressor genes.

Inhaled procarcinogens (incomplete carcinogens) are transformed into carcinogens through the action of cytoplasmic enzymes in bronchial cells exposed to smoke. Inducibility of these enzymes, which are potentially important for carcinogenesis, is genetically determined. It is high in some persons and low in others. These genetic differences could account for the fact that not all smokers develop lung cancer, as well as for the increased predisposition to lung cancer noted in some families.

The chemicals inhaled in tobacco smoke contain several proven carcinogens, but also various irritants that could act as promoters of incipient neoplasia. Histologic studies of respiratory epithelia in smokers indicate that, in most cases, bronchial cancer is associated with a variety of preneoplastic lesions that are most likely caused by the combined action of carcinogens and irritants.

It has been proposed that the sequence of events begins with metaplasia of the bronchial epithelium. This reactive, benign lesion is characterized by a transformation of normal, pseudostratified, cylindrical epithelium into squamous epithelium (Fig. 8-24). Metaplasia is initially a reversible lesion. If smoking is discontinued, the lesion will disappear and the normal structure of bronchial epithelium will be restored. If the carcinogenic stimuli persist, metaplasia will progress into carcinoma in situ, and this will give rise to invasive carcinoma, most of which will be of the squamous type. Initial squamous metaplasia explains the paradoxical appearance of a *squamous cell carcinoma* in an epithelium not normally composed of squamous cells.

If the transformed cells progress and become more anaplastic, the tumor will be histologically classified as an *undifferentiated large-cell carcinoma*. In some bronchial carcinomas, the malignant transformation will primarily involve the neuroendocrine cells, which are normally present in the bronchial mucosa as well as in the foci of squamous metaplasia. These tumors of neuroendocrine cells are called *small-cell carcinomas*. Finally, some bronchial tumors will be composed of cylindrical cells, resembling the normal cells in the bronchus. These cells tend to form irregular glands and are classified as *adenocarcinomas*.

In addition to the centrally located *hilar carcinomas*, which can be of four histologic types, lung carcinomas may originate as *peripheral neoplasms*, most of which have the appearance of adenocarcinomas. These probably arise from small bronchi and bronchioli. Such tumors grow inside the alveoli and are, therefore, called *bronchioloalveolar carcinomas*. Peripheral adenocarcinomas also originate from pulmonary scars, presumably from bronchiolar cells trapped in the fibrous tissue ("scar carcinomas"). Finally, it should be noted that malignant tumors can also originate from pleural lining cells. These are called *mesotheliomas*.

Pathology. Early bronchial cancer—the only form of lung cancer for which there is a high chance for cure—is not readily recognizable by radiographic examination and can be identified only by bronchoscopy. The diagnosis is usually made on the basis of histologic examination of "suspicious" lesions that resemble whitish plaques. Unfortunately, these early cancers are seldom identified in clinical practice.

Most tumors that surgeons or pathologists encounter are grossly visible nodules attached to the bronchi and extending into the adjacent parenchyma or protruding into the lumen (Fig. 8-25). These tumors are moderately soft, and are white or grayish on the cut surface. In clinical practice, these tumors are seen on x-ray studies as nodules. Those that protrude into the bronchi and those that cause ulceration of the overlying bronchial mucosa can be recognized by bronchoscopy.

Histologically, tumors of the lung can be classified into several groups:

- squamous cell carcinoma (30 percent)
- adenocarcinoma (30 percent)
- large-cell undifferentiated carcinoma (10 percent)
- small-cell carcinoma (20 percent)
- tumors of mixed pattern (10 percent)

Each of these tumor types has unique histologic features, although there is some overlap between some of them. For practical purposes, it is sufficient

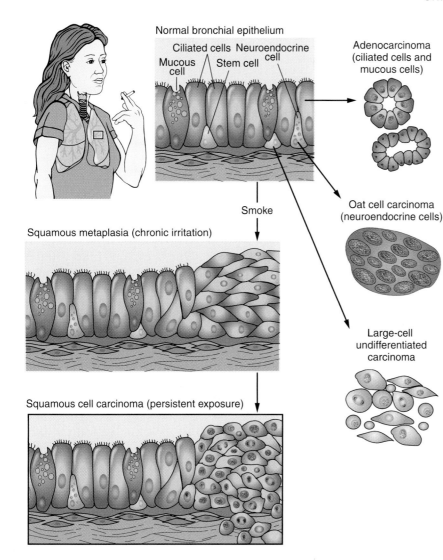

Normal bronchial epithelium

Ciliated cells Neuroendocrine cell

Mucous cell Stem cell

Adenocarcinoma (ciliated cells and mucous cells)

Smoke

Oat cell carcinoma (neuroendocrine cells)

Squamous metaplasia (chronic irritation)

Large-cell undifferentiated carcinoma

Squamous cell carcinoma (persistent exposure)

FIGURE 8-24
Histogenesis of lung carcinoma of the bronchus. Most tumors originate from bronchi and are caused by smoking. The columnar epithelium undergoes squamous metaplasia, which is reversible but can progress to carcinoma in situ and invasive squamous cell carcinoma. Tumors resembling and/or originating from mucous or ciliated cells are classified as adenocarcinomas, whereas those from neuroendocrine cells are classified as oat cell carcinomas. Large-cell undifferentiated carcinomas orginate from stem cells that have become anaplastic and have never differentiated.

FIGURE 8-25
Lung cancer. (A) Centrally located lung carcinoma. (B) Peripheral carcinoma.

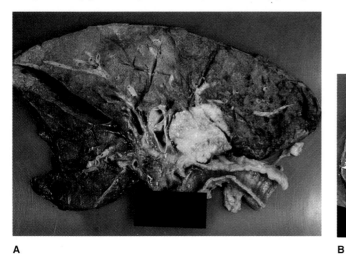

A

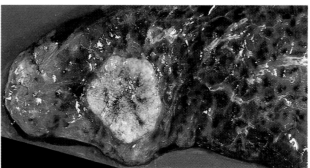

B

to separate small-cell carcinomas from all others, which are grouped under the name of non–small-cell lung carcinoma (NSCLC). Small-cell carcinomas are treated differently and have a worse prognosis than do NSCLCs. Mixed tumors that have a significant small-cell component are treated as pure small-cell carcinomas.

Lung cancer is a highly invasive tumor and it tends to metastasize early. Locally, these tumors extend into the mediastinum and often spread into the pleural cavity. At the time of diagnosis, more than 70 percent of patients already have metastases that are apparent, and many more probably have microscopic metastases that are clinically inapparent. Approximately one half of those with tumors extending beyond the lung parenchyma have metastases to the local lymph nodes.

Distant metastases are most often found in the liver and brain (Fig. 8-26). Lung cancer also has a tendency to metastasize to bones, kidneys, and, for some peculiar reason, to the adrenals.

FIGURE 8-26
Metastases from lung carcinoma.

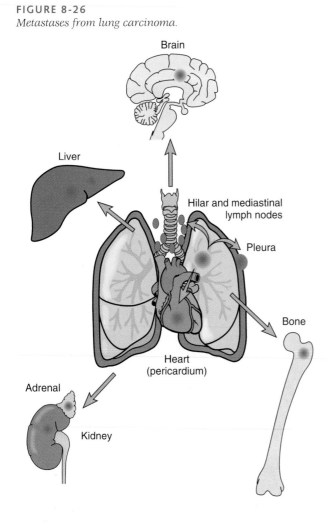

Clinical Features. Symptoms of lung cancer can be classified as being related to

- bronchial irritation or obstruction
- local extension into the mediastinum or pleural cavity
- distant metastases
- systemic effects of neoplasia

Approximately 10 percent to 15 percent of patients with lung cancer have no obvious symptoms, and the tumor is discovered incidentally during routine chest x-ray examination. Among the patients who are symptomatic, approximately one third will report to the physician with symptoms pertaining to local effects of tumor in the chest, one third will present with symptoms pertaining to distant metastases, and one third will present with nonspecific systemic complaints and no localizing symptoms.

Bronchial irritation most often causes coughing; less commonly, it causes respiratory wheezing, dyspnea, and other respiratory symptoms. Hemoptysis is reported in 30 percent of all patients.

Local extension of the tumor into the pulmonary parenchyma tends to obstruct bronchi, cause atelectasis, and predispose the individual to lung infection. Extension to the pleural surface is typically associated with pleural effusion and progressive dyspnea secondary to lung compression. Ingrowth of tumor into the mediastinal nerves causes pain or paralysis of muscles of the diaphragm or vocal cords. Tumor may also extend into the esophagus and cause dysphagia.

Distant metastases produce symptoms that are specific to the organ(s) involved. Liver metastases cause hepatomegaly. Brain metastases result in neurologic symptoms and are associated with high mortality. Bone metastases result in fractures. Adrenal metastases may produce destruction of the glands and cause Addison's disease (i.e., adrenocortical insufficiency).

The *systemic symptoms* of lung cancer do not differ significantly from symptoms produced by other tumors, and include weight loss and cachexia, anorexia, and general malaise.

Lung tumors also produce various *paraneoplastic syndromes*. The most common among these are syndromes caused by oversecretion of

- parathyroid-like polypeptide, which results in hypercalcemia
- adrenocorticotropic hormone (ACTH), which results in overstimulation of the adrenals (Cushing's syndrome)
- antidiuretic hormone, which results in excessive retention of water in the kidneys and dilutional hyponatremia

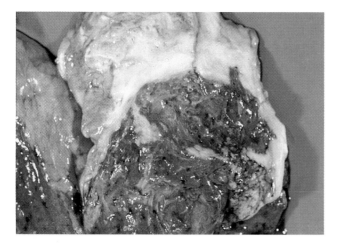

FIGURE 8-27
Mesothelioma. The tumor is on the pleural surface encasing the lung.

Lung cancer is essentially incurable. Treatment includes surgery, radiation therapy, and chemotherapy. The overall 5-year survival is around 10 percent to 15 percent. The only tumors that can be cured are those that are clinically inapparent and were discovered by chance on cytologic examination or bronchoscopy.

Metastatic Cancer

Although lung cancer represents the most common malignant disease in humans today, primary lung carcinomas are less common than lung metastases from other sites. As a large amount of blood circulates through the lungs, any tumor cell floating in the blood could be filtered out while passing through the pulmonary capillaries. Furthermore, the thoracic duct, the main lymphatic vessel, is confluent with the superior vena cava; thus, tumor cells transported in the lymph will also lodge in the lungs.

Pulmonary metastases may present as

- solitary lesions
- multiple lesions
- diffuse lesions replacing large parts of the lung or diffusely covering the pleural surface

Solitary metastases may be resected. If the patient has no other evidence of tumor, such treatment may be beneficial and prolong life. Metastases, recognized by x-ray studies as round nodules ("cannonball lesions"), are incurable.

Other Tumors

All other tumors besides primary lung cancer and metastases are rare. *Carcinoid* is a neuroendocrine tumor of low-grade malignancy. These tumors have a tendency to invade locally and to grow slowly, and they do not metastasize to distant places. Local resection is the treatment of choice. Cure can be achieved in more than 80 percent of cases. *Mesothelioma* is a rare malignant tumor of the pleura (Fig. 8-27). Almost invariably, mesothelioma is related to exposure to asbestos in the workplace. These tumors are invasive locally but do not metastasize outside the thorax until late in the course of the disease. The pleural tumors encase the lung, preventing its expansion during inspiration. Mesothelioma is an incurable neoplasm with an abysmal prognosis.

Pleural Diseases

The pleura forms the outer covering of the lung (visceral pleura) and the inner covering of the chest cage (parietal pleura). The space between the two layers of pleura is called the pleural cavity. It is a virtual space because the two layers of the pleura are tightly apposed to one another and are separated only by a thin film of fluid that keeps the surfaces moist, allowing movement of the lungs during respiration. The negative pressure within the pleural cavity keeps the lungs expanded. If the traction of this negative pressure is lost, the internal elastic forces of the lung tissue will prevail and the lung will collapse toward the hilum.

Entry of air into the pleural cavity is called **pneumothorax** (Fig. 8-28). This typically occurs following stab wounds of the chest wall or rupture of

FIGURE 8-28
Pleural diseases. Pleuritis is usually associated with pleural effusion. Fibrothorax is an encasement of the lungs with fibrous tissue that obliterates the pleural cavity. Pneumothorax denotes the entry of air into the pleural cavity. Empyema involves pockets of pus enclosed in fibrous adhesions.

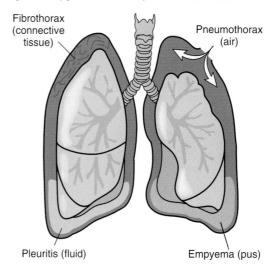

Fibrothorax (connective tissue)

Pneumothorax (air)

Pleuritis (fluid)

Empyema (pus)

emphysematous lung tissue. Pneumothorax causes pulmonary atelectasis. It is a reversible lesion which may heal spontaneously or be cured surgically.

Accumulation of fluid in the pleural cavity is called **hydrothorax** or **pleural effusion.** The fluid can be an *exudate,* caused by inflammation, or a *transudate (hydrothorax).* Exudate is a hallmark of **pleuritis.** Bacterial pneumonias typically produce a fibrinous or purulent pleuritis, whereas viral pneumonias produce serous pleuritis. Tuberculosis and other granulomatous diseases tend to produce serous or fibrinous pleuritis and do not cause exudation of PMNs. Transudate accumulates in the pleural cavity secondary to heart failure or in generalized edema.

Serous pleuritis or hydrothorax tends to resolve without any consequences. Fibrinous or fibrinopurulent pleuritis, especially if associated with inflammation of the pleura or tissue destruction, stimulates the ingrowth of granulation tissue into the pleural cavity. This leads to obliteration of the cavity and the formation of fibrous adhesions between the visceral and parietal pleura, called *fibrothorax.* Partial fibrotic obliteration of the pleural cavity filled with pus results in *empyema.* Empyema resembles an abscess in which the pus may remain for extended periods of time unless surgically removed.

Tumors of the pleura may be primary or secondary. *Primary tumors* (mesotheliomas) are rare, and are, as mentioned earlier, found almost exclusively in people exposed to asbestos. *Secondary tumors* are either pulmonary primaries extending to the pleura or metastases from distant sites. Ovarian and breast cancers often metastasize to the pleura. These tumors are usually associated with pleural effusions, which contain floating tumor cells. The diagnosis can be made by submitting a sample of pleural fluid for cytologic examination. All malignant pleural tumors have a poor prognosis.

Review Questions

1. What kind of epithelia line the respiratory tract?
2. What are the main functions of the respiratory system?
3. Describe the respiratory defense system.
4. What are the main respiratory diseases?
5. Compare the infections of the upper respiratory system with those of the so-called "middle respiratory system."
6. What could cause a "runny nose?"
7. What is croup?
8. Compare epiglottitis and bronchiolitis.
9. Compare alveolar and interstitial pneumonia.
10. List the most common causes of pneumonia and give specific characteristics about each of these forms of lung infection.
11. Compare lobar pneumonia and bronchopneumonia with interstitial pneumonia.
12. Explain complications of bacterial pneumonia.
13. Compare community-acquired pneumonia and hospital-acquired pneumonia.
14. What are the clinical signs of pneumonia and how is this disease diagnosed?
15. Explain the concept of atypical pneumonia and give specific examples of this clinicopathologic entity.
16. Compare primary and secondary tuberculosis.
17. Which fungi cause pneumonia and under what circumstances?
18. Which pathogens cause pulmonary abscesses?
19. Compare chronic obstructive pulmonary disease (COPD) caused by chronic bronchitis and COPD caused by emphysema.
20. What is bronchiectasis and how does it develop?

21. Compare centrilobular and panacinar emphysema.
22. List the most important immune diseases of the respiratory tract.
23. Explain the pathogenesis of asthma.
24. Compare extrinsic and intrinsic asthma.
25. What is sarcoidosis and how does it affect the body?
26. List several important antigens that cause hypersensitivity pneumonitis.
27. Compare acute and chronic hypersensitivity pneumonitis.
28. What is pneumoconiosis?
29. How does inhalation of mineral particles damage the lungs?
30. Explain the effect of air pollutants on the lungs.
31. Explain the pathogenesis of coal-workers' lung disease.
32. What is silicosis and how does it present pathologically?
33. Which lung diseases are related to exposure to asbestos?
34. Explain the pathogenesis of dyspnea caused by various mechanisms.
35. Compare the pathologic findings in wet drowning and dry drowning.
36. List four main pathogenetic mechanisms of ventilatory failure and explain how they affect respiration.
37. List common causes of adult respiratory distress syndrome.
38. Describe the pathology of adult respiratory distress syndrome and explain its pathogenesis.
39. What are the possible outcomes of adult respiratory distress syndrome?
40. What is atelectasis and what are its possible causes?
41. What are the most important neoplasms of the respiratory tract?
42. Correlate the pathology of carcinomas of the larynx with clinical findings and prognosis of the disease.
43. How common is lung cancer?
44. How is tobacco smoking related to lung carcinoma?
45. Explain the histogenesis of various histologic types of lung carcinoma.
46. Compare hilar (central) and peripheral lung carcinoma.
47. Where do lung carcinomas metastasize?
48. What are the clinical signs of lung cancer?
49. What are the common paraneoplastic syndromes caused by lung carcinoma?
50. Compare pneumothorax and hydrothorax.
51. Explain the pathogenesis of pleuritis.
52. What is mesothelioma?

Learning Objectives

After reading this chapter, the student should be able to:

1. Describe the morphology of blood cells and their functions.

2. Define anemia and list three major forms of this disease.

3. Discuss the possible causes of aplastic anemia and the bone biopsy findings in aplastic anemia.

4. Describe the causes and typical findings in iron deficiency and pernicious anemia.

5. List three forms of hereditary anemia and discuss their pathogenesis.

6. Compare hemolytic anemias caused by intrinsic and extrinsic red blood cell defects.

7. Discuss the pathogenesis of hemolytic disease of the neonate due to Rh incompatibility between the mother and the fetus.

8. Compare polycythemia vera with secondary polycythemia.

9. Define leukocytosis-leukopenia and lymphocytosis-lymphopenia, and list the possible causes of these conditions.

10. Define leukemia and lymphoma and discuss the classification of these diseases.

11. List the common pathologic findings in leukemia and lymphoma and relate them to clinical symptoms.

12. Define Hodgkin's disease and compare it with non-Hodgkin's disease.

13. Define multiple myeloma, list the most common sites involved by this disease, and list three laboratory findings.

14. List three congenital bleeding disorders and explain their pathogenesis.

Additional Key Terms and Concepts

Anticoagulants

Disseminated intravascular coagulation (DIC)

Erythropoietin

Hemophilia

Purpura

Chapter Outline

The Hematopoietic and Lymphoid Systems

Chapter 9

nalysis of blood represents one of the most important laboratory tests. It is routinely performed on most, if not all, hospitalized patients, as well as many of those seen in ambulatory health care facilities. The blood reflects the pathologic changes in many internal organs and is thus a valuable source of information about body functions and health in general. General medical practitioners, highly specialized physicians, nurses, and many allied health professionals deal with hematologic data on a daily basis and are trained to interpret such findings.

The discipline concerned with the study of blood is called *hematology* (derived from the Greek words for blood [*haima*] and science [*logos*]). The clinicians treating disorders of blood cells and coagulation factors are called hematologists and hematopathologists.

Expert hematologists are called in as consultants on complicated cases and those patients who do not respond to standard therapy. Hematologists also treat patients with neoplastic diseases of blood-forming tissues, such as leukemia; primary deficiencies of bone marrow, such as aplastic anemia; and bleeding disorders, such as hemophilia. Hematopathologists supervise blood banks and prepare blood and blood components for transfusions.

NORMAL ANATOMY AND PHYSIOLOGY

Blood is a specialized tissue that consists of fluid, known as **plasma**, and cells, including **white blood cells** (*leukocytes*), **red blood cells** (*erythrocytes*), and **platelets** (*thrombocytes*). White blood cells are further divided into granulocytes, monocytes, and lymphocytes. Granulocytes are of three kinds: neutrophils, eosinophils, and basophils.

Hematopoiesis (from the Greek *haima,* meaning blood, and *poiesis,* meaning formation) begins in fetal life from stem cells located in the yolk sac (Fig. 9-1). From the yolk sac, the hematopoietic stem cells migrate to the liver and then to the bone marrow and, to some extent, to the **spleen** and **lymph nodes** and thymus. Extramedullary hematopoiesis in the liver and the spleen subsides after birth, and the **bone marrow** remains the primary blood-forming organ. As the organism matures, the red bone marrow of the long bones is replaced by fat. Only the flat bones (e.g., sternum or pelvic bones) produce blood during adulthood. The thymus and lymph nodes remain sites of lymphocytopoiesis in infancy and adolescence. The thymus usually involutes after puberty. Lymph nodes form lymphocytes, but in adults, these organs do not produce red blood cells or granulocytic leukocytes. However, if the hematopoietic bone marrow is destroyed, *extramedullary hematopoiesis* may resume in the spleen, liver, and lymph nodes.

The mature blood cells are descendants of developmentally pluripotent hematopoietic stem cells. The term pluripotent means that these cells can differentiate and develop into more than one mature cell type. The mother stem cell differentiates into several developmentally committed stem cells, which are the precursors of distinct cell lineages, the ultimate product of which are the mature blood cells. Two major cell lineages are formed: lymphoid and myeloid (Fig. 9-2). The lymphoid stem cell gives rise to B cells, which finally mature into immunoglobulin-secreting plasma cells, and T cells, which assume their function in mediating cell-mediated immune reactions after they have passed through the thymus (T—thymus!). The myeloid stem cell, also known as the trilineage-myeloid stem cell, gives rise to three subsets of stem cells, which are the precursors of mature erythrocytes, megakaryocytes, neutrophils, monocytes, eosinophils, and basophils.

The stem cells of various cell lineages are small, undifferentiated cells that are indistinguishable from one another, yet they differ with regard to their development potential. This developmental potential can be realized only in the presence of specific growth factors, called colony-stimulating factors (CSFs). Most CSFs are produced in the bone marrow, which forms the ideal microenvironment for the growth and development of hematopoietic stem cells. Many other growth factors, such as interleukins produced by macrophages and T lymphocytes, also stimulate blood cell formation. Only the growth factor for the erythroid cell lineages—*erythropoietin*—is produced outside the bone marrow, (i.e., in the kidney).

Peripheral Blood

In living persons, the blood is found in the vessels and the heart. It amounts to 7.5 percent of total body weight, which means that an average person has 5.5 to 6 L of blood. Taller men have more blood than small men, and females typically have less blood than males.

The blood cells circulate through blood vessels

Did You Know?

Isolation of the genes for erythropoietin and other hematopoietic growth factors made it possible for researchers to produce those recombinant growth factors in large quantities. Anemic patients who do not have endogenous erythropoietin because their kidneys have been destroyed by disease can be treated successfully with recombinant erythropoietin.

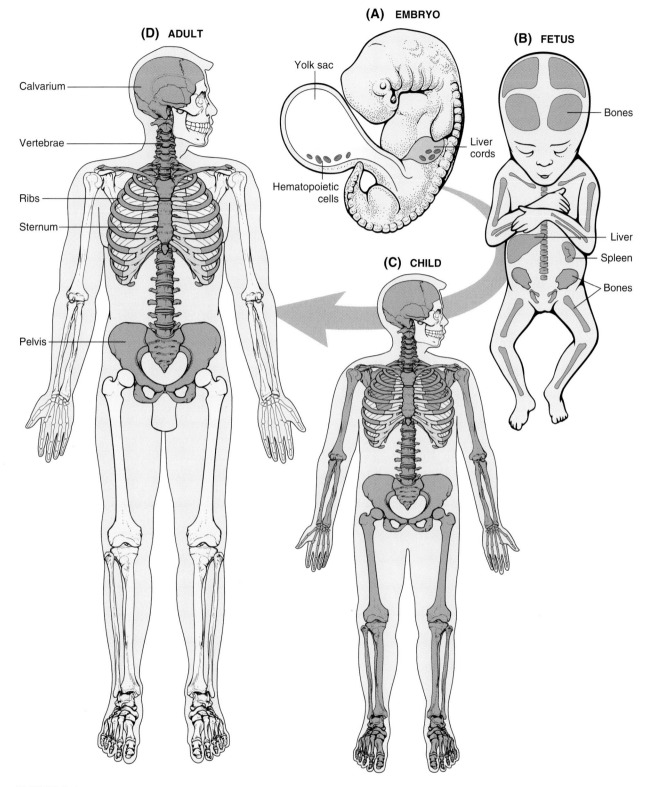

(A) EMBRYO

Yolk sac

Hematopoietic
cells

Liver
cords

(B) FETUS

Bones

Liver

Spleen

Bones

(D) ADULT

Calvarium

Vertebrae

Ribs

Sternum

Pelvis

(C) CHILD

FIGURE 9-1

*Sites of hematopoiesis in various age groups. (A) The first signs of hematopoiesis are in the
fetal yolk sac. (B) Fetus. Hematopoiesis is evident in all the bones, liver, and spleen. (C) Child.
Hematopoiesis is evident in the short bones. (D) Adult. Whereas in the child, essentially all
bones contain hematopoietic bone marrow, in the adult, the hematopoiesis is limited to the flat
and short bones of the axial skeleton (i.e., the calvaria, vertebrae, ribs, and pelvic bones).*

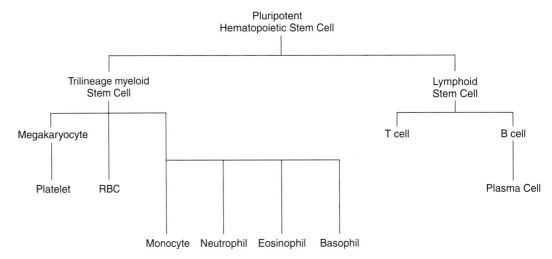

FIGURE 9-2

Hematopoiesis. All cell lineages originate from a developmentally pluripotent stem cell. This common precursor gives rise to developmentally restricted stem cells: erythromyeloid stem cells and lymphoid stem cells. The descendants of these intermediate stem cells are mature T and B lymphocytes, erythrocytes, neutrophils, monocytes, eosinophils, basophils, and megakaryocytes (platelets).

suspended freely in the plasma. Blood cells can be separated from the plasma by allowing the formed elements to form a sediment over a period of several hours at the bottom of a tube coated with anticoagulant. This can be achieved much faster by centrifuging the blood at high speed for 2 to 3 minutes. The volume of packed red blood cells, expressed as a percentage of the total peripheral blood, is called the *hematocrit*. In normal adults, formed blood cell elements constitute 40 percent to 45 percent of the total blood volume, whereas the plasma accounts for 55 percent to 60 percent. Normal peripheral blood parameters are listed in Table 9-1.

The blood withdrawn into a tube that is coated with anticoagulants can be separated by centrifugation into a fluid phase (*plasma*) and a cell-rich phase (Fig. 9-3). Most of this second phase consists of red blood cells except for the top layer, called the "buffy coat," which contains leukocytes and platelets.

Blood cells can be separated from the fluid by allowing the blood to coagulate. The coagulation proteins are consumed in this process, which leads to transformation of plasma into serum. Serum is defined as defibrinated plasma. It contains all the proteins except fibrinogen, prothrombin, and other coagulation factors. Some blood tests can be performed only on plasma, whereas others can be

Table 9-1 Composition of Blood

Plasma (55%)	Cells (45%)
Water (92%)	Red blood cells (erythrocytes): 4.5 million/μL
Proteins (7%) Albumin Immunoglobulins Clotting factors Enzymes Transport proteins	White blood cells (leukocytes): 5,000–10,000/μL
	Granulocytes
Salts	Neutrophils (60–70%)
Lipids Cholesterol	Eosinophils (1–3%)
	Basophils (1%)
Carbohydrates Glucose	Monocytes (4–8%)
	Lymphocytes (20–40%)
Gases Oxygen Carbon dioxide	Platelets (thrombocytes): 150,000–400,000/μL

FIGURE 9-3

Blood drawn into a tube that contains an anticoagulant can be separated by centrifugation into plasma and formed cell elements (red blood cells and a buffy coat that contains mostly white blood cells and platelets). EDTA, ethylenediaminetetraacetic acid.

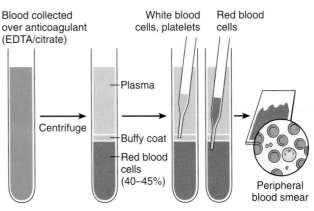

performed on serum. The blood submitted in heparinized ("green top"), ethylenediaminetetra-acetic acid (EDTA)–coated ("lavender top"), or sodium citrate–containing tubes ("blue top") will not clot, and with centrifugation, plasma will be obtained. By contrast, blood collected in "red top" tubes, which do not contain anticoagulants, will coagulate and, upon centrifugation, will yield serum. Plasma is typically used for the study of clotting disturbances. Most other biochemical tests are performed on serum. In general, clinical laboratories specify the requirements for each test, and one must check the hospital manual before drawing blood for a specific test.

OVERVIEW OF MAJOR DISEASES

Hematologic diseases occur as a result of abnormal formation, increased destruction, or abnormal structure and function of blood cells. Principal hematologic diseases include the following:

- Anemia
- Leukemia
- Lymphoma
- Bleeding disorders

Several facts important to an understanding of the hematopoietic system are presented here, before a discussion of specific pathologic entities.

1. *Erythrocytes are ideally suited for their primary function: transport of oxygen from the lungs into the peripheral tissues.* Erythrocytes are red (in Greek, *erythros* means red), biconcave disks that are thinnest in the center (Fig. 9-4) and thickest at the periphery. The red color is derived from hemoglobin, an iron-containing pigment that constitutes 90 percent of the dry weight of each erythrocyte. In peripheral blood smears, the thinner central portion, spanning half of the cell diameter, appears paler than the peripheral part. The erythrocytes are round, but can easily be deformed while passing through small capillaries and other small vessels. Erythrocytes do not have nuclei or organelles that would interfere with their transport function. Because of their biconcave shape, they have a large surface that allows easy diffusion of gases.

2. *Hemoglobin is a complex molecule that consists of four heme groups and four globins.* Heme is composed of four pyrrole rings held together with a centrally placed iron in ferrous form (Fe^{++}). The heme portion of hemoglobin is the oxygen-binding part of the molecule. Heme cannot be synthesized without iron. *Iron deficiency anemia* is thus marked by low hemoglobin (Hb) values.

FIGURE 9-4
Schematic drawing of an erythrocyte and hemoglobin. The cell is biconcave and lacks a nucleus. Hemoglobin is the main component of red blood cells. Note that the molecule consists of globin and heme. The globin consists of four polypeptide chains (α, β, γ, δ). Heme is made up of four pyrrole rings held together by iron in ferrous form (Fe^{++}). Upon degradation of hemoglobin, iron and globin are reutilized immediately. Pyrrole rings give rise to bilirubin.

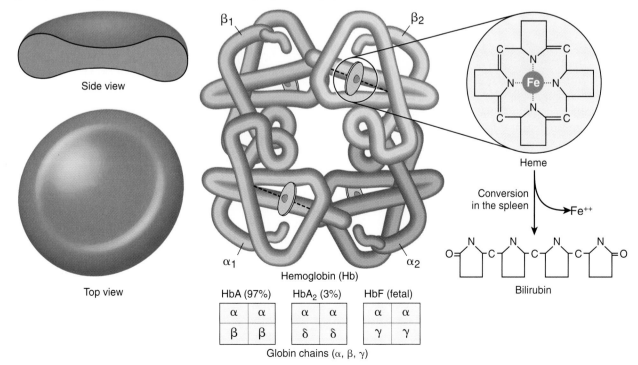

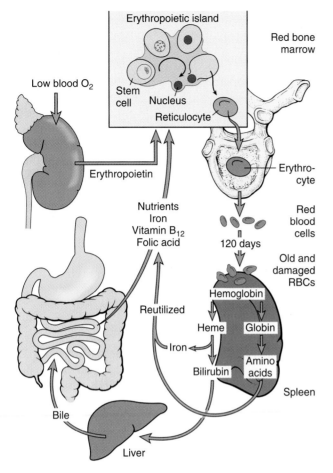

FIGURE 9-5

The events in the life of erythrocytes. Nucleated red blood cell (RBC) precursors, stimulated by erythropoietin, form erythrocytes in the bone marrow. Normal synthesis of hemoglobin occurs only in the presence of nutrients, iron, vitamin B$_{12}$, and folic acid. Mature RBCs are released into circulation. The old or defective RBCs are degraded in the spleen. Iron and globin are reutilized immediately. Bilirubin is released in bile into the intestine.

The globin part of hemoglobin consists of four polypeptide chains designated by the Greek letters alpha, beta, gamma, and delta. Alpha chains are present in all hemoglobins. Two alpha and two beta chains form HbA; two alpha and two delta chains form HbA$_2$; and two alpha and two gamma chains form HbF (see Fig. 9-4).

Each globin chain is synthesized under the control of a specific gene. Mutations of these genes cause hemoglobinopathies marked by abnormal hemoglobins; for example, sickle cell anemia is characterized by an abnormal A chain known as hemoglobin S (HbS).

3. *Hemoglobin synthesis requires iron, vitamin B$_{12}$, vitamin B$_6$, and folic acid.* Deficiency of these nutrients also results in anemia. Anemia may develop because the nutrient is not available in food, because it cannot be absorbed, or because the loss exceeds the intake.

4. *Red blood cells live in the circulation 120 days* (Fig. 9-5). The aging cells are sequestered in the spleen, which removes the old and defective red blood cells from circulation and serves as their primary "graveyard." The phagocytic cells of the spleen digest the main components of the red blood cells and release them into the circulation for reutilization and excretion from the body. Essentially, all protein components and iron are reutilized. Heme is converted to *bilirubin,* which is excreted in bile into the intestine. The intestinal bilirubin is reabsorbed and partially reutilized and/or metabolized, and is excreted in the form of urobilinogen and stercobilinogen in urine and feces.

5. *Objective measurements of red blood cell parameters are done with instruments that estimate the mean size of red blood cells and their hemoglobin content.* Analysis of blood has become highly automated and is performed with highly sophisticated instruments. The following measurements are clinically important:

- *Mean corpuscular volume* (MCV) denotes the mean volume of each red blood cell. Normal values are in the range of 83 to 99 fL. MCV is calculated by dividing the hematocrit value by the red blood cell count. Low values (< 80 fL) indicate microcytic anemia, whereas high values (> 100 fL) indicate macrocytic anemia.
- *Mean corpuscular hemoglobin* (MCH) content denotes the content of hemoglobin per each red blood cell. It is obtained by dividing hemoglobin concentration by the hematocrit value. Normal values are in the range of 28 to 32 pg. Low values indicate hypochromic anemia.
- *Mean corpuscular hemoglobin concentration* (MCHC) denotes the concentration of hemoglobin in red blood cells. It is obtained by dividing the hemoglobin level by the hematocrit value. Normal values are in the range of 32 to 36 g/dL. Low values indicate hypochromic anemia.

6. *White blood cells participate in the body's defense against infections. Neutrophils* are the most numerous white blood cells in the blood, accounting for 60 percent to 70 percent of all nucleated cells. The main function of neutrophils is to defend the body against bacterial infections. Neutrophils are most qualified for this job, as they have remarkable mobility (i.e., they can *migrate* rapidly to the site of infection by ameboid movement), they respond quickly to *chemotactic* stimuli released from the site of inflammation, they are capable of *phagocytosis* (i.e., uptake of bacteria), and finally, they can kill the bacteria with the *bactericidal* substances contained within their cytoplasmic granules. *Eosinophils* form 1 percent to 3 percent, and *basophils* less than 1 percent, of all white blood cells in the blood.

These cells have an important role in allergic reactions. Typically, eosinophils and basophils counteract each other's effects; however, in some reactions, they react synergistically, helping each other. Eosinophils are also the major inflammatory cells in parasitic infections.

7. *Neutrophils are short-lived cells that survive no more than 4 days in the peripheral circulation.* These cells must, therefore, be replaced constantly, and the bone marrow produces new neutrophils at a very fast pace. Because the life span of neutrophils is about 300 times shorter than the life span of erythrocytes, the bone marrow contains three times more white blood cell precursors than erythroid precursors. Technically, this is reported as the myeloid (white cell precursors) to erythroid ratio, or *M:E ratio,* which in normal bone marrow is 3:1.

8. *Monocytes and lymphocytes are long-lived blood cells.* Monocytes account for 4 percent to 8 percent of white blood cells. These cells are precursors of macrophages or histiocytes (i.e., tissue cells, from the Greek *histos,* meaning tissue). Lymphocytes form 40 percent of the white blood cells. Peripheral lymphocytes are predominantly T cells, but there are also B cells, natural killer (NK) cells, and stem cells.

9. *Platelets or thrombocytes are essential clotting factors.* Platelets are cytoplasmic fragments derived from megakaryocytes. Megakaryocytes are very large cells found only in the bone marrow. Abundant cytoplasm of megakaryocytes forms buds which are released into the circulation as platelets. Platelets do not have nuclei but, nevertheless, they survive 8 to 10 days in the circulation.

10. *Malignant transformation of hematopoietic cells may result in solid tumors or leukemia.* Malignant tumors of hematopoietic cells may arise in all hematopoietic organs and even in other sites. The bone marrow and the lymph nodes are the most common primary sites. The malignant cells may be of any of the hematopoietic cell lineages. These cells may remain localized to their site of origin, extend into the adjacent tissues, or enter the circulation. Because of the white color of blood that contains large numbers of malignant leukocytes, the malignancy of circulating white blood cells is called leukemia.

Anemia

Anemia is a reduction of hemoglobin in the blood to below normal levels. In practice, this means 13 g/dL in males and 11.5 g/dL in females. This may be associated with the

- appearance of abnormal hemoglobin
- reduced number of red blood cells
- structural abnormalities of red blood cells

Owing to the reduction of hemoglobin in the circulating blood, the tissues do not receive enough oxygen, and symptoms of *hypoxia* develop. These symptoms vary, as no organs are equally susceptible to oxygen deprivation. In principle, all organs show signs of slower metabolism and a reduced capacity to respond to increased demand for action. For example, hypoxia of the brain causes somnolence, and cardiorespiratory hypoxia causes shortness of breath and easy fatigability. Paleness of the skin is a common feature of anemia, but it has almost no functional consequences.

Classification. There are two ways to classify anemias: (1) *etiologically,* by determining what has caused it; and (2) *morphologically* and biochemically, by assessing the size and shape of erythrocytes and analyzing hemoglobin and other major constituent proteins of red blood cells.

Etiology and Pathogenesis. Anemia may be a consequence of

- decreased hematopoiesis
- abnormal hematopoiesis
- increased loss or destruction of red blood cells

Each of these categories includes several distinct diseases, the most important of which are listed in Table 9-2.

Decreased Hematopoiesis. *Decreased hematopoiesis* may be a consequence of bone marrow failure or a deficiency of essential nutrients. *Bone marrow failure* is also called aplastic anemia. The stem cells disappear from the bone marrow with consequent *pancytopenia* (lack of all blood cells) in the peripheral blood. Bone marrow stem cells may be damaged or replaced by infiltrates of metastatic tumor cells. This is called *myelophthisic anemia.* Similar bone marrow destruction occurs in various forms of leukemia, in which the leukemic cells infiltrate the bone marrow, replacing all normal cell components.

Deficiencies of nutrients also cause anemia. *Deficiency of iron* is the most common form of deficiency anemia. *Deficiency of vitamin B_{12}* and *folic acid*—two vitamins essential for the synthesis of DNA and the maturation of hematopoietic stem cells—causes *megaloblastic anemia. Protein deficiency* results in decreased formation of all hematopoietic cells. Anemia and even pancytopenia are typical features of malnutrition and starvation.

Abnormal Hematopoiesis. *Abnormal hematopoiesis* is usually a consequence of *genetic* abnormalities. These can be inherited as Mendelian traits that affect families, but they may also occur as point mutations in individuals without a previous family history of

Table 9-2 Etiologic Classification of Anemias

Decreased Hematopoiesis

Aplastic anemia (bone marrow failure)

Myelofibrosis

Myelophthisic anemia secondary to bone marrow replacement with tumor cells
  Leukemia
  Multiple myeloma
  Metastatic carcinoma

Deficiency disorders
  Iron deficiency
  Vitamin B_{12} deficiency
  Folic acid deficiency
  Protein deficiency

Abnormal Hematopoiesis

Genetic hemoglobinopathies
  Sickle cell anemia
  Thalassemia

Structural protein defects
  Spherocytosis

Increased Loss or Destruction of Red Blood Cells

Bleeding
  Prolonged menstrual bleeding
  Peptic ulcer

Immune hemolytic anemia

Hypersplenism

Infection
  Malaria

such a disease. The best known among these is probably *sickle cell anemia,* caused by a gene mutation that substitutes a valine for the glutamic acid at position 6 of the beta chain of hemoglobin.

Erythrocytes that contain abnormal hemoglobins (or are abnormally shaped) cannot function properly, and affected patients suffer from chronic hypoxia. Furthermore, the abnormal hemoglobin reduces the life span of erythrocytes, which are destroyed at an increased rate in the spleen as well as within the blood vessels.

Increased Loss and Destruction of Red Blood Cells.

Various conditions may cause increased loss or destruction of red blood cells, including bleeding, intrasplenic sequestration, immune hemolysis, and infections.

Acute blood loss (e.g., bleeding) results in anemia that is only temporary. In order to compensate for the loss of blood and maintain a constant volume of circulating blood, the body mobilizes fluid from the interstitial spaces into the circulation. This restores the volume of blood but dilutes it, changing the ratio of blood cells to fluid. This *temporary dilu-*

tional anemia is usually corrected spontaneously within a few weeks by replenishment of the blood cells from the bone marrow. However, if the bleeding persists, as in patients with a bleeding peptic ulcer, *chronic anemia* will develop.

Normally, old red blood cells are removed from the circulation during their passage through the spleen. The removal of red blood cells may be accelerated in some pathologically altered and enlarged spleens. The best example of this is a condition called *hypersplenism.* This disease of unknown etiology is marked by splenomegaly and increased destruction of red blood cells and suppression of hematopoiesis in the bone marrow.

An important form of red blood cell destruction occurs in various autoimmune disorders and *autohemolytic anemias.* Common to these disorders is an antibody-mediated injury of red blood cell membranes, which leads to their rupture (*hemolysis*) and the release of hemoglobin.

Malaria is the most common infectious cause of hemolytic anemia. It is caused by an infection with the parasite Plasmodium, which invades the red blood cells and causes their lysis. Millions of people are infected with malaria worldwide, but in the United States, the disease is not common.

Morphology of Anemia. Morphologic and biochemical classifications of anemias are based on the study of peripheral blood smears, measurement of hemoglobin content, and chemical analysis of the hemoglobins. These studies utilize various techniques, such as electrophoresis, immunochemistry, and, most recently, DNA analysis (by molecular biology techniques).

The blood smears provide a quick and simple approach to evaluating red blood cells, their size and shape, and hemoglobin content. Normal red blood cells have a uniform biconcave shape that presents as a central pale area and a red peripheral ring (Fig. 9-6). Such erythrocytes are called *normocytic, normochromic* (in Greek, *chromos* means color; in this case, it refers to the normal red color). Small red blood cells are called *microcytic,* whereas the large ones are called *macrocytic.* The variation in size of erythrocytes is called *anisocytosis,* whereas the variation in shape is termed *poikilocytosis.*

On the basis of crucial parameters (i.e., red blood cell count, hemoglobin content, and hematocrit), anemias can be classified into several types, the most important of which are as follows:

- *Normocytic, normochromic anemia.* The red blood cells appear to be normal. Typically, this type of anemia occurs after a massive blood loss ("dilutional anemia"). Chronic infectious and metabolic diseases also cause this type of anemia.
- *Microcytic, hypochromic anemia.* The red blood

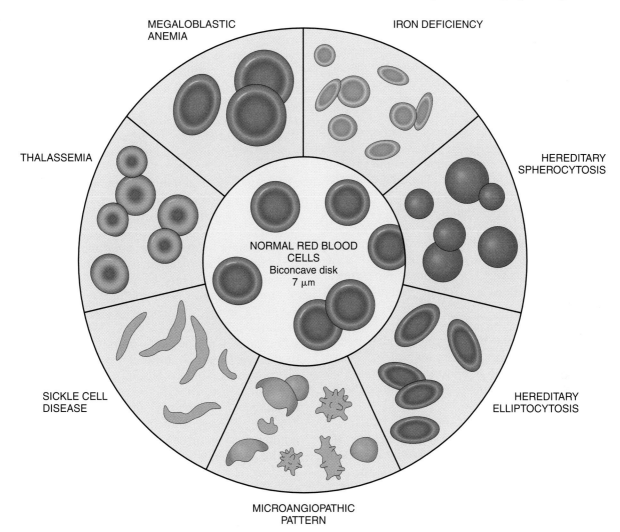

FIGURE 9-6
Morphology of anemias.

cells are small and pale. Most often, this anemia is caused by iron deficiency. It is also seen in thalassemia, a hereditary defect affecting the synthesis of hemoglobin.

- *Macrocytic, normochromic anemia.* The red blood cells are normal in color but are large. Typically, this is caused by a deficiency of vitamin B_{12} and/or folic acid, but it can also occur in chronic liver disease.

- *Anemias characterized by abnormal red blood shapes.* These anemias are descriptively called by the predominant cell shape seen in peripheral smears and include entities such as *elliptocytosis* and *spherocytosis.* The prototype of this form of anemia is *sickle cell anemia,* a disease characterized by the appearance of sickle-shaped erythrocytes.

Morphologic classification of anemias is usually supplemented these days by biochemical data. For example, some microcytic anemias are caused by an iron deficiency, whereas others are a symptom of a

genetic disorder of globin, the gene defect that causes thalassemia. In order to establish the cause of a microcytic hypochromic anemia, one would first have to exclude iron deficiency by measuring the blood iron and estimating the iron stores in the body. Thalassemia, the other cause of microcytic hypochromic anemia, can be diagnosed by demonstrating the abnormal hemoglobin levels typical of this disease. Furthermore, because there are several globin genes, encoding the alpha, beta, or delta chain of this molecule, the diagnosis may be even more specific by demonstrating the gene defect using techniques of molecular biology.

The morphologic-biochemical classification of anemia will, in most cases, point to the cause of the anemia, which then can be assigned to one of the categories within the etiologic-pathogenetic classification system. Once the cause of an anemia is identified, one should try to eliminate the adverse influences or provide substitutional therapy to correct the deficiency. Good response to treatment is the best confirmation of the diagnosis!

Aplastic Anemia

Aplastic anemia is a rare but important disease in which the anemia is usually accompanied by leukopenia and thrombocytopenia. In other words, aplastic anemia is a *pancytopenia,* or generalized bone marrow failure.

Etiology and Pathogenesis. There are two forms of aplastic anemia: idiopathic and secondary. *Idiopathic* cases—those without an identifiable cause—predominate. *Secondary aplastic anemia* is related to bone marrow suppression that is caused by cytotoxic drugs, radiation therapy, or viral infection. Many of these secondary aplastic anemias are reversible, and elimination of the causative agent often allows the bone marrow to recover. The prognosis for recovery in patients with idiopathic aplastic anemia is less favorable.

Pathology. Bone marrow is typically depleted of hematopoietic cells and consists only of fibroblasts, fat cells, and scattered lymphocytes. Anemia, leukopenia, and thrombocytopenia are found in the peripheral blood.

Clinical Features. Uncontrollable infections secondary to leukopenia and a bleeding tendency resulting from thrombocytopenia are usually the first symptoms. Other, general symptoms of anemia, such as chronic fatigue, sleepiness, and weakness, ensue after 4 to 5 weeks. Most patients die of overwhelming infection.

Bone marrow transplantation is the only known treatment for patients with idiopathic aplastic anemia, in whom hematopoiesis does not recover spontaneously. Transplanted new stem cells repopulate the bone marrow and reestablish normal hematopoiesis. Approximately 60 percent of patients so treated will improve and resume a normal life.

Iron Deficiency Anemia

Iron deficiency anemia is the most common form of anemia. In most cases, it is associated with a depletion of body iron stores caused by chronic blood loss. Without iron, which is the essential component of heme molecule, hemoglobin synthesis is impeded. Moreover, newly formed red blood cells are small and contain less hemoglobin than normal.

In order to understand how iron deficiency develops and how it can be corrected, one should first review the metabolism of iron in the body, as well as a few important facts about iron in general (Fig. 9-7).

Iron is an essential nutrient. Many food ingredients, such as meat, liver, beans, and most vegetables and fruits, contain iron. Because iron is added to many packaged and processed foods, the typical American daily diet contains about 15 mg of iron, which is far above the daily requirements for iron.

Iron is absorbed in the intestine through two independent pathways. Iron that is part of heme or respiratory enzymes in animal cells is taken up as part of these molecules by the intestinal cells. The iron is then dissociated from the pyrrole rings within the intestinal cell cytoplasm. Free iron is absorbed through a receptor mechanism. This mechanism is less efficient and only 1 percent to 2 percent of free iron is absorbed from the intestines.

From the intestines, the iron is transported to other sites bound to a transport protein called *transferrin.* Iron delivered to the bone marrow is incorporated into the hemoglobin. Circulating red blood cells contain approximately 60 percent to 80 percent of the total body iron. The rest of the iron is bound to *ferritin,* a storage protein, which aggregates to form granules of brown pigment, known as *hemosiderin.* Hemosiderin is especially prominent in the stroma of the bone marrow, where it can be demonstrated by the Prussian blue reaction.

Iron is lost primarily through cell loss. Aging red blood cells are destroyed in the spleen, but most of the iron released from them is reutilized. Intestinal epithelial cells and skin cells, which also contain iron in the form of ferritin or respiratory enzymes, are shed in large quantities through desquamation. In addition, women lose iron during menstrual bleeding.

Iron deficiency can be caused by

- increased loss of iron (e.g., chronic bleeding)
- inadequate iron intake or absorption (e.g., faulty diet or gastrointestinal disease)
- increased iron requirements (e.g., childhood growth and pregnancy)

The disease is more prevalent among women than men. It has been estimated that 20 percent of women in the United States have iron deficiency. Menstruating women lose 50 to 70 mL of blood every month, and if the iron lost in this blood is not replenished, iron deficiency will develop. Pregnant women may develop iron deficiency if their increased requirements are not satisfied by iron supplements. In adult males, iron deficiency anemia is often caused by occult bleeding. Typically, the origin of the bleeding is a peptic ulcer in the stomach and duodenum, or a carcinoma in the large intestine. Other causes of iron deficiency, such as small intestinal diseases that prevent absorption, are rare.

Iron deficiency causes hypochromic microcytic anemia. Anemia caused by iron deficiency responds well to iron intake. In many cases, anemia is only a symptom of another, more serious disease marked by chronic bleeding or intestinal malabsorption. Such

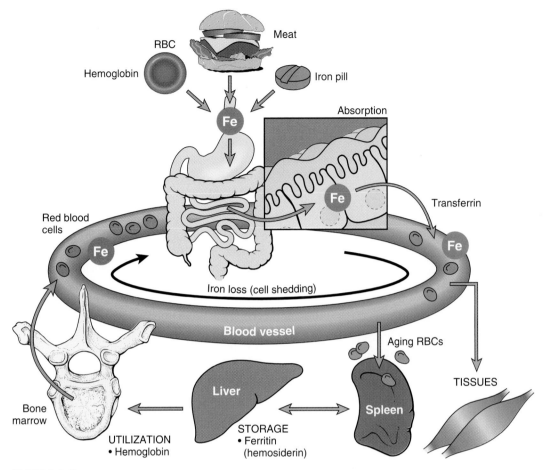

FIGURE 9-7

Iron metabolism. Uptake of heme iron or ferrous iron occurs in the intestine. From the intestine, iron is transported on transferrin to the liver or the bone marrow. Transferrin binds to red blood cell precursors in the bone marrow and delivers iron for incorporation into hemoglobin. Red blood cells (RBCs) in the circulation contain 60 percent to 80 percent of body iron. Old RBCs are destroyed in the spleen. The iron is bound to transferrin for recirculation. Approximately 20 percent to 30 percent of iron is stored in the form of hemosiderin in the spleen, liver, and bone marrow. The remaining iron is in the respiratory enzymes of somatic cells. Iron is lost by desquamation of skin and intestinal cells.

diseases should be treated appropriately, and once the bleeding stops anemia will disappear. Children and pregnant women, who have increased needs, should receive dietary iron supplements.

Megaloblastic Anemia

Megaloblastic anemia is caused by a deficiency of vitamin B_{12} or folic acid, two essential cofactors for DNA synthesis and blood cell production. Both of these deficiencies adversely affect hematopoiesis and delay the normal maturation of blood cells. Red blood cell precursors—normoblasts—do not mature but are instead transformed into *megaloblasts*. In these cells, the nucleus does not mature normally and remains large. Because hematopoiesis is ineffective, many of these megaloblasts are destroyed before they reach maturity. The slow-down of erythro-

poiesis and the loss of megaloblastic cells combine to cause anemia.

The pathologic findings are diagnostic. The bone marrow is hypercellular and contains numerous megaloblasts. The peripheral blood count shows a decreased number of erythrocytes, which are larger than normal (macrocytic anemia). Defective nuclear maturation of leukocytes results in hypersegmentation of neutrophils, which contain five to six nuclear segments instead of the normal three to four segments.

Vitamin B_{12}, also known as cobalamin, is an essential nutrient found in meats, eggs, and dairy products. Because a normal diet usually contains enough vitamin B_{12}, a nutritional deficiency almost never occurs unless absorption is impaired.

The absorption of vitamin B_{12} occurs in several steps. Dietary vitamin B_{12} is released from the food in the stomach, where it binds to an intrinsic factor produced by the gastric parietal cells. The soluble intrinsic factor-B_{12} complex remains in the lumen and is passed into the small intestines. It is absorbed in the terminal ileum, from which it is transferred by blood to the bone marrow. Excess B_{12} is stored in the liver. If any of these phases in the uptake of vitamin B_{12} is disturbed, a deficiency can develop.

The most common form of B_{12} deficiency—*pernicious anemia*—develops as a result of a lack of the gastric intrinsic factor. Although the pathogenesis of pernicious anemia is not completely understood, it is known that these patients have atrophic gastritis. Because of a reduced number of gastric parietal cells, they do not produce sufficient amounts of intrinsic factor. Antibodies to the parietal cells of the stomach can be demonstrated in the serum of most of these patients. Many patients also have antibodies to the intrinsic factor. Presumably, these antibodies destroy the parietal cells or inactivate the intrinsic factor, thereby preventing it from binding to vitamin B_{12}. Antibodies may also inhibit intestinal absorption of the intrinsic factor-B_{12} complex.

Other forms of vitamin B_{12} malabsorption are less common. Resection of the stomach for cancer or peptic ulcer may cause B_{12} deficiency. Conditions that interfere with protein absorption in the small intestine in general, such as celiac disease, will also interfere with B_{12} absorption. Crohn's disease affects the terminal ileum and is typically associated with vitamin B_{12} malabsorption. Finally, some parasites, such as the flat worm *Diphyllobothrium latum,* thrive on vitamin B_{12}. Because these parasites reside in the small intestine, they may compete with the body for this vitamin in the food and cause anemia.

Pernicious anemia caused by B_{12} deficiency is often associated with spinal cord disease. The spinal cord lesions typically involve the posterior and lateral columns. Destruction of these columns results in a loss of the senses of vibration and proprioception, as well as loss of the deep tendon reflexes. Because of these losses, affected patients cannot walk without looking at their legs.

Folic acid deficiency is readily treated by oral intake of folic acid. Vitamin B_{12}, however, must be injected intravenously, as it cannot be absorbed if administered orally. Anemia responds well to treatment, but the neurologic symptoms may persist. Atrophic gastritis cannot be cured by vitamin B_{12}.

Hemolytic Anemias

Hemolytic anemias occur as a result of increased red blood cell destruction, or hemolysis. Hemolysis results from two main abnormalities: intracorpuscular and extracorpuscular red blood cell defects. *Intracorpuscular defects* include structural abnormalities of the red blood cells, as in sickle cell anemia, tha-

Did You Know?

Pernicious anemia was a fatal disease until scientists discovered that the disease can be treated by eating raw liver. Later it was found that liver contains vitamin B_{12}, which was isolated from the liver and then synthesized de novo in the laboratory. Today patients suffering from pernicious anemia do not have to eat raw liver because the synthetic vitamin can be injected intravenously.

lassemia, or hereditary spherocytosis. *Extracorpuscular defects* include antibodies, infectious agents, or mechanical factors. Extracorpuscular causes of hemolysis have been identified in a variety of conditions, such as autoimmune hemolytic anemia, hemolytic disease of the newborn, transfusion reactions, malaria, hemolytic anemia caused by cardiac valve prosthesis, and disseminated intravascular coagulation.

Common to all these conditions are

- anemia (i.e., low erythrocyte count)
- compensatory erythroid hyperplasia of the bone marrow
- hyperbilirubinemia and jaundice

The low erythrocyte count is attributable to the destruction of red blood cells. The erythroid hyperplasia is an attempt of the bone marrow to compensate for the red blood cell loss. Bilirubin released from red blood cells causes hyperbilirubinemia. Jaundice appears when the levels of bilirubin in serum exceed 3 mg/dL.

Sickle Cell Anemia

Sickle cell anemia is caused by a genetic defect in the synthesis of the beta chain of hemoglobin. This defect has been traced to a mutation in the sixth position counting from the N term in a portion of the molecule. Substitution of glutamic acid by valine at this site results in synthesis of an abnormal beta chain. The abnormal beta chain can still combine with alpha chains, but instead of normal HbA, an abnormal hemoglobin (HbS) is formed. In homozygous persons who have two mutated genes for the beta globin, both beta chains are replaced by the product

Did You Know?

Sickle cell anemia was the first human disease linked to a single amino acid substitution. Linus Pauling received the Nobel Prize for this epochal discovery, which changed the way we view genetic diseases.

of the mutated gene. Persons who have less than 40 percent of HbS are asymptomatic; those with 40 percent to 80 percent HbS have mild to moderate disease, and those who have more than 80 percent of HbS show all the typical symptoms of the disease. Thus, although the sickle cell trait is inherited as an autosomal dominant gene, symptoms occur only in homozygotes.

Sickle cell anemia is most prevalent among blacks: 8 percent of African Americans and 30 percent of black Africans have the disease. In the United States, approximately 50,000 persons have sickle cell anemia, which means that approximately 1 percent of all African Americans have symptoms of this disease. The disease also affects some inhabitants of the Mediterranean countries and their descendants in America. However, the prevalence of the mutated gene in these populations is relatively low.

Pathogenesis. HbS undergoes polymerization at low oxygen tension, which causes the red blood cell deformities known as sickling. The aggregates of sickle cells occlude the small blood vessels, causing ischemia in the affected tissue. At the same time, these abnormal blood cells are hemolyzed at an accelerated rate, and the patients develop signs of chronic anemia and jaundice. The bone marrow undergoes compensatory erythroid hyperplasia.

The pathologic findings and the clinical symptoms in patients with sickle cell anemia can be deduced from what is known about the primary defect in this disease. Symptoms usually are first noted in children 1 to 2 years of age, which is the age at which fetal hemoglobin (HbF) is normally replaced by HbA. Affected patients present with signs of chronic anemia, and the course of the disease is marked by typical periodic exacerbations that are clinically classified as *sickling crisis* or *hemolytic crisis*. These may occur spontaneously, but are usually induced or aggravated by fever, respiratory diseases, or some other cause of anoxia. Sickling is accelerated under low oxygen tension, so all situations characterized by reduced oxygen tension can induce a sickling crisis. Thus, these patients should avoid mountain climbing, strenuous exercise, and activities that make them breathless. Pregnancy also may cause sickling.

Pathology. Most of the pathologic findings are related to repeated attacks of sickling crisis, which causes multiple infarcts in various organs (Fig. 9-8). Such infarcts in the brain cause neurologic defects, as well as sharp pain in the bones, spleen, and extremities. Retinal infarcts are common and cause visual problems. As a consequence of repeated infarcts, the spleen becomes fibrotic and shrinks. This process, called autosplenectomy, renders the spleen nonfunctional.

Hemolysis results in hyperbilirubinemia and

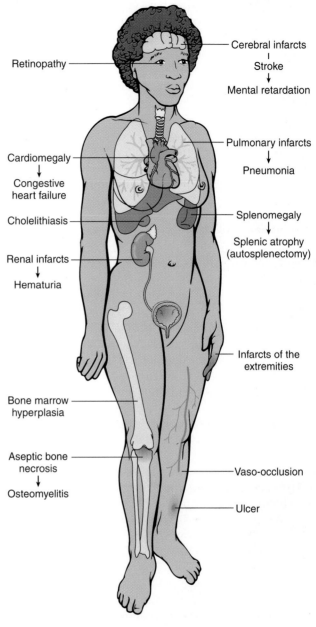

FIGURE 9-8
Clinicopathologic findings in sickle cell anemia. The findings are a consequence of infarctions, anemia, hemolysis, and recurrent infections.

jaundice. Increased excretion of bilirubin in bile leads to the formation of bile stones. Foci of ischemic necrosis, which heal by fibrous scarring, can be detected in all organs.

Clinical Features. Repeated sickling attacks severely damage the vital organs. The most important consequences include the following:

- Retarded intellectual development and neurologic deficits
- Cardiopulmonary insufficiency
- Recurrent infections

Retarded intellectual development is a consequence of brain ischemia and multiple infarcts. Most often, these infarcts are microscopic; however, larger infarcts causing symptoms of stroke can also occur.

The attempt of the heart to compensate for inadequate oxygen transport results in cardiac hypertrophy and, ultimately, heart failure. The occlusion of peripheral small blood vessels with sickle cells and thrombi aggravates the circulatory situation even more by increasing the peripheral resistance. Pulmonary edema is common owing to heart failure, and it tends to predispose the individual to pneumonia.

Other infections are both common and recurrent. These infections typically involve foci of aseptic bone necrosis, infarcts of internal organs, and ischemic skin ulcers. Infections are facilitated by the changes in the spleen and the phagocytic system of the liver. These organs are overloaded with hemosiderin derived from hemolyzed red blood cells. Loss of the spleen, and the overloading of hepatic phagocytic cells with red blood cell fragments, reduces significantly the body's defense system against infection. Moreover, the infections themselves can predispose the patient to even more sickling. The vicious cycle cannot readily be interrupted, and even with the best medical care, sickle cell anemia has a high mortality. Most patients die in early adulthood. No definitive therapy is yet available. The pain and suffering associated with this disease can be reduced only by avoiding conditions that cause sickling and by combating infections.

The diagnosis of sickle cell anemia is indicated by clinical findings, but can be confirmed only by laboratory tests. Severe disease can be recognized by examining peripheral smears, which contain abnormally shaped erythrocytes. The sickling of red blood cells can be induced in a test tube by exposing the blood to low oxygen tension, which is typically done by adding an oxygen-binding chemical, such as metabisulfite. HbS can be demonstrated by electrophoresis because it migrates differently than normal HbA. The complementary DNA (cDNA) probes for the beta chain can be applied to DNA extracted from patients' nucleated cells or the amniotic cells obtained by amniocentesis prenatally. These Southern blots can detect the gene in homozygotes and heterozygotes, and are most useful for genetic counseling.

Thalassemia

Thalassemia is a genetic defect in the synthesis of HbA that reduces the rate of globin chain synthesis. In contrast to sickle cell anemia, no abnormal hemoglobin is produced—that is, the defect is quantitative rather than qualitative.

HbA has four chains: two alpha and two beta chains. There are two genes for the beta chains (one on each chromosome) and four genes for the alpha chain. Each of these genes can be affected. *Thalassemia beta* refers to a reduced synthesis of the beta chain, whereas *thalassemia alpha* indicates reduced synthesis of the alpha chain of globin. The hemoglobin molecule cannot be assembled without alpha or beta chains, and a *hypochromic anemia* develops. In heterozygotes, in whom only one of the four chains is missing, only mild anemia ensues; in this population, the disease is called *thalassemia minor,* or thalassemia trait. Homozygotes develop *thalassemia major,* a severe, usually lethal, form of anemia. Because there are only two genes for the beta chain, compared to four genes for the alpha chain of globin, mutations or deletions of the beta genes produce anemia of greater severity than do mutations of the alpha genes, which can partially be compensated for by the two remaining normal genes.

The deletion of a beta chain gene can be partially compensated for by the gamma chain. The gamma chain may combine with the alpha chain, resulting in the formation of HbF. However, if all four genes for the alpha chain are deleted, the disease is so severe that it causes intrauterine death of the fetus. As may be remembered, the alpha chain is present in all four hemoglobins (α, β, γ, δ), and without it, no species of hemoglobin can by synthesized. Such a condition is incompatible with life, and death occurs in utero or shortly after birth.

Thalassemia beta is more common than thalassemia alpha, and thalassemia minor is more common than thalassemia major. All forms of this disease are most prevalent in Mediterranean peoples; therefore, it is sometimes called Mediterranean anemia. People of North Africa and Southeast Asia can also be affected; in the United States, it is mostly reported in descendants of immigrants from these countries.

Thalassemia minor presents with mild and nonspecific symptoms. Often, the disease is diagnosed only after hematologic examination reveals microcytic hypochromic anemia. In such cases, it is important to distinguish thalassemia from the more com-

Did You Know?

Thalassemia means literally anemia of the sea (derived from the Greek *thalassa,* meaning the sea). Although the ancient Greeks knew many seas, the one with the capital letter was the Mediterranean. Thalassemia is also known as Mediterranean anemia because it is most prevalent around this large water basin.

mon forms of microcytic hypochromic anemia, such as iron deficiency anemia. The latter responds readily to iron supplementation, whereas thalassemia will not. Treatment with iron may even cause signs of iron overload, as the defective globin synthesis hinders its utilization. The mild or subclinical forms of thalassemia require no treatment.

Thalassemia major is a severe and serious disease that has a high mortality in children. Erythrocytes are not produced in sufficient numbers, and those carrying the abnormal hemoglobin are prone to hemolysis. Red blood cell counts are low, and unless transfusions are given, most patients die during childhood. Hemolysis is accompanied by splenomegaly, hemosiderosis, and hepatomegaly (as a result of increased amounts of hemosiderin in the phagocytic cells and hepatocytes). The bone marrow undergoes compensatory hyperplasia and widening. The newly formed bone spicules on the calvarium project perpendicular to the broad basis of the bone, resembling "crew-cut" hair on radiographic study. Hemolysis results in hyperbilirubinemia and jaundice.

Chronic anemia retards the growth of children. Ischemia of the brain impairs their normal intellectual development. Cardiorespiratory insufficiency develops early. These children are always short of breath and tired. Finally, when the heart reserve and its ability to compensate have been exhausted, heart failure occurs.

There is no treatment for thalassemia. Molecular biology probes make it possible to diagnose these diseases in utero, but currently, genetic counseling is the only way to reduce the incidence of this disease among at-risk populations.

Hereditary Spherocytosis

Hereditary spherocytosis is an inborn defect of the red blood cell membrane components. The primary defect has not been fully defined, but most likely involves *spectrin,* a major structural protein in the cell membrane.

Hereditary spherocytosis is the most common hereditary disease of red blood cells in whites. Inherited as an autosomal dominant disease, it affects 1:5000 whites in the United States. Owing to the structural defect of the cell membrane, the erythrocytes "round up" to form spheres, rather than normal biconcave disks. Spherocytosis can be recognized in peripheral blood smears. The red blood cells appear dark red and either do not have a central pale zone or have a very small one. The smears also show marked anisocytosis. The fragility of spherocytes may be demonstrated by suspending them in hypotonic solutions and measuring the rate of their hemolysis. In hypotonic solutions, normal red blood cells swell because of the influx of water across their cell membranes. Spherocytes that are already round cannot

swell much more, and so the abnormal cell membranes rupture faster than do normal erythrocytes. These rounded erythrocytes are less deformable. Owing to the rigidity of their membranes, they do not deform readily and do not adapt to the requirement of microcirculation. During their passage through the spleen, many spherocytes are retained in the sinusoids, where they undergo hemolysis.

The clinical course of spherocytosis, like other hemolytic anemias, is marked by hemolytic or aplastic crises. Symptoms of anemia are, in such instances, accompanied by splenomegaly and jaundice. Splenectomy is currently the preferred treatment for this disease, although clearly, it does not correct the basic cellular defect.

Immune Hemolytic Anemia

Immune hemolytic anemias are mediated by antibodies that destroy red blood cells. These antibodies may be directed to an *autoantigen,* which is normally expressed on a patient's own red blood cells; or an *alloantigen,* which is foreign to the host producing the antibodies. *Neoantigens* are newly formed antigens that are produced by fusion of a normal tissue component with a nonimmunogenic foreign substance that acts as a hapten. Attached to the body's own proteins, haptens may transform such proteins into immunogens.

Mismatched blood transfusion is an example of an immune reaction to a foreign antigen. Red blood cells carry on their surface major blood group antigens of the ABO type (Fig. 9-9). Persons of the A blood group express the A antigen on the surface of their erythrocytes and at the same time have natural antibodies to blood group B antigens. Individuals with blood group B have B antigens on their erythrocytes and antibodies to blood group A in their serum. Mismatched transfusion of B blood into an A person will result in almost instantaneous hemolysis of the donor's B erythrocytes. The natural anti-B antibodies will bind to the red blood cells, forming an antigen-antibody complex. These complexes activate complement in the serum and cause hemolysis of red blood cells. Massive hemolysis may result in shock, and even death.

Hemolytic disease of the newborn is also an immune reaction to foreign antigen. (A detailed description of this disease is presented in Chapter 3.) This neonatal disease is caused by maternal antibodies crossing the placenta and affecting the red blood cells of the fetus in utero or of the newborn infant. Previously, most cases were attributable to the maternofetal Rh factor incompatibility. This form of hemolytic disease can be prevented, and is relatively rare in the United States. Most cases involve some other blood group antigens, which belong to the ABO system, or the so-called minor blood group antigens.

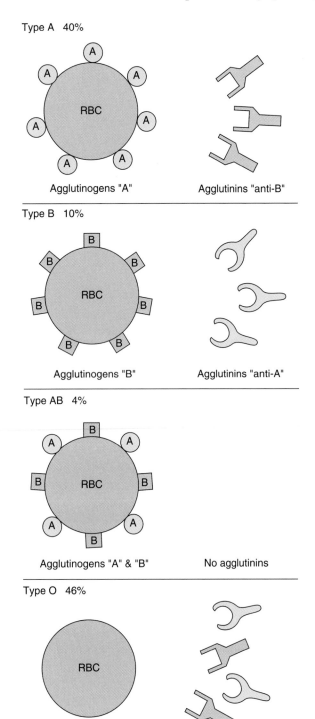

Type A   40%

Agglutinogens "A"   Agglutinins "anti-B"

Type B   10%

Agglutinogens "B"   Agglutinins "anti-A"

Type AB   4%

Agglutinogens "A" & "B"   No agglutinins

Type O   46%

No agglutinogens   Agglutinins "anti-A" & "anti-B"

FIGURE 9-9
Blood group antigens A, B expression results in four blood groups: A, B, AB, and D. (From Applegate EJ: The anatomy and physiology learning system: textbook. Philadelphia: WB Saunders, 1995; 238.)

Autoimmune hemolytic anemias develop as a consequence of an immune reaction to red blood cell autoantigens or neoantigens formed between the body's own proteins and hapten (Fig. 9-10). Red blood cells express numerous blood antigens, but these are not recognized as foreign by the body's immune system and therefore are innocuous. For unknown reasons, some people react to their own red blood cells' antigens, and this causes *autoimmune hemolytic anemia*. This is a typical antibody-mediated immune reaction in which the immunoglobulins bind to the cell surface and form an immune complex with the red blood cell antigen. Antigen-antibody complexes activate the complement, which lyses the cells. In most cases, the reasons for the production of these autoreactive antibodies are not evident. However, because those affected usually have other autoimmune disorders or lymphoma, complex disturbances of the entire immune system may be involved.

Some hemolytic anemias are related to drugs or

FIGURE 9-10
Hemolytic anemias. (A) Autoantigens present on red blood cells (RBCs) are normally not recognized as foreign by the body. In some persons, the body produces antibodies to its own antigens on RBCs. This occurs in some autoimmune disorders for no obvious reasons. (B) Alloantigens are foreign antigens. For example, blood group B RBCs are recognized as foreign by group A persons. (C) Neoantigens are formed from the body's own proteins linked to a nonimmunogenic hapten.

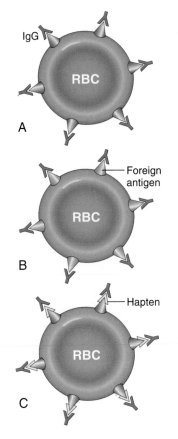

IgG

A

Foreign antigen

B

Hapten

C

environmental chemicals. Ingestion of a drug that is not immunogenic has no effect on red blood cells. However, some of these chemicals may attach to the surface of red blood cells and act as a hapten forming neoantigens that will induce production of antibodies. Drugs rarely cause hemolytic anemia. Nevertheless, it is important to consider this possibility, as drug-induced hemolysis can be prevented by discontinuing use of the drug in question.

Polycythemia

Polycythemia, also called erythrocytosis, denotes an increased number of red blood cells. Typically, affected patients have more than 5.5 million red blood cells per microliter, more than 15.5 g of hemoglobin, and a hematocrit that exceeds 55 percent of the total blood volume.

Polycythemia occurs in two forms: primary and secondary. *Primary polycythemia* or *polycythemia vera* is a neoplastic disease of red blood cell precursors in the bone marrow. It is best to consider it a form of leukemia in which the malignant change involves the red blood cell lineage. In contrast, *secondary polycythemia* denotes an increased red blood cell volume owing to a non-neoplastic, compensatory, or reactive hyperplasia of the erythroid bone marrow. Secondary polycythemia is usually caused by prolonged hypoxia. Living at high altitudes, anoxia secondary to chronic lung disease, and congenital heart disease are all causes of secondary polycythemia.

The symptoms of polycythemia vera are related to the hyperviscosity of blood that contains too many red blood cells. Such blood flows sluggishly and tends to clot more readily than does normal blood. Hypertension is almost always present. Patients appear dark red or flushed in the face, have headaches, visual problems, and neurologic symptoms. Pathologic examination usually reveals disseminated thrombi and foci of bleeding, and splenomegaly is prominent. The bone marrow is hypercellular. The superfluous red blood cells can be removed by phlebotomy (blood-letting from the veins) in both primary and secondary polycythemia. In polycythemia vera, this confers only temporary relief and, as in other leukemias, the disease must ultimately be treated with cytotoxic drugs.

The distinction between primary and secondary polycythemia is made on the basis of clinical findings and laboratory data. In primary polycythemia, the bone marrow cells are neoplastic and appear atypical. In some cases, the proliferation of neoplastic erythroid cells is associated with neoplastic white blood cells which are, then, all part of a myelodysplastic syndrome. In contrast to the neoplastic red blood cell precursors of primary polycythemia, which prolifer-

ate on their own without external stimuli, secondary polycythemia depends on erythropoietin stimulation. Serum erythropoietin levels are invariably elevated in such patients.

Leukocytic Disorders

Disorders of leukocytes include benign reactive disorders characterized by too few or too many leukocytes, as well as malignant diseases, such as leukemias and lymphomas.

Leukopenia

Leukopenia is a reduction in white blood cell count to below normal levels (in Greek, *penia* means lack of). In contrast to the common occurrence of anemias, leukopenia is rare. Several forms of leukopenia are known. The most important of these are *neutropenia,* also known as agranulocytosis, which is marked by low numbers of neutrophils in the peripheral blood, and *lymphopenia,* which is characterized by a reduction in the numbers of lymphocytes. *Selective lymphopenia* is the term used to denote a condition in which a subset of lymphocytes is reduced in number, as in the helper T cell deficiency that occurs in acquired immunodeficiency syndrome (AIDS).

Leukopenia may be induced by many means. In general, any substance that is toxic to the bone marrow cells can provoke leukopenia. The most important among these are various drugs (e.g., the cytotoxic drugs used in cancer therapy) and environmental and industrial chemicals. Radiation therapy and many chronic diseases also damage the bone marrow and cause leukopenia. Deficiency of leukocyte precursors is often combined with a loss of erythroid precursors (*aplastic anemia*). As mentioned earlier, aplastic anemia is a disease affecting the bone marrow stem cells, which are common precursors of both white and red blood cells.

The symptoms of leukopenia relate to the primary function of white blood cells: the body's defense against infections. Neutropenia is typically marked by overwhelming bacterial infections. Lymphopenia deprives the body of its defense against bacterial, as well as viral, fungal, and parasitic pathogens. Short-term leukopenia is treated with antibiotics to prevent massive infections. Long-term leukopenia and the leukopenia of aplastic anemia are often fatal.

Leukocytosis

Leukocytosis is an increased number of white blood cells in the peripheral blood, typically exceeding 10,000 per microliter. The number of all white blood cells can increase proportionally, or some subsets of white blood cells may be increased more than others. *Granulocytosis* (or neutrophilia) is an increased number of granulocytes that typically occurs in response to acute bacterial infection. *Eosinophilic leukocytosis* (or eosinophilia) usually accompanies allergies, such as hay fever, asthma, and some skin diseases or parasitic infections. In many cases, eosinophilia is associated with a normal white blood cell count and an increase only in the number of eosinophils (from 2 percent or 3 percent to 5 percent and more). *Lymphocytosis* is common in viral infections and in chronic infections, such as tuberculosis. It is also a feature of some autoimmune disorders.

Leukocytosis is usually a benign, reactive condition that requires no treatment. Persistent leukocytosis requires thorough investigation as it may represent the first manifestation of a hematologic malignant disease (lymphoma or leukemia).

Reactive leukocytosis is often associated with splenomegaly. In patients with bacterial infection, such an enlarged spleen is called *septic spleen*. Lymphocytosis is often accompanied by a lymph node enlargement, termed *lymphadenopathy* or *lymphadenitis*. Histologically, such lymph nodes show either enlargement of the germinal follicles, widening of the perifollicular (paracortical) cell zone, sinusoidal histiocytosis, or changes in all of these lymph node compartments.

Lymph node enlargement in the neck is especially common in children with upper respiratory diseases. Lymph node enlargement is also common in *infectious mononucleosis*, a disease caused by the Epstein-Barr virus (EBV) (the so-called "kissing disease"). Generalized lymphadenopathy occurs in the early stages of AIDS. As the disease progresses, the lymphoid tissue is depleted and the lymphadenopathy disappears.

It is important to remember that lymph node enlargement is typically one of the most common presenting symptoms of lymphoma. Any persistent lymphadenopathy, especially if unaccompanied by signs of infection, should be evaluated carefully; if persistent for a long time, a lymph node biopsy should be performed. Only lymph node biopsy can definitively confirm the diagnosis and identify reasons for the lymph node enlargement.

Malignant Diseases of White Blood Cells

Malignant diseases of the white blood cells present as *leukemias* and *lymphomas*. Malignant diseases of plasma cells, which are closely related to lymphocytes, are known as *plasmacytomas* or *multiple myelomas*.

Classification. Malignant disease involving white blood cell precursors in the bone marrow, when associated with an increased number of malignant white blood cells in the peripheral blood, are called **leukemias** (in Greek, *leukos* means white; hence, "white blood"). Lymphoid cell malignant diseases predominantly involve the lymph nodes, and thus are called **lymphomas.**

Leukemias can be grouped into two major classes: myeloid (granulocytic-monocytic) and lymphoid (lymphocytic).

Clinically, both myelocytic and lymphocytic leukemia can be classified as acute or chronic. Acute leukemias have a relatively sudden onset and, prior to the modern era of chemotherapy, were frequently fatal within 3 to 6 months. Chronic leukemias have a more insidious onset, and many patients are actually asymptomatic, even though laboratory findings indicate that they have the disease.

Lymphomas occur in several forms, which can correspond to acute and chronic lymphocytic leukemia. A special form of lymphoma is called Hodgkin's disease. Multiple myeloma is a malignant disease of plasma cells. Although related to lymphoma and leukemia, it represents a clinically and pathologically distinct entity.

Etiology and Pathogenesis. The causes of most lymphomas and leukemias, like the causes of most other malignant tumors, are unknown. However, there is considerable evidence that at least some of these malignant diseases are caused by *viruses,* and some are related to the activation of endogenous *oncogens.*

Among the *viruses,* the greatest attention has been devoted to those that infect B or T lymphocytes. Two of these have received special scrutiny: human T-cell leukemia/lymphoma virus-1 (HTLV-1) and EBV.

HTLV-1 is a T-lymphotropic retrovirus from the same family as human immunodeficiency virus (HIV), the virus of AIDS. This virus was originally isolated from a rare form of lymphoma discovered in Japan, but it was found later in other parts of the world as well.

EBV has a predilection for infecting B lymphocytes. This virus has been implicated as the possible cause of Burkitt's lymphoma, but the final proof for its pathogenetic role in this disease is still lacking. EBV is a widespread pathogen which, in most persons, produces only a mild flu-like disease that often passes unnoticed. In others, it causes infectious mononucleosis. Lymphoma develops in a small number of infected persons, most of whom are children or are from sub-Saharan Africa, suggesting that the neoplastic potential of EBV can be realized only under certain conditions.

Endogenous oncogenes probably play an important

role in the pathogenesis of leukemias and lymphomas, as evidenced by the data published daily by various laboratories. Nevertheless, it would be premature to blame endogenous oncogenes for all the malignant diseases of the hematopoietic system. Activation of cellular oncogenes has been related to several chromosomal breaks and translocations noted in hematopoietic malignant diseases. The translocation of fragments of chromosome 8 and 14 seen in Burkitt's lymphoma are good examples of such changes. The *Philadelphia chromosome,* a shortened chromosome 22, is a well-known marker for chronic myelogenous leukemia. The long arm of chromosome 22 is transposed to chromosome 9 and replaced with a fragment of chromosome 9. This leads to juxtaposition of *abl* oncogene (normally present in chromosome 9) and *bcr* oncogene (normally present in chromosome 22). The product of the hybrid *bcr-abl* gene has tyrosine kinase activity and is considered to promote uncontrollable proliferation of leukemia cells.

Leukemias

The term **leukemia** means "white blood." The blood becomes milky white only after the number of white cells has reached approximately 1 million per microliter. This is rarely seen today because patients are usually diagnosed and treated early in the course of the disease.

Clinical Features. All leukemias have several features in common:

- The bone marrow is infiltrated with malignant cells. Thus, a bone marrow biopsy should be performed to confirm the diagnosis.
- The peripheral blood contains an increased number of immature blood cells. Peripheral blood smears may be the first indication that the patient has leukemia.
- Complications common to all leukemias include anemia, recurrent infections, and uncontrollable bleeding. These can be explained by the fact that malignant cells replace the precursors of erythrocytes, white blood cells, and platelets. Owing to these disturbances and normal hematopoiesis, patients exhibit signs of anoxia, cannot effectively combat infections, and develop a bleeding tendency. Overwhelming infection is the most common cause of death in all forms of leukemia.

Leukemia may occur at any age, from birth through old age. However, certain forms of leukemia are more common in certain age groups (Fig. 9-11). Most leukemias (85 percent) affecting children present in an acute form. By contrast, chronic leukemias are more common in adults.

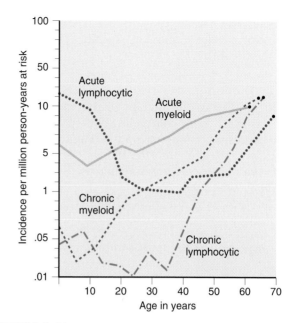

FIGURE 9-11
Age distribution of leukemias. Acute lymphocytic anemia is the most common form affecting children younger than 5 years of age. Acute myelocytic (myeloid) leukemia occurs in all age groups. Chronic myelogenous leukemia is a disease of adulthood. Chronic lymphocytic leukemia is a disease of older persons. (From Upton AC: Comparative aspects of carcinogenesis in ionizing radiation. Natl Cancer Inst Monogr 1964; 14:221.)

Acute lymphoblastic leukemia (ALL) has its peak incidence in children younger than 5 years of age, but the incidence again rises in the elderly population. It accounts for only 20 percent of all leukemias, but is the most common form of leukemia in children.

Acute myelogenous leukemia (AML) is, overall, the most common leukemia (40 percent). It occurs in all age groups, but is most common in older persons.

Chronic myelogenous leukemia (CML) accounts for 15 percent of all leukemias. It rarely occurs before adolescence. It affects adults and its incidence increases with advancing age.

Chronic lymphocytic leukemia (CLL) accounts for 25 percent of all leukemias. It is almost unknown in patients younger than 40 years of age, but its incidence rises progressively thereafter.

Did You Know?

Leukemia was discovered almost simultaneously in 1845 by Rudolf Virchow in Berlin and John Hughes Bennett in Edinburgh. Virchow's name for the disease (*Leukamie,* in German) proved to be more popular than the somewhat convoluted term "leukocythaemia" proposed by Bennett.

Specific Forms of Leukemia

Each form of leukemia has specific clinical and pathologic features.

Acute Lymphoblastic Leukemia. ALL is characterized by massive infiltration of the bone marrow with immature lymphoid cells (blasts). Blast cells, which correspond to precursors of T and B lymphocytes, also spill over into the blood. The peripheral blood, therefore, contains an increased number of malignant lymphoid cells.

The following are most important aspects of ALL:

- Overall, ALL is the most common form of malignant disease in children younger than 5 years of age.
- The disease has a rapid course and is marked by recurrent infections, generalized weakness, and bleeding into the skin and major internal organs. Lymph nodes are enlarged, and there is mild splenomegaly.
- With modern chemotherapy, remission can be induced in essentially all patients, and as many as 50 percent can be cured. Without chemotherapy, ALL is lethal within 3 to 6 months.
- The prognosis is better for children than for adults. This improved prognosis is partially associated with the presence of B cell markers on ALL cells. For some unknown reason, survival in girls is better than in boys.

Acute Myelogenous Leukemia. AML is a heterogenous group of diseases, all with a rapid clinical course. Like ALL, it is characterized by massive infiltration of the bone marrow with immature blasts, which also spill over into the peripheral blood.

On the basis of cell markers, it is possible to classify AML into several categories. The most widely used classification system called the FAB (French-American-British) system, recognizes six forms of AML. These subcategories—known as M1, M2, and so on—reflect the fact that the malignant cells correspond to specific white cell lineages or precursors of various hematopoietic cells. For example, the tumor stem cells of M3 leukemia correspond to promyelocytic; hence, this form of AML is called promyelocytic. Likewise, M6 blasts correspond to erythroblasts, and so this form of AML is called erythroblastic.

The most important aspects of AML are as follows:

- AML is the most common form of acute leukemia in adults.
- AML has an acute course, and without treatment, most patients die within 6 months following the onset of symptoms. Chemotherapy can induce remission, but unfortunately, the long-term results are not encouraging as almost all patients experience a relapse of the disease. Few patients treated with conventional chemotherapy survive 5 years.
- Following high-dose irradiation and chemotherapy, patients undergoing bone marrow transplantation during the first remission have a 70 percent 3-year survival. Clearly, this is the only treatment that offers some hope to patients with AML.

Chronic Myelogenous Leukemia. CML is a malignant disease of myeloid cell precursors that retain their ability to differentiate into more mature forms. The bone marrow is overgrown with malignant stem cells and their descendants, which can be classified morphologically as promyelocytes, metamyelocytes, and so on. These cells are also found in the peripheral blood, which typically shows high white cell counts (Fig. 9-12).

The most important aspects of CML include the following:

- CML is a disease of adulthood; 85 percent of all affected patients are older than 30 years of age.
- Clinically, CML has a slow onset marked by nonspecific symptoms that include mild anemia and signs of hypermetabolism. Patients with CML are tired, lack endurance, and are prone to infections. Splenomegaly and thrombosis secondary to accelerated clotting are common.
- The chronic phase of the disease lasts 2 to 3 years. In about 50 percent of patients, it may then progress into an *accelerated* phase, which usually ends in a *blast crisis* that resembles acute leukemia. In the remaining 50 percent, the onset of the blast crisis is sudden and is not preceded by an accelerated phase. The blast crisis cannot be treated adequately and usually heralds death. Chemotherapy yields unsatisfactory results in patients with CML, and most patients die within 3 to 5 years of the onset of the disease. Bone marrow transplantation, when combined with radiation therapy and chemotherapy, yields a 70 percent chance for 3-year disease-free survival.
- Approximately 90 percent of patients with CML have the Philadelphia (Ph[1]) chromosome. The 10 percent of patients who do not have Ph[1] have a worse prognosis than those who do have this marker.

Chronic Lymphocytic Leukemia. CLL is a malignant disease involving lymphoid cells. CLL cells express a gene called *bcl-2* which counteracts the programmed cell death of normal lymphocytes. This gene immortalizes the CLL cells, which eventually overpopulate the entire body.

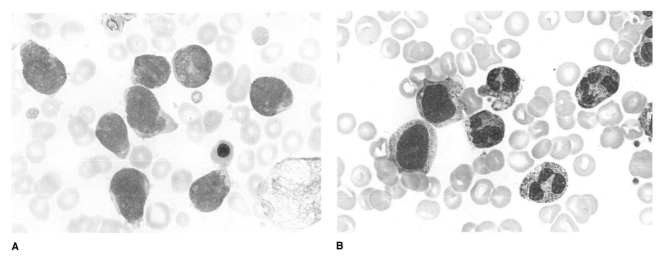

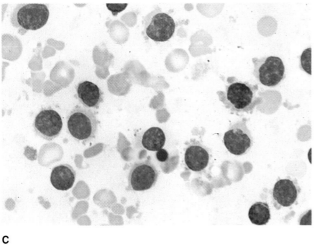

FIGURE 9-12
Leukemia—peripheral blood smears. (A) Acute lymphoblastic leukemia. The peripheral blood contains numerous nonsegmented, immature, atypical white cell precursors. (B) Chronic myelogenous leukemia shows a variety of immature precursors of neutrophils. (C) Chronic lymphocytic leukemia. The cells resemble mature lymphoctyes.

The most important aspects of chronic lymphocytic leukemia are as follows:

- CLL is a disease of older people. Most patients are older than 50 years.
- CLL cells are indistinguishable from normal mature lymphocytes. Normal blood contains less than 4000 lymphocytes per microliter. CLL should be suspected if the number of lymphocytes exceeds 5000/μL. Bone marrow biopsy confirms the diagnosis.
- CLL has many features in common with small-cell lymphocytic lymphoma. Both are slowly progressive diseases. Many patients have only peripheral lymphocytosis or lymph node enlargement and are otherwise asymptomatic. Others may have reduced resistance to infections because the neoplastic abnormal B lymphocytes are not as efficient in combating infections as are normal lymphocytes.
- The course of the disease is prolonged, and most patients survive 7 to 9 years from the time of diagnosis. As CLL cells do not proliferate rapidly,

they are unresponsive to chemotherapy. Thus, chemotherapy is not indicated.

Lymphoma

Lymphoma is a term that can be applied to an entire spectrum of malignant diseases involving lymphocytes and their precursors. There is no need to preface this term with "malignant," as all lymphomas are malignant, and no benign forms are recognized.

Lymphomas comprise approximately 3 percent of all malignant diseases in humans. Pathologically and clinically, they are a heterogeneous group of diseases that can occur in any age group. As stated earlier, lymphomas are closely related to some forms of leukemia. The malignant cells often infiltrate the lymph nodes, spleen, thymus, or bone marrow, but they may also involve any other organ in the body (called *extranodal spread of lymphoma*).

Lymphomas are divided into two large categories: *non-Hodgkin's lymphoma* (NHL) and *Hodgkin's disease*. Both of these can be further subclassified on the basis of histopathologic features, clinical manifestations, and tumor cell biology.

Non-Hodgkin's Lymphomas

Several classifications of NHLs (referred to here simply as lymphomas) have been proposed. The most recent classification, introduced in 1994, is called the Revised American European Classification of Lymphoid Neoplasms (REAL). Nevertheless, the classification developed by the National Cancer Institute (NCI), known as "working formulation," is still the most widely used system. In this classification, three clinical forms of lymphomas are identified:

- Low-grade lymphomas
- Intermediate-grade lymphomas
- High-grade lymphomas

It should be remembered that this classification requires a lymph node biopsy and is dependent on the pathologist's ability to recognize, with the aid of a light microscope, the typical morphologic signs of lymphocytic maturation. Among these features, two are most important: (1) the size and shape of the cell nuclei, and (2) the growth pattern of neoplastic lymphoid cells, which may completely obliterate the normal lymph node architecture or impart to it a nodular (follicular) appearance.

On the basis of nuclear size, the tumor cells are classified as small or large. The shape may be round or irregular, with indentations ("cleaved" nuclei). Remember that normal lymphoid stem cells are small. When activated or stimulated to proliferate, these cells enlarge and transform into lymphoblasts. Lymphoblasts are normally found in the germinal centers of the follicles in lymph nodes, the white pulp of the spleen, and in the bone marrow. Lymphoblasts mature into lymphocytes, which again are usually small. If one follows this normal sequence of events and applies it to the classification of lymphomas, one

can deduce that *well-differentiated* lymphoma cells resemble mature lymphocytes and are, thus, small.

Neoplastic cells may infiltrate the lymph node diffusely or form follicles reminiscent of those formed in the normal lymph node (Fig. 9-13). Morphologically, such well-differentiated lymphomas are therefore termed either *diffuse* or *follicular*. The lymphomas that have features of undifferentiated cells but still show signs of differentiation are considered to be of *intermediate grade*. These lymphomas may be histologically classified as follicular and diffuse. *High-grade lymphomas* are always diffuse and are composed of large lymphoblastic cells or small, undifferentiated, lymphoid stem cells.

Clinical Features. The symptoms of NHL vary. The most prevalent symptoms and clinical findings are as follows:

- *Lymph node enlargement,* which is typically painless, and which may be solitary or diffuse. It may be associated with splenomegaly and lymphocytosis or lymphocytic leukemia.
- *Systemic constitutional symptoms,* including fatigue, malaise, fever, weight loss, pruritus, and sweating. These are attributable to hypermetabolism (i.e., the rapid turnover of proliferating tumor cells); anemia, leukopenia, and associated infections; and autoimmune phenomena that occur with increased frequency in these disorders.
- *Extranodal tumor spread,* whereby tumor cells infiltrate and compress major organs, causing functional disturbances. The best example is lymphoma that infiltrates the brain, causing compression and destruction of parts of the brain.

The diagnosis of lymphoma is made on the basis of histologic findings. To this end, a lymph node is surgically removed and sent to the pathology laboratory for examination. Ideally, the lymph node is di-

FIGURE 9-13

Lymphoma (A and C), compared with a normal lymph node (B). Follicular lymphoma (A) and diffuse lymphoma (C) show a loss of normal lymph node architecture.

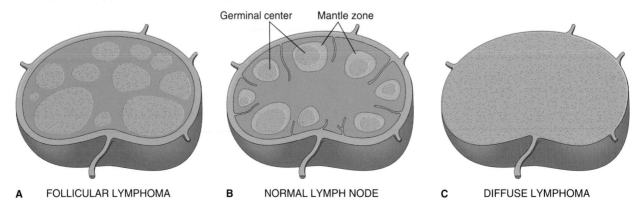

Germinal center   Mantle zone

A   FOLLICULAR LYMPHOMA   **B**   NORMAL LYMPH NODE   **C**   DIFFUSE LYMPHOMA

vided into three parts: one part is fixed immediately for histologic examination, a second part is freshly frozen for cryostat sectioning and marker studies with monoclonal antibodies, and a third part is examined by means of molecular biological techniques. In most cases, an experienced pathologist can provide the correct diagnosis on the basis of light microscopic examination alone; the other studies are performed only for "fine tuning" the diagnosis and subclassifying the tumors. If the pathologists cannot agree on the correct diagnosis, additional immunochemical and molecular biological studies are needed for a definitive diagnosis.

Table 9-3 lists the various lymphomas according to the NCI working formulation. Note that there are several histologic forms, and that the histologic features can predict the clinical course of the disease. A few typical examples of low-grade and high-grade lymphomas will be discussed to describe the salient points.

Follicular lymphoma is the prototype of a low-grade lymphoma. It is the most common subtype of lymphoma, accounting for approximately 40 percent of all cases. It occurs mostly in older people. It shows histologic and cytologic signs of differentiation; that is, the follicular structure of the lymph nodes is partially preserved and the tumor cells resemble mature lymphocytes or follicular center–activated lymphocytes (see Fig. 9-13). Thus, it is a slow-growing tumor, and most patients survive 7 to 9 years after the onset of the disease. Most patients present with long-standing enlargement of the lymph nodes and only mild constitutional symptoms. No chemotherapy is given because the slow-growing tumor cells do not react to cytotoxic drugs. In the terminal stages of this disease, the body becomes overwhelmed with the tumor mass, or a higher grade lymphoma develops that spreads rapidly through the vital organs. Such accelerated forms of lymphoma may temporarily respond to chemotherapy, but overall, they have a rapid downhill course.

Diffuse large cell lymphomas occur in several forms, all of which belong to the intermediate- and the high-grade groups. As a group, these lymphomas constitute 50 percent of all NHLs. Histologically, large cell diffuse lymphomas show complete effacement of the normal lymph node architecture. Instead of normal lymphocyte, the tissue is infiltrated with large lymphoblasts that have irregular nuclear outlines and prominent nucleoli. The tumor cells infiltrate the perinodal tissue, and tumor spread into the parenchyma of major organs is common.

The prognosis is generally poor; those with intermediate-grade lymphomas survive an average of 3 years, whereas those with high-grade lymphomas survive only 1.5 to 2 years. Complete remission can be induced by chemotherapy in 75 percent of patients, and approximately 50 percent of those that respond may be disease-free for several years. The complete cure rate remains low, however.

Burkitt's lymphoma is a highly malignant tumor of lymphoid stem cells. Like normal lymphoid stem cells, Burkitt's lymphoma cells are small and divide rapidly. These cells may originate from the lymph nodes or the bone marrow. Neoplastic lymphoid cells may infiltrate other tissues, and extranodal masses are often more prominent than enlarged lymph nodes.

Burkitt's lymphoma is common in sub-Saharan Africa, where it is endemic among children infected with EBV. The disease presents most often as a tumor involving the mandible and facial soft tissue. Outside the endemic areas, Burkitt's lymphoma is rare, affecting children and young adults, but presenting as an abdominal mass (e.g., ovarian or intestinal mass) rather than involving the orofacial structures. These tumors respond well to chemotherapy, and long-term survival has been reported in 50 percent of patients.

Table 9-3 Classification of the Non-Hodgkin's Lymphomas According to the NCI Working Formulation

Pathology	Clinical Data
Low Grade	Survival: 7–9 years
Small lymphocytic	
Follicular, small cleaved cell	No response to chemotherapy
Follicular, mixed, small cleaved and large cell	
Intermediate Grade	Survival: 2–3 years
Follicular, large cell	
Diffuse, small cleaved cell	
Diffuse, mixed, small cleaved and large cell	
Diffuse, large cell (cleaved and noncleaved)	
High Grade	Survival: 1–2 years
Large cell immunoblastic	
Lymphoblastic (convoluted and nonconvoluted)	
Small noncleaved cell (Burkitt's and non-Burkitt's)	Some patients have a good initial response to aggressive chemotherapy.

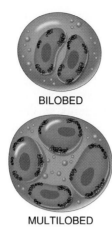

BILOBED

MULTILOBED

FIGURE 9-14
Diagnosis of Hodgkin's disease. Reed-Sternberg cells are binucleated or multinucleated and have prominent nucleoli.

Hodgkin's Disease

Hodgkin's disease is a form of malignant lymphoma that is pathologically distinct from other lymphoid malignant diseases. It affects all age groups. Nevertheless, the age distribution curve is bimodal, with one peak at 25 years and another at 55 years.

Pathologic studies indicate that there are four types of Hodgkin's disease: nodular sclerosis, lymphocyte predominance, mixed cellularity, and lymphocyte depletion. Common to all of these sub-

types are the pathognomonic Reed-Sternberg cells (Fig. 9-14). Typically, the Reed-Sternberg cells have a bilobed or multilobed nucleus and prominent nucleoli surrounded by a clear halo that is reminiscent of an owl's eye. The diagnosis of Hodgkin's disease should not be made unless Reed-Sternberg cells are found.

The histologic subtyping of Hodgkin's disease was important before modern chemotherapy was introduced. Then, as today, in untreated cases, the lymphocyte depletion type of Hodgkin's disease had the poorest prognosis. Today, the prognosis of the disease depends primarily on the extent of spread of the disease throughout the body. Histologic typing of lesions is less important.

To facilitate prognosis determination and treatment, it is important to *stage the disease* accurately. This is done by clinically determining which parts of the body are involved. Multiple lymph nodes are sampled and biopsies of the liver, spleen, or bone marrow are performed.

Stage I disease signifies involvement of a single lymph node region (Fig. 9-15). Stage II disease signifies involvement of two or more lymph node regions on the same side of the diaphragm. Stage III disease signifies involvement of lymph node regions on both sides of the diaphragm, with or without splenic lesions. Stage IV disease signifies widespread dissemination of the disease with involvement of one or

FIGURE 9-15
Staging of Hodgkin's disease.

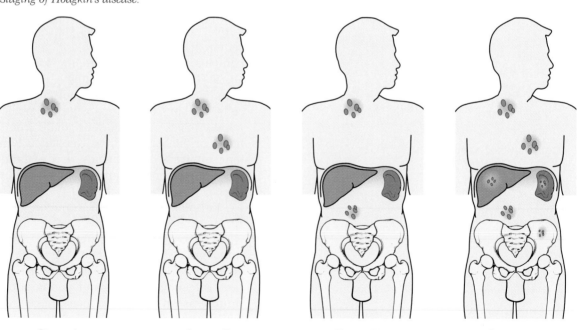

Stage I
Involvement of single lymph node or group of nodes

Stage II
Involvement of two or more sites on same side of diaphragm

Stage III
Disease on both sides of diaphragm. May include spleen or localized extranodal disease

Stage IV
Widespread extralymphatic involvement (liver, bone marrow, lung, skin)

more extranodal tissues and nonlymphoid organs (e.g., liver or intestine). In general, stage I and II tumors are associated with an excellent prognosis and a high rate of cure (close to 100 percent), achieved with chemotherapy. Advanced disease has a less favorable prognosis. Nevertheless, 50 percent of patients with stage IV disease survive 5 years.

The clinical features of Hodgkin's disease are not distinct from those in other lymphomas. Most patients exhibit lymph node enlargement, which may be associated with nonspecific symptoms. The neck nodes are most often involved. Mediastinal lymph nodes are also frequently involved, as the disease seems to spread from one group of lymph nodes to another in continuity. Overall, the central lymph nodes (i.e., those on the body) are more often involved than those on the extremities. Extranodal involvement is generally less common than in other lymphomas and occurs only in advanced disease. Leukemic spread is very rare. Chemotherapy is highly effective, and remission may be induced in almost all patients. Seventy percent of all patients survive 5 years.

Multiple Myeloma

Multiple myeloma is a malignant disease of plasma cells. It is believed that the disease begins with malignant transformation of a single plasma cell. Clonal expansion of the descendants of this malignant cell leads to an overgrowth of the bone marrow by neoplastic cells, all of which share the same features. Because all neoplastic cells are descendant of a single cell that has undergone malignant transformation, the condition is called *monoclonal*. Other lymphomas are probably also monoclonal. The monoclonality of the plasma cell population in multiple myeloma is much more easily detected because plasma cells secrete immunoglobulins, which can be detected in the serum.

In the normal bone marrow, 5 percent of all cells are plasma cells. These cells are descendants of B lymphocytes. With antigenic stimulation, plasma cells proliferate and produce antibodies. Numerous clones of plasma cells are stimulated, with the result that numerous forms of immunoglobulins are produced. Infection causes a polyclonal activation of plasma cells, and the increased immunoglobulins appear as a broad-shaped globin "hump" in the serum electrophoresis pattern. Following malignant transformation of a single plasma cell, as occurs in multiple myeloma, the bone marrow descendants of this malignant cell secrete all the same form of immunoglobulin. This can be detected as a "monoclonal spike" in serum protein electrophoresis. This spike is typical of multiple myeloma.

Multiple myeloma is a disease of old age, with most patients being older than 45 years of age. The malignant plasma cells typically proliferate in the bone marrow, and through this process, destroy the surrounding bone. Punched out holes in the blood-forming bones, such as the calvaria and the vertebrae, can be detected by x-ray studies (Fig. 9-16). Calcium released from the bones contributes to hypercalcemia and the deposition of calcium in many organs, especially the kidneys. In addition, the immunoglobulin secreted by the plasma cells is also excreted in the kidney, where it damages the tubules and contributes to deterioration of renal function. Renal failure ensues. Most other symptoms and complications of multiple myeloma are related to the proliferation of malignant plasma cells in the bone marrow. These cells replace the normal erythroid and myeloid cells, causing anemia and leukopenia. Bone fractures are also common because of widespread bone destruction and weakening.

The diagnosis of multiple myeloma is based on x-ray studies, serum electrophoresis data, and ultimately, bone marrow biopsy. Multiple lytic defects seen on radiographs typically contain numerous plasma cells that can be identified in bone marrow biopsy specimens. The monoclonal spike on electrophoresis supports the diagnosis of monoclonal proliferation of plasma cells.

The course of the disease is variable, but overall, the prognosis is grim. Chemotherapy is ineffective. Most patients die within 3 to 4 years, primarily of kidney failure or infection.

Did You Know?

Dr. Bence Jones reported some 150 years ago that the urine of patients with multiple myeloma contains a peculiar protein. This protein turned out to be a fragment of the immunoglobulin secreted by the neoplastic plasma cells and is still known as the Bence Jones protein. Dr. Bence Jones has entered the history books as the discoverer of the first biochemical tumor marker.

Bleeding Disorders

In order to move through the vessels, the blood must remain fluid. On the other hand, if the integrity of the blood is disrupted, it is in the best interest of the entire organism to prevent unnecessary bleeding. The process that prevents uncontrolled bleeding is called **hemostasis,** whereas pathologic alterations of bleeding are termed **bleeding disorders** or hemorrhagic disorders.

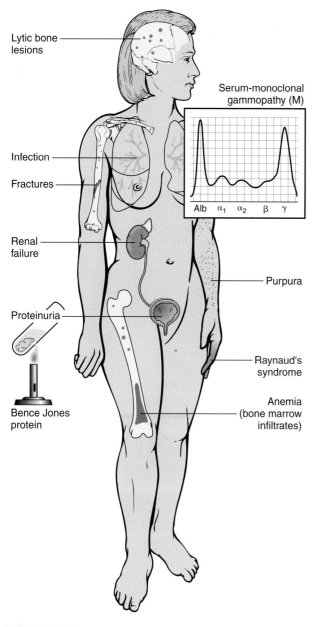

FIGURE 9-16
Multiple myeloma. Radiographs of the skull, ribs, and vertebrae show multiple punched out lesions. There is anemia secondary to bone marrow lesions that replace red blood cell precursors. Kidney failure is the most common cause of death. The urine contains Bence Jones protein.

Normal Hemostasis

Normal hemostasis depends on the closely integrated, coordinated action of

- vascular factors
- platelet factors
- coagulation factors

Following an injury that disrupts the integrity of a vessel wall (e.g., a knife wound), the small arteries supplying blood to the area undergo vasoconstriction. This is mediated by a neural reflex and results

in a slowdown of blood flow. At the same time, the blood extravasated into the surrounding tissue will exert pressure on the damaged vessels, compressing them from outside. The slowdown of the blood flow promotes aggregation of platelets, which leads to the formation of a hemostatic plug. Substances released from platelets act on the circulating coagulation factors of the plasma and initiate the coagulation cascade. Additional clotting factors are released from the damaged endothelium and the surrounding tissue, all of which contribute to the formation of a definitive clot.

The formation of this definitive clot is critically dependent on the activation of the plasma coagulation factors (Fig. 9-17). The salient features of these factors are listed below:

- There are 12 factors (Table 9-4). Note that there is no factor VI! All except factor IV (calcium) are pro-

FIGURE 9-17
Normal hemostasis is accomplished through the interaction of platelets and plasma clotting factors and substances released from endothelial cells and perivascular tissue. (From Applegate EJ: The anatomy and physiology learning system: textbook. Philadelphia: WB Saunders, 1995; 236.)

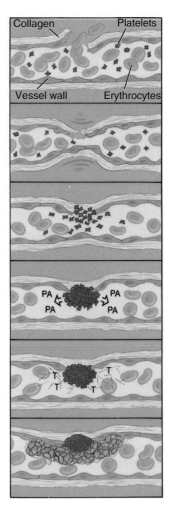

Table 9-4 Coagulation Factors

Factor	Name
I	Fibrinogen
II	Prothrombin
III	Tissue factor
IV	Calcium
V	Proaccelerin
VII	Proconvertin
VIII	Antihemophilic factor
IX	Plasma thromboplastin component
X	Stuart-Prower factor
XI	Plasma thromboplastin antecedent
XII	Hageman factor
XIII	Fibrin stabilizing factor

teins that are produced by the liver. They circulate in plasma as precursors or in an inactive form.

- The activation of factors occurs sequentially through an intrinsic or an extrinsic pathway. These two pathways converge, and both generate the activated factor Xa. In the common pathway of coagulation, factor Xa catalyzes the conversion of prothrombin to thrombin. Thrombin promotes the conversion of fibrinogen to fibrin. Final polymerization of fibrin results in a definitive thrombus.
- The intrinsic pathway is activated through several substances ("intrinsic" to the blood itself) that act on factor XII, also know as Hageman's factor. The extrinsic pathway is activated through the factor VII action of extraneous tissue-derived substances on factor VII. Prothrombin time (PT) is used to measure the extrinsic pathway, whereas the activated partial thromboplastin time (APTT) is used to measure the intrinsic and the common pathway of coagulation (Fig. 9-18).
- The action of clotting factors is counterbalanced by the action of natural anticoagulants, the most important of which are heparin, antithrombin, and plasminogen. *Heparin* acts on several steps of the coagulation cascade and is, therefore, used to prevent clotting in living patients. It is also used to prevent clotting of blood in test tubes. *Antithrombin* inactivates thrombin and prevents its action on fibrinogen. *Plasmin* can lyse fibrin and is, therefore, used to dissolve clots.

Major Bleeding Disorders

Hemorrhage, or the escape of blood from the vessels or the heart, can occur in several forms. It is considered to be *external* if the blood flows outside of the body (wound), or *internal* if the blood enters the tissues or body cavities. Hemorrhages from multiple sites are called *purpura*.

Bleeding disorders occur as a result of defects that are

- vascular
- platelet-related
- clotting factor–related

Frequently, all of these aspects of normal hemostasis are involved.

Vascular Disorders

The most important vascular causes of bleeding are mechanical trauma, vessel wall weakness, and immune injury.

- *Mechanical trauma* to the blood vessels is the most common cause of hemorrhage. It is a feature of everyday life, manifesting as small bruises and wounds or skin hematomas caused by known, as well as unnoticed, minor and major injuries.
- *Vessel wall weakness* is an important cause of spontaneous and trauma-induced hemorrhages.

FIGURE 9-18
Plasma clotting factors are activated in a sequence that corresponds to the intrinsic and extrinsic pathway.

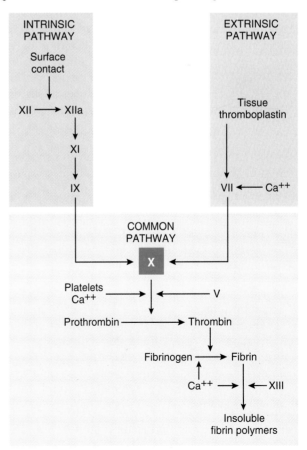

It is well known that some persons tend to bruise more readily than others. Apparently, individuals do not have equally strong connective tissue; therefore, some of us are more prone to bleeding and cannot withstand trauma as readily as others ("devil's pinches"). With aging, the vessels become more fragile, and minor hemorrhages are thus more common in older people ("senile purpura"). Some metabolic disorders, such as Cushing's syndrome, or congenital disorders of connective tissue are characterized by easy bleeding. Hypovitaminosis C (scurvy) is marked by multiple hemorrhages because the intercellular matrix of the blood vessels cannot be formed properly without vitamin C.

- *Immune mechanisms* may damage the blood vessels and cause hemorrhage. Any vasculitis will thus present with hemorrhages, which are, however, most noticeable in the various autoimmune disorders that involve the capillaries and small arteries and veins of the skin. The best example is provided by various allergic drug reactions, the presenting sign of which is skin purpura.

Platelet Disorders

Platelet disorders can be classified as quantitative or qualitative. That is, they may be caused by either a decreased number of platelets or an abnormality in structure and function.

Normal blood contains 150,000 to 300,000 platelets per microliter. A decrease to levels below 70,000 is considered to be abnormal and is called **thrombocytopenia.** A bleeding tendency develops only in severe thrombocytopenia, when the platelet count drops to less than 10,000 to 20,000 per microliter.

Thrombocytopenia develops as a result of decreased production or increased destruction, removal, or utilization of platelets.

Decreased production of platelets occurs in many disorders affecting the bone marrow. Under normal circumstances, the platelets are formed from the megakaryocytes. They represent anuclear fragments of megakaryocytic cytoplasm that survive in the peripheral blood for several days. Any disease or agent that affects megakaryocytes will cause thrombocytopenia. The most important among these are

- aplastic anemia, marked by a loss of all hematopoietic cells
- leukemia, marked by the replacement of normal hematopoietic cells with tumor cells
- drugs that damage megakaryocytes
- infectious agents, such as rubella virus (and probably many others), which affect the megakaryocytes

These patients develop a bleeding tendency and require blood or platelet transfusions.

The primary cause of failure must be identified prior to any treatment. Drug-induced thrombocytopenia may respond to withdrawal of the drug. Virus-related disease may improve upon cure of the infection. In severe thrombocytopenia of aplastic anemia, the only definitive treatment promising survival is bone marrow transplantation.

Increased intravascular destruction of platelets or their increased consumption can also result in thrombocytopenia. Destruction of platelets is a feature of many autoimmune disorders. Antibodies to platelets occur in systemic lupus erythematosus, various forms of hemolytic anemias, and drug-induced hematologic disorders. Such antibodies are also the major features of *idiopathic thrombocytopenic purpura* (ITP), a disease of unknown etiology.

Immune thrombocytopenia also may develop after some blood transfusions because the platelets carry not only the major blood group antigens expressed on the red blood cells, but also some platelet-specific antigens that can induce formation of antibodies.

Thrombocytopenia also develops in some children who are born to mothers immunized with paternal platelet antigens in a manner similar to the hemolytic disorder caused by maternofetal Rh incompatibility.

Increased removal of platelets typically occurs in the spleen. The platelets that have been coated or damaged by antibodies are removed at a faster rate. This occurs in hypersplenism, a syndrome characterized by splenomegaly and pooling of blood in the enlarged spleen. There is also an increased removal of platelets, as well as of other blood cells.

Consumption of platelets occurs at an accelerated rate in various conditions that cause disseminated intravascular coagulopathy (DIC). DIC may be triggered by infection, tumors, or any form of shock. Formation of thrombi in the small blood vessels is typically associated with trapping of platelets and thrombocytopenia. Once the platelets and plasma clotting factors have been used up, the blood cannot coagulate any longer and bleeding ensues.

Disorders of platelet function may be classified as either congenital or acquired. The congenital disorders are rare and involve some of the major platelet functions. These include, for example, defective platelet aggregation (*thrombasthenia*), adhesion to solid surfaces, and the release of biologically active substances. *Acquired disorders* of platelet function are relatively common, but are rarely severe enough to cause clinical problems. Chronic renal failure is the prototype of a metabolic disease associated with abnormal platelet function, probably related to the accumulation of metabolites that are not excreted through the kidney. *Aspirin* prevents platelet aggregation and release of thromboplastin. However, aspirin intake is rarely associated with clinical bleeding problems.

Clotting Factor Deficiencies

Deficiencies of clotting factors can be congenital or acquired. *Congenital clotting factor defects* are relatively common. Each of the proteins that participate in the coagulation cascade is encoded by a distinct gene. Mutation or deletion of these genes results in a bleeding disorder. Although there are many such disorders, only *hemophilia* shall be discussed here, as it is the most important clinical disorder of this type. Acquired clotting factor deficiencies are more common and also deserve to be noted.

Hemophilia is a sex-linked congenital clotting factor deficiency that occurs in two forms: *hemophilia A,* or the deficiency of factor VIII, and *hemophilia B,* or the deficiency of factor IX.

Both of these genes are located on the X chromosome. The gene is recessive, so it cannot be expressed in women who have two X chromosomes. Women who carry the gene (asymptomatic carriers) can transmit the hemophilia gene to their daughters as well as their sons. The daughters will be asymptomatic carriers. The sons whose Y chromosome does not carry the normal allele that could overshadow the recessive hemophilia gene will have the bleeding disease. Note that the sons of hemophiliacs acquire from their fathers the normal Y. They are asymptomatic and do not carry the gene, whereas the daughters of hemophiliac males are always asymptomatic carriers. Hemophilia A affects 1 in 5000 males. Hemophilia B is 10 times less common than hemophilia A and is generally less severe.

The deficiency of factor VIII or factor IX results in uncontrollable bleeding following trauma. Affected males tend to bruise and often develop subcutaneous hematomas or hemarthrosis. Bleeding during surgery cannot be stopped in such individuals, and even minor surgery, such as tooth extraction, can cause profuse blood loss. Joint deformities are common late consequences of repeated hemarthrosis.

The diagnosis of hemophilia may be suggested by the family history. However, it should be noted that at least 20 percent of cases represent newly acquired mutations, and are not associated with a previous family history of hemophilia. Thus, the bleeding disorder must be diagnosed by applying several tests. Typically, the most significant abnormality is a prolonged APPT, an abnormality of the intrinsic pathway. Bleeding time and prothrombin time are normal. Specific tests measuring the functions of factor VIII and IX must be performed to distinguish hemophilia A from hemophilia B. Genetic testing by molecular biology techniques may be used to further characterize the nature of the defect and the extent of the mutation or deletion. The gene for factor VIII is an especially large one, so that different parts of the gene can be affected. Depending on the extent of the genetic defect, the disease may present as a mild, moderate, or severe bleeding disorder. The clinical syndrome develops only if blood levels of factor VIII have been reduced below 1 percent of normal.

Patients with hemophilia need frequent transfusions of fresh blood, which places them at high risk for acquiring various blood-borne infections. Despite careful screening for blood-transmitted pathogens, many hemophiliacs have been infected with hepatitis virus B or C or HIV. Improved screening of blood donors should prevent such untoward reactions in the future.

Acquired clotting factor defects occur in many clinical situations. In general, these are attributable to inadequate production of clotting factors, excessive consumption, or the action of anticoagulants.

Decreased production of clotting factors is typically found in patients with chronic liver disease. Essentially all proteins of the coagulation cascade, except the von Willebrand factor, which is produced by the endothelial cells, are synthesized in liver cells. Chronic liver disease will, therefore, result in a deficiency of these factors. Since fibrinogen represents the most abundant of these factors, this condition is often referred to as *hypofibrinogenemia.*

The synthesis of several clotting factors requires vitamin K. Without vitamin K, the liver cannot synthesize factors II, VII, IX, and X. Vitamin K is a fat-soluble vitamin produced by the bacteria in the intestines. Neonatal hemorrhagic tendency occurs in children in whom the maternally acquired stores of vitamin K have been depleted before their intestines were colonized with bacteria. In adults, hypovitaminosis K occurs if the bacteria that produce vitamin K in the intestines have been eliminated by antibiotics, or if the absorption of fat, which is essential for the uptake of vitamin K, is impaired by biliary or pancreatic disease. Finally, note that vitamin K utilization in the liver can be inhibited medically. The best known of these anticoagulants is coumadin, a drug used to prevent thrombosis in persons at risk for infarcts or thromboemboli.

Increased consumption of clotting factors leads to excessive bleeding. Consumption of coagulation factors occurs during the formation of thrombi of any type, and is most prominent in DIC. This syndrome

Did You Know?

The Babylonian Talmud, the holy Jewish Scripture, contains the first reference to hemophilia, though not under that name. The Scripture quotes Rabbi Judah, a well-known scholar who allowed a boy not to have the ritual circumcision because three of his brothers had bled to death from this procedure. The cause of this familial bleeding disorder remained obscure for more than 2 millenia thereafter.

is typically triggered by thromboplastins released from injured endothelial cells, or from tissue or some substances that are foreign and are "not supposed to be" in contact with the circulating blood. Any form of shock could induce DIC, primarily because the perfusion of the peripheral circulatory system has been compromised. The ischemic endothelial cells themselves promote thrombosis, or they allow the leakage of thrombogenic stimuli from the adjacent tissues into the blood. Infections also damage blood vessels and tissues. On the other hand, many bacteria can themselves initiate formation of clots. Massive tissue injury caused by trauma is yet another source of tissue thromboplastins. Amniotic fluid embolism (i.e., entry of amniotic fluid into the maternal circulation) also can cause DIC. Tumors are often associated with DIC because they release cells or necrotic material into the circulation, thus initiating clotting.

Regardless of the initiating event, DIC is always a consumptive coagulopathy. In the first stages of the disease, the small blood vessels are occluded with numerous thrombi composed of platelets, fibrin, and other coagulation factors. Owing to this increased consumption, the blood is depleted of platelets and clotting factors. Plasminogen activators released from ischemic tissue activate plasmin, which acts as a fibrinolytic agent, dissolving the microthrombi. As the blood rushes through the newly reopened blood vessels whose endothelial cells were damaged by ischemia, bleeding occurs. This bleeding cannot be stopped because the circulating blood does not have any more coagulation factors. These factors must be replenished by transfusions, but often, this is to no avail and the patient dies of exsanguination. Laboratory tests show low values of all coagulation factors and platelets. Fibrin split products are found in the urine of these patients.

Anticoagulants are important causes of acquired clotting factor deficiencies. Some of these anticoagulants are produced by the body itself, whereas others are injected for therapeutic purposes. Many exogenous anticoagulants, such as heparin or warfarin, are widely used in clinical practice. It is important to monitor the effects of these anticoagulants because overdoses can cause uncontrollable bleeding and major mishaps, such as brain bleeding.

Review Questions

1. Describe the sites of hematopoiesis in various age groups.
2. How is hematopoiesis regulated?
3. Describe the pathways of differentiation of pluripotent hematopoietic stem cells.
4. Compare serum and plasma and explain which one you would collect for various blood tests.
5. Explain the molecular structure of hemoglobin.
6. Describe the major events in the life of erythrocytes.
7. Explain the significance of various erythrocytic parameters, like MCV, MCH, MCHC, as well as how they are measured.
8. What are the normal values for a white blood cell count?
9. Compare neutrophils and lymphocytes.
10. What is the function of platelets?
11. What is anemia?
12. Provide an etiologic and a morphologic classification of anemias.
13. Which anemias are caused by decreased hematopoiesis?
14. Which anemias are caused by abnormal hematopoiesis?
15. Which anemias are caused by increased loss or destruction of red blood cells?
16. List typical examples of normocytic, microcytic, and macrocytic anemia.
17. List typical examples of anemias that present with abnormal red blood cell shapes.

18. Explain the pathogenesis and pathology of aplastic anemia.

19. List the causes of iron deficiency anemia.

20. What are the critical events in the metabolism of iron in the human body?

21. Explain the pathogenesis of megaloblastic anemia.

22. Compare anemia caused by vitamin B_{12} with anemia caused by folic acid deficiency.

23. Compare hemolytic anemia caused by intracorpuscular defects with anemia caused by extracorpuscular factors.

24. Explain the pathogenesis of sickle cell anemia.

25. Correlate the pathologic findings in sickle cell anemia with the clinical symptoms of this disease.

26. Explain the pathogenesis of thalassemia.

27. Compare thalassemia minor and thalassemia major.

28. Why are red blood cells spherical (round) in hereditary spherocytosis?

29. Explain the pathogenesis of immune hemolytic anemia.

30. Compare primary and secondary polycythemia.

31. What is leukopenia and what are its causes?

32. What is leukocytosis and what are its causes?

33. What are the possible causes of lymph node enlargement?

34. What is the difference between lymphoma and leukemia?

35. What causes lymphomas and leukemias?

36. What are the common features of all leukemias, and what distinguishes acute from chronic leukemia and lymphocytic from myelogenous leukemia?

37. List the most important features of acute lymphoblastic leukemia and correlate the pathologic findings with the clinical features of this disease.

38. List the most important features of acute myelogenous leukemia.

39. List the most important features of chronic myelogenous leukemia.

40. List the most important features of chronic lymphocytic leukemia.

41. How are non-Hodgkin lymphomas classified?

42. List the most common symptoms and clinical findings of non-Hodgkin lymphomas.

43. Compare follicular lymphoma with diffuse large cell lymphoma and Burkitt's lymphoma.

44. What is Hodgkin's disease?

45. How is Hodgkin's disease classified histologically?

46. How is Hodgkin's disease staged?

47. What is multiple myeloma?

48. How is multiple myeloma diagnosed?

49. How do vascular platelet and coagulation factors interact to ensure normal hemostasis?

50. Compare the mechanism of the activation of the intrinsic and extrinsic pathway of coagulation.

51. What are the three major groups of bleeding disorders?

52. Which bleeding disorders are caused by vascular diseases?

53. What is thrombocytopenia and what is its clinical significance?

54. What are the main causes of thrombocytopenia?

55. What is thrombasthenia?

56. What is hemophilia and how is it diagnosed?

57. Why is hypofibrinogenemia a sign of a chronic liver disease?

58. Why is disseminated intravascular coagulation (DIC) accompanied by a bleeding tendency?

Learning Objectives

After reading this chapter, the student should be able to:

1. Describe the normal gastrointestinal tract and its functions.
2. List the most common alimentary diseases in infants, young adults, and old people.
3. Discuss dental decay and periodontal disease in terms of etiology, pathology, and clinical presentations.
4. Discuss the etiology and clinical presentations of inflammatory diseases of the mouth.
5. Discuss the risk factors for oral cancer.
6. Discuss the main diseases affecting the salivary glands.
7. Discuss the inflammatory diseases of the esophagus.
8. Discuss cancer of the esophagus in terms of etiology, gross and microscopic pathology, and clinical presentation.
9. Discuss the pathogenesis of acute and chronic gastritis and peptic ulcer.
10. List three causes of hematemesis and melena, and explain their pathogenesis.
11. Describe the pathology of various forms of gastric cancer.
12. Describe the pathology and complications of diverticulosis of the colon.
13. Discuss inflammatory bowel disease and compare Crohn's disease and ulcerative colitis.
14. Discuss various causes of diarrhea.
15. Define peritonitis, ileus, and hernia and explain their pathogenesis.
16. Discuss the etiology and pathogenesis of malabsorption syndromes.
17. Describe the pathology of colon cancer and list the most important prognostic factors, comparing the lesions of the right and left colon.

Additional Key Terms and Concepts

Appendicitis
Crohn's disease
Dental caries
Diverticulosis
Gastroenteritis
Hernia
Ileus
Ulcerative colitis

Chapter Outline

The Gastrointestinal System

Chapter 10

NORMAL ANATOMY AND PHYSIOLOGY

The normal gastrointestinal tract, also called the *alimentary* or *digestive tract,* can be divided into two parts: the upper and lower tract. The upper part includes the **mouth, pharynx, esophagus, stomach,** and **duodenum** (Fig. 10-1A). The lower gastrointestinal tract includes the **small** and **large intestine, appendix, rectum,** and **anus.** Clearly, this division is arbitrary, and is based more on current medical practice than on scientific principles. Diseases of the mouth are treated by dentists and otorhinolaryngologists, who also treat the diseases of the salivary glands. Gastroenterologists are concerned with the diseases involving the remainder of the gastrointestinal tract, including the liver and the pancreas. The surgical lesions of the esophagus are in the domain of thoracic surgeons, whereas general surgeons operate on the abdominal parts of the gastrointestinal tract.

The gastrointestinal tract can be perceived as a hollow tube that has essentially the same structural organization from one end to the other (Fig. 10-1B).

Indeed, from the mouth to the anus, the gastrointestinal tract has four layers: mucosa, submucosa, muscularis, and serosa (or adventitia). In the upper gastrointestinal tract, the epithelium of the mucosa is squamous; from the stomach to the anus, it is cuboidal glandular epithelium, and then it again becomes squamous. In the supradiaphragmatic part of the upper gastrointestinal tract, the muscle layer is covered by connective tissue called *adventitia.* The outer surface of the stomach and the intestines is covered with a serosal surface called **peritoneum.** Visceral peritoneum covering the gastrointestinal organs is in continuity with the parietal peritoneum, which covers the rest of the abdominal cavity.

The gastrointestinal tract has a complex blood supply. It is important to remember that the *upper* and *lower mesenteric arteries,* which provide blood to most of the abdominal gastrointestinal organs, receive approximately one-sixth of the arterial cardiac output, and that blood flow can be upregulated or downregulated according to physiological needs. The *portal system* drains most of the venous blood from the small and large intestine.

FIGURE 10-1

Anatomy of the gastrointestinal or alimentary system. (A) The gastrointestinal system may arbitrarily be divided into an upper and lower portion. (B) The gastrointestinal tract has a typical structure. It consists in all parts of four layers: mucosa, submucosa, muscularis, and serosa. Adventitia rather than serosa forms the outer layer of the upper alimentary tracts. (From Applegate EJ: The anatomy and physiology learning system: textbook. Philadelphia: WB Saunders, 1995: 328.)

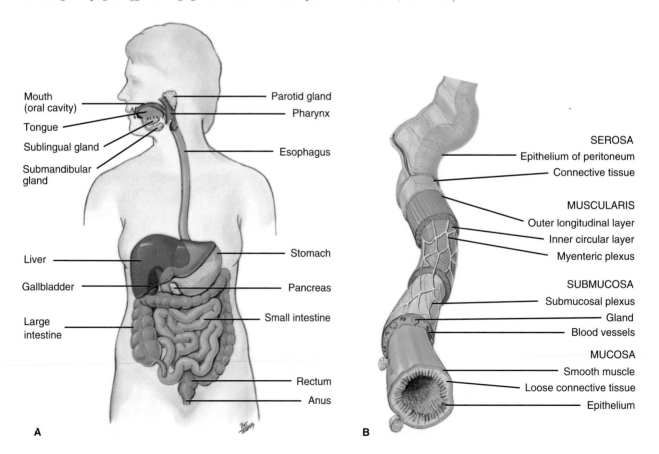

The intestines have a rich supply of lymphatics, which begin as *lacteals* in the mucosal wall and drain into local lymph nodes and larger lymphatic channels that enter into the *thoracic duct*. This lymphatic system is important for the absorption of nutrients from food. Under pathologic conditions, it is the main route for the spread of cancer.

The gastrointestinal tract has a complex innervation that regulates the movements of its various parts. The innervation is mostly derived from the autonomic nervous system and is both vagotonic and sympathomimetic. The autonomic ganglia are located partially outside the gastrointestinal system and partially inside the wall of these organs (*myenteric plexus*).

Developmentally, the gastrointestinal tract is derived from the embryonic gut, which has three parts: foregut, midgut, and hindgut. The foregut gives rise to the pharynx, esophagus, and stomach, as well as to the respiratory tract. The midgut gives rise to the small intestine, but also represents the primordium of the liver and pancreas. The hindgut gives rise to the colon. The mouth and the anus (i.e., the beginning and the end of the gastrointestinal tract) have a complex developmental relationship with adjacent structures, and develop somewhat independently of the remainder of the gastrointestinal tract.

The main functions of the gastrointestinal tract are the digestion of food and alimentation. Each part of the gastrointestinal tract has a specialized role in preparing the food for absorption. Digestion can be divided into the following specific phases:

- *Ingestion.* This takes place in the mouth.
- *Mastication.* Chewing (or *mastication*) is accomplished by the strength of facial muscles compressing the food between the maxilla and the mandible. The *teeth* have a crucial role in mincing of food, which is at the same time mixed with the digestive juices of the *salivary glands*.
- *Deglutition.* Swallowing is a function of the pharyngeal and esophageal muscles. In the begin-

ning, it is voluntary, but once the food enters the esophagus, it is accomplished by *peristalsis* (i.e., contraction of the smooth muscles of the esophagus under the control of autonomic reflexes).

- *Digestion.* *Digestion* begins in the mouth, where the food is mixed with saliva. The food entering the stomach is permeated with hydrochloric acid and gastric enzymes, and it is mechanically propelled into the duodenum. In the duodenum, the food is mixed with bile, pancreatic juice, and intestinal enzymes. Digestive enzymes ensure appropriate lysis of proteins, carbohydrates, and lipids, each of which is absorbed under specific circumstances, and in different parts of the intestines.
- *Absorption.* Chemically digested food components are absorbed, mostly in the small intestine. However, other organs are also involved in the *absorption* of nutrients. For example, alcohol is absorbed in the stomach, and the colon absorbs water and electrolytes.
- *Excretion.* Undigested food, various secretions, and the excretory products of metabolism are passed through the large intestine and extruded as feces. This is called *defecation*.

The processing of food occurs in a highly regulated manner that is under neural and neuroendocrine control. Various neural reflexes regulate salivation, production of gastric juices, and release of bile, as well as the motility of the esophagus, stomach, and intestines. The most important digestive juices and polypeptide hormones secreted by the digestive system are listed in Table 10-1. For example, cholecystokinin that is released from the duodenum, which is distended by food, stimulates the contraction of the gallbladder, release of bile into the intestine, and secretion of bicarbonate in the pancreas. Gastrin, a polypeptide hormone released from the pyloric glandular cells, stimulates the production of hydrochloric acid in the stomach. These polypeptide hormones are secreted by neuroendocrine cells that

Table 10-1 Main Exocrine and Endocrine Products of the Gastrointestinal Tract

Organ	Secretory Product	Function
Salivary gland	Amylase	Digestion of starch
Stomach	Pepsin	Digestion of proteins
	Hydrochloric acid	
	Gastrin	Stimulates secretion of HCl
	Intrinsic factor	Mediates absorption of vitamin B_{12}
Small intestine	Enterokinase	Activates pancreatic enzymes
	Cholecystokinin	Stimulates gallbladder contraction and pancreatic secretion of bicarbonates
	Secretin	Stimulates secretion of pancreatic trypsin and chymotrypsin

are distributed throughout the entire gastrointestinal tract. These cells are loosely integrated into a complex, diffuse network called the *gastrointestinal neuroendocrine system*. Endocrine control of digestion is coordinated neurally and involves several cranial and spinal nerves and the autonomic nervous system.

OVERVIEW OF MAJOR DISEASES

Gastrointestinal diseases are very common. Indeed, approximately 20 million Americans consult their physicians yearly about some problems caused by these diseases. In addition to those diseases that require medical treatment, minor discomforts, such as excessive burping, flatulence (passing of gases), or bad breath, are common.

The most important diseases of the upper and lower gastrointestinal tract are

- dental caries and gum disease
- infectious gastroenteritis
- circulatory disorders and hemorrhagic lesions
- multifactorial disorders, such as peptic ulcer and inflammatory bowel disease
- obstructive disorders, such as hernias and ileus
- functional disorders that result in maldigestion and malabsorption, such as sprue
- neoplasms

Several facts important to an understanding of gastrointestinal disease are presented here, before a discussion of specific pathologic entities.

1. *The function of the normal gastrointestinal tract depends on the normal development of anatomic structures and the functional differentiation of their components.* The development of the gastrointestinal tract occurs at two levels: structural (anatomic) and functional. Structural development of various anatomic parts of the gastrointestinal tract is completed, to a great extent, during the first 3 months of fetal development. It can be disturbed by many external influences that cause complex malformation, and it is often associated with developmental anomalies of other organs. For example, *cleft lip* ("harelip") may be associated with abnormalities of the palate (*cleft palate*) and nose. Likewise, *esophageal atresia* (obliterated lumen) is often associated with abnormalities of the trachea (*esophagotracheal fistula*).

Functional inadequacy of the gastrointestinal cells is usually related to a congenital enzyme deficiency. For example, in *congenital abetalipoproteinemia,* an enzymatic defect in the small intestinal cells prevents the absorption of fats from food, causing steatorrhea.

Abnormal development of the intestinal ganglia, which is a structural defect, may have profound functional consequences. The best example of this is *congenital megacolon* or *Hirschsprung's disease,* in which the intramural ganglia of the rectum do not develop. This leads to spasmodic constriction of the aganglionic segment of the large intestine and the dilatation of the intestine above the obstruction.

2. *The gastrointestinal tract is open-ended and thus is readily accessible to bacteria and other pathogens and allergens.* In contrast to many other organ systems that are sterile, the gastrointestinal tract is, to a large extent, colonized by bacteria. The bacterial flora is site-specific; that is, it is different in the mouth than in the stomach or the rectum. The flora also changes with age, depending on the site, the environment, and the function of the alimentary tract. For example, neonates have a different intestinal flora than do older children and adults. Normally, the host maintains a balance with the saprophytes, but disease may alter that balance. For example, broad-spectrum antibiotics change the colonic flora and facilitate the overgrowth of toxigenic bacteria, such as *Clostridium difficile,* which leads to *pseudomembranous colitis. Candida albicans* infection of the mouth or esophagus is common in debilitated cancer patients.

Many bacteria, protozoa, and parasites that are not normal components of the intestinal flora reach the intestines via the food that is ingested. *Cholera*, a severe watery diarrhea caused by ingested *Vibrio cholerae*, is a good example of such infection.

The immune system of the body, and especially the mucosa-associated lymphoid tract (MALT), may react against foreign pathogens and saprophytes. Immune reactions also occur against various components of food (*food allergy*). Allergens present in the food produce functional or structural changes in the gastrointestinal tract. These are most prominent in children and account for most food allergy in neonates and small children.

3. *The intestinal mucosa is an interface and a barrier between the external and the internal milieu that requires energy to be maintained actively.* The mucosa of the gastrointestinal tract resembles skin in that it protects the body from adverse external influences. Thus, it is essential that the mucosal barrier by kept intact. It can be breached mechanically, by infection, or even chemically. Small defects of the oral mucosa, especially around the teeth, are common sites of bacterial invasion. One infection may lead to another. For example, oral mucosal ulceration caused by herpesvirus may become infected with bacteria. The esophageal mucosal barrier can be breached by hydrochloric acid ingested accidentally, but also by the endogenous hydrochloric acid regurgitated from the stomach. The breakdown of the mucosal defense mechanisms is an important cause of *peptic ulcers* in the stomach and duodenum.

4. *The gastrointestinal tract is a tube that can dilate* *or become obstructed.* Obstruction of the gastrointestinal tube may be anatomic or functional. In *achalasia* of the esophagus, there is a spasm of the lower esophageal sphincter, which prevents the passage of food and causes dilatation of the lumen proximal to the obstruction. A similar obstruction may be caused by *"esophageal webs"* and *"rings"* that protrude into the lumen and are composed of connective tissue and smooth muscles. *Congenital spasm of the pylorus* is a cause of vomiting in neonates and infants, but this condition can be surgically corrected. *Tumors* are probably the most important cause of gastrointestinal obstruction.

The lumen of the gastrointestinal tube may also dilate. *Megacolon* has already been mentioned. *Megaesophagus,* as in achalasia, represents similar dilatation proximal to a structural or functional obstruction. An irregular focal outpouching of the intestinal or esophageal wall is called *diverticulum.*

5. *Gastrointestinal diseases may disturb one or more of the basic functions of the gastrointestinal tract.* Loss of teeth will affect chewing. Diseases of the salivary glands will reduce the moistening of food during mastication and cause "dry mouth" or *xerostomia* (from the Greek *xeros,* meaning dry, and *stoma,* meaning mouth). Stiffening of the esophagus affected by the connective tissue disease scleroderma will cause *dysphagia* (abnormal or strained swallowing). Abnormal secretion of hydrochloric acid can result in *achlorhydria* (lack of hydrochloric acid) or hyperacidity of the gastric content. The term *dyspepsia* is generally used for defective digestion. It has many causes, such as the lack of pepsin that occurs secondary to gastric mucosal atrophy, or the lack of trypsin associated with chronic pancreatitis.

Malabsorption (i.e., abnormal absorption of intestinal contents) may involve carbohydrates, peptides, or lipids, or all the basic food ingredients. Malabsorption of fat is associated with a deficiency of the fat-soluble vitamins: A, D, E, and K. The absorption of essential minerals can also be disturbed.

6. *The movement of the intestines depends on the autonomic contraction of smooth muscles, which is under neural and hormonal control.* Smooth muscle contraction that mediates the swallowing and propulsion of food through the gastrointestinal tract is highly regulated by cranial, spinal, and autonomic nerves. Disturbances of motility result from smooth muscle disease or loss of neural cells in the intestine (e.g., following irradiation). *Carcinoid tumors* secrete polypeptide hormones, which could also cause motility problems owing to neuroendocrine disregulation. Symptoms include *dysphagia* (abnormal swallowing), *constipation* (lack of defecation), *diarrhea* (frequent passing of stools), and *colic* (intestinal spasm).

7. *Abundant blood flow through the gastrointestinal tract and the superficial location of the blood vessels in the mucosa make it prone to hemorrhage or ischemia.* The gastrointestinal tract receives a large amount of blood through large-caliber arteries that originate directly from the aorta. These arteries are prone to atherosclerosis; therefore, with advancing age, the blood supply to the intestine diminishes. This is one of the reasons that the elderly often have problems with digestion and constipation. They often develop ulcerations and ischemic atrophy of the mucosa.

The abundant blood supply irrigates the mucosa of the gastrointestinal tract diffusely, which facilitates absorption of nutrients. This mucosal vascularity makes the stomach and intestines vulnerable to bleeding secondary to mechanical trauma. Furthermore, the mucosal injury of peptic ulcer or other ulcerative diseases is also associated with bleeding, which stems from the sheared mucosal capillaries and even the larger submucosal vessels.

Gastrointestinal hemorrhage may be clinically apparent or occult. Occult hemorrhage may cause iron deficiency anemia secondary to chronic blood loss. Upper gastrointestinal bleeding that leads to a mixing of blood with hydrochloric acid in the stomach will result in *melena* (from the Greek *melas,* meaning black). Massive bleeding from the stomach, duodenum, or esophagus may cause vomiting of blood, called *hematemesis.* Bleeding from the rectum is called *hematochezia.*

8. *The gastrointestinal tract is an important source of enzymes, hormones, and biologically active polypeptides.* Each portion of the gastrointestinal tract produces unique biologically active substances. For example, the intestines secrete *immunoglobulin A* (IgA), which has an important role in mucosal immunity. The stomach secretes the *intrinsic factor,* which is essential for the absorption of vitamin B_{12}. The small intestines synthesize *chylomicrons* and release them into the blood circulation, which is essential for the transport of absorbed food lipids to the liver. Loss of these anatomic parts—i.e., from resection of the stomach or intestine—will affect the well being of the entire body.

Some intestinal secretory products may be used as markers of disease. For example, the fetal intestinal cells secrete a complex glycoprotein called *carcinoembryonic antigen* (CEA), which is not produced by the normal intestine. CEA is produced by adenocarcinomas of the intestine, and it can be measured in the serum. CEA is thus a valuable tumor marker.

9. *The gastrointestinal tract is exposed to environmental carcinogens in food.* Carcinomas of the gastrointestinal tract are among the most common human malignant diseases. It is believed that carcinogens in food play an important pathogenetic role and are directly responsible for most of these malignant diseases. Differences in diet account for many of the differences in the incidence of various cancers in various parts of the world. For example, colon cancer is the most important gastrointestinal cancer in the United States. The incidence of gastric carcinoma, which was very common a century ago in the United States, has decreased here, but it is still high in Japan.

Diseases of the Oral Cavity

The most important diseases of the oral cavity are dental caries, periodontal disease, and cancer. There are also developmental defects that can affect the oral cavity, as well as other inflammatory diseases.

Developmental Abnormalities

Cleft lip is a congenital abnormality that occurs with increased frequency in some families; it is considered to be inherited as a polygenic trait. It results from a lack of fusion of the fetal nasal and maxillary processes that form the upper lip. It may be associated with cleft palate, in which a fissure forms between the mouth and the nasal cavity. Cleft lip is more common in males than in females.

Teeth abnormalities are common. These may involve delayed or irregular dentition and abnormally shaped or abnormally positioned teeth, such as *impacted wisdom teeth*.

Inflammation

Inflammation of the teeth results in *dental caries*. Inflammation of the gums and tissue surrounding the tooth is called *periodontal disease*. Inflammation of the oral mucosa is called stomatitis.

Dental Caries. Dental caries (from the Latin *caries* meaning "dry rot") is one of the most common diseases of humans. It is most prevalent in children and adolescents, but it occurs in older persons as well. Caries has been considered a disease of modern civilization, but archeologists have demonstrated caries in ancient Egyptian mummies and the frozen remains of Neanderthal men as well. Lifestyle and diet probably influence the development of caries, as the disease is less prevalent among Eskimos and some jungle dwellers of South America. Widespread fluoridation of water has decreased the occurrence of caries in the United States.

Dental caries is a multifactorial disease mediated by oral saprophytic bacteria. The predisposition to caries varies from one person to another, and it may have a genetic basis. Resistance to caries can be bolstered by fluoridation of the drinking water. It is thought that fluoride promotes formation of enamel that has increased resistance to bacteria. Saliva that contains various antimicrobial substances, such as lysozyme and lactoferrin, provides additional protec-

tion. Xerostomia is associated with an increased incidence of caries. Dental hygiene, involving regular brushing and flossing of teeth, also reduces caries. This reduction is achieved by removing the bacteria and by preventing the formation of bacterial *plaque*. Sugar-containing food should be avoided, as the bacterial action on teeth is facilitated by lactic acid formed locally from carbohydrates in food.

Caries begins after the bacteria that are forming plaque on the surface of the tooth have eroded the enamel (Fig. 10-2). The defect extends into the dentin, which becomes decalcified and disintegrates, allowing the bacteria to penetrate deep into the tooth and invade the pulp chamber. Because the inside of the tooth contains nerves and blood vessels, pulpitis and inflammation of the root canal are accompanied by pain.

Superficial caries and pulpitis may be treated and the affected tooth salvaged. However, if the infection extends into the root canal, it evokes an inflammatory response in the periodontal tissue known as *periapical granuloma*. Massive suppuration is accompanied by formation of a *periapical abscess,* and this may extend into the jaws, provoking bone infection (*osteomyelitis*). These complications of caries usually require extraction of the tooth and, often, jaw surgery with antibiotic coverage. Less extensive disease may heal spontaneously; in such cases, the periapical granuloma or abscess is transformed into a *pseudocyst* (i.e., a cavity lined by granulation tissue and filled with fluid). The ingrowth of the gum epithelium may transform the granuloma cavity into a cyst lined by squamous epithelium (*radicular cyst*).

Periodontal Disease. Periodontal inflammation is a common disease, accounting for more tooth loss than caries and all other dental diseases combined. It is related to the colonization of periodontal pockets with bacteria. This leads to the formation of plaque, which calcifies and transforms into *tartar*. Bacteria, plaque, and tartar together cause inflammation of the overlying gingiva, which loosens the tooth ligaments and allows bacterial invasion of the tooth socket and the root canal. This impedes the blood supply to the pulp and devitalizes the tooth. The gums are initially swollen and tender, but as the infection progresses, loosening of teeth occurs. Loss of teeth and massive inflammation of the gums predominate in chronic cases. Profuse infection may cause oozing of pus from the gums (*pyorrhea*).

Bacteroides gingivalis seems to be the main cause of periodontal disease. It is not known why this microbe colonizes the mouth cavity of some individuals and spares others, but there seems to be a familial predisposition to periodontal disease. Poor oral hygiene is, however, the most common predisposing factor. Preventive dental care could remarkably re-

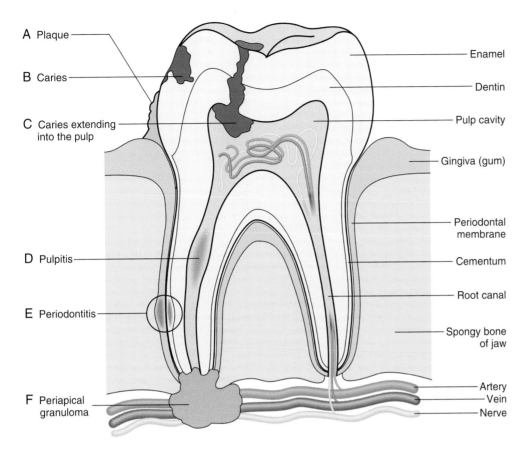

A Plaque
B Caries
C Caries extending into the pulp
D Pulpitis
E Periodontitis
F Periapical granuloma

Enamel
Dentin
Pulp cavity
Gingiva (gum)
Periodontal membrane
Cementum
Root canal
Spongy bone of jaw
Artery
Vein
Nerve

FIGURE 10-2
Dental and periodontal diseases. Caries begins as a bacterial plaque (A), which leads to a defect in the enamel (B). Deeper defects allow the entry of bacteria into the pulp cavity (C). Pulpitis is a bacterial infection that may extend into the root canal (D). Periodontal disease is caused by bacteria that colonize the gingival pockets (E). Extension of infection into the periapical bone leads to the formation of periapical granuloma (F).

duce the incidence of this disease and prevent tooth loss.

Stomatitis. Stomatitis is an inflammation of the mouth. It often occurs during the course of systemic disease, but it may also represent the only sign of infection. It is caused by various viruses, bacteria, and fungi. *Herpesvirus infection* typically causes vesicles on the lips that may extend into the mouth. *C. albicans stomatitis* (thrush) is common in debilitated cancer patients and those with acquired immunodeficiency syndrome (AIDS). It is marked by white surface layers covering the mucosa. *Aphthous stomatitis* (canker sores) are painful, recurrent, superficial, oral ulcers of unknown etiology that cause considerable distress but heal spontaneously.

Oral Cancer
Oral cancer is common and may involve the lips, tongue, soft palate, or just about anywhere else in the mouth (Fig. 10-3). It is a well-known complication of smoking, especially pipe smoking. Chronic alcoholism is also a risk factor. Males predominate among patients with lip carcinoma (10:1) and those with carcinoma of the oral cavity (2:1). The average age at diagnosis is 55 to 60 years.

Carcinoma of the lips and oral cavity presents in the form of mucosal abnormalities, such as

FIGURE 10-3
Carcinoma of the lip. On gross examination, the tumor appears to be ulcerated.

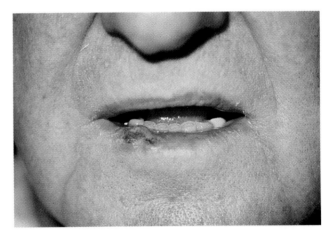

- *leukoplakia,* a white, slightly elevated plaque that covers the mucosal surface
- *erythroplakia,* a red plaque that appears distinct from the surrounding mucosa
- *ulcer,* which appears as a shallow defect
- *crater,* which appears as a defect with raised margins
- *nodule or plaque,* an induration that protrudes from the mucosal surface

Tumors may be multifocal, simultaneously originating in several places. On histologic examination, almost all are squamous cell carcinoma. They tend to invade the underlying tissue and metastasize to local lymph nodes on the neck. The prognosis is good for early lesions, which can be treated with radiation therapy or surgery. Advanced lesions have a poor prognosis. Unfortunately, many patients are still diagnosed with advanced cancers, and the overall 5-year survival rate is only 25 percent.

Salivary Gland Diseases

Saliva is produced by major and minor salivary glands. There are three major salivary glands: the parotid, the submandibulary, and the sublingual—each of which is paired and readily identifiable by palpation or gross examination during surgery. The small salivary glands are scattered throughout the oral cavity, mostly on the floor of the mouth.

The most important diseases of the salivary glands are inflammations and tumors.

Sialadenitis

Inflammation of the salivary glands is called *sialadenitis.* It can be infectious or immunologically mediated. Infections usually spread from the mouth. *Staphylococcus aureus* and *Streptococcus viridans* are the most common causes of suppurative sialadenitis. *Mumps* is the most common viral infection. Enlargement of the salivary glands in children is a typical feature of mumps. Mumps is less common in adults.

Infections cause pain and enlargement of the salivary glands, the latter usually being asymmetrical. Functionally, the disease may present with *sialorrhea* (i.e., overproduction of saliva) or *xerostomia* (dry mouth). Acute sialadenitis typically heals on its own and has few residual effects. Chronic sialadenitis of infectious origin is rare and usually represents a complication of salivary duct obstruction. This may be caused by periductal fibrosis or ductal stones, a condition known as *sialolithiasis* (from the Greek *sialos,* meaning saliva, and *lithos,* meaning stone).

Immunologically mediated sialadenitis is a typical feature of *Sjögren's syndrome.* This autoimmune disease presents with systemic symptoms, but invariably involves the salivary or the lacrimal glands. *Xerostomia* and *xerophthalmia* (dry eyes) are thus typical symptoms. Enlargement of the glands is attributable to infiltrates of lymphocytes and plasma cells, which slowly replace the normal acinar cells and ultimately cause glandular insufficiency. In the later stages of the disease, the glands become fibrotic and shrink in size. An increased incidence of lymphoma has been reported in patients with salivary glands affected by Sjögren's syndrome.

Neoplasms

Tumors of the salivary glands are not common. Nevertheless they constitute 3 percent to 4 percent of all head and neck neoplasms. Their peak incidence is in patients who are 40 to 60 years of age.

Histologically, the tumors can be classified as benign or malignant, and can be assigned to several subtypes, such as pleomorphic adenoma, monomorphic adenoma (a subtype of which is called Warthin's tumor), mucoepidermoid carcinoma, acinic cell carcinoma, adenoid cystic carcinoma, and several other variants. These tumors may originate from either the major or minor salivary glands. The parotid gland, which is the largest of all, is involved most often. Among the other important facts about such tumors are the following:

- Tumors of the major salivary glands are more often benign than malignant. Only 25 percent of these tumors are malignant, whereas 50 percent of the tumors in the minor salivary glands are malignant. However, even the benign tumors are often difficult to remove without mutilating surgery or transection of nerves. If incompletely removed, they tend to recur. Follow-up is thus important for all patients with salivary gland tumors.
- *Pleomorphic adenoma* is the most common histologic tumor type, accounting for 70 percent of all tumors in the major salivary glands and 50 percent of tumors in the minor salivary glands. It is benign and composed of epithelial and myoepithelial cells and areas resembling cartilage (hence, the name pleomorphic adenoma). In a small number of cases, pleomorphic adenoma may evolve into carcinoma. All other tumors, with the exception of monomorphic adenomas, are low-grade malignant lesions.

Salivary gland tumors present as slow-growing masses, compressing the normal facial structures and often causing pain. Surgery is the treatment of choice. Although recurrences are common, the overall prognosis is excellent. The 5-year survival rate exceeds 85 percent.

Diseases of the Esophagus

The most important diseases of the esophagus are esophagitis, circulatory disturbances, and neoplasms (Fig. 10-4). Typical symptoms of esophageal disease include the following:

- *Dysphagia,* or difficulty in swallowing. This includes an inability to initiate swallowing, as well as the sensation that the swallowed food cannot pass. Some patients have true obstruction to the passage of food.
- *Esophageal pain.* This may present as a colic (a spasmodic substernal pain) that occurs spontaneously, presumably owing to muscular spasm; or it may present as retrosternal burning ("heartburn").
- *Aspiration* and *regurgitation* of food and liquids. Food or liquid may reenter the oral cavity from the esophagus and reach the lower respiratory tract.

Developmental Abnormalities

The most important developmental anomaly involving the esophagus is congenital *atresia* (lack of lumen), an abnormality that presents shortly after birth and is often associated with abnormal connections between the esophagus and trachea (*esophago-tracheal fistula*). Because food cannot pass into the stomach, affected babies vomit ingested milk. If the defect is not repaired, these babies die of hunger or aspiration pneumonia.

Esophagitis

Esophagitis, or inflammation of the esophagus, may be caused by

- infection
- reflux of gastric juice ("peptic esophagitis")
- exogenous irritants, chemicals, and drugs

FIGURE 10-4

Non-neoplastic esophageal diseases. (A) Esophagotracheal fistula is usually a defect, but may be caused by cancer. (B) Hernias occur in two forms: sliding hernias or paraesophageal hernias. (C) Achalasia is marked by a stenosis of the lower esophageal sphincter and consequent dilation of the esophagus proximal to it. (D) Varices are the most important circulatory disturbance of the lower esophagus.

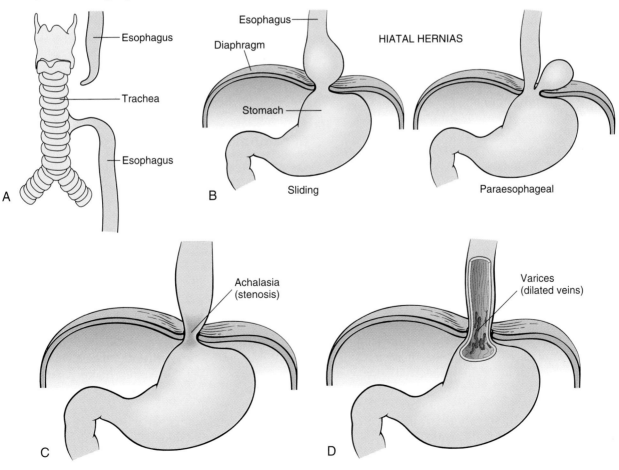

Infectious esophagitis is typically caused by viruses or fungi, and it occurs usually in immunosuppressed or debilitated persons. Normal squamous epithelium is resistant to pathogens, and the rapid passage of food through the esophagus does not favor contact between the pathogens and the mucosa, so that infections usually do not take place. However, if the general health or the immune response of the patient has been compromised, infections may occur. Such infections are caused by viruses, such as herpesvirus or cytomegalovirus, or fungi, such as *C. albicans*. These infections produce superficial lesions (shallow ulcers). Bacterial infections are uncommon in the intact esophagus, but may become superimposed on viral or fungal ulcerations.

Peptic esophagitis is caused by a reflux of gastric juice into the esophagus. Normally, the lower esophageal sphincter (LES) prevents the reflux of gastric juices into the esophagus. However, if the function of the sphincter is compromised, reflux may occur and ulcerations of the esophagus mediated by pepsin and hydrochloric acid may develop.

Peptic esophagitis is histologically characterized by nonspecific inflammation and ulceration of the squamous epithelium. The defects are often repaired by metaplastic epithelium that appears glandular and resembles the columnar epithelium of the stomach or intestine. Foci of esophageal mucosa, composed of metaplastic glandular epithelium, are called *Barrett's esophagus*. This mucosa is more sensitive to injury than normal squamous epithelium, and may give rise to peptic ulcers, which are indistinguishable from similar ulcers in the stomach. Furthermore, Barrett's esophagus is a risk factor for cancer, which develops in a significant number of patients.

Chemical esophagitis, caused by accidental swallowing of inorganic acids or lyes, is typically encountered in children. Suicide attempts are another cause of such changes. Esophagitis may also be caused *mechanically* by permanently placed nasogastric tubes that are used for feeding terminally ill patients.

Hiatal Hernia

There are several conditions that predispose individuals to gastroesophageal reflux. The most common cause of reflux esophagitis is hiatal hernia. It occurs in several forms (e.g., *sliding hiatal hernia* or *paraesophageal hernia*), all of which lead to displacement of the cardia and the adjacent portion of the stomach from the abdominal cavity into the thoracic cavity through the diaphragmatic hiatus. Hiatal hernia alters the function of the LES and facilitates reflux of gastric juice into the esophagus. The tone of the LES also may be reduced by smoking and caffeine. Heartburn is common in pregnancy, which causes physiologic relaxation of the LES.

Motility Disorders of the Esophagus

A large number of functional motility problems affect the esophagus. These disorders have no visible pathologic substrate, but can be diagnosed by measuring the pressure inside the esophagus (by manometry) or by barium swallow examination with x-ray studies. The best known of these disorders is the *"nutcracker esophagus,"* named so because of its typical wavy appearance on radiographs. Scleroderma, a connective tissue disease characterized by replacement of the smooth muscle of the esophagus with fibrous tissue, also causes motility problems.

Achalasia (from the Greek term meaning "lack of relaxation") is the antithesis of LES insufficiency. Achalasia is marked by a spasm of the LES, a dilatation of the esophagus proximal to the site of the spasm, and an inability to swallow food (*dysphagia*). In most instances, achalasia is idiopathic.

Circulatory Disturbances

Circulatory disturbances of the esophagus are important because they may cause hematemesis. **Esophageal varices,** typically caused by cirrhosis of the liver and other diseases marked by portal hypertension, are among the most common causes of upper gastrointestinal bleeding and are associated with high mortality. Laceration of the small blood vessels at the gastrointestinal junction are typical of the *Mallory-Weiss syndrome,* a clinical syndrome marked by hematemesis. Mallory-Weiss syndrome is caused by tears in the mucosa that occur during strenuous vomiting. Understandably, it is most often encountered in alcoholics.

Carcinoma of the Esophagus

Carcinoma is the most important neoplasm of the esophagus. Benign tumors of the esophagus, such as leiomyoma or neurofibroma, are rare and thus do not warrant detailed consideration.

Carcinoma of the esophagus accounts for 4 percent of all malignant neoplasms in the United States. Although less common than carcinoma of the large intestine or the stomach, it is still an important malignant lesion because of its extremely unfavorable prognosis. There are 8000 new cases every year, and 95 percent of these patients will die within 2 years of diagnosis. In certain parts of the world, such as China, Iran, and South Africa, the incidence of esophageal cancer is 10 to 15 times higher than in the United States. In those countries, it is one of the most common cancers.

The etiology and pathogenesis of esophageal cancer are poorly understood. The best clues about the origin of esophageal cancer are derived from epidemiologic studies. Interesting epidemiologic data include the following:

- *Geographic differences.* The high incidence of esophageal cancer in China, Iran, and South Africa points to a possible carcinogen in the soil or food. In China, even the domestic fowl have a high incidence of esophageal cancer, a fact that further points to some potential environmental carcinogens in the soil.
- *Racial differences.* For unknown reasons, esophageal cancer is three times more common in blacks than in whites in the United States.
- *Sex differences.* The male to female ratio is 4:1 in the United States. In China and South Africa, males and females are affected equally.
- *Correlation with tobacco and alcohol abuse.* In the United States, a large number of patients with esophageal cancer have a documented history of chronic alcoholism and tobacco use.

Pathology. Most carcinomas originate from the middle or lower portion of the esophagus. Early cancer limited to the mucosa is barely visible during esophagoscopy. Most early tumors are discovered by biopsy, performed during an investigation of nonspecific upper gastrointestinal discomfort. Tumors tend to grow into the lumen as endophytic masses, or infiltrate the wall as a result of exophytic growth. The part of the esophagus that is infiltrated with tumor is usually indurated and ulcerated (Fig. 10-5), which accounts for the associated pain on swallowing, dysphagia, and bleeding.

Esophageal tumors are locally invasive. By the time of diagnosis, most tumors have already spread through the adventitia into the lymph nodes and the surrounding mediastinal organs. Distant metastases are a late event. Histologically, almost all upper and middle esophageal cancers are squamous cell carcinomas. In the lower third, adenocarcinomas originating in Barrett's esophagus predominate, but even here, approximately 40 percent of cancers are squamous cell carcinomas.

Clinical Features. The clinical symptoms of esophageal cancer include dysphagia, pain, and occasionally, bleeding or malodorous breath. Patients have pain upon swallowing and, as the obstruction becomes more severe, they are unable to ingest any solid food at all. The diagnosis is established by barium swallow x-ray examination or esophagoscopy accompanied by biopsy. The prognosis is dismal. Less than 5 percent of patients survive 2 years.

Diseases of the Stomach and Duodenum

The most important diseases of the stomach are gastritis, peptic ulcer, and carcinoma. The symptoms of gastric diseases include the following:

- *Pain.* This is typically related to ulceration of the mucosa, the caustic action of hydrochloric acid, and the enzymatic action of pepsin in the gastric juice.
- *Vomiting.* Obstruction of the exit portion of the stomach (pylorus) or irritation and disturbed motor function of the gastric musculature result in vomiting. Vomiting is based on a reflex, and although it is an important and common finding in gastric diseases, it may occur in other diseases of the upper gastrointestinal tract and in many systemic and central nervous system disorders, and it may even be initiated voluntarily.
- *Bleeding.* Gastric ulceration may lead to hematemesis or melena.
- *Dyspepsia.* Abnormal function of the stomach may result in digestive problems, such as the inability to digest food. This may be associated with nausea, loss of appetite, or aversion to food.
- *Systemic consequences.* For example, chronic bleeding ulcers may cause iron deficiency anemia. Lack of intrinsic factor, a gastric protein essential for the absorption of vitamin B_{12}, results in *pernicious anemia.*

FIGURE 10-5
Carcinoma of the esophagus appears as an indurated mucosal defect.

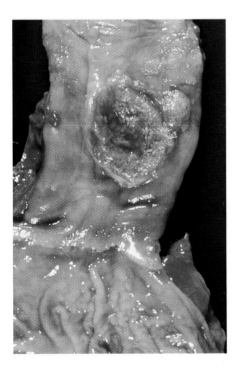

Developmental Abnormalities

Developmental abnormalities of the stomach and duodenum are rare. The most important is *congenital stenosis of the pylorus.* Symptoms appear early in the neonatal period. Boys are affected four times more often than girls. Stenosis prevents emptying of the stomach and results in projectile vomiting. Surgical incision of the contracted gastric muscle will usually relieve the symptoms and permanently cure the disease.

Gastritis

Gastritis may be classified as acute or chronic. *Acute gastritis* (**erosive gastritis**) is a self-limiting disease of short duration that usually heals spontaneously. In contrast, chronic gastritis, which is also known as *nonerosive gastritis,* lasts longer.

Acute gastritis is characterized by shallow mucosal defects limited to the upper layers of the epithelium. They are called *erosions* if they are superficial, or *ulcers* if they are somewhat deeper and extend through the entire thickness of the mucosa.

Mucosal erosions and ulceration of the stomach develop under a variety of circumstances, the most important of which are circulatory disturbances and exposure to exogenous irritants. Circulatory disturbances, such as shock, typically change the blood flow through the gastric mucosa, rendering the superficial parts of the mucosa ischemic, and thus making them susceptible to the adverse effects of gastric juices. This may result in multiple superficial bleeding erosions (acute erosive gastritis) or deeper ulcerations. *Stress-related ulcers* that are associated with various forms of shock, called *Curling's ulcers,* extend through the entire mucosa and are often associated with profound bleeding. *Cushing's ulcers* (named after the famous neurosurgeon who described them in patients with brain tumors) are large stress ulcers. These ulcers heal if the circulatory disturbances that have caused them are cured. On the other hand, they may persist in terminally ill patients, and are often found at autopsy.

Exogenous irritants that cause gastritis include several drugs, alcohol, and chemicals ingested by accident or suicidally. The most important among these is *aspirin,* which often causes superficial erosions in the stomach.

Chronic gastritis is a term used to describe several pathologic processes with differing pathogenesis. The disease is characterized by mucosal atrophy, metaplasia of the gastric glands into intestinal epithelium (*intestinal metaplasia*), and mild, chronic inflammation.

The cause of chronic gastritis is not known. The disease is more common in older persons. In some cases, as in pernicious anemia, it is probably mediated by an immunologic mechanism. In others, it may be related to infection with *Helicobacter pylori.* The disease is much more common in natives of Japan, Finland, and Hungary than in the United States. Even the immigrants from these countries who are living in the United States have a higher incidence of gastritis than other Americans. This suggests that genetic factors and diet may play pathogenetic roles.

Chronic gastritis produces mild digestive symptoms related to gastric atrophy and reduced secretion of pepsin and hydrochloric acid. The symptoms are usually nonspecific and are labeled as *dyspepsia* ("indigestion"). Immune-mediated gastric atrophy results in reduced production of the intrinsic factor and impaired absorption of vitamin B_{12}. Vitamin B_{12} deficiency results in pernicious anemia and a variety of neurologic symptoms. Immune-mediated gastric atrophy and concomitant gastric metaplasia also predispose affected individuals to gastric cancer.

Peptic Ulcer

Peptic ulcer is a chronic multifactorial disease characterized by mucosal ulceration that extends through the entire gastric epithelial layer and into the muscularis. It can occur in any part of the gastrointestinal tract exposed to peptic juice. Most often, it is located in the duodenum or the stomach; less frequently, it involves the esophagus and small intestine. Peptic ulcer is a very common disease, affecting, at any one time, approximately 4 million people in the United States. It accounts for 10 percent of all the money spent for the treatment of gastrointestinal diseases. Approximately 1 percent to 2 percent of all Americans have a peptic ulcer during their life span.

Etiology and Pathogenesis. The etiology and pathogenesis of peptic ulcer are poorly understood, although there is general agreement that several factors play a crucial role. These include the following:

- *Gastric juice.* Peptic ulcer develops only in parts of the gastrointestinal tract that are exposed to pepsin and hydrochloric acid. The dictum "no acid, no ulcer" still holds true. Inhibition of gastric secretion with H-2 blockers, such as cimetidine, promotes ulcer healing.
- *Mucosal barrier.* The normal gastric and duodenal mucosa are resistant to the chemical and enzymatic action of gastric juice. Reduced resistance and frank breakdown of the mucosal barrier occur under a variety of conditions, such as shock and even prolonged psychological stress. Smoking and alcohol also have adverse effects. Drugs, such as aspirin or nonsteroidal anti-inflammatory drugs (NSAIDs), cause mucosal erosions and shallow ulcers.

- H. pylori *infection. H. pylori* is found in the stomach or duodenum of most patients with peptic ulcer. Eradication of the infection cures ulcers in most instances.

In patients who are genetically predisposed (50 percent of duodenal patients have a family history), the disease can evolve under a variety of circumstances. For example, hyperacidity of the gastric juice, coupled with rapid emptying of the stomach, may overburden the duodenum. Because the acid cannot be neutralized, it destroys the mucosa, causing duodenal ulcer. Atrophy of the gastric mucosa in antral gastritis also predisposes the patient to ulceration. A stressful lifestyle, smoking, and chronic intake of aspirin and other NSAIDs promote ulcer formation. Corticosteroids are ulcerigenic if taken as medication, and they are probably also important when internally oversecreted. Gastrin, a polypeptide hormone that stimulates the secretion of hydrochloric acid, is a well-known cause of ulcers in some patients. Psychological stress and vagal stimulation of gastric secretions and motility can also have an adverse effect. *Thus, it is best to consider peptic ulcer as an imbalance between the adverse influences that could damage the mucosal barrier and the protective forces that preserve its integrity.*

Pathology. All peptic ulcers have the same typical appearance, regardless of their location. They appear as sharply punched out, round defects of the mucosa extending into the deep layers of the stomach or duodenum. The bottom of the ulcer consists of glandular amorphous material formed from tissue destruction by hydrochloric acid and, occasionally, larger blood vessels that have an eroded wall and appear gaping (Fig. 10-6). The caustic action of the hydrochloric acid keeps the bottom of the ulcer "clean" and devoid of necrotic tissue. The margins of the ulcer seem to be sharp, in contrast to ulcerated carcinomas of the stomach, which have irregular margins and a necrotic shaggy surface.

Histologically, the ulcers vary in appearance, which usually reflects the duration of the disease. Acute ulcers and those of short duration are more shallow and show little healing. On the other hand, chronic ulcers extend deeper into the muscle layer where they evoke tissue response. In a cross-sectioned ulcer, one can actually recognize several layers, including, from top to bottom: (a) surface composed of necrotic tissue, (b) a zone of acute and chronic inflammation, (c) vascular granulation tissue, and (d) fibrous scar tissue (Fig. 10-6B).

Peptic ulcers can be cured with appropriate medication, especially in the early stages of the disease. In some cases, the disease is resistant to treatment. The most important complications of such chronic ulcers are as follows:

- *Hemorrhage.* Hemorrhage is common in all peptic ulcers. However, it is usually mild, causing melena rather than hematemesis. Large ulcers may erode arteries in the wall of the stomach and duodenum, causing massive, and, occasionally, even lethal bleeding. Such arterial bleedings represent an emergency, and require gastroscopic or even open surgical intervention.
- *Penetration.* Peptic ulcers of the duodenum can erode the entire wall and penetrate into the pan-

FIGURE 10-6
Peptic ulcer. (A) Gross appearance of the ulcer as seen by endoscopy. (B) Histologically, the bottom of the ulcer replacing the mucosa consists mostly of granulation tissue and admixed necrotic cell debris and inflammatory cells. Peptic ulcer may bleed from eroded mucosal blood vessels. The tissue underlying the ulcer shows fibrosis and scarring.

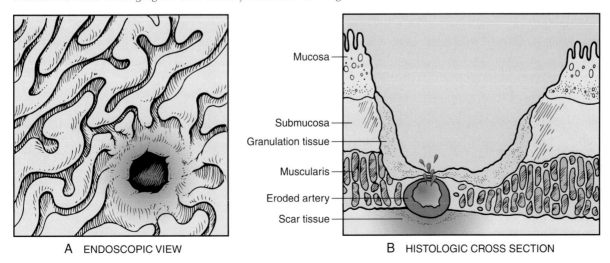

A ENDOSCOPIC VIEW

B HISTOLOGIC CROSS SECTION

Mucosa
Submucosa
Granulation tissue
Muscularis
Eroded artery
Scar tissue

creas. This is typically associated with intractable pain and reactive, smoldering pancreatitis.

- *Perforation.* Duodenal ulcers may extend through the intestinal wall and form a hole. Intestinal contents pass through this hole into the peritoneal cavity and cause *peritonitis*. This is also a surgical emergency. Such perforations can be sutured and cured.
- *Cicatrization.* Healing of duodenal ulcers is occasionally associated with extensive scarring, which may cause intestinal stenosis (narrowing) or obstruction.

Clinical Features. Most peptic ulcers (98 percent) are located in the distal portion of the stomach and the proximal duodenum. Duodenal ulcers are four times more common than peptic ulcers. Gastric ulcers affect persons older than 50 years of age, whereas duodenal ulcers can occur any time during adult life and affect younger persons as well. The disease typically presents with pain 1 to 3 hours after a meal or during the night. The patient can typically point to the site of the maximum pain, which is usually in the midline of the epigastrium. The pain can be alleviated with alkaline agents or food, but often recurs at regular intervals. Other symptoms are nonspecific and include nausea, vomiting and loss of appetite or weight. Melena and associated iron deficiency anemia are common in chronic disease. Hematemesis and peritonitis are complications that could lead to death and so require vigorous treatment.

The treatment of peptic ulcer is based on eradication of *H. pylori* infection and suppression of gastric acid secretion with H-2 antagonists, such as cimetidine. Peptic ulcers have a tendency to recur, but overall, the prognosis for cure is excellent and major complications requiring surgery are rare.

Gastric Neoplasms

Carcinoma of the stomach is the most important neoplasm of the stomach, and it accounts for 90 percent of all tumors. Benign epithelial tumors account for 5 percent of neoplasms. Other neoplasms, such as lymphoma and smooth cell tumors (leiomyoma and leiomyosarcoma), represent the remaining 5 percent of tumors.

Benign epithelial tumors, known as hyperplastic and adenomatous polyps, are mostly asymptomatic. These tumors are usually discovered only at autopsy or during gastroscopy performed for some other, unrelated reason. Although gastric polyps are rare, their significance is twofold:

- These benign tumors may progress to carcinoma and are actually 10 times more common in patients with pernicious anemia (another condition that predisposes to cancer) than in the population at large.
- Gastric polyps may be associated with cancer. The discovery of a polyp warrants a detailed search for carcinoma!

Carcinoma of the Stomach

Carcinoma of the stomach is an important malignant lesion that affects 25,000 Americans and causes 14,000 deaths yearly. The incidence of gastric cancer has decreased significantly in the United States over the last 70 years. In the United States, the incidence is now 10 per 1,000,000, which is approximately 8 times lower than the incidence in Japan or Chile. The fact that U.S. immigrants from these high-prevalence areas have a lower incidence of gastric cancer than their relatives or predecessors in the country of their origin suggests a possible role for environmental carcinogens. Most likely, the exogenous carcinogens are in the food. However, none of these has yet been identified.

Etiology and Pathogenesis. Most of the studies of possible environmental carcinogens have concentrated on *nitrosamines,* which are known to produce cancer in animals. It has been proposed that the current American diet contains less nitrosamines than before. Previously, when most food was not refrigerated, bacterial overgrowth could indeed have generated excessive nitrosamines in such food. Smoked fish, consumed in some of the countries with a high incidence of gastric cancer, contains more nitrosamines than most cooked fish eaten in the United States. Furthermore, the current methods of food processing in the United States eliminate many potentially dangerous bacteria. Bacteria can convert nitrates to nitrites which, in turn, are the source of carcinogenic nitrosamines. Prevention of bacterial growth and proper food processing may be instrumental in gastric cancer prevention.

Environmental carcinogens probably act in concert with several endogenous factors that are poorly understood. Atrophic gastritis, pernicious anemia, and gastric adenomatous polyps carry an increased risk, but the pathogenic chain of events linking these conditions to cancer has not been elucidated.

Pathology. Most carcinomas are found in the distal stomach (i.e., pylorus and antrum). Cardia is involved in 25 percent of cases. Early gastric carcinoma begins as a gastric lesion that may be raised, indented, or at the same level as the normal mucosa. Four types of invasive carcinoma are recognized (Fig. 10-7):

- polypoid
- fungating

- ulcerating
- diffusely infiltrating

Polyoid tumors protrude into the lumen of the stomach. Ulcerating tumors resemble peptic ulcer, but are usually more irregular in shape and larger. Ulcerating-infiltrating tumors resemble craters and have indurated margins and a central ulceration. Diffusely infiltrating tumors permeate the gastric wall and transform it into a leather-bottle-like, stiff organ. This type of cancer is also called *linitis plastica*.

Histologically, all gastric carcinomas are adenocarcinomas. Some tumors are well differentiated, whereas others are poorly differentiated. Some produce mucin and are called signet-ring carcinomas because the cells filled with mucin displace the nucleus onto the periphery, which resembles a signet ring.

Gastric carcinomas metastasize to regional lymph nodes and to the liver. Through the thoracic duct, gastric carcinoma often reaches the supraclavicular lymph nodes on the right, which are called *Virchow's nodes,* in honor of the German pathologist who recognized these metastases as a characteristic sign of gastric carcinoma. Carcinoma of the stomach can also spread to other abdominal organs and to the lungs. Bilateral involvement of the ovaries, occasionally recognized by gynecologists as *Krukenberg's tumor,* is a rare but characteristic presenting sign of gastric carcinoma that has metastasized to the ovaries.

Clinical Features. Carcinoma of the stomach presents with nonspecific symptoms. Because patients do not usually seek medical assistance early, by the time of diagnosis, most tumors are in advanced stages and thus are inoperable. Symptoms include nonspecific signs of tumor growth, such as weight loss, anemia, and weakness. Local tumor growth provokes gastric irritation, vomiting, loss of appetite, and dysphagia. Ulceration leads to bleeding. Sometimes the tumors are diagnosed on the basis of distant metastases, such as to the supraclavicular lymph nodes or ovaries.

Gastric carcinoma has a very poor prognosis. The 5-year survival rate for these patients is 10 percent to 15 percent in most Western countries. Active screening for gastric cancer, involving systematic gastroscopies combined with gastric brushing and cytologic examination, is widely used in Japan with most encouraging results. Early detection of gastric cancer by these techniques and an early gastrectomy seem to be the only way to combat this cancer.

Gastrointestinal Lymphoma

Lymphomas may involve the gastrointestinal tract in the course of dissemination of disease that usually begins in the lymph nodes or the bone marrow. In contrast to these *secondary gastrointestinal lymphomas,* there are tumors that begin in the stomach or the intestines, which are, therefore, called *primary gastrointestinal lymphomas*. These tumors originate in the MALT and typically present as localized masses, which can be resected surgically. Most often, such tumors are found in the stomach (60 percent); less commonly, they involve the small intestine (25 percent) or colon (10 percent).

Gastrointestinal lymphomas are a late complication of several diseases that affect the immune system. The gastrointestinal tract is often involved by AIDS-related lymphomas. Long-standing *malabsorption syndromes,* such as sprue, are also associated with an increased incidence of intestinal lymphoma. Lymphomas of the small intestine appear at an increased rate in the Middle East and are part of the so-called *immunoproliferative small intestinal disease*. It has been speculated that such lymphomas occur as a result of malignant transformation of lymphoid cells that are stimulated to proliferate by foreign antigens prevalent in that part of the world. In the United States, most gastrointestinal lymphomas are not related to any preexisting or environmental pathogenetic cause.

Diseases of the Small and Large Intestine

The most important diseases of the intestines are infections, idiopathic inflammations, vascular disturbances, obstructions of the lumen or changes in the wall of the intestine (e.g., diverticulosis), various forms of malabsorption, and tumors.

FIGURE 10-7
Gastric cancer. Tumors may present as superficial, polypoid, ulcerated, or diffuse carcinoma.

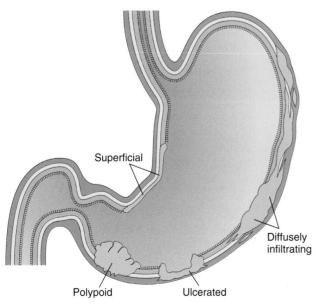

Developmental Abnormalities

In view of the length of the intestines, it is remarkable that developmental abnormalities do not occur more often; of those that do occur, only a few are clinically significant.

Atresia of the intestine—i.e., complete obstruction of the lumen—can occur in any part of the intestine. It can be surgically resected, with end-to-end anastomosis of uninvolved intestinal segments. *Atresia of the anus* prevents defecation, but also can be corrected surgically.

Hirschsprung's disease is an abnormality in the innervation of the rectum and the sigmoid colon. Because the intramural ganglion cells do not develop, the segment of the intestine lacking innervation remains in a permanent spasm. This spasm prevents the passage of feces that accumulate proximal to the obstructed segment, causing dilatation of the large intestine (*megacolon*). The aganglionic segment must be resected with an end-to-end anastomosis of the proximal and distal normal intestine. Such operations usually relieve all symptoms.

Congenital diverticula are outpouchings of the intestine. The best known of these is the *Meckel's diverticulum,* which represents an incompletely obliterated embryonic connection between the intestine and the umbilicus (*omphalomesenteric duct*). Like other diverticula, it may become filled with food and rupture, or it may become infected. Symptoms of Meckel's diverticulitis resemble those of acute appendicitis, except that the pain has its epicenter in the left lower quadrant (i.e., on the opposite side of appendicitis).

Diverticula

Diverticula are outpouchings of the intestinal wall. They may be solitary or multiple, congenital or acquired. Diverticula occur in all parts of the gastrointestinal tract, but from a clinical point of view, the most important are those involving the sigmoid colon.

Diverticula of the sigmoid colon are protrusions of the mucosa and submucosa through a hole in the weakened wall of the large intestine (Fig. 10-8). This usually occurs at the point where the arteries penetrate through the muscle wall from the subserosal space along the teniae coli. Diverticula typically occur in older persons, especially those with chronic constipation. The weakening of the intestinal wall at the point of arterial entry through the muscle layer, combined with increased intraluminal pressure generated by straining during defecation, contributes to evagination of the mucosa between the muscle fibers. Such outpouchings, which typically measure less than 1 cm in diameter, are easily obstructed with fecal material. Obstruction may cause bleeding or inflammation (*diverticulitis*).

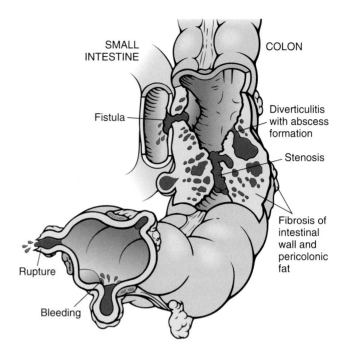

FIGURE 10-8
Diverticulosis of the colon. Complications include bleeding, abscess formation, perforation and rupture, fistula formation with adjacent structures (e.g., small intestine), and fibrosis extending into the pericolonic fat.

Perforation of diverticula may lead to the formation of pericolonic abscesses, fistulae, or pericolonic fibrosis, all of which are common complications of extensive diverticulitis. Massive pericolonic inflammation may encase the affected sigmoid colon and cause symptoms indistinguishable from those of carcinoma. Intestines that are severely deformed by diverticulitis may require surgical resection, which is often the only way to relieve intestinal obstruction.

Intestinal Vascular Diseases

Of the many vascular disorders of the intestine, only three prototypical diseases shall be discussed, exemplifying venous, arteriovenous, and arterial lesions. These include hemorrhoids, angiodysplasia, and ischemic bowel disease, respectively.

Hemorrhoids, or *piles,* are varicosities of the anal and perianal region that affect approximately 5 percent of all adults. Lesions of the lower hemorrhoidal plexus (i.e., below the anorectal line) are called *external,* whereas those above the line are termed *internal* hemorrhoids. The pathogenesis of hemorrhoids is complex. A congenital, hereditary predisposition may be based on the looseness of connective tissue. For example, hemorrhoids are more common in persons whose parent also had hemorrhoids. An association between hemorrhoids and varicose veins of the lower extremities and inguinal hernias has also been noted. The increased pressure in the hemorrhoidal plexus plays an important role. This may be related to constipation, and is often seen in pregnant women. Cirrhosis of the liver and other causes of portal hypertension also cause hemorrhoids because the veins of the hemorrhoidal plexus represent the site of anastomosis between the portal and the systemic circulation.

On gross examination, hemorrhoids appear as dilated veins, or nodules filled with blood and thrombi. The mucosa overlying the thrombosed hemorrhoids may ulcerate, and bleeding is common. Protruding hemorrhoids may become strangulated and infarcted. Surgical resection, previously the treatment of choice, is rarely done today because the lesions respond well to conservative medical therapy.

Angiodysplasia is a localized vascular lesion of the colon that may cause unexplained bleeding in the elderly. It consists of dilated, thin-walled blood vessels that serve as an anastomosis between the arterial and venous circulation in the mucosa and submucosa of the colon. The reasons for the formation of dilated vascular channels are not known, and it is also not known why they occur preferentially in the cecum and the ascending colon. Recurrent bleeding from foci of angiodysplasia may be difficult to control, and resection of the involved intestine may be the only way to stop it.

Ischemic bowel disease includes several disorders that compromise blood flow through segments of the intestine. Such ischemic changes may involve the entire thickness of the intestine and result in transmural infarction, or they may be limited to the mucosa.

Clinically, these disorders are classified as chronic or acute. *Chronic ischemia* secondary to atherosclerosis of intestinal arteries is very common,

but often remains undiagnosed because it usually produces only nonspecific, mild symptoms. *Acute obstruction* is less common, but is usually of sudden onset and associated with high mortality.

Pathologically, ischemic bowel disease can be classified as *occlusive* or *nonocclusive*. Occlusive disease is caused by thrombi or emboli, whereas nonocclusive disease is caused by atherosclerotic narrowing of arteries.

Thrombosis of the mesenteric arteries, usually a common complication of atherosclerosis, is the most important cause of transmural infarction. It typically affects the small intestine. The thrombus is most often found in the superior mesenteric artery. Under normal circumstances, occlusion of one artery is compensated for by collateral anastomoses from other arteries. However, if these are not able to compensate for the cessation of blood flow because they are extremely narrowed by atherosclerosis, a transmural infarction of the entire small intestine can occur. The intestinal loops appear bluish red and edematous. Histologically, the entire intestinal wall is necrotic and permeated with extravasated blood. This catastrophic event is accompanied by high mortality.

Mucosal ischemia is caused by hyperfusion of the intestines, attributable either to vascular narrowing or to central circulatory insufficiency. The narrowing of arteries is usually caused by atherosclerosis. Repeated episodes of hypotension secondary to heart failure can cause similar changes. These *"nonocclusive" intestinal infarcts* are typically multiple, limited to the mucosa and submucosa, and scattered through parts of the small or large intestine. Initially, they appear as small hemorrhagic patches that subsequently ulcerate and undergo fibrosis. *Ischemic colitis* or enteritis is common in the elderly, accounting, in part, for the intestinal problems affecting this population.

Inflammatory Bowel Disease

Inflammatory bowel disease (IBD) is a term used for two closely related but nevertheless distinct diseases: *Crohn's disease,* or regional enteritis, and *ulcerative colitis*. These diseases are characterized clinically by recurrent inflammation of the intestines and a chronic, unpredictable course. In the classical form, each of these diseases is easily distinguished from the other. However, in many cases, the symptoms and findings overlap, and in 20 percent of cases, it is not possible to tell them apart on the basis of clinical, radiologic, or pathologic findings. Ulcerative colitis is two or three times more common than Crohn's disease, with a prevalence of 70 to 150 per 100,000. Crohn's disease has a prevalence of 20 to 40 per 100,000 in Western countries.

Etiology and Pathogenesis. The etiology and pathogenesis of IBD are not known. It has been suggested that these diseases have a strong emotional basis and that they may have a genetic basis. The pathogenetic role of immune factors and bacteria, postulated by some authorities, has not been elucidated.

It is not known whether Crohn's disease and ulcerative colitis are distinct pathogenetic entities or only variants of a single disease that might take different forms under different conditions. Some authorities consider Crohn's disease and ulcerative colitis to be part of a spectrum, whereas others maintain that they are two distinct diseases.

In favor of a single pathogenetic entity are the following facts:

- Both diseases affect the same population; that is, they are more common among whites than blacks or Asians, and are especially common among Jews of East European origin. Both diseases have a peak incidence in the third decade (i.e., between 20 and 30 years of age).
- Both diseases show a familial predisposition. Actually, in some families, some members have typical Crohn's disease, whereas others have ulcerative colitis.
- Both diseases have the same extraintestinal complications.
- Both diseases have an immunologic component.
- Morphologic changes in the mucosa are often indistinguishable from one another, especially in the early stages of the disease.

Keeping in mind these similarities, we shall nevertheless try to differentiate between these two diseases, limiting our description to the classical manifestations of each.

Crohn's Disease

Crohn's disease is a chronic inflammation of the gastrointestinal tract that most often involves the terminal ileum and the colon. In about 50 percent of cases, the disease affects both the terminal ileum ("terminal ileitis") and colon; in 30 percent of cases, it is limited to the ileum; and in 20 percent of cases it is limited to the colon. The appendix is involved in most cases, and occasionally, Crohn's disease even may present clinically as acute appendicitis. In a small number of cases (1 percent to 2 percent), the disease involves the esophagus, stomach, or other abdominal organs, such as the fallopian tubes. Approximately one third of all patients also have extraintestinal inflammatory lesions in the joints, skin, liver, or eyes.

Pathology. The earliest pathologic changes in typical Crohn's disease involve the terminal ileum and are known under the name of *aphthous ulcers* (an oxymoronic term because *aphthous* means ulcerative in Greek). These shallow mucosal defects typically overlie the lymphoid aggregates forming the Peyer's patches, which suggests that immune cells may be involved in their pathogenesis. The inflammation does not remain limited to the mucosa, but extends through the entire wall of the intestine (*transmural inflammation*). This is often associated with the formation of granulomas (50 percent of cases). Chronic inflammation is also associated with fibrosis of the muscularis and serosa. The wall of the intestine is thickened and rigid (Fig. 10-9). The mucosa has a cobblestone appearance in which the fibrotic defects appear as "seams" surrounding the remaining patches of mucosa ("the cobbles"). The fibrotic intestine may be narrowed (*intestinal strictures*). The inflammation of the serosa leads to adhesions with adjacent intestinal loops and the formation of *fistulas*.

FIGURE 10-9

Crohn's disease. (A) A thickened intestinal wall and a narrowed lumen are shown. (B) The mucosa has a cobblestone-like appearance.

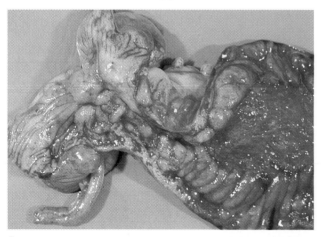

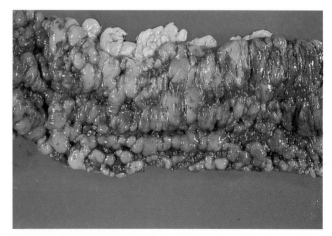

A

B

Anal involvement is often associated with formation of *fissures.*

Clinical Features. The clinical presentation of Crohn's disease is variable. The initial symptoms are often so nonspecific that the diagnosis may be delayed by several months. The most common symptoms are diarrhea, abdominal pain, and weight loss. Bleeding is more common with rectal involvement. Fever occurs in one third of patients. In later stages of the disease, there might be constipation because of intestinal narrowing, fistulas, and adhesions. Weight loss, vitamin deficiency, and anemia secondary to malabsorption are common in the chronic stages of the disease. The most common extra-abdominal manifestations, found in one third of patients, are arthritis, skin lesions, liver disease, and eye lesions. The diagnosis is established by colonoscopy, x-ray studies, and mucosal biopsy. Crohn's disease has a chronic course. Cases that are resistant to medical therapy require surgical treatment, which includes resection of the involved intestine.

Ulcerative Colitis

Ulcerative colitis is an intestinal inflammation of unknown etiology that most often involves the large intestine. The rectum is invariably affected. From initial rectal lesions, the inflammation spreads proximally, ultimately involving the entire colon. In contrast to Crohn's disease of the colon, which is typically segmental, ulcerative colitis is a diffuse disease. Furthermore, it does not extend into the ileum, although 10 percent of patients will show mild inflammation in the terminal ileum, called *backwash ileitis.* The appendix, however, is involved in about 30 percent of patients.

Pathology. Ulcerative colitis is a disease principally limited to colonic mucosa. The earliest lesions seen by rectoscopy appear like flattened edematous patches involving the entire circumference of the rectum. Clinicians observing the intestine through the endoscope describe the mucosa as "sandpapered," and prone to bleeding, especially if wiped gently. This fragile mucosa appears edematous and inflamed on histologic examination. These changes are nonspecific, though, and the diagnosis is not easily made. As the disease progresses, the mucosal lesions become more prominent. On rectoscopy, the mucosa appears flattened and pitted, like pig skin or a football. Histologically, such mucosa shows atrophy of crypts and aggregates of leukocytes in the bases of the crypts (*crypt abscesses*). Ulcerations begin appearing in the colon proximal to the initial rectal lesions, which themselves rarely ulcerate in early stages of the disease. The ulcerated mucosa bleeds easily and is often infected. Colonic ulcerations spread through the entire colon and become confluent (*serpiginous ulcerations*), leaving behind only small remnants of mucosa (Fig. 10-10). The remnants of inflamed mucosa that have not been destroyed appear to be elevated over the base of the surrounding ulcerations and are *inflammatory polyps.* Pseudopolyps would be a more appropriate term because they are not tumors, but consist of residual, heavily inflamed mucosa. Some polyps represent foci of mucosal regeneration. Regeneratory foci of epithelium may undergo malignant transformation, which is the most significant late complication of ulcerative colitis.

Clinical Features. Ulcerative colitis usually begins with mild symptoms that evolve into bouts of diarrhea, rectal bleeding, and pain. In 70 percent of all

FIGURE 10-10

Ulcerative colitis. There is diffuse involvement of the intestine, but the colon shows marked ulceration and pseudopolyposis, which account for the irregularity of the internal intestinal surface.

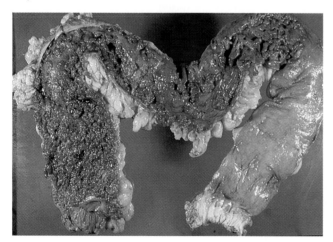

A

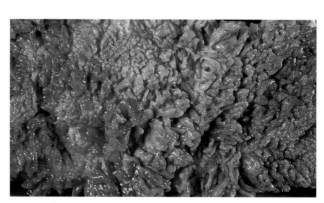

B

patients, the disease has a chronic course, with alternating periods of recrudescence and asymptomatic intervals. In about 10 percent of cases, the disease has only a single episode and heals spontaneously. In about 20 percent of cases, the disease has a fulminant course and is resistant to medical treatment. These patients often require surgical treatment, and only colectomy—resection of the entire large intestine—is life-saving.

The diagnosis of ulcerative colitis is based on clinical, radiographic, and pathologic data. Several criteria are useful for distinguishing ulcerative colitis from Crohn's disease (Table 10-2). Ulcerative colitis predominantly affects the left side of the colon, whereas Crohn's disease tends to involve the right side of the colon and the ileum. The patterns of involvement also differ: the lesions of ulcerative colitis are diffuse, whereas Crohn's disease presents with numerous skip areas. Ulcerative colitis is limited to the mucosa, whereas Crohn's disease is transmural. Granulomas are diagnostic of Crohn's disease, but unfortunately, they occur only in 50 percent of cases. Mucosal ulcers in ulcerative colitis are wide, leaving few small patches of uninvolved mucosa that protrude as inflammatory polyps; by contrast, in Crohn's disease, the ulcers are linear and resemble cobblestones. The broad ulcers of ulcerative colitis tend to bleed more.

Table 10-2 Features of Crohn's Disease and Ulcerative Colitis

	Crohn's Disease	Ulcerative Colitis
Clinical Features		
Familial predisposition	+ +	+ +
Jewish ancestry	+ +	+ +
Peak age (years)	15–25	15–25
Immune disturbances	+	+
Extraintestinal complications	+	+
Treatment efficacy	+	+
Pathology		
Diffuse (colon)	0	+ +
Segmental		
Colon	+ +	0
Ileum	+ +	0
Transmural inflammation	+ +	0
Granuloma	+ + (50%)	0
Fistulas, fissures	+	0
Megacolon	–	+
Cancer	+	+ +

The transmural inflammation of Crohn's disease contributes to thickening of the intestinal wall and peri-intestinal fibrosis, as well as formation of adhesions and fistulas. The thinner wall of the colon in ulcerative colitis predisposes the patient to intestinal dilatation and "megacolon." *Toxic megacolon,* a sudden dilatation of the large intestine, is a dangerous complication of ulcerative colitis; it occurs only exceptionally in Crohn's disease. Anal lesions are found in 80 percent of patients with Crohn's disease, but only 20 percent of patients with ulcerative colitis. The extraintestinal complications of ulcerative colitis are identical to those of Crohn's disease and are, therefore, not useful in the differential diagnosis of these two diseases.

Gastrointestinal Infections

The gastrointestinal system contains in its lumen saprophytic bacteria which live in equilibrium with the host. Diseases may develop under the following conditions:

- When the balance between the host and the intestinal flora has been lost and the ecosystem has been perturbed. The best example of this is *pseudomembranous colitis,* caused by an overgrowth of *C. difficile* in the colon of patients treated with broad-spectrum antibiotics.
- When new pathogens have been introduced into the system. This is typical of several *diarrheal diseases* caused by viruses (*rotavirus infection*), bacteria (*cholera*), or protozoa (*amebiasis*).

Gastrointestinal infections are very common and vary from mild "stomach upset" to severe "food poisoning" and debilitating diarrhea. For practical purposes, it is useful to consider diarrheal disease as either small intestinal or colonic (Table 10-3). It would be almost impossible to cover all the gastrointestinal infections systematically. Instead, only a few of the more common ones, along with their underlying pathology, will be discussed.

Bacterial Diarrhea

Bacterial diarrhea may be caused, as illustrated in Fig. 10-11, by the following:

- *Bacterial toxins.* These may be ingested preformed in food, as in food poisoning, or released by bacteria growing inside the intestine.
- *Lytic action of bacteria.* This follows colonization of the intestines by bacteria that have the capacity to invade the intestine and destroy tissue.

Preformed bacterial toxins account for typical *food poisoning.* This occurs following ingestion of food contaminated with *Staphylococcus aureus* or *Escherichia coli.* For example, food poisoning occurs fol-

Table 10-3 Comparison of Diarrhea in Small Intestinal and Large Intestinal Diseases

	Pathologic Lesions/Involvement	
	Small Intestine	Large Intestine
Cause		
Bacteria	*Escherichia coli* *Vibrio cholerae*	*Escherichia coli; Shigella sp.*
Viruses	Rotavirus	Norwalk virus
Parasites	*Giardia lamblia*	*Entamoeba histolytica*
Stool Characteristics		
Volume	Large	Small
Appearance	Watery	Mucoid
Blood	Rare	Common
Leukocytes	—	+/−, +, or ++
Proctoscopic findings		
	—	+ (ulcers, hemorrhage)

lowing ingestion of unrefrigerated leftovers or "spoiled" fish. A rare but highly lethal food poisoning is *botulism* caused by the ingestion of canned food contaminated with *C. botulinum.*

Enterotoxigenic bacteria produce enterocolitis by colonizing the intestinal lumen. This is typical of so-called "traveler's" diarrhea, which is most often caused by enterotoxigenic strains of *E. coli* consumed in contaminated food or water. Tourists in Mexico call it "Montezuma's revenge." *V. cholerae* is another enterotoxigenic bacterium that causes epidemic diarrheal disease in parts of Asia.

Invasive bacteria, such as Shigella and Salmonella, produce intestinal ulcerations that are often associated with bleeding, mucopurulent inflammation, and even intestinal perforation. Such bacteria may enter the blood or lymphatics and may cause a systemic infection ("typhoid fever").

Pseudomembranous Colitis

Pseudomembranous colitis is an acute infectious disease marked by the formation of pseudomembranes on the surface of the intestinal mucosa. It predominantly involves the colon. In more than 90 percent of cases, it is caused by *C. difficile.* Clostridial overgrowth usually follows broad-spectrum antibiotic therapy, which wipes out the normal intestinal flora, allowing pathogens to expand over the intestinal mucosa. Other toxigenic bacteria, such as Staphylococcus and Shigella, are less common causes. In a small number of cases, pseudomembranous colitis is not related to antibiotic therapy but to some other predis-

posing cause, such as vascular insufficiency, debilitating diseases of the elderly, or abdominal surgery.

In typical cases, pseudomembranous colitis is a complication of antibiotic treatment. Broad-spectrum antibiotics, such as clindamycin, eradicate the normal bacterial flora and allow the intestine to be overgrown with *C. difficile.* The exotoxin produced by *C. difficile* acts on epithelial cells of the intestine, causing foci of necrosis and superficial ulcers. These ulcers are covered with a layer consisting of exudated fibrin, inflammatory cells, remnants of destroyed cells, and mucin (see Fig. 10-13). The pseudomembranes adhere firmly to the mucosa but can also be shed, leaving behind bleeding mucosal ulcerations.

Pseudomembranous colitis presents as an acute diarrhea that may contain blood. The diagnosis may be made on the basis of a history of recent broad-spectrum antibiotic treatment. Rectoscopy is indicated only in less obvious cases. Biochemical tests for *C. difficile* toxin in bloody feces are useful in questionable cases. Eradication of *C. difficile* with antibiotics, such as vancomycin, yields good results, except in debilitated patients and those with persistent extraintestinal problems.

Viral Gastroenteritis

Viral infections of the gastrointestinal tract occur more often than one would assume from health statistics, because most of these infections are unreported. The gastrointestinal disease is usually mild, and the pathogens are rarely isolated. The most frequently documented causative agents are rotavirus and Norwalk virus.

Rotavirus is a common cause of viral gastroenteritis in infants and children. In those younger than 2 years of age, it is responsible for a least 50 percent of acute diarrheal diseases in this country. *Norwalk viruses* are common causes of acute viral gastroenteritis in adults. The disease tends to occur in small epidemics. These viral infections produce minimal tissue damage and heal without consequences.

Protozoal Enteritis

Giardia lamblia is a noninvasive protozoan that infests the small intestine. The infection is typically acquired by swallowing the cysts in contaminated food or water. It presents as diarrhea or malabsorption secondary to heavy colonization of the duodenum and the proximal small bowel.

Amebiasis is an infection with *Entamoeba histolytica.* This protozoan is widespread in the tropics. Most infected persons are asymptomatic, and the clinical disease occurs only under exceptional circumstances, which are not fully understood. Tourists traveling to southern countries are probably at greater risk than natives. Amoebas invade the colonic mucosa and form "flask-shaped" ulcers extending into the submu-

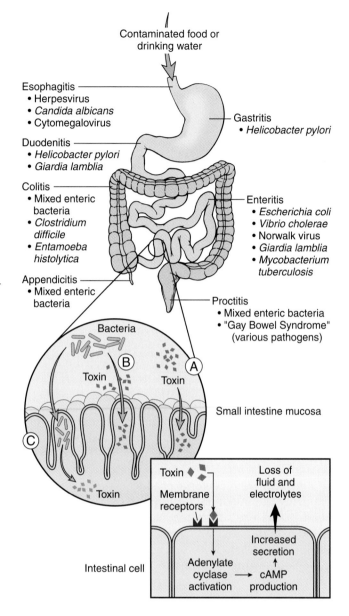

FIGURE 10-11

Bacterial diarrhea may be caused by an ingested toxin (A), toxins formed by bacteria colonizing the intestine (B), or bacteria that invade the wall of the intestine (C). Cyclic adenosine monophosphate (cAMP) is essential for transduction of toxic signals that lead to watery diarrhea.

cosa. Ulcers are surrounded by normal, uninvolved mucosa. Because of histolytic properties, amoebas can penetrate into even deeper layers of the intestine and cause pericolonic abscesses, or they can invade vessels and spread to the liver, where they produce metastatic abscesses. Amebiasis responds well to chemotherapy.

Acute Appendicitis

Bacterial infection of the appendix is one of the most common acute intestinal infections, and the only one that requires prompt surgical intervention. It may occur at any age, but is most common in children and adolescents.

Acute appendicitis is usually caused by enterogenic bacteria of the normal intestinal flora that become pathogenic following an obstruction of the lumen of the appendix. This may be caused by a hardened piece of feces, a worm, or enlarged lymph nodes or intramural lymphoid tissue of the appendix. The bacteria trapped inside the appendix multiply and reach a critical number, at which time they become noxious, causing ulceration and invading the wall of

Did You Know?

Patients suffering from AIDS often have symptoms pertaining to the gastrointestinal tract, and all parts of the gastrointestinal tract may be involved. Such diseases may be caused by viruses, bacteria or fungi, or protozoa. Some infections, such as enteritis and intestinal malabsorption caused by *Mycobacterium avium intracellulare*, are found almost exclusively in AIDS patients.

the appendix. This usually evokes a purulent inflammation (Fig. 10-12). The swollen and inflamed appendix may necrotize (*gangrenous appendicitis*), or rupture and cause *peritonitis*. This may be diffuse or localized to the right lower quadrant. The inflammation may become encapsulated, leading to an accumulation of pus around the appendix (*perityphlitic abscess*).

Acute appendicitis is marked by sudden fever, leukocytosis, and abdominal pain. The pain is typically strongest in the lower abdominal quadrant (*McBurney's point*) but may be referred to the umbilical area. Tenderness and rebound pain on palpation may be found in patients who have already developed localized peritonitis. Appendectomy in the hands of an experienced (or even not so experienced) surgeon is the treatment of choice, and should be performed in a timely fashion to prevent gangrene and potentially serious complications of rupture, such as purulent peritonitis.

Peritonitis

Acute **peritonitis,** an inflammation of the peritoneal lining of the abdominal cavity, can be localized or diffuse. It is usually caused by bacteria, most of which are of enteric origin. Chronic tuberculous peritonitis was common previously, but is rare today.

Etiology and Pathogenesis. Peritonitis is classified as *infectious* or *sterile*. Infectious peritonitis is caused by bacterial invasion of the abdominal cavity. This is usually secondary to

- rupture of the stomach (e.g., peptic ulcer) or intestines (e.g., acute appendicitis)
- spread of infection from the fallopian tubes (e.g., gonococcal salpingitis)
- rupture of an abscess (e.g., subphrenic abscess)
- infection of preexisting ascites (e.g., in alcoholic cirrhosis)

Sterile peritonitis is mediated by chemical irritation. This occurs in

- acute pancreatitis, due to a spill of pancreatic enzymes
- rupture of the gallbladder secondary to entry of bile into the peritoneum
- postsurgical peritonitis caused by talc or chemicals used during operation

Pathology. In acute peritonitis, the serosal surface of the intestines and the parietal peritoneum are congested and edematous. This is associated with exudation of fluid into the abdominal cavity. The fluid may be cloudy or markedly purulent and thick yellow-green. In acute pancreatitis, the fluid is typically brownish yellow owing to hemorrhage and enzy-

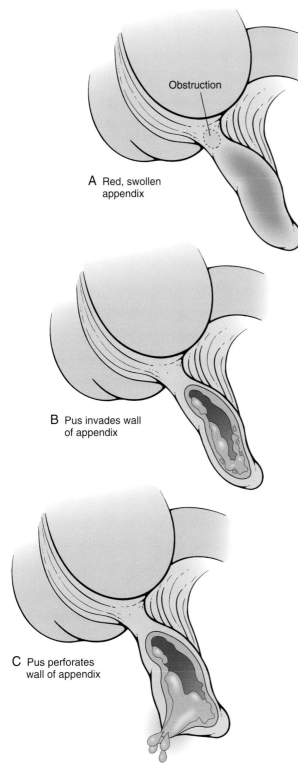

FIGURE 10-12
Acute appendicitis. (A) The disease is caused by an obstruction of the appendix. (B) The trapped bacteria invade the wall of the intestine, causing transmural inflammation. (C) Rupture of the appendix leads to localized or diffuse peritonitis.

A   Red, swollen appendix

B   Pus invades wall of appendix

C   Pus perforates wall of appendix

Obstruction

Table 10-4 Causes of Intestinal Obstruction

Paralytic ileus

Mechanical ileus
   Atresia
   Stenosis

Strictures

Intussusception

Volvulus

Hernia

Adhesions

Neoplasms

matic tissue digestion. In biliary peritonitis, the fluid may be greenish from biliverdin.

Histologically, acute peritonitis is characterized by inflammatory exudates containing polymorphonuclear leukocytes and fibrin. Prolonged inflammation is marked by granulation tissue extending into the fibrinopurulent inflammatory exudate. The healing of acute inflammation results in fibrous adhesions between the intestines, which may cause obstruction (ileus).

Clinical Features. Symptoms of acute peritonitis are typical and include sharp abdominal pain, rebound tenderness, and voluntary guarding of the abdominal muscles. Intestinal peristalsis slows down until the intestines become paralyzed. Treatment of peritonitis usually requires surgical exploration to remove pus and to repair the site of rupture. All forms of peritonitis still have a high mortality.

Intestinal Obstruction

Intestinal obstruction, also called **ileus** (from the Greek *eilo,* meaning to roll up), may be of two basic types: adynamic and obstructive. Various causes of intestinal obstruction are listed in Table 10-4.

Adynamic or *paralytic ileus* results from neuromuscular paralysis, usually related to inflammation or the disruption of innervation. Thus, paralytic ileus is a common feature of acute peritonitis and spinal cord injury.

Obstructive ileus may be caused by intraluminal material (e.g., gallstones, fecaliths, or inspissated meconium in children with cystic fibrosis) or abdominal adhesions secondary to peritonitis. Ileus may also be caused by hernia, intussusception, or volvulus (Fig. 10-13).

A *hernia* is a protrusion of the abdominal contents through the abdominal wall. Pathogenetically,

hernias relate to a weakness or a defect in the abdominal wall. The best known are

- *inguinal hernia,* which protrudes through the inguinal canal and extends into the subcutaneous tissue or into the scrotum
- *femoral hernia,* which occurs through the femoral canal in the groin
- *periumbilical hernia,* which protrudes through the anterior abdominal wall, around the umbilicus
- *diaphragmatic (hiatal) hernia,* which occurs through the hiatus of the diaphragm and extends into the thoracic cavity

FIGURE 10-13
Intestinal obstructions. (A) Hernia. (B) Intussusception. (C) Volvulus.

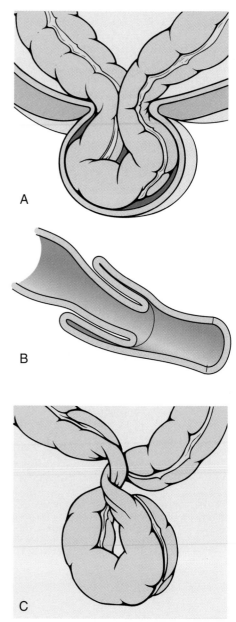

Inguinal hernia is the most common of these. The intestinal contents are easily repositioned surgically and the abdominal wall defect is repaired. However, an untreated hernia may lead to the formation of adhesions between the hernia sac contents and the pouch in which they are located, with subsequent *incarceration*. The neck of the hernia may compromise blood flow, causing strangulation and gangrene of the intestinal loop.

Intussusception is an invagination of one segment of the intestine into another. The blood flow to the invaginated segment may be compromised because of constriction by the outside segment, and this could lead to necrosis. In children, intussusception is usually caused by hyperactive peristalsis or enlarged lymphoid tissue in the wall of the intestine that is propulsed into the loop distal to it. In adults, the leading margin of the intussuscepted intestine usually contains a tumor. Obstruction caused by intussusception can be repaired by repositioning the intestinal loops. If the inside loop is necrotic, it may need to be resected, followed by an end-to-end anastomosis of viable intestinal segments.

Volvulus is a rotation of the intestine around its mesenteric attachment site. This leads to twisting of the arteries and veins and an infarction of the rotated intestinal loop. Most often, volvulus involves the loops of the small intestine or the sigmoid colon.

Malabsorption

Malabsorption, or the inability of the intestines to absorb nutrients from food, results from abnormalities involving

- intraluminal digestion of the food
- uptake and processing of nutrients within the intestinal cells
- transport of the nutrients from the intestine to the liver

Malabsorption is usually caused by more than one mechanism (Fig. 10-14). For the sake of simplicity, we shall classify malabsorptions on the basis of the predominant pathogenetic mechanism (Table 10-5).

The *intraluminal digestion* of food depends upon the proper secretion of digestive juices, most notably gastric and pancreatic juice and bile. It may be disturbed in many conditions. Atrophic gastritis from resection of the stomach will reduce the gastric production of hydrochloric acid and pepsin. Chronic pancreatitis or cystic fibrosis of the pancreas reduces the output of pancreatic enzymes and bicarbonate. Lack of lipase affects the absorption of lipids, and the lack of peptidases, such as trypsin and chymotrypsin, affects the absorption of proteins. Reduced bile flow from the liver because of obstructive jaundice also impairs absorption of lipids. In patients with Crohn's disease, or in those undergoing small bowel resection, the normal enterohepatic circulation is interrupted, also interfering with lipid absorption.

The *uptake of nutrients* and their further processing inside the intestinal epithelial cells is markedly affected in primary intestinal diseases. The best examples are celiac sprue and Crohn's disease. Another example is congenital abetalipoproteinemia, a deficiency of betalipoprotein synthesis that prevents the passage of lipids from the intestinal cells into the circulation. Such patients cannot form chylomicrons and, therefore, cannot prepare the absorbed intestinal lipids for transport to the liver.

The *transport of nutrients* from the intestine to the liver may be obstructed in the intestinal wall. This occurs, for example, in gastrointestinal lymphoma that infiltrates the intestinal wall and prevents its normal function. Congestive heart failure and intestinal ischemia could adversely affect the portal circulation, thus impeding the transport of nutrients from the intestine.

Pathology. Pathologically, it is possible to divide the malabsorption syndrome into three major groups:

- Those that have characteristic pathologic findings involving the intestine, including diseases of unknown origin, such as celiac sprue or Crohn's disease; congenital metabolic defects, such as abetalipoproteinemia; infection with bacteria or protozoa, such as *G. lamblia, Cryptosporidium parvum;* and tumors, such as lymphoma.
- Those that have nonspecific pathologic findings involving the intestine, including a variety of systemic diseases, such as atherosclerosis, diabetes, scleroderma, radiation enteritis, and others.
- Those that have no pathologic findings involving the intestines; these functional disorders could be caused by intestinal bacterial overgrowth, oversecretion of hormones that alter intestinal motility (e.g., vasoactive intestinal polypeptide [VIP]), or pancreatic insufficiency.

Celiac Sprue. Celiac sprue, also known as gluten-sensitive enteropathy, is an intestinal disease characterized by hypersensitivity to gliadin in dietary grains. Gliadin, or its breakdown products, may be directly toxic to the intestine, or it may act as an allergen. Symptoms appear in early childhood, after the child is exposed to cereals. There is a familial clustering of cases that suggests a genetic predisposition, but the inheritance pattern seems to be complex. The diagnosis is based on a perceived sensitivity to grains in the diet. Symptoms can thus be

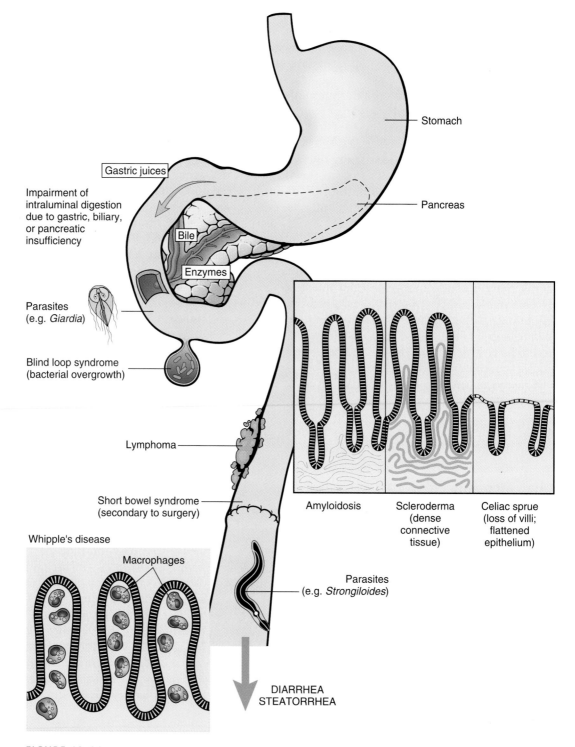

FIGURE 10-14

Pathophysiology of malabsorption. Intraluminal digestion may be impaired owing to a gastric, biliary, or pancreatic insufficiency or bacterial overgrowth and parasites. Uptake of the nutrients in the intestine may be affected by intestinal diseases, such as celiac sprue or Whipple's disease, or systemic diseases, such as scleroderma and amyloidosis. Partial resection of the intestine also causes malabsorption. Transport of nutrients from the intestine may be affected by gastrointestinal lymphoma.

Table 10-5 Causes of Malabsorption Syndromes

Inadequate Intraluminal Digestion
Exocrine pancreatic insufficiency
Chronic pancreatitis
Cystic fibrosis
Reduced intestinal bile salt concentration or impaired micelle formation
Liver disease
Cholestasis (intrahepatic or extrahepatic)
Abnormal bacterial proliferation in the small bowel (blind loop syndrome)
Postgastrectomy states
Primary Mucosal Absorptive Defects
Celiac sprue
Enteritis
Abetalipoproteinemia
Intestinal resection
Endocrine and metabolic disorders
Impeded Transport of Nutrients
Lymphatic obstruction (e.g., lymphoma)
Congestive heart disease
Intestinal ischemia

induced by a diet containing grain, and they disappear upon removal of grains from the food.

Small intestinal biopsy is useful in diagnosis because it shows typical changes. These include mucosal atrophy with flattening of villi. There is also marked inflammation of the mucosa, which is infiltrated with IgA-containing plasma cells and lymphocytes. Following withdrawal of gliadin from the diet, the mucosa returns to normal. Follow-up of patients is important because of the risk of lymphoma, which develops in 10 percent to 15 percent of patients.

Tropical Sprue. Tropical sprue is caused by bacteria that typically affect visitors to the tropics. More than one pathogen has been implicated. Morphologic changes in the intestine may be indistinguishable from those in celiac sprue, but are often milder. In contrast to celiac sprue, which affects the proximal intestine more than the distal intestine, tropical sprue is more pronounced distally. Furthermore, it responds favorably to broad-spectrum antibiotic treatment, which presumably eradicates the offending pathogens. Because tropical sprue is not caused by hypersensitivity to gliadin, there is no need to restrict the intake of cereals in these patients.

Whipple's Disease. *Whipple's disease* is malabsorption caused by *Trophyrema whippelii,* a bacterium that invades the small intestinal mucosa. The disease affects predominantly middle-aged males and shows typical familial clustering. Small intestinal biopsy is diagnostic. It shows accumulation of bacteria-laden macrophages in the lamina propria mucosae. The bacteria can be seen by electron microscopy. Treatment with antibiotics cures the malabsorption.

Clinical Features of Malabsorption Syndromes. All malabsorption syndromes are characterized by a deficiency of nutrients that evolves over variable periods of time. The most prominent are deficiencies of protein and lipids. Protein deficiency results in anemia. This may be accentuated owing to abnormal iron absorption, which occurs concomitantly in small intestinal diseases. Hypoalbuminemia may be severe enough to cause edema. In the most severe cases, there might even be growth retardation in children and weight loss in adults. Amenorrhea, impotence, and general muscle weakness may also be present. Malabsorption of fat results in bulky, fatty stools (*steatorrhea;* from the Greek *steatos,* meaning fatty, and *rheo,* meaning to flow) and deficiency of fat-soluble vitamins A, D, K, and E. Owing to small stores of vitamin K, *bleeding disorders* caused by vitamin K deficiency appear the earliest. Vitamin D deficiency results in metabolic bone disorders (*osteomalacia*) and hypocalcemia, which is also caused, in part, by reduced intestinal uptake of calcium.

Intestinal Neoplasms

Neoplasms of the intestines are important causes of morbidity and mortality in the United States and the entire Western world. These tumors are less common in underdeveloped countries and the Far East. The significance of intestinal tumors can be illustrated by the following statistical data:

- Cancer of the intestines is one of the three most common malignant diseases, exceeded in incidence only by lung tumors in men and lung and breast tumors in women.
- Approximately 190,000 new cases of intestinal cancer are diagnosed yearly in the United States.
- Benign intestinal tumors outnumber malignant tumors twofold to threefold. Because the benign tumors may progress to cancer, they must be removed as soon as detected. Early diagnosis and regular surveillance of persons at risk are the only currently available means of combating colon cancer.

Two additional facts are worth remembering about intestinal neoplasia:

- In more than 95 percent of the cases of epithelial origin, the tumors protrude into the lumen of the intestine and can be seen by endoscopy or on x-ray examination with barium enema. Even more importantly, tumors of the rectum can be detected by anal digital palpation. This procedure should be performed during routine physical examination, as it is an important way of diagnosing these tumors. The intraluminal location of intestinal tumors makes them vulnerable to mechanical trauma by the intestinal contents, and accounts for the frequent bleeding that is a common presenting sign of these tumors. Surveillance for blood in the stools is an effective approach to early diagnosis of intestinal cancer.

- Most tumors are located in the large intestine; indeed, the small intestine is involved in only 1 percent of all cases of gastrointestinal cancer. Even more important to remember is the fact that more than one third of all tumors involve the rectum, and can be detected by digital examination.

Etiology and Pathogenesis. Any discussion of etiology and pathogenesis of intestinal tumors must take into consideration two important sets of potential carcinogenic influences: genetic factors and nutritional factors.

Genetic factors play an important role in the pathogenesis of intestinal tumors. It has been estimated that at least 20 percent of all intestinal cancers have a genetic basis. This is most evident in families with *polyposis syndromes,* such as *familial adenomatous polyposis* (FAP) or *Gardner's syndrome.* In these rare autosomal dominant diseases, the colon shows multiple adenomas which predictably evolve into adenocarcinomas. More common are the families with *hereditary nonpolyposis colorectal cancer* (HNPCC), which accounts for about 5 percent of all colorectal cancers. In these patients, colonic cancers do not evolve from preexisting polyps but rather from apparently normal mucosa. In some families with HNPCC, colon carcinoma occurs in association with carcinoma of the ovary, uterus, and pancreas. This association, called *Lynch syndrome I,* suggests that these patients harbor some oncogenes or lack tumor suppressor genes, and that their genetic predisposition to cancer is not limited to the intestine.

Dietary factors are considered to be important in the pathogenesis of intestinal cancer. All aspects of dietary carcinogenesis are not fully understood, but there is enough circumstantial evidence to incriminate several key aspects of the typical Western diet as major causes. What one eats is as important as what one does not eat. A typical Western diet—rich in red meat, fat, and refined carbohydrates and low in vegetable fibers—is considered to be most damaging. It is not known why red meat consumption carries this high risk. Fat presumably can be degraded to potential carcinogens during food processing or during intestinal digestion. Red meat that is barbecued on a charcoal grill apparently contains more carcinogens than white meat cooked in the same manner. Fried fat is presumably degraded to potential carcinogens, which act on intestinal epithelial cells. Fat in the food also stimulates the release of bile, which is a potential source of intestinal carcinogens, presumably derived from degraded bile acids.

Foods that are rich in refined carbohydrates and low in vegetable fibers produce low-volume waste. Because colonic peristalsis depends on the volume of feces in the lumen, the transit time of the feces in the large intestine is prolonged. This allows for longer contact between the potential carcinogens in the intestinal contents and the intestinal mucosal cells. In favor of this explanation, there are several observations and a vast volume of epidemiologic research. The fact that the food passes through the small intestine much faster than the large intestine probably accounts in part for the 50 times lower incidence of tumors in the jejunum and ileum than in the colon and rectum. It is also worth noting that the rectosigmoid area—the site where feces are retained the longest—is the most common site of intestinal cancer.

Intestinal tumors develop from epithelial cells lining the crypts and villi. It has been proposed that the epithelial cells undergo malignant transformation through the action of oncogenes or because of a loss of tumor suppressor genes. The most attractive hypothesis actually combines these two pathogenetic mechanisms, suggesting that the tumors evolve through several sequential events. Accordingly, a loss of the tumor suppressor gene on chromosome 5, or hypomethylation of the tumor suppressor gene DNA in this area could deregulate the normal proliferation–maturation sequence of the epithelial cells. Normally, these cells multiply in the intestinal crypts and then migrate toward the tip of the villi until they are shed at the end of their life span. Mitoses are limited to the crypts. In neoplastic mucosa, the cell divisions may be seen not only in the crypts but also in higher zones of the epithelium. At the same time, programmed cell death (*apoptosis*) does not occur. All this results in an irregular accumulation of cells that form benign adenomas. Initially, the lesions are flat, but as they evolve, the tumors begin to protrude into the lumen of the intestine as villous or tubular polyps. These *polyps* (in Greek, literally meaning "with many feet" because of their attachment to the mucosa) are benign tumors. A "second hit" must occur to transform the polyp into a malignant tumor. This could involve activation of an oncogene, such as *ras,* or deletion and/or inactivation of a tumor suppressor gene. Most current evidence implicates the tumor *suppressor gene p53* as the crucial factor in colonic neoplasia.

Molecular biologists have discovered several genetic changes that apparently occur during the transformation of polyps into carcinoma. These have been most extensively studied in patients with FAP, who develop cancer in a predictable manner. Such tumors develop as a consequence of a germ line mutation involving the so-called *adenomatous polyposis coli* (APC) gene mapped to the long arm of chromosome 5. The polyps appear early in life, and by the time the patient is 20 years of age, some of them already contain malignant cells. This probably occurs as a result of a "second hit," which is not well defined and could involve oncogenes, tumor suppressor genes, or chemical carcinogens. It is not known whether nonfamilial colon cancer evolves in a similar polyp-to-cancer sequence, but one can assume that there is a common pattern of development of malignant disease in both familial and nonfamilial cases.

Pathology. Tumors of the intestine can be subdivided into three groups: non-neoplastic polyps, benign neoplasms, and malignant neoplasms (Table 10-6).

Non-Neoplastic Polyps. This group of lesions includes hyperplastic, hamartomatous, and inflammatory or lymphoid polyps.

Hyperplastic polyps are the most common non-neoplastic polyps. These innocuous, benign lesions are usually discovered accidentally during endoscopy or at autopsy. More than 80 percent are located in the rectosigmoid area. On gross examination, they appear as dew droplet–like protrusions on the mucosa and measure less than 5 mm in diameter. They are often multiple, but may be solitary as well. Histologically, the polyps are composed of hyperplastic glands made up of well-differentiated absorptive and mucin-rich goblet cells surrounded by stroma. Hyperplastic polyps are considered to be "cosmetic defects" or "minor imperfections" that do not progress to true neoplasia.

Juvenile polyps are hamartomas; that is, they are developmental abnormalities in which the normal components of the tissue aggregate in an abnormal manner. As one might expect, most of them are found in children younger than 5 years of age. Most are solitary, with diameters of 1 to 3 cm, and are located in the rectum. These lobulated sessile lesions are composed histologically of glands lined by normal epithelium and a well-developed stroma. The glands tend to dilate cystically because of the obstructed flow of mucus—hence, the name *retention polyps*. These polyps are often inflamed and ulcerated, giving rise to symptoms, such as rectal irritation and bleeding. Juvenile polyps have no malignant potential.

Peutz-Jeghers polyps are also hamartomatous. These histologically distinct polyps may occur in any part of the intestine and are often multiple. These polyps are part of an autosomal dominant hereditary disease, which also includes melanotic pigmentation around the mouth, genitals, and palmar surface of the hand. The polyps are not preneoplastic. However, Peutz-Jeghers syndrome predisposes individuals to malignant disease in general; thus, some patients may even develop colon cancer, albeit unrelated to preexisting polyps.

Inflammatory polyps, also known as pseudopolyps, are encountered in inflammatory bowel disease, especially ulcerative colitis. They represent multiple fragments of normal or regenerating mucosa surrounded by broad ulcers. Inflammatory polyps consist, on histologic examination, of colonic glands and granulation tissue.

Lymphoid polyps are small mucosal protrusions composed of hyperplastic lymphoid tissue arranged into follicles. These polyps also do not have any malignant potential.

Neoplastic Polyps. In contrast to non-neoplastic polyps, which are composed of normal glandular and stromal cells, neoplastic polyps are composed of neoplastic epithelium that shows no evidence of normal differentiation. On the basis of gross and microscopic features, the neoplastic polyps are classified as tubular, villous, and tubulovillous adenomas (Fig. 10-15). Although distinct from one another, these polyps are best considered as premalignant because all of them can progress to adenocarcinomas. For tubular adenomas, this risk is around 20 percent; for tubulovillous adenomas and villous adenomas, it is between 20

Table 10-6 Classification of Intestinal Tumors

Non-Neoplastic Polyps
Hyperplastic polyp
Inflammatory polyp
Juvenile polyp
Peutz-Jeghers polyp
Lymphoid polyp
Benign Neoplasm
Tubular adenoma
Villous adenoma
Tubulovillous adenoma
Malignant Neoplasms
Adenocarcinoma
Carcinoid
Lymphoma
Sarcoma

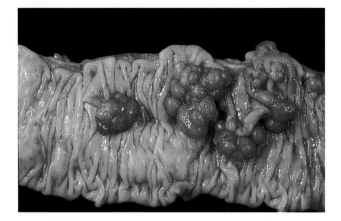

FIGURE 10-15
Multiple polyps of the large intestine. The polyps are round and protrude into the lumen of the intestine.

percent and 50 percent and greater than 50 percent, respectively.

Common to all polyps are the following:

- Their incidence increases with age.
- They are more common in males than females (2:1 ratio).
- They are often multiple.
- Seventy percent of the large polyps are located in the rectosigmoid part of the colon.

Tubular adenomas are the most common benign tumors, accounting for 75 percent of all neoplastic polyps. They may occur in any part of the intestine—small or large—but approximately one half are located in the rectosigmoid colon. They are typically attached to the mucosa by a stalk. In addition to these pedunculated polyps, which have a slender stalk and a lobulated "head," the smaller polyps tend to be sessile. The size of polyps and the length of the stalk vary, but most are less than 2.5 cm in diameter and have a short stalk measuring less than 5 mm in length.

Histologically, tubular adenomas are lined by cuboidal epithelium that shows neither differentiation nor obvious nuclear atypia. Malignant transformation can be histologically recognized by nuclear atypia, piling up of nuclei, and abnormal mitotic figures. The malignant glands are more crowded and show a back-to-back arrangement, with intratubular proliferation of cells. Invasive cancer can be recognized by its tendency to invade the stalk.

Tubular adenomas can readily be resected through an endoscope. Tumors measuring less than 1 cm have a 2 percent chance of being malignant, those measuring 1 to 2 cm have a 10 percent chance, and those exceeding 2.5 cm in diameter have a 50 percent chance of being malignant.

Tubulovillous adenomas are defined as predominantly tubular tumors that appear villous on at least 25 percent of their surface. These tumors tend to be sessile and larger-than-typical tubular adenomas. Histologically, the tumors contain tubular and villous elements. Histologically confirmed malignant disease is found in 25 percent to 50 percent of tubulovillous adenomas.

Villous adenomas are sessile, broad-based tumors composed of epithelial cells aligned into elongated villi. These project into the lumen of the intestine, forming finger-like protrusions. On gross examination, they have a velvety appearance. Most villous adenomas measure more than 2 cm in diameter, and many are quite large. Histologically, the neoplastic villi are reminiscent of the normal villi of the small intestine. In contrast to normal small intestinal mucosa that contains several cell types, tumorous villi are lined with a single cell type that cannot be classified and does not show signs of differentiation. Invasive carcinoma is found in almost 50 percent of these tumors. Owing to their size and broad base, these tumors cannot be resected through the endoscope. A segmental resection of the involved intestine is curative if performed before the malignant transformation takes place.

Adenocarcinoma. Adenocarcinoma accounts for 95 percent of malignant tumors of the intestine; the remaining 5 percent comprise carcinoids, sarcomas, and lymphomas. Adenocarcinomas are 50 times more common in the large intestine than the small intestine, which contains less than 2 percent of these tumors. For practical purposes, only colorectal adenocarcinomas shall be considered here.

The incidence of colorectal cancer has remained stable in the Western world for the last 100 years. Great geographic variation has been noted, however. Tumors are 10 times more common in the United States and Western countries than in Asia and Africa. The peak incidence is during the ages of 50 to 70 years. Rectal cancer is twice as common in men than in women, but the incidence of colonic cancer does not show such sex-related difference. Most cases occur spontaneously without any identifiable risk factors. A small number of cases (5 percent) occur in persons with a familial predisposition, called HNPCC. A very small number of adenocarcinomas also occur in persons with the autosomal dominant hereditary polyposis syndromes, such as FAP and Gardner's syndrome. The risk factors of these were discussed earlier.

Pathology. Approximately 50 percent of intestinal cancers develop in the rectosigmoid area, whereas the remaining tumors are evenly distributed through the other parts of the colon. Most adenocarcinomas of the intestine originate in neoplastic polyps, and many are actually found only upon histologic examination of surgically removed polyps. Established invasive carcinomas can present also as mucosal plaques, ulcerations, or endophytic protruding masses. The tumors of the right colon tend to grow as fungating masses or ulcerated, shallow, crater-like lesions (Fig. 10-16). In contrast, adenocarcinomas of the sigmoid and rectum tend to infiltrate the intestine circumferentially, producing so-called *napkin-ring* concentric narrowing (see Fig. 10-16).

Adenocarcinomas are staged morphologically into four categories (A to D) according to the system devised by Dukes, and modified by many other surgeons (e.g., the Astler-Coller modification). Patients with Dukes' A lesions have an 85 percent chance for 5-year survival, but this drops to 55 percent in those with B lesions, to 30 percent in those with C lesions, and to about 10 percent in those with D lesions. Obviously early detection is the only viable approach to colon cancer.

Clinical Features. Symptoms of intestinal cancer vary depending on the location, size, and shape of the lesion. Early cancer may produce no symptoms at all. Such lesions are typically diagnosed by endoscopy followed by biopsy, or by screening of feces for occult blood. Adenocarcinoma of the right colon and cecum tend to be clinically silent, producing only nonspecific signs, such as weakness and fatigue. Chronic blood loss may cause anemia. The left-side lesions, especially those in the rectum, tend to narrow the intestine and obstruct the passage of feces.

> **Did You Know?**
>
> Occult blood—that is, blood that is not visible by the naked eye—is an important early sign of colonic cancer. The test can easily be performed by smearing a small amount of feces onto a test strip that changes color on contact with blood. Early detection is the only efficient way to combat carcinoma of the intestines.

Constipation; narrow, pencil-like feces; and blood in the feces are the characteristic findings. Hematochezia may also occur, although it is usually a sign of far-advanced lesions.

The diagnosis of intestinal cancer depends on visualizing the tumor by colonoscopy or rectoscopy, x-ray studies combined with barium enema, and computerized axial tomography. The final diagnosis depends on histologic examination of the tissue (Fig. 10-17).

Most adenocarcinomas of the intestine release into circulation a glycoprotein called CEA. CEA is normally produced by the embryonic intestines, but is not found in the intestinal cells of the adult except in special circumstances, such as in the regenerating epithelium of ulcerative colitis. CEA produced by

FIGURE 10-16
Carcinoma of the colon. (A) Carcinoma of the right colon forms intraluminal fungating or ulcerating masses. (B) Carcinoma of the left colon produces "napkin-ring" stenotic lesions.

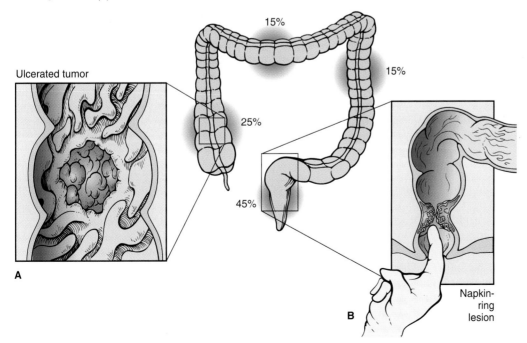

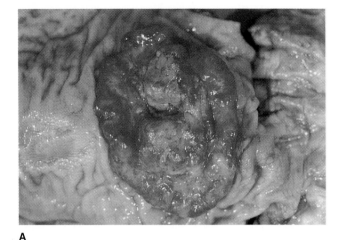

A

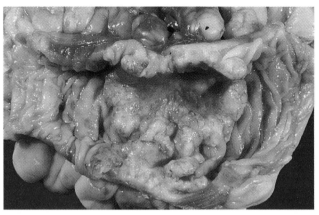

B

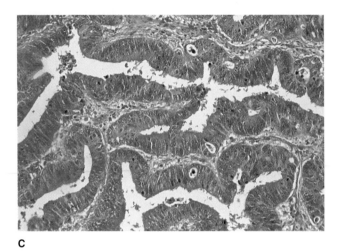

C

FIGURE 10-17
Surgically resected carcinomas of the large intestine. (A) This carcinoma of the cecum appears ulcerated. (B) This carcinoma of the sigmoid colon has diffusely infiltrated the entire circumference of the intestine. (C) Histologically, these tumors are adenocarcinomas.

tumor cells enters the blood circulation and can be measured in serum. Unfortunately, CEA cannot be used for early detection or for the screening of populations at risk because it is also elevated in chronic ulcerative colitis and other nonspecific intestinal inflammations. The test is useful in the follow-up of patients whose carcinoma has been resected. A rise in serum CEA level in these patients usually heralds a recurrence of tumor.

Carcinoid. The term carcinoid is used for neuroendocrine tumors of low malignancy, meaning that they are malignant but not so malignant as true carcinomas. The gastrointestinal tract is the major site of origin of carcinoid tumors, 90 percent of which originate in the intestines. The most common sites of carcinoids, in order of frequency, are the appendix, terminal ileum, rectum, the remainder of the colon, and the small intestine and stomach.

Pathology. Carcinoids are typically located in the submucosa, where they form small nodules elevating the overlying mucosa. Most carcinoids are small, measuring less than 2 cm, and are often found acci-

dentally in surgically resected tissue or at autopsy. Tumors larger than 2 cm may be symptomatic and also tend to metastasize to local lymph nodes and to the liver. Carcinoids, especially those in the terminal ileum and the stomach, are often multiple.

Histologic examination reveals that carcinoids are composed of small neuroendocrine cells arranged into islets or cords and trabeculae. The neuroendocrine nature of the tumor cell is best demonstrated by immunohistochemical or electron microscopy studies. By immunohistochemical methods, it is possible to demonstrate that these cells contain polypeptide hormones, such as secretin, gastrin, or VIP, and biogenic amines, such as histamine and serotonin. Electron microscopy reveals that the tumor cells contain neuroendocrine granules, which have a dense central core surrounded by a clear halo and a limiting membrane.

Clinical Features. Carcinoids are malignant tumors. This is evident histologically because tumor cells typically invade the normal tissue, often metastasizing to local lymph nodes. The propensity to metastasize correlates with the size of the tumor and its location.

Metastases are most common with tumors larger than 2 cm in diameter, especially those localized in the right colon, small intestine, or stomach. Carcinoids of the appendix tend to remain localized. Clinical symptoms of carcinoid tumors include those related to local growth, which are not different from the symptoms produced by other malignant tumors, and those related to their secretory neuroendocrine activity. Secretory products of intestinal carcinoid tumors that are released into the portal circulation are detoxified during their passage through the liver. Carcinoids that have metastasized to the liver release their secretory product into the venous blood; this causes a systemic disease known as *carcinoid syndrome.* Symptoms, which are probably caused by a release of serotonin, bradykinin, and histamine, include episodes of facial blushing, bronchial wheezing, attacks of watery diarrhea, and abdominal colic. In long-lasting carcinoid syndrome, there is also endocardial fibrosis of the right ventricle and tricuspid valve. Carcinoids are slow-growing neoplasms, and the 5-year survival rate of treated patients exceeds 80 percent.

Review Questions

1. Compare the structure and function of the upper and the lower digestive tract.
2. List the main exocrine and endocrine products of the gastrointestinal tract and their functions.
3. How do developmental anomalies affect the function of the digestive tract?
4. What is dental caries and how can it be prevented?
5. What are the main complications of dental caries?
6. What causes periodontal disease?
7. What is stomatitis and what are its causes?
8. What is the significance of oral leukoplakia and erythroplakia?
9. What are the risk factors for oral cancer?
10. How does oral cancer present clinically?
11. What is sialadenitis and what are its causes?
12. How does Sjögren's disease affect the salivary glands?
13. Are salivary gland tumors mostly benign or malignant?
14. What is the most common salivary gland tumor?
15. What are the clinical signs and symptoms of esophageal disease?
16. What is dysphagia and what are its causes?
17. What is esophagitis and what are its causes?
18. What is a hiatal hernia and how does it present clinically?
19. What is achalasia and what are its causes?
20. What is the most common cause of esophageal varices?
21. What are the risk factors for esophageal cancer and how do they account for the differences in the incidence of this disease in various parts of the world?
22. Correlate the pathologic and clinical features of esophageal carcinoma.
23. What are the main forms of gastritis?
24. What causes gastritis?
25. Explain the pathogenesis of peptic ulcer, placing special emphasis on the role of gastric juice, the mucosal barrier, and *Helicobacter pylori.*
26. Describe the gross and microscopic pathology of peptic ulcer and correlate these morphologic findings with the clinical signs and symptoms of the disease.
27. What are the main complications of peptic ulcer?
28. How common is gastric cancer in the United States in comparison with the incidence of this neoplasm in other parts of the world?
29. How does gastric carcinoma present on macroscopic (naked eye) examination?
30. Where do gastric carcinomas metastasize?
31. What are the clinical signs and symptoms of gastric carcinoma?
32. How is gastric lymphoma related to MALT?
33. Compare atresia of the small intestine with Hirschsprung's disease.
34. Describe diverticula of the large intestine and their complications.
35. Compare hemorrhoids and intestinal angiodysplasia.
36. Compare occlusive and nonocclusive ischemic bowel disease.
37. How common is inflammatory bowel disease?

38. Compare Crohn's disease and ulcerative colitis.

39. What is pseudomembranous colitis?

40. List the most important bacterial and protozoal infections of the intestines.

41. Compare diarrhea caused by small intestinal disease with diarrhea caused by large intestinal disease.

42. What are the clinical and pathologic features of acute appendicitis?

43. Compare infectious and sterile peritonitis.

44. Describe the pathogenesis and pathology of acute peritonitis.

45. List the most common causes of intestinal obstruction.

46. What are the best known types of hernia?

47. Compare intussusception and volvulus.

48. Classify malabsorption syndromes according to their pathogenesis.

49. Compare iliac sprue and tropical sprue.

50. What are the clinical features of malabsorption syndrome?

51. How common are intestinal neoplasms and where are they most often located?

52. Classify intestinal neoplasms.

53. What are the risk factors for intestinal neoplasms?

54. What are polyps and how are these intestinal lesions classified?

55. Compare neoplastic and non-neoplastic polyps.

56. What are the clinical features of large intestinal cancer?

57. Compare adenocarcinomas of the right and left colon.

58. What is CEA and what is the clinical value of this tumor marker?

59. How do carcinoids differ from adenocarcinoma of the large intestine?

60. What is carcinoid syndrome?

Learning Objectives

After studying this chapter, the student should be able to:

1. Describe the normal liver and biliary tract.

2. List the cells of the hepatobiliary tract and describe their primary functions.

3. Describe the formation of bile and explain the main disorders that can cause jaundice.

4. Describe the principal biochemical changes typical of acute liver disease.

5. Describe the principal clinical, biochemical, and pathologic findings in chronic liver disease.

6. Describe the pathologic changes induced by hepatitis virus and compare the effects of hepatitis virus A, B, and C.

7. Define cirrhosis and describe the most important pathologic findings in this disease.

8. Describe three forms of alcohol-induced liver disease.

9. Compare predictable and nonpredictable drug-induced liver disease.

10. Describe three hereditary diseases affecting the liver.

11. Discuss the pathogenesis of immunologic liver diseases and compare primary biliary cirrhosis with primary sclerosing cholangitis.

12. Describe typical infectious liver diseases caused by bacteria, protozoa, and parasites.

13. Describe the morphology of gallstones and discuss their pathogenesis.

14. List the symptoms and biochemical findings caused by biliary tract diseases and relate these to pathologic changes in the gallbladder and extrahepatic biliary ducts.

15. List three malignant liver tumors and compare their features.

16. Compare the features of gallbladder cancer and cancer of the extrahepatic bile ducts.

17. Describe the benefits and hazards of liver transplantation.

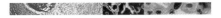

Additional Key Terms and Concepts

Alpha-fetoprotein

Ascites

Autoimmune (lupoid) hepatitis

Cholangitis

Cholecystitis

Hepatitis viruses

Portal hypertension

Chapter Outline

The Liver and Biliary Tract

Chapter 11

NORMAL ANATOMY AND PHYSIOLOGY

The **liver** is the largest parenchymal organ in the body, weighing about 1500 g. It is located in the right upper abdominal quadrant in a space delimited cranially by the diaphragm, anteriorly by the rib cage, and posteriorly by bones and muscles of the abdominal wall. The normal liver has a smooth surface and is firm. The anterior lower edge of the liver can be palpated below the right costal margin, at the peak of deep inspiration, when the entire liver is pushed caudally by the diaphragm. Owing to its anatomic relationship to the chest cage, the liver can be reached by a biopsy needle inserted through the intercostal muscles.

On the inferior side, the liver is attached to the **gallbladder** and the **extrahepatic bile ducts,** which connect it to the duodenum (Fig. 11-1). The point at which the bile ducts exit from the liver is called the hilus. Through the hilus, the liver receives its dual blood supply—arterial oxygenated blood through the **hepatic artery,** and venous blood rich in nutrients absorbed from food through the **portal vein.** The portal circulation is separate from the systemic circulation, to which it is interconnected with narrow, nonfunctioning anastomoses. These carry little blood, but are able to expand if the pressure in the portal system increases as a result of portal hypertension. The **hepatic vein** drains into the inferior vena cava.

The liver is primarily composed of liver cells, also known as **hepatocytes,** which constitute 90 percent of the total mass. The other cells are **bile ductal cells** and the vascular cells lining the sinusoids, veins, and arteries (Fig. 11-2). Connective tissue forms the capsule of the liver (Glisson's capsule) and portal tracts.

The hepatocytes are arranged into functional units called **lobules** (see Fig. 11-2). Blood enters the lobules from the periphery through the *portal tract* and flows through the **sinusoids** toward the central vein. The portal tract is also called the portal triad because it contains a small branch of the hepatic artery, portal vein, and bile duct. The lobular blood spaces and the sinusoids are lined by Kupffer cells and a discontinuous basement membrane. This allows easy passage of nutrients and metabolites from the blood into the liver cells and vice versa. The **Kupffer cells** are fixed phagocytes and serve as the main scavengers for foreign and internal particulate material (e.g., bacteria and blood cell fragments).

The **liver** has several **major functions** which can be classified as

- excretory
- metabolic
- storage
- synthetic

Bile is the main excretory product of the liver. Bile is a complex mixture of bilirubin, bile salts, lipids, and many other minor components. It is produced by liver cells and excreted through the bile ducts into the intestine or stored in the gallbladder. Upon reaching the intestine, the bile is mixed with food and pancreatic and intestinal enzymes. The bile that is not used up during intestinal digestion is transformed into urobilinogen, which is reabsorbed into the portal circulation and returned to the liver (*enterohepatic circulation* of bile).

The liver has multiple metabolic functions. It is

FIGURE 11-1

Normal liver. (From Applegate EJ: The anatomy and physiology learning system: textbook. Philadelphia: WB Saunders, 1995:340.)

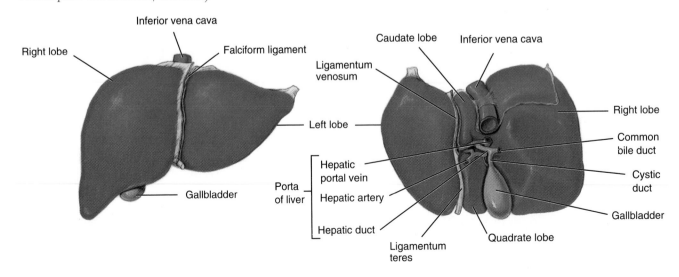

Did You Know?

Bile was considered by ancient physicians to be an important body fluid. The term melancholy (in Greek, meaning black bile), which is used to denote a form of depression, attests to those ancient beliefs. It was thought that pessimistic and depressed people had black bile that influenced their mood. Modern psychiatry does not subscribe to such views, but it still uses the term melancholy.

proteins except the immunoglobulins. **Albumin,** the most copious plasma protein, as well as the coagulation proteins, and all the transport proteins essential for the transfer of hormones, vitamins, and other biologically active substances, are synthesized in the liver.

OVERVIEW OF MAJOR DISEASES

The most important diseases affecting the liver and the biliary tract are the following:

- *Jaundice syndromes.* These include abnormal formation, processing, or excretion of bilirubin.
- *Hepatitis.* Inflammation of the liver can be caused by viruses, as well as drugs, alcohol, and immune mechanisms.
- *Toxic/metabolic hepatic injury.* Liver cells may be injured by exogenous chemicals or endogenous metabolites.

considered the main "processing factory" for all food components, and its normal function is essential for the intermediary metabolism of carbohydrates, fats, and proteins. The liver is also the major storage site of carbohydrates and lipids.

Liver is the site of synthesis of all major plasma

FIGURE 11-2
Fine structure of the normal liver. (From Applegate EJ: The anatomy and physiology learning system: textbook. Philadelphia: WB Saunders, 1995:341.)

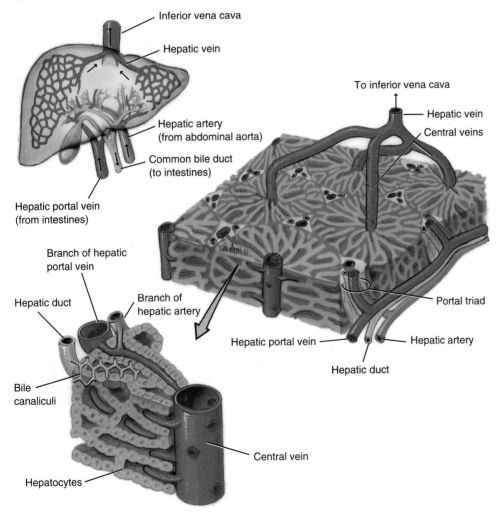

- *Cirrhosis.* This condition may result from a variety of liver diseases. The term cirrhosis is used as a synonym for end-stage liver disease.
- *Diseases of the extrahepatic bile ducts and gallbladder.* The most important among these diseases are those that are caused by gallstones.
- *Tumors.* Tumors of the liver and the biliary tract can be classified as benign or malignant, primary or secondary.

Several facts important to an understanding of liver disease are presented here, before a discussion of specific pathologic entities.

1. *The liver is a part of the digestive tract, to which it is connected by two important links: the portal veins and the bile ducts.* The liver is involved in processing nutrients that are absorbed in the intestines. These nutrients reach the liver through the portal vein. The portal vein circulation is a low-pressure venous system that is self-contained and does not have functional communications with the systemic blood flow. However, if the blood flow through the liver is obstructed owing to liver disease, such as cirrhosis, the increased pressure in the portal system will open up the nonfunctioning anastomoses between the portal and the systemic circulation. Through these anastomoses, the portal blood will bypass the liver and enter the systemic circulation. This has two important consequences: (1) the blood that has bypassed the liver contains various metabolites and toxic substances that may have deleterious effects on other organs; and (2) at the same time, such blood lacks the essential metabolites formed in the liver. For example, the blood concentration of ammonia absorbed from the intestine might be high, whereas the blood glucose level, which is not released from the liver, might be low.

Portal hypertension widens the venous channels connecting the portal and systemic circulation. Increased pressure in these anastomoses results in the formation of varicosities (i.e., tortuous, dilated veins). These varicosities, which are prone to rupture and tend to bleed profusely, are typically located in the esophagus, in the hemorrhoidal venous plexus of the rectum, and the umbilical venous plexus of the anterior abdominal wall (Fig. 11-3).

Portal hypertension has two other important consequences. Because the portal vein receives venous blood from the spleen, portal hypertension causes chronic passive congestion in the spleen and *splenomegaly.* The transudation of fluid into the abdominal cavity will contribute to the formation of *ascites.*

The *bile ducts* connect the liver to the duodenum and serve as the main route for the excretion of bile into the intestine. Obstruction of the bile ducts results in jaundice. Lack of bile in the intestines ad-versely affects digestion, particularly, the absorption of fats and fat-soluble vitamins (A, D, E, and K). The bile ducts may also serve as the site of entry of ascending bacterial infections. Even worms, such as Ascaris, or the liver fluke *Opisthorcis sinensis,* may reach the liver through the bile ducts.

The terminal portion of the bile duct passes through the head of the pancreas, where it becomes confluent with the main pancreatic duct, entering into the wall of the intestine at the papilla of Vater. Diseases of the duodenum or the pancreas may also obstruct the extrahepatic bile ducts. Obstructive jaundice is an important symptom of carcinomas involving the head of pancreas.

2. *The liver is an encapsulated, self-contained organ that is loosely attached to adjacent structures.* This is important to bear in mind, especially today when the diseased liver can easily be removed and replaced with a newly transplanted organ. As mentioned before, the liver moves down with each inspiration and can be palpated underneath the right costal margin. The external surface of the normal liver is smooth and covered with Glisson's capsule. Glisson's capsule contains nerves. Distention of this capsule secondary to chronic passive congestion, which is typical of congestive heart failure, causes pain that is usually dull and diffuse over the entire liver. Tumors and hepatitis also can distend Glisson's capsule and cause pain.

3. *The liver is essential for the uptake, processing, and excretion of bilirubin released from aged red blood cells.* Bilirubin is the degradation product of heme, the principal component of hemoglobin in red blood cells (RBCs). Bilirubin released from senescent RBCs is taken up by the liver and excreted in bile. Hyperbilirubinemia (i.e., a serum bilirubin level exceeding the normal concentration of 1.2 mg/dL) is one of the most common biochemical abnormalities in liver diseases. Retained bilirubin diffuses into tissues and binds to connective tissues in various organs. In the skin and mucosa, this is recognized as jaundice.

4. *The liver is the major source of most plasma proteins.* Essentially all major plasma proteins, except the immunoglobulins, are produced by the liver. Liver diseases result in *hypoproteinemia.* Lack of albumin, which is the most abundant plasma protein, reduces the oncotic capacity of the plasma, resulting in *edema.* Decreased production of coagulation factors, such as fibrinogen, prothrombin, and factors VIII, IX, X, XI, and XII, which are all synthesized in the liver, results in a *bleeding tendency.*

5. *Liver cells are rich in enzymes, which are released into the circulation upon liver cell injury.* Liver cell injury results in a release of aspartate aminotransferase (AST) and alanine aminotransferase (ALT) into the circulating blood. AST and ALT are ubiquitous enzymes whose levels are elevated in

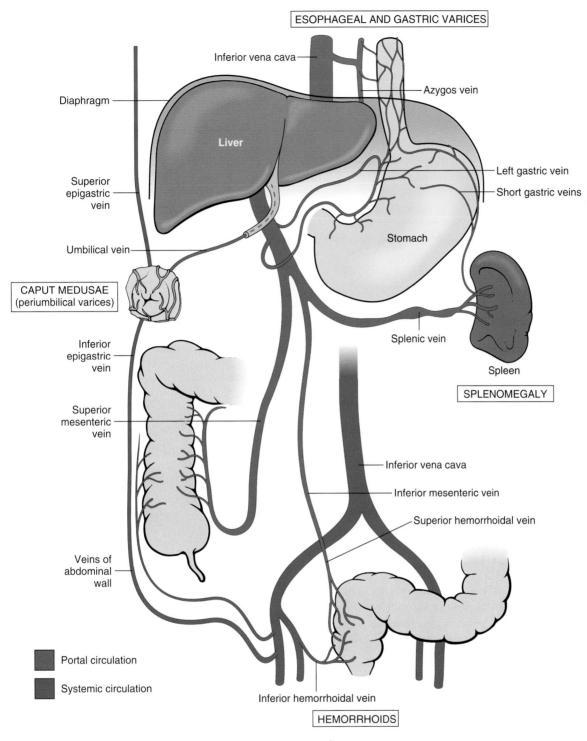

ESOPHAGEAL AND GASTRIC VARICES

Inferior vena cava

Azygos vein

Diaphragm

Liver

Left gastric vein

Short gastric veins

Superior epigastric vein

Stomach

Umbilical vein

CAPUT MEDUSAE (periumbilical varices)

Splenic vein

Spleen

Inferior epigastric vein

SPLENOMEGALY

Superior mesenteric vein

Inferior vena cava

Inferior mesenteric vein

Superior hemorrhoidal vein

Veins of abdominal wall

Portal circulation

Systemic circulation

Inferior hemorrhoidal vein

HEMORRHOIDS

FIGURE 11-3

Anastomoses form between the portal and systemic circulation as a result of portal hypertension.

blood following injury of many other organs, as well as in the case of myocardial infarction. Because the liver represents the major source of AST and ALT, these enzyme levels are commonly used as indicators of liver function. Alkaline phosphatase, another enzyme that is also not restricted to liver, is used as a marker of bile duct obstruction.

6. *The liver removes from circulation, metabolizes, and detoxifies or modifies many drugs, hormones, cytokines, and biologically active metabolites.* The liver removes from circulation various metabolites, such as carbohydrates, lipids, and proteins, derived from the food or peripheral storage sites; immunoglobulins and various other proteins; hormones, such as androgens and estrogens; biogenic amines, such as histamine or serotonin; and many other substances. If uptake into the liver cells is blocked or cannot take place because of liver cell insufficiency, these substances persist in the blood in high concentrations and may have adverse effects on other tissues. The best example of such a condition is the accumulation of ammonia and other presumptive neurotoxins in the intestines; upon absorption, these substances may act on the brain and even cause coma (*hepatic encephalopathy*).

Chronic liver disease is associated with disturbances in the metabolism of sex hormones. Excess estrogen that has not been removed appropriately from the circulation is considered to be the cause of dilated arterioles surrounded by dilated capillaries, known in the skin as *spider nevi.* Testicular atrophy and loss of libido and gynecomastia, which are seen in some alcoholics with cirrhosis, have also been attributed to hyperestrinism.

7. *Certain viruses have exclusive tropism for the liver.* The liver may be affected by various bacterial, viral, protozoal, fungal, and parasitic infections that reach this organ via the blood or through the bile ducts. Most of these pathogens cause disease in other organs as well. Certain viruses, such as hepatitis virus A, B, C, D, and E, show hepatotropism (i.e., they preferentially affect the liver). The reasons for this tropism are not known, but apparently, the liver cells provide an ideal environment for their growth and replication.

8. *Liver cells can regenerate.* Liver cells are facultative mitotic (labile) cells, and lost liver cells are readily replaced by new hepatocytes derived from the remaining healthy cells. For example, a liver lobe that is injured in a car accident can be resected because it will regenerate; within a few days, the liver will regain its normal size. Regeneration takes place in cirrhotic livers as well. However, because of concomitant fibrosis, this results in formation of nodules rather than the restoration of normal parenchyma.

9. *The liver can give rise to tumors, but it is even more often involved by tumor metastases.* Hepatocellular carcinoma is common in parts of the world in which hepatitis B viral infection is endemic, such as the Far East or sub-Saharan Africa. Worldwide, it is probably the most common human malignant disease, with more than one million new cases reported every year. In the United States, the liver is more often affected by metastatic cancer than by primary liver cell tumors. Because the liver receives blood from two sources, and thus serves as a major blood thoroughfare, it is a common site of metastasis of tumors originating in other organs.

10. *Bile can form gallstones.* Gallstones are formed, under a variety of circumstances, from the normal components of bile. These stones may cause

obstruction or inflammation and are the most important cause of pathologic changes in the biliary tract.

Jaundice

Jaundice (*icterus* in Latin) is a symptom and not a disease. It is characterized by yellow discoloration of the skin and mucosa caused by hyperbilirubinemia, that is, elevation of blood bilirubin levels above the upper limit of normal, which is 1.2 mg/dL. In practical terms, jaundice becomes apparent only after the concentration of bilirubin has exceeded 3 mg/dL.

Pathogenesis. As shown in Figure 11-4, jaundice may be classified as

- prehepatic or hemolytic
- hepatic
- posthepatic or obstructive

FIGURE 11-4
Jaundice may be attributable to prehepatic (A), hepatic (B), or posthepatic (C) causes.

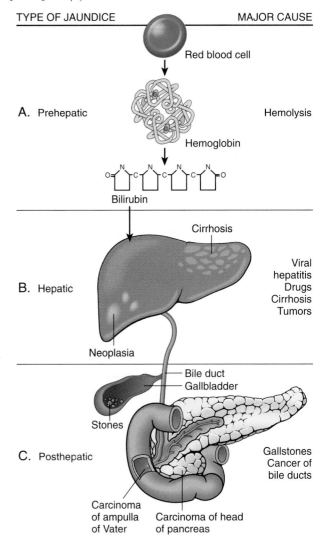

TYPE OF JAUNDICE   MAJOR CAUSE

Red blood cell

A. Prehepatic   Hemolysis

Hemoglobin

Bilirubin

Cirrhosis

B. Hepatic   Viral hepatitis
Drugs
Cirrhosis
Tumors

Neoplasia

Bile duct
Gallbladder

Stones

C. Posthepatic   Gallstones
Cancer of bile ducts

Carcinoma of ampulla of Vater   Carcinoma of head of pancreas

Bilirubin is derived mostly from the heme portion of hemoglobin; 70 percent of hemoglobin is of RBC origin, whereas the remaining 30 percent stems from the respiratory enzymes in various tissues or the precursors of the hemoglobin in bone marrow that are not utilized (owing to "inefficient hematopoiesis").

The senescent RBCs are taken up by the phagocytic cells of the spleen and the Kupffer cells of the liver. Within these cells, the hemoglobin is degraded into heme and globin. Heme loses the iron and is transformed into yellow pigment bilirubin. Bilirubin is released into the blood, where it binds to albumin. This unconjugated bilirubin, which is not water-soluble, is taken up by the liver cells and conjugated to glucuronide. Bilirubin bound to glucuronide becomes water-soluble. This conjugated bilirubin is excreted in bile and into the intestine, where it participates in the digestion of dietary fats. Bilirubin that is not used up in the intestine is converted by bacteria into urobilinogen, which is reabsorbed. Most of it is recirculated into the liver, whereas a small portion is excreted in urine.

Hyperbilirubinemia is biochemically classified as *conjugated, unconjugated,* or *mixed* (Table 11-1). *Unconjugated hyperbilirubinemia* is prehepatic and mostly caused by excessive bilirubin formation secondary to hemolysis. Gilbert's disease, an autosomal dominant defect in the hepatic uptake of bilirubin, can also cause mild unconjugated hyperbilirubinemia. *Conjugated hyperbilirubinemia* reflects disturbances in the excretion of bilirubin that has been conjugated to glucuronide in liver cells. Typically, this occurs as a result of obstruction of bile flow, usually at the level of the common bile duct. Gallstones that are impacted in the extrahepatic bile ducts or tumors of the bile ducts, pancreas, or duodenum are the most common causes of such obstructions.

In obstructive jaundice, the bile does not reach the intestine and the feces appear tan-colored, rather than their normal brown color. Such stools are called *acholic* and are associated with *steatorrhea.*

Mixed conjugated and unconjugated hyperbilirubinemia is a feature of various diseases marked by liver

Did You Know?

Jaundice is best recognized on the sclera. The sclera is normally white, even in blacks and orientals, but in those with jaundice it becomes yellow.

If the blood is allowed to clot in a test tube, the RBCs separate from the plasma. Plasma, which consists of water and solutes, is yellow because it normally contains small amounts of bilirubin. In cases of jaundice, the plasma becomes even more yellow or turns brown.

Bilirubin excreted in the urine of jaundiced persons makes the urine appear brown and bubbly. Bilirubin is a surface active substance, like detergents. Urine that contains bilirubin is similar to bubble bath and could be used for cleansing. In ancient times, bathing in animal urine was a part of certain religious rituals and beautification rites. Bilirubin-rich urine would have been more efficient!

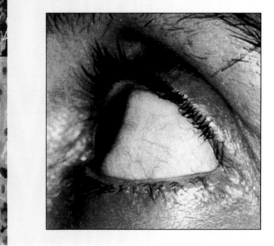

cell necrosis and destruction of liver parenchyma. It occurs in viral hepatitis or drug-induced hepatitis, as well as in various metabolic liver diseases, alcoholic hepatitis, and cirrhosis.

Clinical Features. Bilirubin, both conjugated and unconjugated, binds to connective tissue and stains it yellow. This is best seen on the sclera, which is normally white. Other mucous membranes and the skin become yellow as well. Jaundice is usually accompanied by itching, but otherwise, it has few serious consequences.

The unconjugated bilirubin is bound to albumin. Thus, it does not cross the blood–brain barrier and does not appear in the cerebrospinal fluid or in the brain. It does not filter into the urine either. In hemolytic jaundice, urine is thus of normal color. However, conjugated bilirubin, which is water-soluble, is excreted in urine. Because of its high bilirubin con-

Table 11-1 Common Causes of Jaundice

Prehepatic	Hepatocellular	Posthepatic (Obstructive)
Hemolysis	Viral hepatitis	Gallstones
Hematoma	Alcoholic liver disease	Carcinoma of the pancreas or bile ducts
Gilbert's disease	Drug-induced liver disease	
	Cirrhosis	

tent, the urine of patients with viral hepatitis will appear brown and foamy. Brown urine is frequently reported as the first sign of viral hepatitis.

As mentioned earlier, jaundice is not a disease but a symptom of several liver diseases. The underlying cause of jaundice can be identified by establishing whether the jaundice is attributable to unconjugated or conjugated hyperbilirubinemia; whether the liver disease is acute or chronic; whether there are other signs of liver cell injury; and whether there is evidence of obstruction of the bile ducts. In viral hepatitis, jaundice is usually short-lived and disappears on its own. In cirrhosis, the jaundice is usually mild but persistent. In primary biliary cirrhosis, the jaundice may be mild or severe; severe jaundice usually predicts an unfavorable outcome. Obstructive jaundice caused by biliary stones is associated with spastic contractions (known as *colic*), which abate upon surgical removal of the stone. Jaundice caused by carcinoma of the pancreas may be surgically relieved by shunting the bile flow into the intestine, but the patient has almost no chances of surviving because carcinoma of the pancreas has an abysmal prognosis.

Acute Viral Hepatitis

Acute **viral hepatitis** is a clinical syndrome of variable severity caused by one of several hepatotropic viruses known as hepatitis A, B, C, D, and E. It is the most prevalent liver disease in the world. In the United States, hepatitis affects, on average, 2 persons per 1000 every year. The disease is often asymptomatic, which is attributable to the fact that 40 percent of all Americans have antibodies to hepatitis A virus and 5 percent to 10 percent have antibodies to hepatitis B virus, even though most of these individuals do not remember ever having had hepatitis.

Acute hepatitis may also occur in the course of several systemic diseases. These "other" forms of hepatitis must be distinguished from hepatitis caused

> **Did You Know?**
>
> Jaundice is a symptom characterized by yellow skin and mucosa. Yellow skin can also be a consequence of hypercarotenemia, an excess of the yellow pigment—carotene—found in carrots and other yellow fruits and vegetables. Overindulgence in these foodstuffs can cause yellowing of the skin, which must be distinguished from clinical jaundice. Beware of people who are overly fond of pumpkins, mangos, or paw paws!

by hepatotropic viruses. The best known examples of nonspecific hepatitis are infectious mononucleosis, caused by the Epstein-Barr virus, herpesvirus, and cytomegalovirus infection. All of these viruses and many others cause hepatitis, especially in immunosuppressed patients with acquired immunodeficiency syndrome (AIDS). Childhood viral diseases (measles, rubella, varicella) may also affect the liver, although such hepatitis is usually overshadowed by other symptoms. The virus of yellow fever is an important cause of acute hepatitis in the tropics, but is rare in the United States. In clinical practice, the term *viral hepatitis* is reserved for the disease caused by hepatitis A, B, C, D, and E viruses.

Etiology and Pathogenesis. The main features of hepatitis viruses are listed in Table 11-2. From this table, one may see that hepatitis viruses vary in size and belong to several viral families. Hepatitis B virus (HBV) is a DNA virus, whereas all the others are RNA viruses. The duration of viremia, the mode of infection, the duration of incubation, and the clinical presentation are distinct for each virus. Three viruses (HBV, HCV, HDV) can also cause a chronic disease, and at least two of these (HBV and HCV) predispose the infected individual's liver cells to malignant transformation. At the present time, vaccines exist for hepatitis A virus (HAV) and HBV, and these can be used for preventive immunization of persons who are at increased risk. For example, travelers to tropical countries are immunized against HAV. Additionally, health professionals are usually immunized against HBV because they are at increased risk of infection through exposure to blood or blood products.

Forms of Hepatitis

Hepatitis A

HAV is a 27-nm, nonencapsulated RNA virus similar to other picornaviruses, such as poliovirus and some enteric viruses. The infection is transmitted by the fecal-oral route, and it may occur in a sporadic or epidemic form. The sources of the virus are sewage, contaminated food and drinks, and shellfish. The disease is most prevalent among children in underdeveloped countries. Tourists traveling to southern countries are also at risk.

Symptoms usually develop after a short incubation period of 15 to 50 days. Clinically, HAV infection is characterized by short-lived, mild, enteric fever with vomiting, loss of appetite, and jaundice. Recovery occurs within days, usually without any long-term consequences. Transition to chronic hepatitis or cirrhosis never occurs. The fulminant form of the disease, accompanied by hepatic failure, is extremely rare. HAV infection thus has a favorable prognosis.

Table 11-2 Features of Known Human Hepatitis (A, B, C, D, and E) Viruses

Feature	HAV	HBV	HCV	HDV	HEV
Family	Picorna	Hepadna	Flavi	(Viroid)	Calici
Genome	RNA	DNA	RNA	RNA	RNA
Size	27 nm	42 nm	30–60 nm	35 nm	32 nm
Viremia	Brief	Long	Long	Like HBV	Brief
Transmission	F/O	Par/sex	Par/sex	Par/sex	F/O
Incubation (days)	15–45	40–180	15–150	30–50	14–60
Fulminant hepatitis risk (%)	0.1	1	0.1	10	1–2 (if pregnant, 20)
Chronicity	No	10%	50%	10%	No
HCC association	No	Yes	Yes	No	No
Chronic carrier state	No	Yes	Yes	Yes	No
Vaccine available	Yes	Yes	No	No	No

F/O, fecal/oral; Par/sex, parenteral/sexual; HCC, hepatocellular carcinoma.

Hepatitis B

HBV is an encapsulated DNA virus that is species-specific for humans and higher primates. Nevertheless, it is closely related to other Hepadna family viruses that cause hepatitis in woodchucks, ducks, and ground squirrels. The DNA of HBV is partially double-stranded and contains four partially overlapping genes that encode the message for the synthesis of the protein components of the virion, colloquially known as the Dane particle. These include hepatitis B *surface* antigen (HBsAg), hepatitis B *core* antigen (HBcAg), and hepatitis B *e* antigen (HBeAg). These antigens are important for serologic diagnosis and monitoring of the disease.

HBsAg is secreted and released into circulation early in the disease, and can be detected in the serum 1 week after the onset of infection (Fig. 11-5). HBsAg disappears from the blood during the convalescent period, which is marked by the appearance of antibody to HBsAg (anti-HBs). HBsAg persists in circulation only in patients who develop chronic hepatitis. These patients do not produce anti-HBs, and apparently cannot clear the virus from the body.

HBeAg appears in the serum during acute infec-

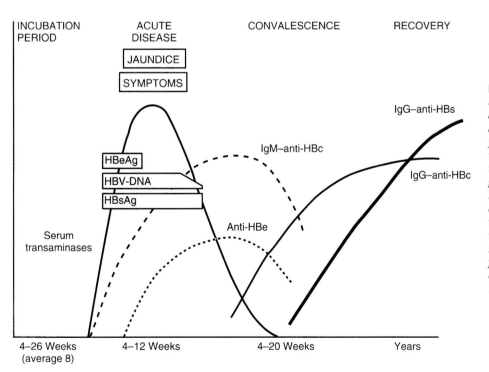

INCUBATION PERIOD — ACUTE DISEASE — CONVALESCENCE — RECOVERY

JAUNDICE
SYMPTOMS

HBeAg
HBV-DNA
HBsAg

Serum transaminases

IgM–anti-HBc

Anti-HBe

IgG–anti-HBs

IgG–anti-HBc

4–26 Weeks (average 8)   4–12 Weeks   4–20 Weeks   Years

FIGURE 11-5
Serologic findings in acute hepatitis B viral infection. Viral antigens can be detected even before the onset of jaundice. Convalescence is characterized by the disappearance of viral antigens and the appearance of antibodies to the virus. Recovery is characterized by a strong immunoglobulin G (IgG) antibody response. (From Cotran RS, Kumar V, Robbins SL: Robbins' pathologic basis of disease, 5th ed. Philadelphia: WB Saunders, 1994:846.)

tion, but disappears faster than HBsAg, usually during the icteric stage of the disease. Persistence of HBeAg in serum is found in patients with chronic hepatitis, and its presence is a good marker of infectivity of such serum.

HBcAg and viral DNA are not released into the blood. However, antibodies to this antigen (anti-HBc) appear in all infected persons, usually a few days before the onset of jaundice. Initially, the antibodies are IgM, after which IgG appears. Patients with chronic hepatitis also have anti-HBcAg. This antibody may be the only serologic evidence of viral infection in such patients.

Clinical Features. Symptoms of HBV appear 40 to 180 days after infection. Infection follows transfusion of blood, exposure to contaminated blood or blood products, or sexual contact. The disease has three phases: preicteric, icteric, and convalescent. In the preicteric phase, there is weakness, nausea, and vomiting, which are occasionally associated with mild enlargement and tenderness of the liver. Some patients develop a measles-like skin rash. Darkening of the urine, which contains bilirubin, is a useful diagnostic finding. Jaundice, a symptom found in less than 30 percent of affected patients, usually appears 2 months after exposure, and is associated with worsening of clinical symptoms and laboratory findings. Typically, these include elevated serum levels of bilirubin, ALT, and AST. The jaundice persists for several weeks and, in most patients, disappears spontaneously. The more profound the jaundice the more likely it is that the disease will enter into an uneventful period of recovery. Mild jaundice may herald a protracted course of the disease and a transition to chronic hepatitis.

The outcome of HBV infection is outlined in Figure 11-5. The disease may be symptomatic (icteric) or asymptomatic (subclinical). HBV produces clinically recognizable symptoms in one third of infected persons. The remaining two thirds have subclinical disease, which is recognized only by the subsequent appearance of antibodies to HBs and HBc. Most infected patients (90 percent) recover completely. Acute *fulminant hepatitis* develops in 1 percent, and chronic hepatitis in less than 10 percent of those with clinically evident infection. Chronic hepatitis may develop even without an acute icteric phase. *Chronic hepatitis* is subclinical in 75 percent of cases. These patients have no symptoms. HBsAg in the serum of affected patients and mild portal tract inflammation seen on liver biopsy are the only signs of disease. These persons show histologic signs of mild *chronic persistent hepatitis* and are classified as asymptomatic HBsAg carriers. *Chronic active hepatitis*, which develops in about 25 percent of patients with serologic evidence of chronic hepatitis, is a more serious form and may progress to cirrhosis. *Hepatocellular carcinoma* is a rare but well-known late complication of chronic HBV and posthepatitic cirrhosis.

Hepatitis D

HDV is an incomplete RNA virus (viroid) that requires HBV for its own replication. Infection with these two viruses can occur simultaneously (*coinfection*), or the HDV infection may occur as a *superinfection*, following a pre-existing HBV infection. Coinfection produces symptoms that are indistinguishable from HBV hepatitis, although the symptoms may be more prominent and there is a greater likelihood of fulminant hepatic necrosis. Superinfection of asymptomatic HBV carriers may activate the disease, and in those with active chronic hepatitis, progression to cirrhosis may be accelerated. HDV infection is best documented by demonstrating antibodies to HDV. The HDV antigen appears only briefly in the blood, so it is impractical to search for it.

Hepatitis C

HCV, a flavivirus, is an RNA virus of variable size (30 to 60 nm) that encodes a single polypeptide, which, upon post-translational cleavage, gives rise to the typical HCV proteins. Antibodies to these proteins are used to diagnose HCV infection.

HCV infections are acquired by blood transfusion or sexual contact. In times before the antibody test to HCV became available, HCV caused 90 percent of all cases of post-transfusion hepatitis. Nevertheless, more than 50 percent of those with antibodies to HCV have no history of blood transfusion or any intimate contact with another HCV-infected person. It is not known how these patients became infected.

The clinical presentation of HCV infection is indistinguishable from that of HBV infection. Generally, however, the disease is less severe. It is often anicteric, and it is commonly associated with mild abnormalities in laboratory test results. Despite the mild course associated with the acute infection, HCV

Did You Know?

Hepatitis viruses are the most common cause of jaundice in clinical practice. Do not neglect to ask a jaundiced patient whether he or she has recently traveled abroad (HAV) or had a blood transfusion from or sexual intercourse with an unknown person (HBV and HCV). Information regarding drug use should also be elicited for two reasons: jaundice could be drug- induced, or it could also be the result of a viral infection transmitted by shared hypodermic needles.

has a tendency to progress to chronic hepatitis in 50 percent of affected individuals, many of whom develop cirrhosis. Hepatocellular carcinoma develops in some persons as a late complication. Some estimates indicate that as many as one half of all patients with HCV-related cirrhosis develop cancer, but such claims have not yet been documented.

Hepatitis E

Hepatitis E virus (HEV) is an RNA virus transmitted by the fecal-oral route. The virus is endemic in parts of Asia, Africa, and South America, and even as close to the United States as Mexico. It tends to cause water-borne epidemics, especially during the rainy season. HEV resembles HAV in many aspects. The infection is usually asymptomatic or mild and transient. It heals without serious consequences. Chronic hepatitis and chronic carrier states do not develop following HEV infection, and the virus does not promote liver carcinogenesis. For unknown reasons, HEV infection during pregnancy has a poor prognosis, and up to 20 percent of acutely infected pregnant women develop fulminant hepatic necrosis.

Pathology. All hepatitis viruses produce similar changes in the liver. It is, therefore, impossible to distinguish one viral infection from another on the basis of histologic findings, although certain features occur more often in some infections than in others, and certain lesions do not develop in some forms of viral hepatitis. For example, HAV and HEV infections do not cause chronic hepatitis, and cirrhosis does not develop in affected individuals.

Hepatitis viruses are hepatotropic and invade liver cells, damaging them and disrupting their normal functions. This process is usually associated with obvious morphologic changes, which are evident on histologic examination of liver biopsy specimens (Fig. 11-6). These changes include the following:

- *Reversible hepatocellular changes.* Affected liver cells have normal nuclei and a well-preserved cell membrane, but show cytoplasmic changes, such as granularity, or vacuolization ("ballooning degeneration"). Intracellular and intercellular bile stasis may be prominent.
- *Irreversible hepatocellular changes.* Necrotic liver cells lose their nuclei and are transformed into round, anuclear, cytoplasmic fragments called eosinophilic or Councilman bodies. In many instances, the necrotic cells cannot be identified because they are phagocytized by scavenger cells.
- *Inflammatory infiltrates.* Damaged and dead liver cells are phagocytized by macrophages that invade the liver lobule, forming small foci within the disrupted strands of liver cells. Kupffer cells

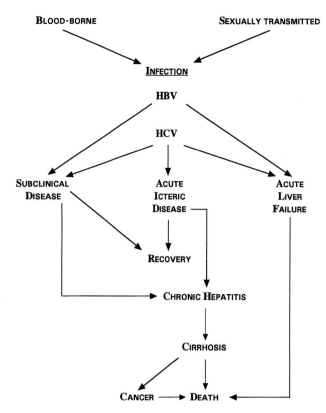

FIGURE 11-6
Outcome of hepatitis B and C virus infections.

also proliferate, and enlarged polymorphonuclear leukocytes (PMNs) are not seen in acute viral hepatitis.

- *Regeneration of hepatocytes.* Liver cells have a high capacity for regeneration, and any loss is usually accompanied by regeneration, which occurs at random. The newly formed liver cells are relatively smaller and have more basophilic cytoplasms.

Acute hepatitis may resolve without any consequences or, in a small number of patients with HBV and HCV infections, it may progress to *chronic hepatitis.*

Histologically, chronic hepatitis may be classified as mild, moderate, or severe. Mild inflammation is limited to the portal tracts. There is very little, if any, intralobular inflammation. In chronic carriers of HBV, the cytoplasm of scattered liver cells appears finely granular, like ground glass, owing to an accumulation of HBsAg. In chronic HVC, the portal tracts usually contain prominent lymphoid infiltrates that obliterate and destroy bile ducts. Severe chronic hepatitis is characterized by disruption of the lobular architecture secondary to an aggressive inflammation that spreads from the portal tracts across the limiting plate into the liver lobule. Necrotic liver cells along the limiting plate of the portal tract are replaced by inflammatory cells and fibrous tissue extending from the portal tracts in between the preserved liver cells. This is called *piecemeal necrosis* or interface hepatitis. The fibrosis that accompanies liver cell necrosis may form connective tissue bridges between portal tracts. This so-called bridging necrosis may progress to cirrhosis.

Cirrhosis

Cirrhosis is a chronic liver disease characterized by a loss of normal liver structure and function. The term cirrhosis is a synonym for end-stage liver disease; it is irreversible and incurable except by liver transplantation. Morphologically, it is characterized by fibrosis and liver cell nodules replacing the normal parenchyma.

Etiology. The most important causes of cirrhosis are listed in Table 11-3. In the United States, cirrhosis is a finding in 5 percent of the autopsies performed in general hospitals or medical examiner's offices. A large number of these cases are related to abuse of alcohol. Alcoholic cirrhosis is the fourth most common cause of death in men 40 to 60 years of age. Viral hepatitis B and C are also important causes of cirrhosis. HCV is currently the most common viral cause of hepatitis in the United States. Recent studies have shown that many alcoholics have been infected with HCV, and in such cases, it would appear that the cirrhosis has a dual etiology. Alcohol abuse and hepatitis virus infections probably account for 65 percent of all cases of cirrhosis in this country. Hereditary metabolic diseases, autoimmune diseases, drugs, and biliary obstruction account for a small number of cases. In approximately 30 percent of cases, the etiology of cirrhosis cannot be established. Such cirrhosis is thus labeled *cryptogenic*.

Pathogenesis. The exact pathogenesis of cirrhosis is not known. It is, however, generally accepted that the main pathologic processes include

- necrosis of liver cells
- repair by fibrosis
- regeneration

Morphologically, there are two basic patterns of cirrhosis: portal cirrhosis and biliary cirrhosis. **Portal cirrhosis** is believed to result from liver cell necrosis followed by an ingrowth of fibrous tissue from the portal tracts (Fig. 11-7). Experimentally, it is possible to produce portal cirrhosis in laboratory rats by treating them with carbon tetrachloride (CCl_4). CCl_4 produces liver cell necrosis, which is repaired by regeneration. Continuous exposure to this toxin impairs the ability of liver cells to regenerate, and parenchymal losses caused by liver cell necrosis are replaced by fibrous scars. With time, the fibrous tissue increases in amount, encircling parts of the remaining liver parenchyma and thus inhibiting its ability to regenerate. This dual repair by regeneration and fibrosis alters the normal architecture of the liver. The liver becomes irregularly shaped, shrunken, firm and nodular. Such pathogenetic mechanisms probably cause the human disease as well, although in the latter, the course might be much more protracted. It takes 10 to 20 years of alcohol abuse before symptoms of cirrhosis develop. Viral hepatitis–induced liver injury requires less time, but on average, cirrhosis secondary to viral hepatitis becomes evident 10 to 15 years after the infection. Occasionally, cirrhosis develops within months or a few years following massive necrotizing hepatitis.

Hereditary inborn errors of metabolism, such as Wilson's disease or alpha$_1$-antitrypsin deficiency, produce cirrhosis over a period of 10 to 20 years. However, because these diseases are congenital, the first signs of liver failure usually appear early (i.e., in the second or third decade of life).

Biliary cirrhosis results from diseases of the biliary tree. It may be primary or secondary. *Primary biliary cirrhosis* is an autoimmune disease affecting the bile ducts. *Secondary biliary cirrhosis* develops following prolonged partial or complete obstruction of bile flow. The obstruction is most often caused by biliary stones in the common bile duct. Such stones may mechanically occlude the duct, or they may cause chronic inflammation and fibrosis that eventually leads to obliteration of the ductal lumen. Other causes of secondary biliary cirrhosis are chronic pancreatitis and tumors of the pancreas and biliary tree. Other, less common causes of bile obstruction have the same effect. For example, in cystic fibrosis, the

Table 11-3 Causes of Cirrhosis

Alcohol
Hepatitis virus (B, C, D)
Hereditary metabolic diseases
Hemochromatosis
Wilson's disease
Alpha$_1$-antitrypsin deficiency
Autoimmune diseases
Primary biliary cirrhosis
Sclerosing cholangitis
Autoimmune (lupoid) hepatitis
Drugs
Biliary obstruction
Cystic fibrosis
Gallstones
Cryptogenic

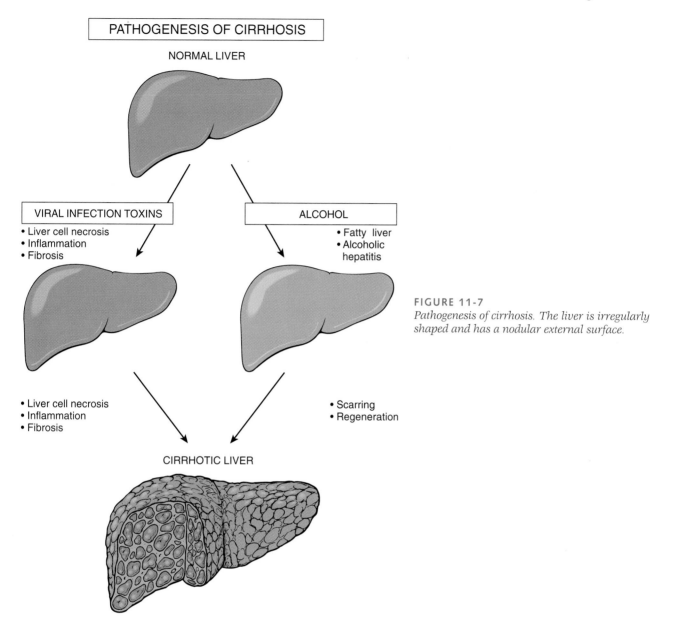

FIGURE 11-7
Pathogenesis of cirrhosis. The liver is irregularly shaped and has a nodular external surface.

viscous mucus plugs inside the bile ducts cause biliary obstruction. Primary sclerosing cholangitis, a disease of unknown etiology characterized by destruction of the larger bile ducts and fibrosis, also leads to secondary biliary cirrhosis. In the tropics, secondary biliary cirrhosis develops as a result of bacterial cholangitis and infections with parasites, such as *Clonorchis sinensis* or *Schistosoma mansoni*.

Chronic bile stasis leads to extravasation of bile inside the liver. Bile destroys liver cells and intrahepatic bile ducts, which are replaced by fibrous strands that separate the liver parenchyma into irregular lobules. Secondary biliary cirrhosis resembles other forms of cirrhosis. However, it is most often associated with bile stasis, which causes yellow or green discoloration of the liver. Clinical symptoms are also similar to those caused by portal cirrhosis, but the lab-

oratory data show prominent signs of biliary obstruction, such as a marked elevation in alkaline phosphatase and conjugated bilirubin levels in the blood.

Pathology. Cirrhosis of the liver can be diagnosed on gross examination at autopsy, during surgical exploration of the abdomen, or by laparoscopy, a procedure that allows inspection of the abdominal organs through a needle-sized optical instrument called a laparoscope. The final diagnosis is made on the basis of histologic findings. In order to make the correct diagnosis, the observer must record the following:

- Size of the liver
- Size and shape of the nodules
- Distribution of the nodules and fibrous scars
- Color of the parenchyma

The cirrhotic liver may be larger or smaller than the normal liver. In cirrhosis secondary to alcohol abuse, hemochromatosis, or autoimmune disorders, the liver is usually enlarged and can be palpated beneath the right costal margin. Massive hepatic necrosis secondary to fulminant hepatitis results in a shrunken liver. In late stages of the disease, all cirrhotic livers tend to be small. Enlargement of a shrunken liver is an ominous sign, and usually heralds the development of hepatocellular carcinoma.

Cirrhosis is termed *micronodular* if the nodules are smaller than 5 mm in diameter and *macronodular* if the nodules are larger than 5 mm. Most often, cirrhosis is of mixed type and contains both small and large nodules. If the nodules are uniformly distributed throughout the entire liver, the cirrhosis is called *regular*. However, if there are large scars alternating with nodules of variable size, the cirrhosis is called *irregular*. Generally speaking, alcoholic cirrhosis is micronodular and regular, whereas postnecrotic cirrhosis secondary to viral infection or drug injury is macronodular and irregular and contains wide scars. Alcoholic cirrhosis is marked by fat accumulation, and the nodules are, therefore, yellow (Fig. 11-8). By contrast, posthepatitic cirrhosis is characterized by brown nodules similar to normal liver. In hemochromatosis, the nodules have a rusty brown appearance ("pigmentary cirrhosis"). In biliary cirrhosis, the nodules may be yellow or green owing to accumulation of bilirubin and biliverdin, respectively.

Histologic findings are diagnostic of cirrhosis, although they rarely provide a reliable clue about the causes of the disease. The normal liver architecture is lost. Instead, the parenchyma consists of liver cells arranged into nodules separated from each other by dense connective tissue strands (Fig. 11-9). The presence of fat in liver cells and alcoholic hyaline (Mallory's bodies) favors the diagnosis of alcoholic cirrho-

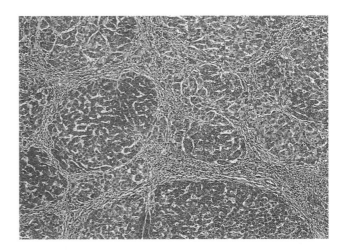

FIGURE 11-9
Histology of cirrhosis. The parenchyma consists of nodules of liver cells surrounded by strands of connective tissue.

sis. The presence of cytoplasmic granules in hepatocytes is a feature of alpha$_1$-antitrypsin deficiency. Iron accumulation favors the diagnosis of hemochromatosis.

Complications. Complications of cirrhosis may be seen in the liver, the abdominal organs, and in extraabdominal sites. Cirrhosis is a progressive disease that relentlessly destroys the liver cells. If the patient does not die of extrahepatic complications, the liver will, in most instances, shrink. Instead of the normal 1500-g liver, autopsy will disclose a small, shriveled liver one third its normal size (weighing 500 to 700 g).

Fibrosis and nodularity of the liver impede blood flow and cause portal hypertension. Portal hypertension has three major anatomic consequences:

- ascites
- splenomegaly
- anastomoses between the portal and systemic circulation

Ascites (from the Greek *askos,* meaning bag) is an accumulation of fluid in the abdominal cavity. As it can also be considered a peritoneal transudate or edema limited to the abdominal cavity, it is also called hydroperitoneum. Ascites develops as a result of the interaction of several mechanisms, the most important of which are portal hypertension and hypoproteinemia (Fig. 11-10). Back pressure in branches of the portal vein results in the transudation of fluid from the serosal surfaces of the intestines, liver, and peritoneal surfaces lining the abdominal cavity. Reduced oncotic pressure of the plasma secondary to hypoalbuminemia facilitates the passage of fluids from the circulation into the abdominal cavity. This results in relative hypovolemia (i.e., reduced volume of circulating blood), which triggers the release of al-

FIGURE 11-8
Alcoholic cirrhosis. The normal liver parenchyma has been replaced by nodules that are yellow because of their high fat content.

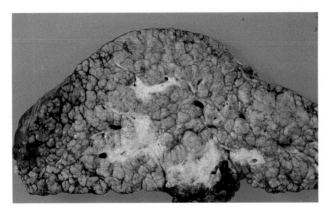

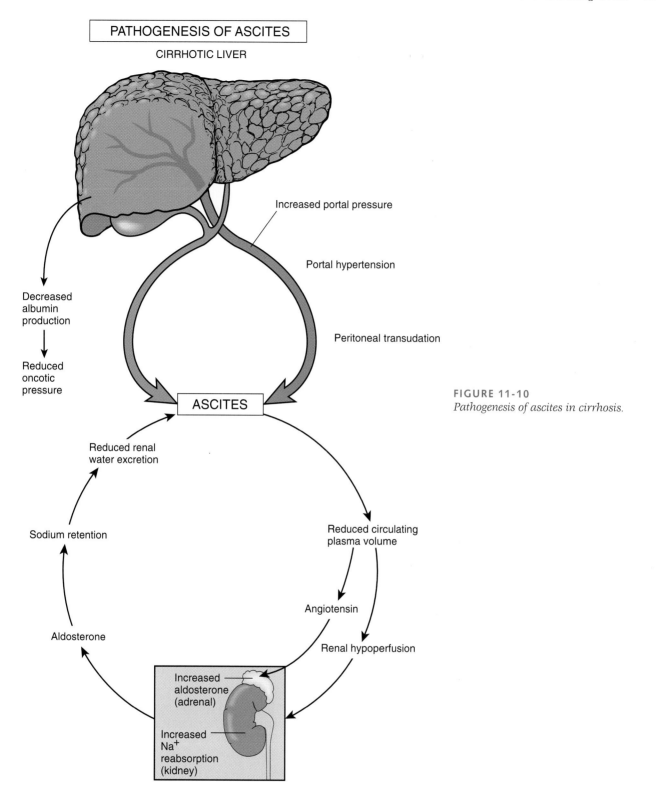

PATHOGENESIS OF ASCITES

CIRRHOTIC LIVER

Increased portal pressure

Portal hypertension

Peritoneal transudation

Decreased albumin production

Reduced oncotic pressure

ASCITES

Reduced renal water excretion

Sodium retention

Aldosterone

Reduced circulating plasma volume

Angiotensin

Renal hypoperfusion

Increased aldosterone (adrenal)

Increased Na$^+$ reabsorption (kidney)

FIGURE 11-10
Pathogenesis of ascites in cirrhosis.

dosterone from the adrenal cortex. Aldosterone acts on the kidneys, causing sodium and water retention, which further compounds the problem. All this adversely affects the kidneys, which eventually stop producing urine. The patient becomes anuric and develops a *hepatorenal syndrome*.

Ascites is resistant to treatment, and drainage of the fluid from the abdominal cavity does not have any beneficial effects. The hepatorenal syndrome is also resistant to treatment, even though the kidneys appear normal and will resume normal function if transplanted to another individual after the death of the patient. Ascites may become infected, which will lead to bacterial peritonitis.

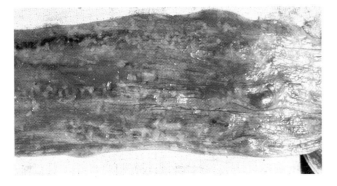

FIGURE 11-11
Esophageal varices. The submucosa of the esophagus contains dilated veins filled with blood.

Splenomegaly is very common in cirrhosis. The spleen, which normally weighs 150 g, enlarges three to six times to a weight of 500 to 1000 g. The affected patient will perceive the enlarged spleen as heavy and painful. The enlarged spleen has a tendency to sequester and destroy blood cells, which results in anemia, leukopenia, or thrombocytopenia. These hematologic consequences are aggravated by *hypersplenism*, a poorly understood syndrome characterized by inhibition of hematopoiesis in the bone marrow.

Anastomoses between the portal and systemic circulation develop as a result of shunting of the portal blood into systemic veins in the lower esophagus, hemorrhoidal plexus, and periumbilical venous plexus. The most important of these vessels are the veins of the lower esophagus, which undergo dilatation and transform into *varices* (Fig. 11-11). Esophageal varices are prone to bleeding, which results in hematemesis or melena. Massive hemorrhage is one of the most common causes of death in patients with cirrhosis.

Shunting of blood from the portal to the systemic circulation is accompanied by serious metabolic consequences and corresponding clinical symptoms. The most important of these is *hepatic encephalopathy*, a syndrome marked by clouded mentation and distinct neurologic symptoms. Cerebral dysfunction is thought to be caused by ammonia and putative neurotoxins absorbed from the intestine. Because the shunts allow the enteric venous blood to bypass the liver, neurotoxic substances are not detoxified and, therefore, act directly on susceptible cells in the brain. The diseased brain shows edema and altered astrocytes, but no other morphologic changes that would explain the pathogenesis of neurologic symptoms. Hepatic coma is associated with a high mortality rate, and the patient's life can be saved only by emergency liver transplantation.

Clinical Features. The diagnosis of cirrhosis is made on the basis of clinical findings, but it must be confirmed by laboratory studies and liver biopsy. Associated symptoms and findings reflect the following:

- *Liver cell injury and necrosis.* This is usually marked by an elevation in serum liver enzymes. ALT and AST levels are the best markers of liver cell injury.
- *Loss of liver cell function.* Decreased output of albumin leads to hypoalbuminemia, which contributes to the formation of ascites and edema. Decreased synthesis of coagulation proteins results in a bleeding tendency. Defective excretion of bilirubin may result in jaundice, which is usually mild.
- *Portal hypertension.* The principal consequences of portal hypertension are ascites, splenomegaly, and anastomoses between the portal and systemic circulation (which tend to bleed). The blood from ruptured esophageal varices is a major source of ammonia. Ammonia formed from degraded blood proteins is absorbed in the intestines and, thus, contributes to hepatic encephalopathy.

In addition to these most important signs of cirrhosis, affected patients also have numerous other symptoms involving the cardiorespiratory, renal,

Did You Know?

Ascites causes bulging of the anterior abdominal wall. Portal hypertension may be associated with dilated periumbilical veins, known in the medical literature as caput medusae (i.e., Medusa's head). In Greek mythology, Medusa was a woman who had snakes emanating from her head instead of hair. The tortuous veins on the abdomen reminded a literary physician of Medusa's head. The term is still used, although the comparison with snakes is a bit far-fetched. (Photograph courtesy of Dr. Olav Hilmar Iversen. From Basic Text in Pathology, Universitetsforlaget, Oslo, Norway, 1974.)

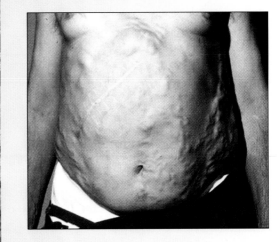

endocrine, and hematopoietic systems. Ascites and secondary hyperaldosteronism and hypernatremia cause a fluid overload, with consequent *cardiopulmonary failure* and *pulmonary edema*. Hypoperfusion of the kidneys and sodium retention secondary to the action of aldosterone may precipitate renal failure (*hepatorenal syndrome*). Endocrine symptoms, such as *impotence* or *gynecomastia* in males, and *anovulation* in females, reflect abnormal metabolism of sex hormones. *Osteodystrophy* is related to abnormal vitamin D metabolism and calcium homeostasis, whereas *hypothyroidism* may result from a deficiency of thyroid hormone–binding protein and abnormal metabolism of thyroglobulins. *Anemia* is very common in cirrhosis, owing in part to a subnormal supply of metabolites from the liver, and in part to splenomegaly.

Cirrhosis has an unfavorable prognosis, and unless a liver transplantation is performed, all affected patients die 5 to 15 years after diagnosis. After the onset of ascites, only 20 percent of affected patients survive 5 years. The others die of massive esophageal bleeding from esophageal varices, hepatic encephalopathy, hepatorenal syndrome, or complex metabolic disturbances.

Drug- and Toxin-Induced Liver Diseases

The liver is the primary site for the metabolic conversion and inactivation of drugs and various toxins. In this process, the liver cells may be injured by the chemical that is metabolized or by the toxic derivatives formed inside the liver cells. For example, carbon tetrachloride, a chemical component of brass polish and a cause of accidental poisoning in children, is metabolized into carbon trichloride, a toxic radical that may cause liver cell necrosis, as discussed in Chapter 1.

Drug reactions can be classified either as *predictable* (those that are dose-related) or *unpredictable* (those that occur without obvious explanation) (Table 11-4). An example of the former can be found in the pain-killer acetaminophen (Tylenol). This drug, which occasionally is ingested in suicide attempts, always produces liver necrosis if ingested in a dose exceeding 15 g. Likewise, tetracycline, an antibiotic widely used for acne, invariably produces fatty changes in liver cells, fortunately without any serious consequences. Predictable liver cell injury can be prevented by avoiding the possibly toxic substance.

Unpredictable drug reactions can take place in any setting and can induce a variety of histologic changes. In some sensitive persons, the anesthetic halothane will induce an acute febrile jaundice resembling that associated with acute hepatitis. Isoni-

Table 11-4 Drug-Induced Liver Disease

Pathology	Drug
Predictable (Dose-Related) Reaction	
Necrosis	Acetaminophen
Fatty changes	Tetracycline
Unpredictable Reaction	
Viral hepatitis-like changes	Halothane
Cholestasis	Chlorpromazine
Chronic hepatitis-like changes	Methyldopa
Granuloma	Phenylbutazone
Tumor	Estrogens

azid, used for the treatment of tuberculosis, is a well-known cause of a mild hepatitis–like disease that most often occurs in older persons. Chlorpromazine, a psychoactive drug, occasionally causes intrahepatic bile stasis and conjugated hyperbilirubinemia. Methyldopa, used for the treatment of Parkinson's disease, may induce chronic hepatitis–like changes. Phenylbutazone, an anti-inflammatory drug used for arthritis, may induce granulomas. Estrogens (and even oral contraceptives) appear to promote formation of liver cell tumors. Today, in the era of "minipills" that contain small amounts of estrogen, such hormone-induced tumors are rare. Furthermore, most of the reported tumors are benign (liver cell adenomas).

Alcoholic Liver Disease

Alcohol is an important cause of liver diseases. Chronic alcohol abuse may cause the following hepatic lesions:

- Fatty liver
- Alcoholic hepatitis
- Cirrhosis

Alcohol is imbibed in large quantities in most Western countries, primarily because of its mind-altering effects. However, it is also an important source of calories (7 calories per gram) and has complex metabolic and potentially toxic effects on many cells in the body. Alcohol affects the liver, inhibiting some enzymes and stimulating others, as discussed in Chapter 1. It also alters the fluidity and function of cell membranes, as well as the intracellular transport of organelles and metabolites. Because of increased fatty acid synthesis, decreased fatty acid oxidation, and decreased export of fats in the form of lipoproteins, alcohol invariably produces fatty changes in liver cells in a dose-dependent manner. The liver becomes enlarged, but without any metabolic consequences or symptoms. These changes are completely reversible, disappearing after the patient stops drinking.

A small number of patients with alcoholic fatty liver (10 percent to 15 percent) develop signs of *alcoholic hepatitis*. These signs usually include fever, leukocytosis, abdominal pain, and jaundice. Histologic examination of the liver shows fatty change of hepatocytes, as well as focal necrosis of liver cells associated with leukocytic infiltrates and bile stasis. The cytoplasm of hepatocytes often contains eosinophilic aggregates of intermediate cytoskeletal filaments, which form so-called alcoholic hyaline or Mallory's bodies (Fig. 11-12).

Cirrhosis is the most serious complication of alcohol abuse. It is not known why some alcoholics develop cirrhosis whereas others do not. In some cases,

it is preceded by alcoholic hepatitis. In others, it may be attributable to the additive effects of alcohol and other toxins or viruses. In most instances, it is not possible to sort out all the factors that contribute to the progression of the disease, particularly if the cirrhosis evolves insidiously over a long period of time.

As stated earlier, alcoholic cirrhosis does not differ clinically from other forms of cirrhosis. However, certain morphologic features occur more often in alcoholic cirrhosis than in cirrhosis caused by other toxins or viruses. The best telltale sign of an alcohol abuser is fatty liver change, which contributes to the enlargement of the liver and imparts a yellow, greasy appearance to the liver on gross examination. The histologic findings of fat droplets and Mallory's bodies in liver cells also provide supportive evidence of alcohol abuse. However, as many other hepatic diseases can present with similar changes, the diagnosis of al-

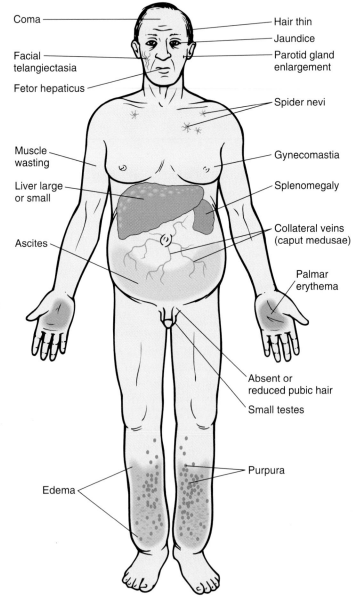

FIGURE 11-12
Clinical features of cirrhosis.

coholic liver disease can be made only in the appropriate setting, taking into consideration the patient's personal history and a documented intake of alcohol.

Hereditary Diseases of the Liver

Essentially all **hereditary metabolic diseases** affect the liver. However, the symptoms of liver cell injury are usually overshadowed by symptoms pertaining to other organs. Only a few examples of hereditary diseases that present primarily as hepatic disorders or induce significant changes in the liver are presented here. These hepatic lesions may vary from mild to severe.

Gilbert's Disease

Gilbert's disease is an autosomal dominant disorder of bilirubin metabolism that affects about 5 percent of the total population. The disease causes intermittent jaundice that usually begins after puberty and that is most common in male subjects. Unconjugated hyperbilirubinemia, which is typical of this disorder, reflects a defect in the uptake of bilirubin from blood into liver cells. The nature of the enzyme defect that causes this hereditary jaundice is not known. Except for jaundice, these patients have no other symptoms and thus require no treatment.

Hemochromatosis

Hereditary **hemochromatosis** is an autosomal recessive defect of iron absorption that results in excessive accumulation of iron in the liver and several other organs. This accumulation of iron stores, which can be increased by up to 50 times the normal level, damages liver cells and induces cirrhosis. The cirrhotic liver is typically enlarged, heavy, and micronodular. Because of the rusty red-brown appearance of the tissue, it is often called pigmentary cirrhosis. Excess amounts of the iron pigment hemosiderin can be demonstrated in the liver by the Prussian blue histochemical reaction.

The gene for hemochromatosis is extremely prevalent. Approximately 10 percent of the general population are heterozygous and 0.4 percent are homozygous for this gene. However, the symptoms occur in only a small proportion of homozygous persons. In addition to cirrhosis, they show pigmentation of the skin and diabetes mellitus, a combination of symptoms referred to as "bronze diabetes." Other endocrine organs may also be affected, and congestive heart failure is a common cause of death. The diagnosis of hemochromatosis is established by demonstrating a high concentration of iron in the blood, high saturation of *transferrin* (the main iron transport

protein of the plasma), and the presence of iron deposits in the cirrhotic liver. Therapy for hereditary hemochromatosis is directed at reducing the iron stores, which is best accomplished by blood-letting. Weekly phlebotomies have a most beneficial effect and significantly prolong the lives of these patients.

Wilson's Disease

Wilson's disease, also known as hepatolenticular degeneration, is an autosomal recessive disorder of copper metabolism that produces lesions in the liver, brain, and eye. Heterozygotes are found at a rate of 1 percent, but the disease, which occurs only in homozygotic persons, has a much lower prevalence (3 per 100,000 persons).

The gene for Wilson's disease has been identified, but the mechanisms underlying the disease remain obscure. It is thought that the defect lies in the inability of liver cells to excrete copper in bile. As this is the primary means for preventing copper overload, the defect results in excessive copper storage in the liver. The concentration of the copper carrier protein *ceruloplasmin* is also decreased in serum, which leads to compensatory binding of copper to albumin. This albumin-bound copper has a tendency to precipitate in the brain and the eyes.

The symptoms of Wilson's disease may be related to the toxic effect of copper, which is deposited in the liver, the eyes, or the brain. In the liver, excess copper causes cirrhosis. This form of cirrhosis has an early onset, and may even be diagnosed in children. Additional findings include Kayser-Fleischer ring of the eye, which appears as a brownish discoloration of the iris; reddish-brown discoloration and degeneration of striatum and closely related basal ganglia of the brain; and acute hemolytic episodes. Wilson's disease can be treated with chelating (metal binding) agents, like D-penicillamine, which bind copper and remove it from the body. Chelating agents can be used not only to prevent the disease, but also to alleviate symptoms in patients who have already developed signs of copper toxicity.

Alpha$_1$-Antitrypsin Deficiency

Alpha$_1$-antitrypsin (α_1-AT) **deficiency** is an autosomal recessive disorder that is related to the presence of the PiZ allele of the gene that encodes for α_1-AT. As mentioned in Chapter 8 on the lung, this mutation of the Pi gene is found in about 5 percent of the population, and in homozygous PiZ mutants, it may cause emphysema and cirrhosis of the liver. α_1-AT is synthesized in the liver; in PiZ homozygotes, it accumulates in the form of cytoplasmic globules inside the liver cells. The exact mechanism for liver cell injury is not known. A significant number of affected persons develop childhood cholestasis and chronic hepatitis, which progress to cirrhosis in about 20 percent of affected individuals.

α_1-AT deficiency is one of the most common causes of childhood cirrhosis, which has a high mortality. Children who survive are at a great risk for the development of liver cell cancer.

Immune Disorders

An immunologic origin has been proposed for several liver diseases, including autoimmune (lupoid) hepatitis, primary biliary cirrhosis, and primary sclerosing cholangitis, although it has not been conclusively proven that any liver disease is primarily an immune disorder. The features of these three diseases are summarized in Table 11-5.

Autoimmune Hepatitis

Autoimmune or **lupoid hepatitis** is a form of chronic hepatitis. It is thought to be immune-mediated because, like systemic lupus erythematosus, it is associated with other autoimmune phenomena. The disease predominantly affects young women and is serologically characterized by antinuclear antibodies and other autoantibodies (e.g., to smooth muscle cells and even mitochondria). Clinically and pathologically, the disease resembles other forms of chronic hepatitis, but has a more favorable diagnosis. It responds very well to steroid treatment.

Primary Biliary Cirrhosis

Primary biliary cirrhosis (PBC) is a disease of unknown etiology that is characterized by destruction of intrahepatic bile ducts and progression to cirrho-

sis. This "nonsuppurative destructive cholangitis," as it is also known, resembles the T-cell–mediated destruction of bile ducts associated with hepatic transplants and the graft-versus-host disease that often follows bone marrow transplantation. Hence, it has been proposed that PBC is an immune disease mediated by type IV hypersensitivity reactions. The appearance of T lymphocytes within the lesions and the formation of granulomas also suggest that the disease is a cellular immune response, but the nature of the antigen evoking this response remains unknown. Most patients also have antibodies to mitochondria. Although this could mean that the humoral immune system is involved, the appearance of antibodies could be secondary to tissue destruction and, therefore, of limited pathogenetic significance.

PBC predominantly affects women (the ratio of females to males is 9:1). The disease begins as an inflammation of the intrahepatic bile ducts. Infiltrates of lymphocytes and macrophages subsequently destroy the bile ducts (Fig. 11-13). Occasionally, the portal tracts also contain granulomas. The destruction of bile ducts is accompanied by intrahepatic cholestasis and fibrosis, which ultimately leads to cirrhosis.

Clinically, biliary cirrhosis has an insidious onset. It affects middle-aged women who present with nonspecific symptoms, such as fatigue and loss of appetite. Itching related to jaundice, enlargement of the liver, and biochemical signs of liver disease are prominent features. The diagnosis is confirmed by demonstrating antimitochondrial antibodies and by liver biopsy findings. Other immunologic findings may also be present, and many women have signs of some other immune disorder, such as mild hemolytic anemia, atrophic gastritis, and thyroiditis. As the bile duct destruction proceeds, obstructive jaundice become more pronounced, the stools become

Table 11-5 Liver Diseases of Presumptive Immune Origin

	Autoimmune (Lupoid) Hepatitis	Primary Biliary Cirrhosis	Primary Sclerosing Cholangitis
Sex predominance	Females	Females	Males
Age (years)	20–30	30–60	20–40
Bile duct lesions			
Intrahepatic	+/–	+ +	+
Extrahepatic	–	–	+ +
Hepatitis (intralobular)	+/–	+/–	–
Antibodies to:			
Mitochondria	–/+	+ +	–
Nuclear antigens	+ +	+/–	–
Smooth muscle	+ +	–	–
Steroid therapy	+ +	–	–

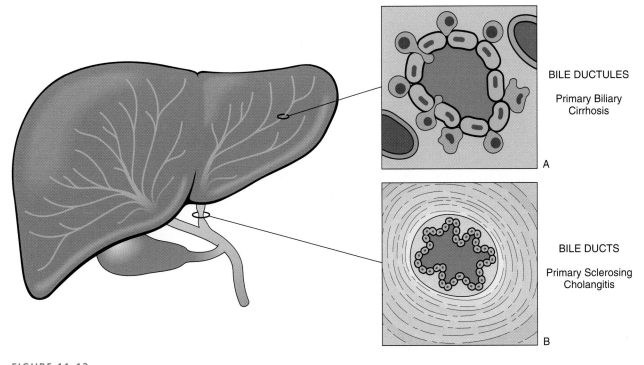

FIGURE 11-13
Primary biliary cirrhosis and primary sclerosing cholangitis. (A) Primary biliary cirrhosis leads to destruction of intrahepatic ductules. (B) Primary sclerosing cholangitis constricts extrahepatic and intrahepatic ducts.

acholic, and steatorrhea develops. Biliary obstruction impedes the excretion of cholesterol, which is often deposited in the subcutaneous connective tissue in the form of small yellow nodules called *xanthomas* (from the Greek *xanthos*, meaning yellow). These are not true neoplasms, but rather infiltrates of macrophages loaded with lipid. Ultimately, affected patients develop cirrhosis, which is lethal unless a suitable donor is found for liver transplantation.

Primary Sclerosing Cholangitis

Primary sclerosing cholangitis is a disease of unknown origin that also may have an immune pathogenesis. In contrast to PCB, it primarily affects young males. The associated destruction of intrahepatic and extrahepatic bile ducts by lymphocytes and macrophages is consistent with a cell-mediated immune reaction, but the original antigen inciting the cellular infiltrates remains obscure. The cellular phase of the disease is followed by fibrosis that obliterates the bile ducts inside and outside the liver (see Figure 11-13). The disease is typically segmental; therefore, the larger bile ducts appear to be beaded and composed of alternating narrowed fibrotic and dilated segments. Similar, if not identical, changes occur as a complication of ulcerative colitis and Crohn's disease, and many patients show evidence of other immune disorders. Ultimately, the disease causes ob-

structive jaundice and secondary biliary cirrhosis. Cholangiocellular carcinoma develops from affected bile ducts in 10 percent of patients. The overall prognosis of primary sclerosing cholangitis is unfavorable, but liver transplantation may save the life of an affected patient.

Bacterial, Protozoal, and Parasitic Infections

The liver is resistant to bacterial infections, presumably because of the protective role of phagocytic Kupffer cells. Thus, all infections except viral hepatitis are rare in the United States. Bacterial, protozoal, and parasitic pathogens may reach the liver by

- *an ascending route*, via the bile ducts, from the duodenum (typical of *ascending bacterial cholangitis*)
- *blood flowing to the hepatic artery or portal vein*, causing portal vein infection, also known as *pylephlebitis*
- *direct inoculation* (as in wounds)
- *direct extension* from adjacent abdominal organs or from a perihepatic or subphrenic (subdiaphragmatic) abscess

Ascending cholangitis is most often caused by gram-negative enteric organisms, such as *Escherichia coli*, Proteus, and *Streptococcus fecalis*. Most protozoal

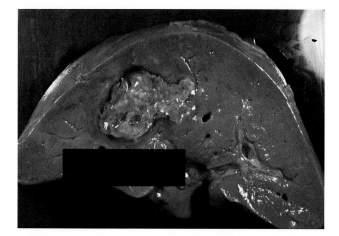

FIGURE 11-14
Amebic abscess. This cavitary lesion contains yellow, paste-like material.

infections are caused by *Entamoeba histolytica. S. mansoni, S. japonicum, O. sinensis,* and *Echinococcus granulosus.* These are parasites that infect millions of persons in tropical countries and the Far East, but are uncommon in the United States. For reasons that are not entirely clear, all such infections occur more commonly in males than in females. Infections usually promote suppuration, but the pus remains localized to bile ducts or encapsulated within hepatic parenchyma in the form of abscesses.

Cholangitic abscesses of the liver may be solitary or multiple. Most of these are associated with biliary obstruction caused by ascending infection with enteric bacteria. *E. coli* and other aerobic and anaerobic bacteria are easily cultured from the pus, but in 25 percent of patients, the fluid appears sterile and no bacteria can be isolated, presumably because of their removal by phagocytic liver cells.

Pylephlebitic abscesses (i.e., those that develop owing to the entry of bacteria into the liver through the portal vein) may be solitary or multiple. In the preantibiotic era, pylephlebitic abscesses of the liver were common complications of acute appendicitis. Today, they are less common, usually affecting patients with inflammatory bowel disease or infected diverticula of the sigmoid colon.

Amebic abscess is a tropical disease (Fig. 11-14). It is almost invariably a complication of intestinal infection with *E. histolytica* that reaches the liver through the portal circulation. Treatment with amebicidal drugs yields excellent results.

Cholelithiasis (Gallstones)

Gallstones—concretions composed of chemicals normally formed in bile—are extremely common. In the United States, more than half a million people undergo biliary surgery for gallstones each year. An estimated 20 percent of people older than 65 years of age have gallstones. Women are especially at risk, as the incidence of gallstones is three times higher in women than in men. Because of some metabolic deficiency, Native Americans, such as Pima Indians, are at an extremely high risk for developing gallstones. Indeed, 75 percent of the women in this population develop gallstones by the age of 25 years. The incidence of gallstones is higher in whites than in blacks, which further underscores the genetic predisposition for this disease.

Pathogenesis. There are two types of gallstones: cholesterol stones and pigmentary stones. More than 75 percent of the gallstones that develop in patients in the United States are cholesterol stones, whereas the remainder are either brown or black pigmentary stones (Table 11-6). Each of these stones is formed as a result of a distinct mechanism, although it is not uncommon to have mixed stones, which shows that these pathogenetic mechanisms may be interrelated.

Cholesterol stones are formed in bile that is supersaturated with cholesterol and, at the same time, contains decreased amounts of bile acids and lecithin. Bile acids and lecithin are secreted together by the liver cells, but independently of cholesterol. In the gallbladder, these substances form water-soluble micelles with cholesterol. These micelles form only if the three substances are present in appropriate concentrations. If the normal ratio of bile components is altered, the bile becomes *lithogenic* (i.e., capable of stone formation). This occurs typically in obese persons who excrete large amounts of cholesterol in the bile, but also may occur in patients with certain metabolic disorders, such as diabetes. Pregnancy, estrogen therapy, use of oral contraceptives, and certain drugs used for the treatment of hypercholesterolemia, such as clofibrate, also promote cholesterol excretion in the bile. Such bile is prone to accelerated nucleation of cholesterol crystals, which is most apparent during the concentration of bile in the gallbladder. The slower bile flow that occurs with age also predisposes such individuals to gallstone formation. It is thus understandable that most cholesterol gallstones are located in the gallbladder, and that the typical risk factors include the so-called four Fs: **f**emale, older than **f**orty, **f**ertile, and **f**at.

Pigmentary stones are composed of calcium bilirubinate and are either black or brown. The *black stones,* which are most common in Western countries, also contain bilirubin polymers, calcium phosphate and carbonate, and glycoproteins. These stones form in the gallbladders of patients with chronic hemolytic anemia (e.g., sickle cell anemia) and those with cirrhosis. In such patients, the stones form presumably because of supersaturation of bile

Table 11-6 Types of Gallstones

| | Cholesterol | Pigmentary | |
		Black	Brown
Major components	Cholesterol	Calcium bilirubin	Calcium bilirubin
		Cholesterol	Calcium salts
		Calcium soaps	Glycoproteins
Location	Gallbladder	Gallbladder	Bile ducts
Incidence in the U.S.	75%	20%	5% (more common in Far East)
Shape/pattern	Solitary, round	Multiple, faceted	Multiple, irregularly shaped
Radiopaque	30%	>50%	10%
Risk factor(s)	Female	Hemolysis	Infection
	Obese	Cirrhosis	
	Fertile	(Most have no risk factors)	
	Older than 40 years of age		

with bilirubin. Indeed, most patients with black gallstones excrete increased amounts of unconjugated bilirubin in bile. The reasons for the hypersecretion of unconjugated bilirubin are not clear.

Brown stones are often laminated and consist of alternating layers of calcium bilirubinate and cholesterol admixed with calcium soaps. These stones occur more commonly in individuals living in the Far East than in those from the West, and are often associated with biliary infections or infestations with liver flukes, such as *O. sinensis*. Brown stones are most often located in the extrahepatic bile ducts and tend to recur after removal. It is believed that these stones form as a result of the action of bacteria and parasites, which change the biochemical composition of bile.

Pathology. Cholesterol stones are typically solitary, measure 1 to 5 cm in diameter, and are round, yellow, and firm. On cross-sectioning, they have a glistening, radiating, crystalline appearance. Black pigmentary stones, which measure 5 to 10 mm in diameter, are multiple, jet black, ovoid or polygonal, and often faceted (Fig. 11-15). They are soft and can be crushed between the fingers. Brown pigmentary stones are irregularly shaped and vary in size from 1 to 3 cm. On cross-sectioning, they are often laminated (i.e., they show darker and lighter layers around a central core).

The gallbladder harboring the stones usually shows signs of inflammation (cholecystitis). This develops because the gallstones may mechanically injure the mucosa, allowing entry of enteric bacteria into the wall of the gallbladder. Acute cholecystitis may evolve into a chronic inflammation. Severe infection, especially if associated with obstruction of

the biliary outflow tract, may cause *gangrene of the gallbladder*. The necrotic wall of the gangrenous gallbladder may then rupture, leading to bacterial peritonitis. Alternatively, the inflamed serosa of the gallbladder may stimulate adhesion with the intestinal loops and the formation of a *cholecystoenteric fistula*. This fistula may serve as a conduit through which the gallstones may be discharged into the intestine. Obstruction of the intestine with gallstone causes *gallstone ileus*.

Chronic obstruction of the cystic duct will interrupt the normal circulation of bile through the gallbladder. Bile in an obstructed gallbladder may become resorbed and may be replaced with clear, watery fluid by a process called *hydrops of the gallbladder*. If the hydrops persists, the wall of the nonfunctioning gallbladder may become thickened and fibrotic, and ultimately will undergo dystrophic calcification (also called *porcelain gallbladder*).

The obstruction of the cystic ducts prevents normal flow of bile into and out of the gallbladder, but

FIGURE 11-15
Gallstones.

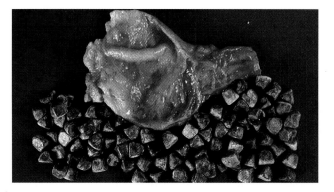

does not affect the flow of hepatic bile into the intestine. Gallstones forming in the common bile duct or small gallbladder stones that are discharged through the cystic duct may obstruct the common bile duct and produce obstructive jaundice. Approximately 50 percent of all cases of extrahepatic jaundice are attributable to gallstones in the common bile duct. Long-standing obstruction of the common bile duct may cause secondary biliary cirrhosis. Gallstones also predispose individuals to ascending infections of the biliary tract and are well-known causes of ascending bacterial cholangitis. Gallbladders that are removed to treat cholelithiasis occasionally contain cancerous lesions, but these are rare, and there is no proof of a pathogenetic link between gallstones and cancer.

Clinical Features. Most gallstones are asymptomatic or produce minor nonspecific symptoms that require no treatment. Many gallstones are incidentally discovered during routine x-ray examination; indeed, only 20 percent of all patients with gallstones present with clinical symptoms, which are usually related to cholecystitis, or obstruction of the cystic duct or the common bile duct (Fig. 11-16).

Histologic signs of chronic cholecystitis are found in almost all gallbladders that contain stones. Such cases of chronic cholecystitis usually are associated with only minor discomfort. Obstruction of the cystic duct is typically associated with smooth muscle cell contraction and bouts of excruciating spasmodic pain (*colic*). Obstruction of the cystic duct may lead to exacerbation of cholecystitis, and also to reinfection. Such cases of superimposed acute cholecystitis usually present with fever.

The gallstones released into the common bile duct or those formed in the major ducts may obstruct the bile flow from the liver and cause *jaundice*. These stones also predispose the affected individual to ascending cholangitis.

The diagnosis of gallstones, suggested by the typical symptoms of obstruction of bile flow and biliary colic, is usually confirmed by x-ray studies. Gallstones that contain radiopaque calcium salts can be seen on plain x-ray films. Approximately 30 percent of cholesterol stones and more than 50 percent of black stones can be seen on plain x-ray studies. The remaining gallstones cannot be seen on routine radiographs and are best visualized by ultrasonography.

The treatment of gallstones may take several forms. Asymptomatic gallstones usually do not require treatment, whereas acute impaction and biliary colic require prompt treatment with antispasmodic and analgesic drugs. Biliary stones may be removed surgically or dissolved by extracorporeal shock wave therapy (*lithotripsy*). Recently, good results have been reported for the chemical dissolution of stones with appropriate drugs.

Hepatobiliary Neoplasms

The primary tumors of the liver may be benign or malignant (Table 11-7). *Benign tumors* of the liver and the biliary tract are of limited clinical significance. The most common tumor is *cavernous hemangioma*, which is present in 5 percent of livers at autopsy. These hemangiomas are usually small (less than 2 cm in diameter) and cause no symptoms.

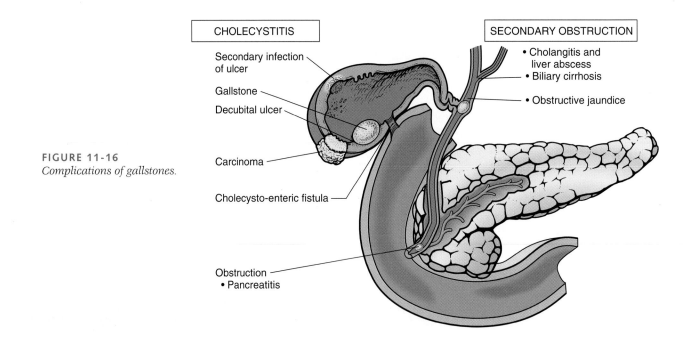

FIGURE 11-16
Complications of gallstones.

CHOLECYSTITIS

Secondary infection of ulcer

Gallstone

Decubital ulcer

Carcinoma

Cholecysto-enteric fistula

Obstruction
• Pancreatitis

SECONDARY OBSTRUCTION

• Cholangitis and liver abscess
• Biliary cirrhosis

• Obstructive jaundice

Table 11-7 Primary Hepatobiliary Neoplasms

Tumor	Incidence	Risk Factors	Markers
Liver cell adenoma	F:M = 9:1 Rare	Oral contraceptive use	—
Hepatocellular carcinoma	M:F = 5:1 Rare in USA/Europe Common in Asia/Africa	Cirrhosis, HBV, HCV, hemo-chromatosis, α_1-antitrypsin deficiency	AFP
Cholangiocellular carcinoma	M:F = 5:1 Rare in USA Common in China	*Opisthorchis sinensis* infection Primary sclerosing cholangitis	NS (CEA)
Gallbladder carcinoma	F:M = 2:1 Rare in USA Common in Pima Indians and Mexicans F:M = 4:1	Cholelithiasis	NS (CEA)

F:M, female:male ratio; M:F, male:female ratio; AFP, alpha-fetoprotein; NS, nonspecific; CEA, Carcinoembryonic antigen.

Benign *hepatocellular adenomas* are tumors composed of cells resembling normal hepatocytes. These tumors appear almost exclusively in women, which suggests that the female sex hormones may play an important pathogenetic role. Indeed, more than 90 percent of all hepatocellular adenomas have been diagnosed in women taking oral contraceptives. In view of the widespread use of oral contraceptives and the fact that only 1 in 20,000 of these women will develop a benign liver tumor, one must postulate that some additional factors play a role in tumorigenesis. For unknown reasons, these hepatocellular adenomas are highly vascular and tend to bleed, sometimes profusely; if not recognized and treated, they can cause death secondary to exsanguination.

Malignant tumors can originate in liver cells, bile ducts, the gallbladder, and Kupffer cells (see Fig. 11-7). *Hepatocellular carcinomas* are the most important primary liver tumors, causing more than 1 million deaths worldwide. In the United States and Western countries, these tumors have an incidence of 5 per 100,000 and account for 2 percent of cancer deaths. By contrast, the incidence is 100 per 100,000 in the Far East and Africa and other parts of the world in which HBV is endemic. *Gallbladder cancer* is less common worldwide than hepatocellular cancer, and in the United States accounts for 1 percent of all cancer deaths. Tumors involving the intrahepatic bile ducts are even less common, representing only 1 percent of all hepatobiliary tumors. *Kupffer cell sarcomas* are extremely rare, although a mini-epidemic of Kupffer cell sarcoma was reported in the 1970s among vinylchloride workers in the rubber tire industry, suggesting that vinylchloride may have been the causative carcinogen. Except for this historical episode, though, Kupffer cell sarcomas are of limited practical significance.

Hepatocellular Carcinoma

Hepatocellular carcinoma is a highly malignant tumor composed of neoplastic liver cells. The tumor occurs in adults and has a male predominance. The male to female ratio is 5:1. Most tumors originate in cirrhotic livers. The highest incidence of cancer has been reported in individuals with cirrhosis secondary to HBV and HCV infection, hemochromatosis, and α_1-AT deficiency. In patients with other forms of cirrhosis, such as alcoholic or primary biliary cirrhosis, the risk of malignant disease is lower; however, the risk is still higher in these individuals than in those with structurally normal livers.

In the Far East and sub-Saharan Africa, where HBV is endemic, such tumors often appear in adults 30 to 50 years of age. In the United States and other nonendemic areas, these tumors occur most often in the elderly. Hepatoblastoma, a liver cell cancer affecting children, is rare worldwide.

Pathology. Hepatocellular carcinoma presents in three forms: (1) as a diffuse infiltrative lesion, (2) as a solitary mass limited to one lobe of the liver, or (3) as multiple nodules (Fig 11-17). These lesions may be yellow because they contain glycogen and lipid, brown like normal liver, or green because of discoloration with bile. On histologic examination, the tumor is composed of cells resembling, to some extent, normal liver cells. Well-differentiated tumors may even produce bile, whereas the poorly differentiated tumors are composed of small epithelial cells that show few signs of differentiation. Tumor cells often synthesize alpha-fetoprotein (AFP), a protein that can be demonstrated in the cytoplasm by immunohistochemical methods and in the serum by biochemical means. AFP is useful for early diagnosis of primary malignant liver cell tumors.

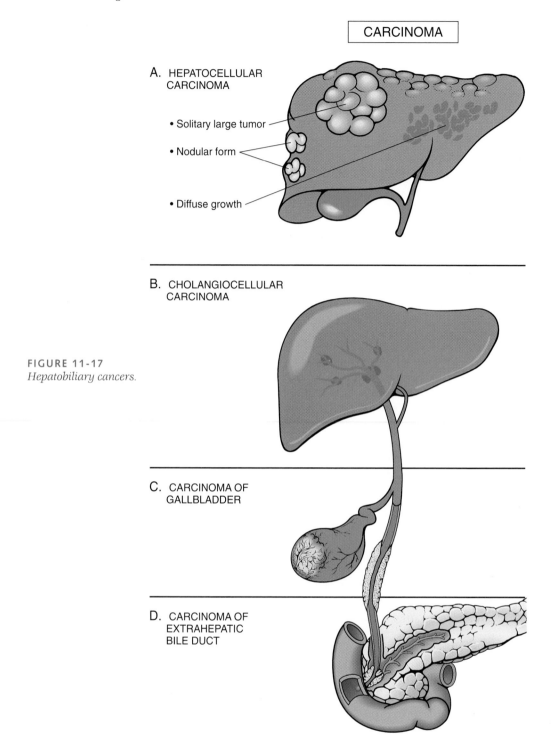

CARCINOMA

A. HEPATOCELLULAR CARCINOMA

• Solitary large tumor

• Nodular form

• Diffuse growth

B. CHOLANGIOCELLULAR CARCINOMA

C. CARCINOMA OF GALLBLADDER

D. CARCINOMA OF EXTRAHEPATIC BILE DUCT

FIGURE 11-17
Hepatobiliary cancers.

Clinical Features. Clinical symptoms of hepatocellular cancer include nonspecific signs of malignant disease, such as weight loss, loss of appetite, and nausea, and symptoms that are directly related to tumor growth within the liver. The enlarged liver is tender and even painful, compressing adjacent abdominal organs. Portal hypertension with bloody ascites and splenomegaly are common and often develop quickly following invasion of the portal vein by tumor or tumor-related thrombosis of the portal vein. Tumor may obstruct the hepatic vein, cause intravenous thrombosis, and impede the outflow of venous blood from the liver. This is called *Budd-Chiari syndrome*, and it is typically associated with massive liver enlargement secondary to venous congestion.

Hepatocellular carcinomas are associated with a number of *paraneoplastic syndromes* reflecting the synthetic and metabolic functions of tumor cells.

These tumors may store glycogen and secrete insulin-like growth factors, causing hypoglycemia. Tumors that produce erythropoietin can cause erythrocytosis. Hyperestrinism, hypercholesterolemia, and hypercalcemia are also noted in some patients.

Metastases of hepatocellular carcinomas occur relatively late and usually involve lymph nodes and adjacent abdominal organs. Hematogenous spread to the lungs may occur as well. Overall, the 5-year survival is 10 percent.

Bile Duct Cancer

Cholangiocellular carcinoma is a malignant tumor of the bile ducts. In the United States, these tumors are rare, but they are more common in other parts of the world. An association of bile ductal cancer with infection with the liver fluke, *O. sinensis*, has been noticed in China. Primary sclerosing cholangitis is a rare but well-known risk factor.

Pathology. Bile ductal carcinomas are adenocarcinomas that have no special histologic features that distinguish them from other gastrointestinal adenocarcinomas. The tumors may originate from intrahepatic or extrahepatic bile ducts (see Fig. 11-17). The prognosis for all such tumors is poor, regardless of their location.

Clinical Features. Intrahepatic tumors cause few symptoms, grow insidiously, and are incurable by the time of diagnosis. Tumors of the extrahepatic duct produce jaundice early in the course of their development and can, therefore, be diagnosed earlier. Such tumors have a somewhat better chance of being detected while still operable. The 5-year survival for intrahepatic cholangiocarcinoma is 10 percent whereas it is 35 percent for those involving the common bile duct and the papilla of Vater.

Carcinoma of the Gallbladder

Carcinoma of the gallbladder originates from the surface epithelium of the gallbladder. The tumor occurs in older patients and is two times more common in females than in males. This correlates with the higher prevalence of gallstones in females, and the fact that most carcinomas develop in gallbladders harboring stones. Native Americans, such as the Pima Indians, and Mexicans—both of whom often have gallstones—have the highest incidence of gallbladder cancer in the entire world.

Pathology. The tumor, which is initially localized to the gallbladder, eventually grows through the wall of the gallbladder, infiltrating the liver. In later stages of

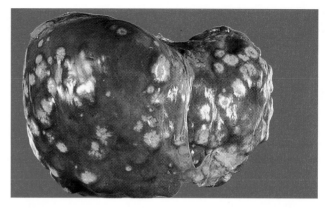

FIGURE 11-18
Metastatic carcinoma of the liver. The liver contains multiple nodules that have a depressed central area. This umbilicated appearance (resembling the belly button) is typical of metastatic tumor nodules

disease, the tumor may invade the extrahepatic bile ducts and cause jaundice, or it may infiltrate the duodenum and cause intestinal obstruction. Metastases are most prominent in local lymph nodes and adjacent abdominal organs.

Clinical Features. Gallbladder carcinoma produces few symptoms, and most of those, such as local discomfort or pain in the gallbladder area, may remain unnoticed or may be overshadowed by symptoms of cholelithiasis. Because of the delay in diagnosis, most tumors are discovered too late for surgical resection. By the time a tumor has caused jaundice or intestinal obstruction, it is usually too advanced to be resected. The prognosis for these lesions, therefore, is abysmal, and the 5-year survival rate is only 5 percent.

Metastases to the Liver

Secondary liver tumors (i.e., metastases) are much more common in the United States than are primary liver tumors. These metastases, which reach the liver through the portal or arterial circulation, are most often related to primary tumors of the gastrointestinal tract, lungs, and breast. The metastases are typically multiple, and appear as round nodules with a central softened or indented necrotic area (Fig. 11-18).

Clinical features. Metastases are the most common causes of hepatic enlargement. The liver is tender and may extend several fingerbreadths below the right costal margin. Jaundice, ascites, and splenomegaly are common symptoms. The diagnosis is typically made by computed tomography studies (CT) and is confirmed by liver biopsy. The appearance of liver metastases is an ominous sign; most patients die within months after these metastases have been identified.

Liver Transplantation

End-stage liver disease (cirrhosis) has invariably proved fatal until recently, when it became possible to replace a terminally damaged liver with a new liver from a healthy donor. Today, thousands of liver transplantations are performed worldwide, and the results are most encouraging.

The indications for liver transplantation are broad and include all forms of cirrhosis, as well as acute liver necrosis caused by viruses, toxins, or drugs. Liver transplantation is the treatment of choice for cirrhosis secondary to metabolic disorders, such as α_1-AT deficiency, Wilson's disease, or hemochromatosis.

Transplantation of the liver is technically easy to perform. Owing to antigenic differences between the host and the donor, though, the liver will invariably show signs of transplant rejection. This immune response of the host can be suppressed by corticosteroids and immunosuppressive cytotoxic drugs. Despite treatment, the host's T cells may damage the transplant and ruin its function. The most important consequences of immune rejection are the destruction of the bile ducts and intrahepatic blood vessels. Recurrence of HBV or HCV infection in patients suffering from chronic viral hepatitis is also common. Liver transplant recipients are at increased risk for various nosocomial diseases, such as cytomegalovirus, herpesvirus, or fungal infections. Nevertheless, most liver transplant patients survive with appropriate treatment for at least 5 to 10 years, and often much longer.

Review Questions

1. How is the liver connected to the intestine and the great vessels?
2. Which cells form liver lobules?
3. What are the main functions of the liver?
4. What are the consequences of portal hypertension?
5. How is bilirubin formed and excreted?
6. Which enzymes are released into the circulation from damaged liver cells?
7. What are three principal forms of jaundice and what causes each of them?
8. Compare the biochemical laboratory findings in prehepatic, hepatic, and posthepatic jaundice.
9. What are the causes of viral hepatitis?
10. Compare viral hepatitis A with viral hepatitis B and C.
11. Explain the significance of serologic tests for the diagnosis of viral hepatitis.
12. Compare the findings in acute and chronic hepatitis.
13. What is cirrhosis and how does this disease present clinically?
14. What are the most common causes of cirrhosis?
15. Compare portal and biliary cirrhosis.
16. Describe the gross and microscopic features of a cirrhotic liver.
17. Why are some cirrhotic livers yellow and some others are rusty brown?
18. What is the pathogenesis of ascites and splenomegaly in chronic liver disease?
19. What is the pathogenesis of hepatic encephalopathy and how does it present clinically?
20. What is hepatorenal syndrome?
21. Which endocrine abnormalities are found in patients with cirrhosis?
22. Why do patients with cirrhosis bleed?
23. Compare predictable and unpredictable liver injury caused by drugs.
24. How does alcohol affect the liver?
25. What is Gilbert's disease?

26. Compare hereditary hemochromatosis and Wilson's disease.

27. How does alpha$_1$-antitrypsin deficiency affect the liver?

28. What is autoimmune hepatitis?

29. Compare primary biliary cirrhosis and primary sclerosing cholangitis.

30. How do bacteria, protozoa, and parasites infect the liver?

31. What is the difference between cholangitic and pylephlebitic abscesses?

32. How are gallstones formed?

33. Compare cholesterol stones with pigmentary gallstones.

34. What is the pathogenesis of cholecystitis?

35. List the most important complications of cholelithiasis and cholecystitis.

36. List the most important primary tumors of the hepatobiliary tract.

37. Compare hepatocellular carcinoma with cholangiocellular carcinoma.

38. Compare cholangiocellular carcinoma with gallbladder carcinoma.

39. Compare the pathology of primary and metastatic liver tumors.

40. What are the indications for liver transplantation?

Learning Objectives

After studying this chapter, the student should be able to:

1. Describe the gross and microscopic anatomy of the pancreas.
2. Describe the main functions of the exocrine pancreas and list the main components of pancreatic juice.
3. List three main hormones produced by the islets of Langerhans and describe their function.
4. Discuss the pathogenesis of acute pancreatitis.
5. List three biochemical changes and three symptoms caused by acute pancreatitis.
6. List three main complications of acute pancreatitis.
7. Explain the pathogenesis of chronic pancreatitis.
8. List the main clinical symptoms of chronic pancreatitis and relate them to the pathologic changes in the pancreas.
9. Discuss the gross and microscopic features of pancreatic carcinoma.
10. Compare the clinical symptoms of carcinoma involving the head and the tail of the pancreas.
11. List three syndromes caused by islet cell tumors.
12. Describe the gross and microscopic features of islet cell tumors and relate these to the clinical course of the disease.
13. Discuss the pathogenesis of type I and type II diabetes.
14. Compare the essential features of type I and type II diabetes.
15. List the main complications of diabetes.

Additional Key Terms and Concepts

Amylase

Gastrinoma

Hyperglycemia

Insulinoma

Lipase

Malabsorption

Chapter Outline

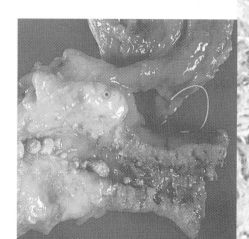

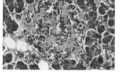

The Pancreas
Chapter 12

NORMAL ANATOMY AND PHYSIOLOGY

The pancreas is a gland composed of an exocrine and an endocrine part (Fig. 12-1). It is located in the retroperitoneal space of the upper abdomen, and is closely attached to other retroperitoneal structures, most notably, the ganglia and nerves of the celiac plexus. Because of this close relationship between the pancreas and the retroperitoneal nerves, pain radiating into the back is one of the common features of pancreatic diseases.

The **pancreas** can be divided into three parts: the **head,** which lies within the loop of duodenum; the mid-portion, which is called the **body;** and the **tail,** which extends laterally and left to the hilus of the spleen (see Fig. 12-1). More than 98 percent of the entire pancreas consists of exocrine tissue—**acini, ductules,** and **ducts.** The *endocrine* cells are arranged into **islets of Langerhans** that are scattered through the entire organ but are most prominent in the tail.

The digestive juices produced by the exocrine pancreatic cells drain through the *main pancreatic duct* into the duodenum. The terminal part of the main pancreatic duct is confluent with the common bile duct, with which it shares the common entry into the duodenum called the *papilla of Vater.* There is often an *accessory duct* entering the duodenum as well, which is unrelated to the bile duct. This close relationship of the head of the pancreas and the duodenum, as well as the common bile duct, is important for an understanding of the obstructive symptoms caused by tumors of the head of the pancreas. Reflux of bile into the pancreatic duct as a result of

obstruction of the papilla of Vater may be important in the pathogenesis of pancreatitis, as shall be explained later. Hormones produced by the endocrine cells are released into the blood circulation; therefore, there is no need for endocrine excretory ducts.

The exocrine pancreas is the main source of **digestive enzymes,** the most important of which include

- **amylase,** which is essential for the digestion of starch
- **lipase,** which is essential for the digestion of lipids
- **peptidases,** such as trypsin and chymotrypsin, which are essential for the digestion of proteins

All these enzymes are synthesized in the acinar cells and released into the ductal system in an inactive form (i.e., like proenzymes). Pancreatic juice also contains bicarbonate and small amounts of mucin, which are released from the ductal cells.

The secretion of pancreatic juices is controlled by the vagus nerve and the polypeptide hormones *cholecystokinin* and *secretin.* These hormones are released from the duodenum in response to the entry of acidic and fat-rich food into its lumen from the stomach. Cholecystokinin stimulates the secretion of enzymes, whereas secretin stimulates the release of bicarbonate. The **pancreatic juices** that contain proenzymes and bicarbonates are mixed with the duodenal content. This results in activation of enzymes through the action of intestinal enteropeptidase, and the alkalization of the luminal content through the action of bicarbonates. **Bicarbonates** act as buffers to neutralize the gastric hydrochloric acid,

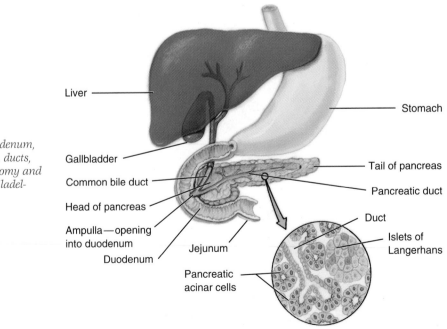

FIGURE 12-1
The pancreas in relation to the liver, duodenum, and stomach. The insert shows the acini, ducts, and islets. (From Applegate EJ: The anatomy and physiology learning system: textbook. Philadelphia: WB Saunders, 1995:343.)

Liver

Gallbladder

Common bile duct

Head of pancreas

Ampulla—opening into duodenum

Duodenum

Jejunum

Pancreatic acinar cells

Stomach

Tail of pancreas

Pancreatic duct

Duct

Islets of Langerhans

and by raising the pH in the intestine, they provide optimal conditions for the action of pancreatic digestive enzymes. It should be noted that cholecystokinin also stimulates contraction of the gallbladder and secretin stimulates production of bile in the liver. Because bile and pancreatic juices have a common terminal outflow tract, it is easy to see how heavy meals, especially those rich in lipids, can overburden the pancreaticobiliary ductal system and cause potentially harmful consequences.

The endocrine pancreatic cells secrete several polypeptide **hormones,** the most important of which are **insulin, glucagon,** and **somatostatin.** The excess or deficiency of these hormones produces distinct clinical symptoms, which will be discussed later.

OVERVIEW OF MAJOR DISEASES

The most important diseases affecting the exocrine pancreas are

- pancreatitis
- tumors

The most important disease caused by dysfunction of the endocrine pancreas is diabetes mellitus. Tumors of the endocrine pancreas are relatively rare and thus receive only mention.

Several facts important to an understanding of pancreatic diseases are presented here, before a discussion of specific pathologic entities.

1. *The pancreas is anatomically and functionally a part of the digestive tract.* Pancreatic juice is produced at a rate of 100 mL per hour, or at a rate of 2 to 3 L per day. The production of pancreatic juice is hormonally controlled and is coordinated with the production of other digestive enzymes. Improper diet, overeating, consumption of a fat-rich diet, and alcohol abuse strain the pancreas and biliary system. A loss of pancreatic parenchymal cells or inadequate drainage of juices into the duodenum profoundly affects digestion. Incomplete absorption of digested food results in *malabsorption* and *diarrhea* (loose and frequent stools), which are the most important consequences of pancreatic diseases.

2. *Many symptoms of pancreatic diseases can be understood in terms of basic anatomic facts.* In this context, it is essential to remember that the pancreas is in close contact with the duodenum, the common bile duct, and the retroperitoneal nerves of the celiac plexus. Because tumors of the head of pancreas often occlude the common bile duct, obstructive jaundice is a common symptom. Duodenal obstruction is usually found in more advanced cases. Invasion of the retroperitoneal nerves is a common cause of back pain in patients with pancreatic cancer, but nerve involvement can also occur in those with chronic pancreatitis as well.

3. *Pancreatic juice contains inactive proenzymes which are activated in the intestine.* Proenzymes, such as trypsinogen or prolipase, are kinetically inactive while passing through the pancreas and are, therefore, innocuous to ductal cells. Premature activation of proteolytic or lipolytic enzymes in the ducts, or even worse, in the parenchyma of the pancreas, may result in enzymatic tissue destruction secondary to enzyme action. Once released into the tissue, the enzymes become autocatalysts and it is very difficult to interrupt their destructive action. This process may result in large tissue defects known as pseudocysts. Pancreatic enzymes can be activated inside the pancreas chemically, or by trauma (even by surgical scalpel or needle). It is no wonder, then, that surgeons do not like to operate near the pancreas or perform pancreatic biopsies.

4. *Under normal circumstances, pancreatic enzymes are found in trace amounts in the circulating blood.* Pancreatic necrosis typical of acute pancreatitis results in a release of enzymes from damaged acini and disrupted ducts. Proteolytic enzymes, such as elastase, further destroy not only the pancreatic parenchyma, but the vessel wall, which makes it possible for enzymes to enter the circulation. As pancreatic enzymes can be detected in blood, blood tests are useful in the diagnosis of pancreatic disease. Likewise, because these enzymes pass from the blood into the urine, urinalysis is also a valuable source of diagnostic data.

5. *The anatomic location of the pancreas accounts for most symptoms and, to a great extent, for the poor prognosis of pancreatic cancer.* Carcinoma of the pancreas is the fourth most common cause of cancer-related death in males and the fifth most common cause in females. This tumor is essentially incurable because, in most cases, it is detected too late to allow surgical resection. Because of their location, pancreatic tumors are clinically silent for extended periods of time and produce no early warning signs. There are presently no screening techniques that allow early detection of these tumors at a stage when they are still operable.

6. *Endocrine tumors are composed of slowly dividing endocrine cells that are biologically less aggressive than exocrine malignant lesions.* For reasons that are unknown, endocrine tumors of the pancreas grow slowly. In this respect, these tumors resemble carcinoids, the neuroendocrine tumors of the intestines. Histologically, too, pancreatic islet cell tumors and carcinoids resemble one another. Endocrine tumors produce hormone-related symptoms, permitting earlier detection. Unfortunately, endocrine tumors account for only 5 percent to 10 percent of all pancreatic neoplasms.

7. *Insulin is the most important hormone secreted by the pancreas.* Insulin regulates the intermediary metabolism of carbohydrates and lipids. A deficiency of insulin results in diabetes mellitus. Diabetes is the most prevalent endocrine disease, affecting millions of people worldwide. In the past, it was a lethal disease. Even today—at a time when the disease can be treated with animal insulin and drugs that stimulate release of insulin from islet cells—its long-term prognosis is unfavorable. Diabetes is one of the most important risk factors for atherosclerosis.

Pancreatitis

Pancreatitis is an inflammation of the pancreas. It can occur in an acute or chronic form. In contrast to the inflammations in other organs, which are typically caused by infectious agents, pancreatitis is, in most cases, a sterile chemical inflammation. The inflammation is a secondary reaction to tissue destruction caused by digestive enzymes released from damaged exocrine pancreatic cells.

There are three important forms of pancreatitis:

- acute edematous pancreatitis
- acute hemorrhagic pancreatitis (acute pancreatic necrosis)
- chronic pancreatitis

Acute edematous pancreatitis is a mild form of pancreatic injury; its incidence cannot be determined because most patients do not require hospitalization and the disease is not registered for statistical purposes. Histologic evidence of mild pancreatic inflammation is found in 0.5 percent of autopsies, indicating that such pancreatitis occurs more often than it is clinically diagnosed. *Acute hemorrhagic pancreatitis* is a serious disease that still has a high mortality and can have serious sequelae. It is encountered in one of every 500 hospital admissions. The incidence of *chronic pancreatitis* has been estimated to be 3 to 5 per 100,000 adults.

Acute Pancreatitis

Acute pancreatitis is an acute response to tissue necrosis caused by digestive enzymes released from exocrine pancreatic cells. As acute edematous pancreatitis is rarely diagnosed clinically, we shall concentrate on acute hemorrhagic pancreatitis, a medical emergency characterized by typical symptoms and laboratory findings.

Etiology and Pathogenesis. Pancreatic exocrine cells forming the acinus secrete digestive enzymes into the ductules, where the enzymes enter the larger ducts. In the pancreatic ducts, the enzymes are mixed with bicarbonates and mucins secreted by the ductal cells. From the ducts, the pancreatic juices reach the duodenum through the papilla of Vater. Within the pancreas, the enzymes remain in an inactive form (i.e., as proenzymes), becoming activated only upon entry into the duodenum. Premature activation of proenzymes within the pancreas results in *autodigestion:* tissue lysis caused by the action of pancreatic enzymes.

Experimental data show that pancreatic autodigestion can be induced in a number of ways, including the following:

- Obstruction of the main pancreatic duct
- Injection of bile or other chemicals into the pancreatic duct
- Mechanical disruption of the pancreatic acinar cells
- Chemical injury of pancreatic acinar cells
- Overstimulation of pancreatic acinar cells

In all these experimental models of acute pancreatitis in animals, it is possible to provoke an acute pancreatic cell necrosis, typically followed by acute inflammation. However, the clinical relevance of experimental data remains questionable, and our understanding of the human disease is still incomplete. Nevertheless, good arguments have been advanced that the experimental models have their clinical equivalents, as illustrated in Fig. 12-2.

Obstruction of the main pancreatic duct is a potentially important cause of pancreatitis, and it can occur in association with biliary disease. As noted before, the main pancreatic duct and the common bile duct are confluent in their terminal part, and both discharge their contents into the duodenum through the papilla of Vater. Obstruction of the papilla of Vater or the pancreatobiliary duct by gallstones is an important factor in the pathogenesis of acute pancreatitis, as evidenced by the fact that at least 50 percent of patients have gallstones. The obstruction could also lead to the *reflux of bile* into the pancreas. Bile normally activates pancreatic proenzymes in the intestine and, presumably, it could activate the enzymes prematurely in the pancreatic ducts as well.

Mechanical disruption of pancreatic cells has been documented in patients who develop acute pancreatitis following abdominal trauma, such as that caused by seat belt trauma in car accidents. *Chemical injury* of pancreatic cells can be induced by various drugs, such as cytotoxic anticancer drugs. However, drugs rarely precipitate acute pancreatic necrosis. *Overstimulation of pancreatic cells* by secretin could be the cause of pancreatitis in obese persons indulging in fatty foods. It is believed that alcohol also stimulates pancreatic secretion. An increased incidence of acute pancreatitis has been reported in alcoholics.

In clinical practice, acute pancreatitis is related

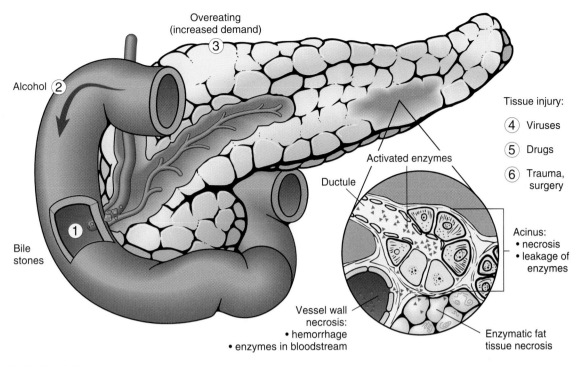

FIGURE 12-2
Hypothetical pathogenesis of acute pancreatitis.

to gallstones and alcohol abuse in about 80 percent of the cases. Other rare causes account for 5 percent of the cases, whereas the remaining 15 percent of cases are idiopathic (i.e., without an obvious external cause) (Table 12-1). Reflux of bile into the pancreas can also increase intrapancreatic pressure and can activate the proenzymes, thus causing autodigestion. Alcohol can cause spasm of the sphincter of Oddi in the papilla of Vater, likewise increasing intrapancreatic pressure. Although alcohol is known to be toxic to cells and could presumably damage and disrupt acinar cells directly, the exact mechanism for alcoholic injury of the pancreas is still unknown. Alcohol could also stimulate pancreatic acinar cells, directly or through its effects on the intestine and the action

of secretin, which is the primary secretagogue for acinar cells.

Regardless of the precipitating cause of acute pancreatitis, the tissue damage occurs in a predictable manner and is always mediated by pancreatic digestive enzymes. Proteolysis caused by activation of trypsinogen, the inactive form of trypsin, leads to necrosis of tissues. Elastase acts on the elastic tissue, forming large gaps in the blood vessel wall that result in massive hemorrhage. The action of lipase on fat cells inside the pancreas and the peripancreatic fat tissues results in fat necrosis. Other hydrolytic enzymes, more than 100 of which are present in the pancreatic juice, act on other tissue components, including carbohydrates, DNA, and RNA.

Enzymatic tissue destruction is accompanied by liquefaction of the digested pancreas. This fluid accumulates also in cystic spaces within the pancreas. These spaces are called *pseudocysts* because they are not lined by an internal epithelial cell layer, as are regular cysts. Necrotic tissue foci tend to attract calcium salts and undergo dystrophic *calcification*. Free fatty acids formed through the hydrolysis of triglycerides also bind calcium ions, thus forming *calcium soaps* which can be seen as whitish specks underneath the peritoneum and wherever the fat cells have undergone enzymatic necrosis.

Pathology. Acute pancreatitis is marked by massive edema, hemorrhage, and necrosis of the pancreas (Fig. 12-3). The pancreas appears swollen and is per-

Table 12-1 Causes of Acute Pancreatitis

Common (95%)		Rare (5%)
Alcohol	} 80%	Trauma (as from a car accident)
Bile stones		Surgery
Unknown	15%	Partial resection of pancreas
		Biopsy of pancreas
		Drug-induced
		Diuretics
		Oral contraceptives
		Metabolic
		Hyperlipidemia
		Infection
		Mumps

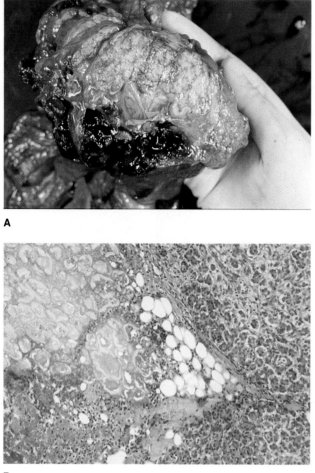

A

B

FIGURE 12-3
*Acute pancreatitis. (A) Gross appearance of the pancreas.
Note the massive hemorrhage into the pancreas. (B) Necrotic
foci are scattered throughout the parenchyma.*

meated with blood. Yellow or smudgy brownish-yel-
low areas of necrosis appear 2 to 3 days after the
onset of the attack. The leakage of digestive enzymes
into the abdominal cavity may cause peritoneal irritation, and a chemical peritonitis may ensue. Areas
of fat necrosis appear as grayish yellow discol-
orations that gradually calcify and become whitish.
By the end of the first week, pseudocysts appear as
small cavities filled with liquefied tissue and pancreatic enzymes. These small cavities coalesce into
larger pseudocysts which are typically found in patients who survive the initial attack.

Histologically, the hallmarks of normal pancreatic tissue are lost as a result of necrosis. The necrotic
pancreatic cells are transformed into amorphous
granular material. The fat cells, which are normally
vacuolated and filled with fat, lose their outlines and
transform into washed-out "ghosts" composed of col-
lapsed cell membranes.

Complications. Acute pancreatitis commonly
causes complications. As already mentioned, the
spilling of digestive enzymes into the peritoneal cavity causes peritonitis. Small cystic spaces resulting
from the destruction of the parenchyma of the pancreas may become confluent, resulting in large
pseudocysts. These large pseudocysts resemble bags
filled with fluid. They may replace large portions of
the pancreatic parenchyma or may distend the pancreas, compressing and displacing the duodenum or
the stomach. The content of pseudocysts, as well as
the remaining necrotic pancreatic parenchyma, may
become infected by enteric bacteria. This bacterial
infection leads to the formation of *abscesses.* In contrast to pseudocysts, which contain liquefied tissue
debris and enzymes, pancreatic abscesses contain
pus. However, the capsule of the pseudocyst resembles the wall of an abscess. In both of these structures, the capsule is composed of fibrotic granulation
tissues formed in an attempt to delimit the spread of
tissue destruction and/or inflammation. As time
passes, such granulation tissue becomes more and
more fibrotic until finally, these cystic structures assume the appearance of leather bags.

Chronic pancreatitis is a late complication of
acute pancreatitis. Destruction of pancreatic tissue in
acute pancreatitis may result in exocrine pancreatic
insufficiency, which is typically found in persons
who have had recurrent bouts of the disease. It has
been estimated that chronic pancreatitis develops in
20 percent of patients who survive acute pancreatitis.

Diabetes mellitus is an uncommon consequence
of pancreatic tissue destruction associated with
acute pancreatitis. Acute hyperglycemia, which is
usually mild, may be seen in many patients during
the initial attack. Massive destruction of the islets of
Langerhans, resulting in permanent diabetes, is less
common.

Did You Know?

Pseudocysts that form in the pancreas following an
attack of acute pancreatitis contain digestive enzymes that prevent healing of the pseudocyst. To
allow tissues to heal, surgeons drain the pancreatic
juices through a pouch made by attaching the
opened pseudocyst to the external abdominal wall.
The name for this procedure, **marsupialization**, is
derived from the Latin word for "pouch." The same
word is used for the animal order Marsupialia, which
includes kangaroos and opossums. To most patients
marsupialization probably sounds less intimidating
than kangaroozation or possumization!

Clinical Features. Acute pancreatitis is a disease of sudden onset. Typically, it occurs in patients with a history of gallstones or alcoholism. Characteristic symptoms include abdominal pain and distention, nausea, and vomiting. Affected patients display apprehensiveness, are in great distress, and sweat profusely. The pain is often uncontrollable. Syncope and rapidly developing shock are typical of severe disease. Peritoneal rigidity signals the onset of peritonitis, which is usually accompanied by paralytic ileus.

The diagnosis of acute pancreatitis can be corroborated by laboratory data. In addition to leukocytosis, which develops in response to acute inflammation, serum tests typically reveal a marked elevation in amylase and lipase levels. Pancreatic enzymes are also found in the urine. Peritoneal fluid may contain the same enzyme. Biochemical signs of pancreatitis appear 24 to 72 hours after the onset of the attack.

X-ray findings are also useful. Computed tomography (CT) scans may be used to demonstrate swelling in the pancreas. In patients with rapidly developing peritonitis, x-ray studies can help rule out other catastrophic abdominal events, such as perforation of the intestines. In later stages of disease, radiographs may demonstrate calcification.

There is no effective treatment for acute pancreatitis; however, efforts should be directed at containing the damage and preventing the systemic consequences of shock. The overall mortality rate of acute pancreatitis is still in the range of 20 percent. Death is usually the consequence of circulatory shock. Elderly patients with acute respiratory failure, hypotension, and peritonitis have the highest risk of all populations, with a mortality rate near 50 percent.

Patients who survive the acute attack are at a risk for recurrence. This can be prevented by removing gallstones, eliminating alcohol, and avoiding a high-fat diet. Symptoms of chronic pancreatitis occur in about 20 percent of surviving patients.

Chronic Pancreatitis

Chronic pancreatitis is characterized by irregular fibrosis replacing portions of the normal pancreatic parenchyma. These changes are progressive and irreversible, and produce exocrine as well as endocrine pancreatic insufficiency. The disease is found in 4 per 100,000 adults and is more common in males than in females, the male:female ratio being 3:1.

Chronic pancreatitis has an insidious onset, so it is very difficult to determine either its cause or pathogenesis. However, a history of alcohol abuse can be elicited in most patients. It is, therefore, believed that alcohol accounts for more than 70 percent of cases. Because chronic alcoholism is much more widespread than chronic pancreatitis, it is difficult to

explain why only some chronic alcoholics develop this disease while others are spared. In a few cases, chronic pancreatitis is preceded by acute pancreatitis, but in most instances, the onset of the disease is slow and imperceptible. In a few patients, chronic pancreatic insufficiency follows trauma or pancreatic surgery, or occurs during the course of systemic metabolic and endocrine diseases. It is most puzzling that 20 percent of patients have no risk factors or preexisting disease and present with idiopathic chronic pancreatitis.

Pathology. On gross examination, the pancreas does not show the typical lobulation, but appears fibrotic and firm. The main pancreatic duct is usually dilated and often contains stones (Fig. 12-4). Fibrous tissues may extend from the pancreas into the surrounding structures and cause constriction of the common bile duct, duodenum, or the pylorus. Histologically, there is marked fibrosis, with scattered foci

FIGURE 12-4
Chronic pancreatitis. (A) Gross appearance of the atrophic pancreas. Note the calculi in the dilated duct. (B) Histologic examination reveals that the acini have been replaced by fibrous tissue.

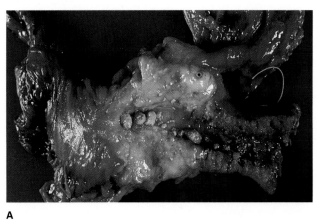

A

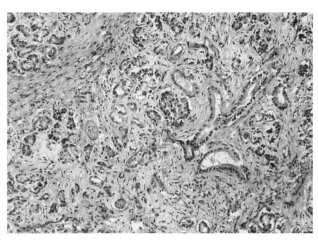

B

of chronic inflammation replacing the acini. The ducts and islets of Langerhans tend to persist longer, but in advanced cases, they, too, are destroyed and obliterated by fibrosis. Calcifications of the fibrous tissue are common.

Clinical Features. The symptoms of chronic pancreatitis develop insidiously. All of the symptoms can be explained in terms of the underlying pathology (Fig. 12-5). Typically, they include the following:

- *Pain.* This is related to the entrapment of nerves in the fibrous tissue, which often extends into the celiac plexus. Fibrosis may cause stenosis of the duodenum, which impedes the passage of food from the stomach into duodenum, causing pain after eating.
- *Exocrine pancreatic insufficiency.* Destruction of acinar cells reduces the capacity of the pancreas to produce digestive enzymes, which results in malabsorption and steatorrhea. Lack of trypsin and chymotrypsin results in malabsorption of proteins. Lipase deficiency accounts for the fatty stools and inappropriate absorption of fat and fat-soluble vitamins (A, D, K, and E). Most patients lose weight and feel weak. Signs of vitamin deficiency, such as night blindness secondary to avitaminosis A, or a bleeding tendency, secondary to avitaminosis K, are seen in severe cases.
- *Endocrine insufficiency.* Destruction of the islets of Langerhans occurs at a slower rate than does the loss of exocrine pancreatic cells. Nevertheless, in later stages of the disease, more than 70 percent of patients have signs of diabetes.

The diagnosis of chronic pancreatitis is based on a typical history, which usually includes alcohol abuse, and the typical complaints. Pain, which is usually epigastric, tends to radiate into the back and is commonly exacerbated by drinking and the ingestion of fatty meals. Bulky fatty stools are an important tell-tale sign. Weight loss is common.

The work-up of the patient must include abdominal x-ray studies which will usually show numerous calcifications in the pancreas. Laboratory findings may disclose mild elevations in amylase and lipase levels in serum, but they often yield normal values and are noncontributory. Most patients with advanced disease show hyperglycemia and other features of diabetes. The course of pancreatitis is relentless. It cannot be stopped or reversed, but some improvement may be noticed if the patient stops drinking. Malabsorption can be treated symptomatically by enzyme supplementation, but the commercial enzyme preparations are of low potency. Most patents compensate for low absorption by eating increased amounts of high-calorie food. With such adjustments, quality of life may not be quite normal, but it is not shortened substantially. These patients tend to be at an increased risk for developing pancreatic cancer, which develops approximately three times more often in this population than in age-matched controls.

Pancreatic Neoplasms

Neoplasms of the pancreas can be classified clinically as benign or malignant. On gross examination, they may appear solid or cystic. On the basis of their origin, the tumors may be classified as being derived from either exocrine or endocrine cells. The tumors may show secretory activity, or they may be functionally inactive.

It is important to remember that most—more than 95 percent—pancreatic tumors are

- malignant epithelial neoplasms (e.g., adenocarcinomas)
- solid, rather than cystic, with cystadenomas and cystadenocarcinomas occurring only rarely (2 percent of all tumors)
- derived from the pancreatic ducts (i.e., originating from the exocrine part of the pancreas)
- functionally silent (i.e., arising from ductal cells and secreting neither hormones nor enzymes)

Adenocarcinoma of the Pancreas

Carcinoma of the pancreas, the most important tumor involving this organ, is the fourth major cause of cancer-related deaths in males and the fifth in females in the United States. Approximately 25,000 new cases are recorded every year in the United States, and essentially all of them die within 12 to 24 months of diagnosis.

FIGURE 12-5
Chronic pancreatitis may be caused by stones, pseudocysts, calcification, or fibrosis that entraps nerves.

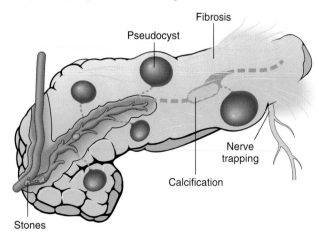

The risk factors for pancreatic tumors have not been clearly delineated. The strongest epidemiologic association noted has been smoking, which increases the risk threefold. It has been proposed that dietary factors, such as a high-fat diet and alcohol abuse, predispose individuals to pancreatic cancer, but this hypothesis has not been definitively proven. Chronic pancreatitis has been associated with a twofold to threefold higher incidence of pancreatic cancer. However, this disease is relatively rare and can be implicated as a possible cause for only a minority of pancreatic carcinomas.

For all practical purposes, carcinoma of the pancreas is a disease of old age. The tumors rarely occur before the age of 40 years, but thereafter, their incidence increases steadily. The incidence of tumors in males equals that in females, except in the group younger than 50 years of age, in which males outnumber females 3 to 1.

Pathology. Adenocarcinoma of the pancreas is an epithelial malignant lesion originating from ducts. Among the tumors diagnosed clinically, approximately 60 percent are located in the head of the pancreas (Fig. 12-6). This is understandable because the head forms the bulk of the pancreas and contains most of the ducts. Furthermore, because these tumors of the pancreatic head tend to obstruct the bile ducts and cause jaundice, they are diagnosed more readily than are tumors of the body or the tail of the pancreas, which account for 15 percent of all pancreatic carcinomas. Approximately 25 percent of cancers involve the pancreas diffusely.

Microscopic examination reveals that most tumors are adenocarcinomas that may be well differentiated or undifferentiated. Well-differentiated tumors usually secrete mucus, whereas undifferentiated tumors are usually desmoplastic (i.e., they show prominent dense connective tissue stroma). Histologically, such tumors do not differ from other adenocarcinomas of the gastrointestinal tract. Adenocarcinomas displaying unique histologic features, such as acinar cell carcinomas or cystadenocarcinomas, are rare.

Metastases occur early in the course of the disease. At the time of diagnosis, grossly visible metastases are found in the local lymph nodes of 40 percent of patients, and distant metastases are noted in yet another 40 percent. These metastatic lesions are most often in the liver, but also occur commonly in the lungs and bones. Only 20 percent of affected patients have cancer that is strictly limited to the pancreas.

Clinical Features. Symptoms of pancreatic carcinoma depend on the location of the tumor, its size, and the extent of spread. Most often, the symptoms are nonspecific and include weight loss, loss of appetite, nausea, and vomiting. Upper abdominal pain may suggest the pancreas as the cause of these cancer-related symptoms. Tumors located in the head of the pancreas tend to obstruct the common bile duct and cause jaundice. The gallbladder may be dilated, and may even be palpable on physical examination (*Courvoisier's sign*). Tumors of the tail tend to invade the celiac plexus. Tumors of the body and tail of the pancreas do not cause jaundice, but tend to invade the celiac plexus and cause pain. Splenomegaly may occur owing to obstruction of the splenic vein.

Metastases and local spread of the tumor into the duodenum cause intestinal obstruction. Liver metastases cause enlargement of the liver. Peritoneal seeding is associated with ascites and a protruding abdomen, which are the presenting findings in one third of all patients. Distant metastases are also common.

The diagnosis of carcinoma of the pancreas is based on a combination of physical findings and X-ray findings. The CT scan is the most reliable technique for visualizing pancreatic tumors. Many tumors are diagnosed during laparoscopy that is performed to relieve intestinal or biliary obstruction. Endoscopic retrograde cholangiopancreatography or percutaneous transhepatic cholangiography are special radiographic techniques that are sometimes used to distinguish carcinoma from chronic pancreatitis. During these procedures, it is also possible to obtain cells for cytopathologic analysis. Pancreatic tumors can also be sampled by thin-needle aspiration biopsy or incisional biopsy during surgical exploration.

Carcinoma of the pancreas is an incurable disease. Surgical resection may be attempted, but the results are not encouraging. Radiation therapy and chemotherapy are also ineffectual. The 5-year survival rate is less than 5 percent. Most patients die within the first year of diagnosis.

FIGURE 12-6
Carcinoma of the pancreas. The tumor is located in the head of the pancreas in 60% of cases, but may also involve the body (10%) or the tail (5%). Diffuse infiltration of the entire organ by tumor occurs in 25% of cases.

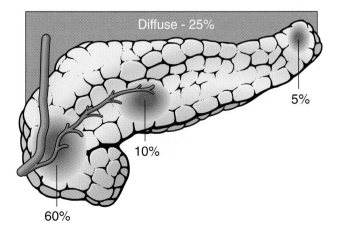

Diffuse - 25%

5%

10%

60%

Tumors of the Endocrine Pancreas

Tumors of the endocrine pancreas are called **islet cell tumors,** as all of them originate from the endocrine cells in the islets of Langerhans. Endocrine tumors are rare, being 10 times less common than carcinomas of the exocrine pancreas and having an incidence of 1 per 100,000 per year. Nevertheless, it is important to distinguish endocrine tumors from the more common adenocarcinomas for several reasons:

- Endocrine pancreatic tumors are benign or low-grade malignant lesions with a better prognosis than exocrine adenocarcinomas.
- Endocrine pancreatic tumors are usually hormonally active and cause systemic symptoms that vary depending on the cell of origin and the predominant hormone released from the neoplastic cells. Hormones produced by these tumors are useful in establishing the diagnosis.
- Endocrine tumors may be multiple and are also associated with tumors of other organs, as in multiple endocrine neoplasia syndrome type I (MEN1).

Endocrine tumors may originate from any of the four cell types in the normal islets of Langerhans. The most common tumors are *insulinomas,* which are composed of insulin-secreting beta cells. *Glucagonomas, somatostatinomas,* and *vipomas* are less common.

Insulinomas, or beta cell tumors, are typically small, solitary, benign tumors measuring 1 to 3 cm in diameter. These tumors secrete insulin, which can be detected in blood by radioimmunoassay. Hyperinsulinemia may cause hypoglycemia, syncope, and profuse sweating, especially after prolonged fasting. These symptoms can be reversed promptly by infusion of glucose. Insulinomas can be easily resected, which results in a permanent cure of the patient's hypoglycemic episodes.

The pancreas is also the most common site of *gastrinomas,* which constitute 25 percent of pancreatic endocrine tumors. The normal pancreatic islets of Langerhans do not contain gastrin-secreting cells, and it is believed that gastrinomas originate from developmentally pluripotent cells that are the common fetal precursors of pancreatic islet cells and normal gastric and intestinal G cells. Clinically, gastrinomas present as the *Zollinger-Ellison syndrome.* This syndrome is marked by gastric hypersecretion and intractable peptic ulcers. Ulcers may be multiple, located in unusual sites, and resistant to standard medical therapy. Gastrinomas are usually malignant, and they may be multiple; in some families affected by MEN1, gastrinomas are associated with tumors of the pituitary and parathyroid glands.

Diabetes Mellitus

The islets of Langerhans contain several endocrine cell types. Alpha cells, which secrete glycagon, account for 20 percent; beta cells, which secrete insulin, account for 70 percent; and the remaining 10 percent are delta cells, which secrete somatostatin.

Functional insufficiency of the islets of Langerhans, caused by a destruction of islets or a selective loss of beta cells, results in **diabetes mellitus.** An anatomic or functional defect in the endocrine pancreas is, however, only one of the causes of diabetes. Other causes of diabetes, which are unrelated to the pancreas, are also discussed here.

Definition and Classification. The term diabetes is derived from a Greek term, the literal meaning of which is "to pass through." It was coined to denote *polyuria*—the production of large amounts of urine—which is the most common sign of the disease. The adjective "mellitus" was added to indicate that the urine was sweet (i.e., contained sugar), in contrast to diabetes insipidus, a pituitary polyuria in which the urine is insipid (i.e., tasteless). Because pituitary polyuria is rare and polyuria secondary to diabetes mellitus (DM) is very common, it has become customary to call the more common disease simply "diabetes." The adjective, diabetic, has come to refer exclusively to DM and thus does not need to be followed by the adjective mellitus.

DM is a heterogeneous group of systemic disorders characterized by hyperglycemia; complex disturbances of carbohydrate, lipid, and protein metabolism; and a variety of organic changes resulting primarily from blood vessel pathology. Diabetes is a consequence of absolute or relative insulin deficiency or an abnormal response of target tissues to insulin.

Diabetes is a very common disease, affecting between 1 percent and 2 percent of humans. The symptoms vary from mild to severe, and although

> **Did You Know?**
>
> The common form of diabetes characterized by elevated blood sugar and sugar in urine is called diabetes mellitus, in contrast to diabetes insipidus, which is caused by pituitary diseases. Ancient physicians tested urine by wetting a finger and licking it. If the urine was sweet, the disease was called diabetes mellitus; if the urine had no taste, the disease was called diabetes insipidus, from the Latin insipid, meaning "tasteless."

Table 12-2 Classification of Diabetes Mellitus (DM)

Primary DM	Secondary DM	Special Forms of DM
Type 1 (insulin-dependent)	Pancreatic diseases	Gestational
Type 2 (non–insulin-dependent)	Chronic pancreatitis	Impaired glucose tolerance
	Tumors	
	Endocrine diseases	
	Acromegaly	
	Cushing's syndrome	
	Pheochromocytoma	
	Drugs	
	Corticosteroids	
	Diuretics	
	Antihypertensive drugs	
	Insulin receptor deficiency	
	Genetic syndromes	
	Hemochromatosis	
	Hyperlipidemia	

most people have a mild form of the disease, the cumulative effects of long-standing diabetes account for approximately 35,000 deaths per year in the United States.

The classification of diabetes is based on pathogenetic principles. The most common forms of DM are listed in Table 12-2. *Primary diabetes,* which accounts for most cases of DM, is a multifactorial disease caused by the interaction of hereditary and environmental factors. It includes insulin-dependent DM (IDDM), also known as type 1 diabetes, and non–insulin-dependent DM (NIDDM), also known as type 2 diabetes. *Secondary diabetes* is the form of the disease that can be traced to some other documented disease, such as chronic pancreatitis or disturbances of carbohydrate and lipid metabolism (e.g., as a result of pituitary or adrenocortical hyperactivity). Insulin receptor abnormalities also cause secondary DM. As gestational diabetes is difficult to classify, it is in a category by itself. Patients who have impaired glucose tolerance (IGT) have a subclinical form of diabetes, which is distinct from the major forms of clinically overt diabetes.

Type 2 diabetes accounts for more than 90 percent of all cases. In the United States, there are approximately 6 million people who have type 2 diabetes. The incidence of type 1 diabetes is much lower (50 persons per million). However, it occurs more often in children and adolescents. In persons younger than 20 years of age, the incidence of type 1 diabetes is three times higher than that in the general population (i.e., 150 per million). Overall, 15,000 persons develop type 1 diabetes every year in the United States. Other forms of diabetes are less common.

The salient features of type 1 and type 2 diabetes are presented in Table 12-3.

Pathogenesis. Diabetes may develop in the presence of several conditions, all of which are characterized by abnormal regulation of the intermediary metabolism of carbohydrates, lipids, and protein by insulin (Fig. 12-7). The most important causes of these metabolic disturbances are

- an absolute deficiency of insulin (e.g., lack of beta cells secondary to islet cell destruction)

Table 12-3 Typical Features of Type 1 and Type 2 Diabetes

Characteristic	Type 1	Type 2
Age of onset (years)	Usually < 30	Usually > 30
Speed of onset	Sudden	Gradual
Body build	Normal	Obese (90%)
Family history	< 20%	60%
Twin concordance	Low	High
Antibodies to islet cells	+	–
Histology of islets	Loss of beta cells	Normal
Serum insulin level	Low	Normal
Treatment	Insulin	Diet Oral hypoglycemics or insulin

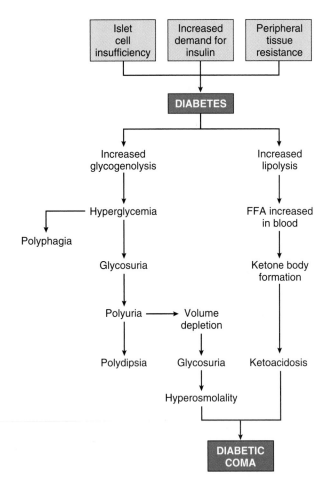

FIGURE 12-7
Pathogenesis of hyperglycemia and other metabolic and pathologic changes associated with diabetes mellitus. FFA, free fatty acids.

- a relative deficiency of insulin (e.g., when the demand for insulin exceeds the supply)
- interference with insulin binding to target tissues (e.g., tissue resistance to insulin owing to faulty insulin receptors or antibodies to insulin or insulin receptor)

In order to understand the pathogenesis of DM, it is important to realize that insulin plays a crucial role in the intermediary metabolism of carbohydrates, lipids, and amino acids. Insulin is produced by the beta cells in the islets of Langerhans. Normal beta cells store insulin in neurosecretory cytoplasmic granules, which are released into the circulation after appropriate stimulation. The major stimulus for insulin secretions is *hyperglycemia* (i.e., high serum glucose level). Insulin reduces the level of serum glucose by promoting its influx into the liver, where it is catabolized (*glycolysis*) and transformed into storage form (glycogen) by *glycogenesis*. Insulin stimulates the influx of glucose into the striated muscle cells as well. Insulin deficiency results in hyperglycemia, whereas an excess of insulin causes hypoglycemia.

Insulin has other functions as well. It stimulates the synthesis of proteins from amino acids, mainly in striated muscles, and fat formation from triglycerides in fat cells (*lipogenesis*). All these effects of insulin are mediated through the activation of the cellular insulin receptors, expressed on liver, muscle, and fat cells, and several other cell types. Insulin bound to the receptor triggers several cytoplasmic responses, in addition to glucose influx.

The effects of insulin are partially counteracted by glucagon, a polypeptide hormone secreted by the alpha cells in the islets of Langerhans, and pituitary growth hormone, steroid hormones, and epinephrine. Lack of insulin, inhibition of its action (e.g., by antibodies to insulin), blockade of insulin receptors (e.g., by antibodies to insulin receptors), or inadequate cell response to insulin (the so-called *postreceptor defect*) can result in hyperglycemia, the first and foremost sign of DM. Excess glucose in the blood spills over into the urine, causing glucosuria. Glucose leads to osmotic diuresis and causes polyuria.

The utilization of glucose in striated muscle cells, including the heart, is impaired in DM. Anaerobic glycolysis, instead of oxidative aerobic glycolysis, is used for energy production, resulting in the formation of excessive amounts of lactic acid. This may cause lactic acidosis, a serious complication of untreated diabetes. Inadequate utilization of fats and reduced lipogenesis lead to the accumulation of free fatty acids, which are oxidized into ketones. Ketogenesis is still another cause of acidosis in advanced diabetes (*ketoacidosis*).

Hyperglycemia also leads to the deposition of glucose tissues that do not require insulin receptor for the uptake of glucose, such as the blood vessels, nerves, lens, and kidney tubules. In these tissues, glycose is metabolized to osmotically active compounds (sorbitol and fructose). This stimulates the influx of fluids into the affected tissue. Sorbitol is a polyol, or alcohol, that inhibits enzymes involved in the maintenance of cell homeostasis and probably has direct toxic effects on cells in various tissues.

The pathogenesis of the various forms of diabetes has not been fully elucidated. Overall, however, there is agreement that:

- *Diabetes has a genetic predisposition.* This predisposition is stronger for type 2 than for type 1 diabetes. For example, type 1 is concordant in 50 percent of monozygotic twins, whereas the concordance of type 2 is much higher (over 90 percent). The inheritance does not follow the rules of mendelian genetics, and the disease is probably polygenic.
- *Diabetes develops under the influence of some environmental factors.* In some cases of type 1 diabetes, sudden onset of the disease may be related

to viral infection, such as measles or Coxsack-ievirus B infection. Seasonal occurrences of type 1 diabetes, suggestive of "miniepidemics," are also consistent with an infectious pathogenesis, although the suspected virus has not yet been isolated.

Antibodies to beta cells can be detected in the blood of patients with type 1 diabetes. In early stages of the disease, the islets of Langerhans are infiltrated with lymphocytes and macrophages, which apparently destroy the endocrine pancreatic tissue. In later stages of type 1 diabetes, the islets show a depletion of beta cells, which are replaced by hyalinized fibrous tissue. All this suggests an autoimmune reaction which may be triggered by a virus or some other exogenous stimulus. However, in most instances, the causative agent remains unidentified, and the pathogenesis of the disease is unknown.

Exogenous factors contributing to type 2 diabetes are obscure. Because type 2 diabetes occurs often in obese persons, a pathogenetic link between these two conditions has been postulated. However, not all obese persons have diabetes and not all diabetics are obese, which indicates that other factors may be important as well.

Pathology. The pathologic basis of diabetes is highly variable. In type 1 diabetes, there is ample evidence of islet destruction and beta cell loss. In early stages of type 1 diabetes, there is *insulitis* (i.e., mononuclear cell infiltration of the islets of Langerhans). Most of the cells involved in the destruction of islets are cytotoxic T lymphocytes and macrophages. This insulitis is short-lived, but the damage is irreparable. The damaged islets show interstitial fibrosis and hyalinization (Fig. 12-8). The hypoinsuline-mia that ensues correlates directly with the extent of islet cell destruction.

In patients with type 2 diabetes, the islets of Langerhans are usually of normal size and contain a normal or even an increased number of beta cells. This probably reflects the body's attempt to compensate for the relative deficiency of insulin under conditions in which the demand is not met by the output. The same happens when the target tissues are resistant to the action of insulin.

Metabolic changes caused by diabetes affect many organs. Many, if not most, of these changes are a consequence of hyperglycemia, which adversely alters the metabolism of basement membranes and damages the small blood vessels. Diabetes also accelerates the development of atherosclerosis. *Microangiopathy* and *atherosclerosis* could, thus, be considered common denominators for most of the pathologic changes in diabetes. Diabetics are prone to infection, which is yet another cause of pathologic changes.

The extent of pathologic changes in diabetes depends on the type of diabetes, the duration of disease, and the coexistence of other diseases, but it primarily reflects the degree and duration of hypoglycemia. Patients whose disease is well controlled show fewer pathologic changes than those who have uncontrollable disease or those who have not been treated adequately.

Complications

The most prominent changes caused by uncontrolled or inadequately controlled diabetes involve the following:

- Cardiovascular system
- Kidneys
- Eyes
- Nervous system

The complications of diabetes are outlined in Figure 12-9.

The *cardiovascular complications* of diabetes account for most of the morbidity and mortality associated with the disease. Diabetes promotes the development of atherosclerotic lesions in the large arteries. The consequences include coronary disease, cerebrovascular diseases, and atherosclerosis of the aorta with formation of aneurysms. The arteries of the lower extremities are often affected, and their narrowing or occlusion frequently results in *gangrene* of the toes or of the entire foot.

The *renal complications* of diabetes include *glomerulosclerosis, pyelonephritis,* and *papillary necrosis.* The glomerular capillaries show signs of diabetic microangiopathy and appear to be thickened. The mesangial areas are widened by the increased amounts of basement membranes, and the entire

FIGURE 12-8

Histologic appearance of the islets of Langerhans in a patient with type 1 diabetes mellitus. Fibrous tissue replaces islet cells that have been lost.

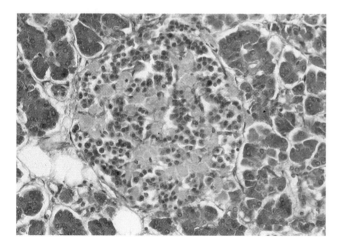

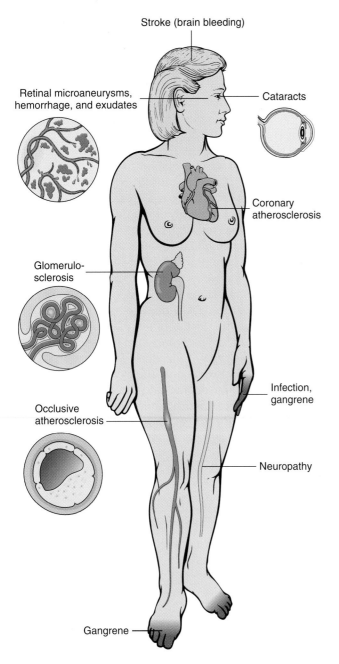

Stroke (brain bleeding)

Retinal microaneurysms, hemorrhage, and exudates

Cataracts

Coronary atherosclerosis

Glomerulo-sclerosis

Occlusive atherosclerosis

Infection, gangrene

Neuropathy

Gangrene

FIGURE 12-9
Complications of diabetes mellitus.

glomerulus ultimately becomes hyalinized and afunctional. Microangiopathy involving the arterioles (hyaline arteriosclerosis) causes renal ischemia, which results in tubular atrophy and interstitial fibrosis. Affected kidneys are also prone to infections, and bacterial pyelonephritis occurs frequently. Ischemic changes in the renal papilla (the part of the renal medulla that protrudes into the renal pelvis) may cause infarcts, which typically result in papillary necrosis. Necrotic papillae are sloughed off and dis-

charged in the urine, usually obstructing the urethra and ultimately causing renal colic.

The *eyes* are often affected by diabetes, which is the leading cause of blindness in this country. *Diabetic microangiopathy* affects the retinal vessels, causing microaneurysmal dilatations, microinfarcts with hemorrhage, and (in most severe cases) reactive proliferation of vascular sprouts. Vascular changes may also obstruct the outflow of vitreous fluid and cause *glaucoma*. Diabetes also causes *cataracts*. These opacities of the lens are related to the deposition of sorbitol and fructose in the lens matrix and subsequent swelling caused by the osmotic action of these carbohydrates.

Both the central and peripheral *nervous systems* are often affected by diabetes. Most of the pathologic changes are related to diabetic *microangiopathy*, which leads to widespread focal ischemia. Diabetes usually affects the autonomic nerves, causing symptoms that vary from mild to severe urinary incontinence or impotence. *Peripheral neuropathy*, a common complication of diabetes, is partially a consequence of diabetic microangiopathy and partially related to the deposition of sorbitol and fructose in the axons and myelin sheaths. Clinically, it presents with both sensory and motor deficits.

Clinical Features. The symptoms and clinical findings of diabetes are related to

- hyperglycemia and abnormalities of intermediate metabolism related to insulin deficiency
- vascular changes caused by diabetes
- increased susceptibility to infection

The most common symptoms of diabetes are polyuria and *polydipsia* (excessive thirst). Because of an excessive loss of water in urine, the patients feel thirsty and tend to drink a lot of fluids. Abnormal utilization of carbohydrates, proteins, and lipids generates a negative energy balance that results in muscle wasting, which is compensated for by an increased appetite. Affected patients tend to eat large amounts of food (*polyphagia*). Hyperglycemia predisposes individuals to bacterial infections, which are common. Cardiovascular and cerebrovascular changes account for the fact that diabetics have a life span that is shorter (by 7 to 9 years) than their age-matched peers.

Treatment of diabetes depends on the type of disease, its duration and severity, and the presence or absence of complications. Patients with type 1 require insulin for the rest of their lives. Maturity-onset NIDDM, when associated with obesity, may improve with weight loss and appropriate dietary modifications. Hypoglycemic drugs or insulin are prescribed for those who do not respond to dietary measures.

Review Questions

1. How is the pancreas attached to the intestine?
2. Compare the exocrine with the endocrine portion of the pancreas.
3. List the main secretory products of the pancreas.
4. List the main causes of acute pancreatitis.
5. Correlate the pathologic findings in acute pancreatitis with the clinical features of this disease.
6. What are the most important complications of acute pancreatitis?
7. What is chronic pancreatitis and how does this disease present clinically?
8. How common are tumors of the pancreas?
9. Compare adenocarcinoma of the pancreas with tumors of the endocrine pancreas.
10. How common is diabetes mellitus?
11. Classify diabetes mellitus.
12. Compare type 1 (insulin-dependent) with type 2 (non–insulin-dependent) diabetes mellitus.
13. Explain the pathogenesis of hyperglycemia in diabetes mellitus.
14. Explain the pathogenesis of diabetic ketoacidosis.
15. Explain the cardiovascular, renal, ocular, and neurologic complications of diabetes mellitus.
16. What is the pathogenesis of polydipsia, polyphagia, and polyuria in diabetes mellitus?

Learning Objectives

After reading this chapter, the student should be able to:

1. Describe the gross and microscopic anatomy of the urinary tract, as well as the principal functions of the kidneys and the urinary bladder.

2. List two congenital renal malformations and explain the significance of adult polycystic kidney disease.

3. Discuss the pathogenesis, clinical course, and outcome of poststreptococcal and crescentic glomerulonephritis.

4. Discuss three causes of the nephrotic syndrome.

5. Compare the pathogenesis of acute and chronic renal failure.

6. Describe the pathologic changes in the kidney caused by diabetes.

7. List four types of renal stones, explain their pathogenesis, and describe the clinical symptoms they produce.

8. List five causes of urinary obstruction.

9. Compare the pathology and clinical symptoms of acute and chronic pyelonephritis.

10. Discuss the etiology and pathogenesis of cystitis in men and women.

11. Define acute tubular necrosis and describe its pathogenesis and outcome.

12. Describe the pathology and clinical features of renal cell carcinoma, Wilms' tumor, and transitional cell carcinoma of the renal pelvis.

13. Describe the pathology and clinical features of bladder cancer.

Additional Key Terms and Concepts

Cystitis

Goodpasture's syndrome

Hematuria

Nephrotic syndrome

Proteinuria

Pyelonephritis

Uremia

Chapter Outline

The Urinary Tract
Chapter 13

The urinary tract comprises the kidneys, the ureters, the urinary bladder, and the urethra (Fig. 13-1). Diseases affecting the kidneys are usually treated by *nephrologists,* whereas *urologists* generally treat renal tumors and most of the diseases of the lower urinary tract.

NORMAL ANATOMY AND PHYSIOLOGY

The primary function of the urinary tract is the formation and excretion of urine. Urine is formed by ultrafiltration of blood in the kidneys. From the **kidneys,** the urine flows into the renal collecting system (renal calices and **pelvis**) and passes through the **ureters** before it reaches the urinary bladder. The **urinary bladder** serves as a receptacle for the urine. The urine is stored in the urinary bladder for several hours and then discharged from the body through the **urethra.**

The formation of urine in the kidneys is accomplished in the **nephron,** which represents the basic functional unit of each kidney. The kidneys contain approximately 2.5 million nephrons, each of which consists of a **glomerulus, tubules,** and **collecting ducts** (Fig. 13-2). The glomerulus consists of specialized capillaries that are modified so that they allow selective passage of fluids and solutes from the blood into the lumen of the nephron. This "primary filtrate" is modified during its passage through the tubular parts of the nephron, which are known as the proximal and distal tubules, loop of Henle, and collecting ducts. The contents of the primary filtrate are partially resorbed and partially enriched by substances that are secreted into the nephron. Most of the fluid filtered in the glomeruli is actually resorbed and returned to the circulation. Because the primary filtrate is concentrated in the tubules, only a small portion of it is excreted as urine. Approximately 1.5 L of urine are excreted daily, which represents less than 10 percent of the blood volume filtered through the glomeruli.

In contrast to the complex histology of the kidneys, the excretory portion of the urinary tract is relatively simple, reflecting its simple function. The calices, pelves, ureters, and urinary bladder, and most of the urethra, are lined by **transitional epithelium.** The transitional epithelium is "waterproof" and can withstand prolonged exposure to urine. External to this epithelial layer, these organs consist of connective tissue and smooth muscle cells. Transitional epithelium and the smooth muscular wall can expand, allowing the bladder to store urine. The smooth muscle in the bladder wall is important for extrusion of urine during micturition.

As mentioned, the urinary tract primarily has an excretory function. In addition, the kidney has secretory functions: it secretes *renin,* a hormone that raises blood pressure, and *erythropoietin,* the growth factor that stimulates the production of red blood cells (RBCs) in the bone marrow.

FIGURE 13-1

The urinary tract consists of the kidneys, ureters, urinary bladder, and urethra. (From Applegate EJ: The anatomy and physiology learning system: textbook. Philadelphia: WB Saunders, 1995:372.)

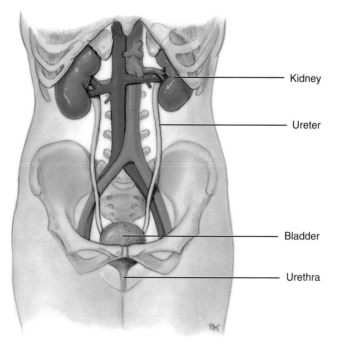

Kidney

Ureter

Bladder

Urethra

OVERVIEW OF MAJOR DISEASES

The most important diseases of the urinary tract are

- immunologic disorders (e.g., glomerulonephritis)
- metabolic disorders (e.g., diabetic nephropathy)
- circulatory disturbances (e.g., prerenal renal failure secondary to shock)
- bacterial infections (e.g., cystitis, pyelonephritis)
- tumors

Several facts important for the understanding of urinary tract pathology are presented here, before a discussion of specific pathologic entities.

1. *The primary function of the urinary tract is to form and excrete urine.* It goes without saying that the kidneys must be anatomically normal to perform their normal function. However, the formation of urine depends also on sufficient blood flow and adequate hydration of the body. Several polypeptide and steroid hormones also regulate renal function. The most important hormones are the *antidiuretic hormone* (ADH), which is secreted by the posterior pituitary; the *atrial natriuretic hormone* (ANH), which is

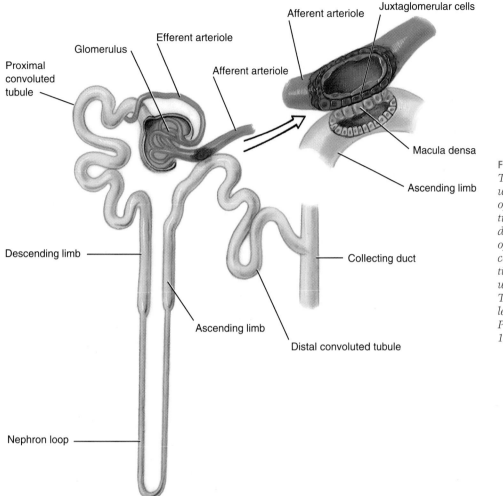

Proximal convoluted tubule

Glomerulus

Efferent arteriole

Afferent arteriole

Afferent arteriole

Juxtaglomerular cells

Macula densa

Ascending limb

Descending limb

Ascending limb

Collecting duct

Distal convoluted tubule

Nephron loop

FIGURE 13-2
The nephron is the functional unit of the kidney. It consists of the glomerulus, convoluted tubules, and the collecting ducts. The close positioning of blood vessels allows concentration of urine and selective excretion of minerals and water. (From Applegate EJ: The anatomy and physiology learning system: textbook. Philadelphia: WB Saunders, 1995:375.)

derived from the atria of the heart; and *aldosterone,* which is from the zona glomerulosa of the adrenal cortex. Once the urine is formed, it can be discharged only if the urinary passages are patent. Any obstruction of the ureters (e.g., owing to urinary stones) or of the urinary bladder (e.g., owing to an enlarged prostate secondary to hyperplasia) will result in retention of urine.

Failure of the urinary tract to produce normal amounts of urine may be classified as *prerenal, renal,* or *postrenal. Prerenal renal failure* is most often caused by shock or heart insufficiency (e.g., myocardial infarction). Prerenal failure is usually reversible, and if its cause is cured, normal renal function can be restored. *Intrarenal causes of acute renal failure,* such as tubular necrosis, are also reversible. Although chronic renal failure previously was lethal, modern technology has made it feasible to treat even irreversible renal failure by dialysis machines or renal transplantation. *Postrenal causes of renal failure,* such as prostatic disease or stones in the bladder, can be treated by surgery.

2. *The urinary tract is extremely sensitive to bacter-*

ial infections. The kidneys are perfused constantly by a high volume of blood which is filtered in the glomeruli. Bacteria found in the circulation thus have a good chance of entering and colonizing the kidneys and causing a urinary tract infection (UTI). Moreover, because the urethral opening lies external to the body, bacteria may easily enter the urinary tract through it as well. UTIs that are acquired from bacteremia are called *descending* or *hematogenous infections,* whereas those attributable to upstream bacterial spread are called *ascending infections.*

3. *The specialized capillaries of the glomeruli are a ready target for blood-borne antibodies.* The glomeruli filter large amounts of blood. During this process, their basement membranes are exposed to potentially noxious plasma components—most notably, antibodies and antigen-antibody complexes. Glomeruli are thus frequently involved in many systemic autoimmune diseases mediated by antibodies. Antibody-mediated disease of the glomeruli is known as *glomerulonephritis.*

4. *Glomerular capillaries, even though they are highly specialized, are, nevertheless, part of the circula-*

tory system and arterioles. The glomeruli are affected by many diseases that involve the vasculature. Although atherosclerosis, which is a disease involving the larger arteries, does not affect the glomeruli directly, the narrowing within atherosclerotic renal arteries and their branches produces secondary changes in the glomeruli and their obsolescence (*glomerulosclerosis*). Renal arterioles and glomeruli are often pathologically altered by hypertension, which may damage the kidneys irreparably. Diabetes mellitus, a common metabolic disorder of intermediate metabolism, affects the capillaries and arterioles in many organs. Hence, it is no surprise that this microangiopathy frequently damages the glomeruli as well (*diabetic glomerulosclerosis*).

5. *Renal tubules are composed of highly specialized cells that are very sensitive to a lack of oxygen, as well as to the adverse action of toxins.* Like all other highly specialized cells, such as neurons, renal tubular cells require a constant supply of oxygen and nutrients. Even a short interruption of blood supply or a hypoperfusion of the kidneys, as typically occurs in shock or heart failure, results in *tubular necrosis.* Because the proximal tubular cells have the most complex function and require the most oxygen, they are most susceptible to hypoxia or anoxia. Many drugs, poisons, heavy metals, and endogenous waste products that are filtered through the glomeruli are taken up by the proximal tubular cells, and may adversely affect them. For example, mercury salts inactivate the enzymes of the proximal tubules and, if ingested in large amounts (e.g., in suicidal mercury poisoning), can cause necrosis of the proximal tubules.

6. *The urinary tract consists of many mitotic or facultative mitotic cells that may undergo malignant transformation.* Tumors of the urinary tract develop most often in the urinary bladder, which is lined by regularly cycling (mitotic) cells. As with most other tumors, the causes of urogenital tumors are not known. However, because the urinary tract serves as a route for the excretion of chemicals, many of which are potential carcinogens, it is possible that some tumors are chemically induced. It has also been postulated that some tumors originate from the interaction of chemical carcinogens and endogenous proto-oncogenes. In support of this hypothesis is the finding of chromosomal changes in many renal cell and urinary bladder carcinomas. *Wilms' tumor,* the most common urinary tract tumor of infancy that shows a familial preponderance, has been linked to a deletion of a specific tumor suppressor gene in about 15 percent of cases (Wilms' tumor gene—*WT-1*).

7. *Diseases of the urinary tract may present with local or systemic symptoms.* Diseases of the urinary tract produce a variety of symptoms that may either be localized to the urinary tract or may be systemic, affecting the entire body. The best-known local symptom is the flank pain that occurs with kidney

infection (*pyelonephritis*) or renal tumors. Painful urination (*dysuria*) is the best known symptom of *cystitis.* Urinary *colic* is a symptom associated with urinary stones impacted in the ureters. Colics are attacks of spasmodic pain that occur as the ureteral smooth muscles contract in an effort to propel the stone and relieve the urinary obstruction.

Localized Symptoms. The local symptoms and findings are best exemplified by a variety of changes reflected in the urine itself. The *volume* of urine may be altered so that too much or too little urine is produced. *Polyuria* indicates an increased amount of urine, whereas *oliguria* means a decreased daily output of urine. *Anuria* is a state in which no urine is produced.

The *chemical composition* of urine may be determined and a microscopic analysis of urinary sediment is routinely performed in the clinical laboratory. *Proteinuria* and *glucosuria* refer to increased excretion of protein or glucose in the urine, respectively. *Hematuria,* which is blood in the urine, may present as a grossly visible change in the color of urine (e.g., the brown or red urine typical of macroscopic hematuria) or be detectable only by microscopic analysis of urine (microscopic hematuria refers to RBCs in urine). *Pyuria* is the appearance of pus in urine. Such urine contains a large number of viable and dead polymorphonuclear leukocytes and appears turbid. Urine normally contains few bacteria, most of which are from the terminal urethra, which is normally colonized by bacteria. Infections of the urinary tract are associated with an increased number of bacteria in urine, which can be documented by quantitating bacteria in urine. Typically, the results are expressed as the number of bacterial colonies per milliliter of urine. More than 100,000 colonies per milliliter is evidence of infection.

Systemic Symptoms. *Systemic symptoms* and findings caused by urinary tract disease vary depending on the underlying pathology. Bacterial infection affecting the kidneys, such as acute pyelonephritis, or acute cystitis affecting the urinary bladder may cause *fever, shivering,* and *malaise,* like any other infection. Renal failure may cause complex metabolic changes, mostly because of the accumulation of substances that cannot be excreted from the body through the urinary tract. This condition, called *uremia,* is, in simplified terms, equivalent to "poisoning with urine." It is characterized by retention of water; minerals (e.g., sodium, potassium, chloride, calcium, and phosphate); organic substances, such as creatinine or uric acid; and other nitrogen-rich substances, such as ammonia, which are measured in the clinical laboratory as blood urea nitrogen (BUN). Hypercalcemia or hyperkalemia endanger life because these metabolic changes may cause cardiac arrest. Chronic uremia is marked by profound neurologic changes and depression of the central nervous system, which initially presents as somnolence and fatigue, and ultimately results in coma and death. Fortunately, by an act of Congress introduced in the 1970s, all Americans are entitled to free treatment of chronic renal failure; therefore, chronic uremia is a condition that is rarely seen today.

Developmental Disorders

Developmental disorders of the urinary tract are very common. Fortunately, most of these anomalies do not produce symptoms and are often discovered only by chance. For example, 1 in 800 people is born with only one kidney (one-sided *renal agenesis*) or with a solitary *horseshoe kidney* formed by the fusion of the kidneys in the midline. Patients with such anomalies are usually asymptomatic and the congenital defect is often noted on routine x-ray examination for some other disease, or if the affected person is being considered for kidney donation. Clearly, these individuals cannot donate their solitary kidney for transplantation.

Polycystic Kidney Disease

The most important developmental disorder of the urinary tract is *autosomal dominant polycystic kidney disease* (ADPKD), which is inherited as a mendelian trait at a rate of 1:1000. ADPKD affects the kidneys bilaterally. Both kidneys are enlarged, contain numerous cysts, and weigh 3000 to 4000 g, which is 20 times more than the normal weight (150 to 200 g). These cysts, which are derived from obstructed tubules, contain fluid (Fig. 13-3). The reasons for the obstruction of tubules are unknown. Cystic change in the tubules gradually impairs renal function. Most affected patients develop renal failure by the age of 30 to 40 years.

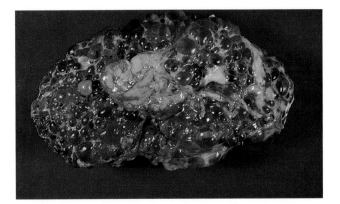

FIGURE 13-3
Autosomal dominant polycystic kidney disease. Note the numerous cysts.

ADPKD must be distinguished from several other congenital kidney diseases, most of which present during infancy and childhood. The most important of these is *cystic renal dysplasia.* In contrast to ADPKD, cystic renal dysplasia is usually unilateral. The enlarged abnormal kidney may be palpated by either a parent or the pediatrician. This condition should be distinguished from renal tumors of infancy (Wilms' tumor) or adrenal nephroblastomas, which are two other causes of abdominal masses in that age group. Unilateral renal lesions can easily be removed without consequences, and if the kidney is normal, the patient has an excellent chance for complete recovery.

Glomerular Diseases

Classification. The classification of glomerular diseases may be based on morphology, pathogenesis, or clinical presentation of the diseases. On the basis of pathogenesis, glomerular diseases can be classified into several categories (Fig. 13-4):

- immunologic diseases
- metabolic disorders
- circulatory disturbances

Immunologic Diseases. Immunologic injury is most often mediated by antibodies and can be classified as a type II (cytotoxic) or type III (immune complex) hypersensitivity reaction. Pathologic studies reveal that such injury is marked by deposits of immunoglobulins in the glomeruli. If the deposition of immunoglobulins evokes an inflammatory reaction, the disease is classified as glomerulonephritis. Those glomerulopathies that have an immunologic pathogenesis or a presumptive immunologic pathogenesis, but that do not show signs of inflammation, carry names without the suffix *-itis* (which is re-

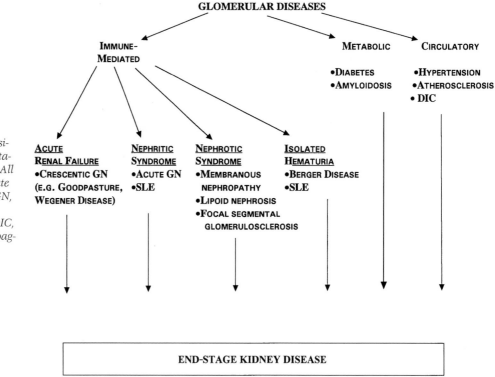

FIGURE 13-4
Glomerulopathies can be classified as immune-mediated, metabolic, or circulatory diseases. All of these diseases may terminate in end-stage kidney disease. GN, glomerulonephritis; SLE, systemic lupus erythematosus; DIC, disseminated intravascular coagulation.

served for inflammatory disease). Within this category, the most important diseases are *lipoid nephrosis, membranous nephropathy,* and *immunoglobulin A (IgA) nephropathy (Berger's disease).*

Immune-mediated glomerulonephritis can occur in an isolated form (*primary*) or in the course of a systemic disease (*secondary*), as in systemic lupus erythematosus or Wegener's granulomatosis. Primary glomerulonephritis is often limited to the glomeruli, whereas secondary glomerulonephritis is usually associated with tubulointerstitial renal inflammation.

Metabolic Disorders. *Metabolic glomerulopathy* occurs in the course of systemic metabolic disorders. The best example is diabetes mellitus, which typically presents with polyuria and glycosuria and leads to chronic renal failure in about 5 percent to 10 percent of affected patients. Diabetes causes biochemical changes in the composition of the basement membranes, which become thickened, glomerulosclerotic, and lose their semipermeability. Diabetic glomerulosclerosis, like other metabolic glomerulopathies, is also associated with pathologic changes involving other parts of the kidney.

Circulatory Disturbances. Circulatory disturbances affect glomeruli in several ways. Atherosclerosis of the renal arteries is typically associated with hypoperfusion, which leads to involution and hyalin-

ization of glomeruli. The sudden onset of hypertension may cause fibrinoid necrosis of the glomerular capillaries. Shock is often associated with disseminated intravascular coagulation (DIC) and the formation of microthrombi in the glomerular capillaries.

Multiple Mechanisms. The border between immunologic, metabolic, and circulatory glomerular diseases is not always sharp. This is best illustrated by diabetes. The metabolic changes of diabetes cause thickening of the glomerular basement membranes. Diabetes is also a systemic *microangiopathy* (i.e., disease of small vessels), and is often associated with atherosclerosis and hypertension, both of which affect the glomeruli, producing additional changes. Moreover, diabetes is usually accompanied by deposition of IgG in the glomerular basement membranes and increased permeability. These deposits of IgG probably do not cause an immunologic glomerular injury, but we do not know for sure.

Clinical Features. Glomerular diseases can present clinically with a set of symptoms, which collectively are recognized as particular syndromes. The most important of these syndromes are

- acute renal failure
- nephritic syndrome
- nephrotic syndrome
- isolated hematuria and/or proteinuria

The term *acute renal failure* is self-explanatory. The disease has a sudden onset and, in either a few days or weeks, renal excretory function ceases, resulting in anuria or severe oliguria. As mentioned earlier, acute renal failure may be prerenal, renal, or postrenal. Prerenal failure accompanies shock or heart failure caused by myocardial infarction. Renal failure may be a consequence of glomerular destruction in individuals with glomerulonephritis or tubular necrosis. Sudden obstruction of excretory pathways (e.g., such as that caused by enlargement of the prostate obstructing urine outflow from the urinary bladder) is a cause of postrenal failure.

Nephritic syndrome is diagnosed on the basis of typical clinical and laboratory findings. These include generalized edema, hypertension, hematuria, proteinuria, and hypoalbuminemia.

Nephrotic syndrome is characterized by generalized edema, proteinuria, hypoalbuminemia, and often, hyperlipidemia and lipiduria.

The syndrome of *isolated glomerular hematuria,* with or without *proteinuria,* is usually not accompanied by constant clinical symptoms and generally can be diagnosed only on the basis of abnormal urinary findings. This syndrome, as typically seen in Berger's disease, may, however, progress to chronic renal failure like any other immune-mediated glomerulonephritis.

Acute Glomerulonephritis

Acute glomerulonephritis is an immune-mediated inflammatory glomerulopathy that occurs 1 to 2 weeks after an acute infection, most often a streptococcal upper respiratory disease ("strep-throat"). The disease typically affects children. Previously, before the era of antibiotics, poststreptococcal glomerulonephritis was very common. Today, it is uncommon in the United States, but is still prevalent in underdeveloped countries and even some countries as close as the Caribbean islands.

Acute poststreptococcal glomerulonephritis is caused by the antibodies produced in response to infection with certain streptococcal strains. The antigen-antibody complexes are trapped in the glomerular basement membranes, where they activate complement, and thus attract inflammatory cells into the kidney (Fig. 13-5). On histologic examination, the glomeruli appear hypercellular because they contain an increased number of mesangial cells and numerous inflammatory cells (Fig. 13-6). These cells compress or occlude the capillaries, thereby preventing blood flow through the glomeruli.

Acute glomerulonephritis presents with a nephritic syndrome. The damaged basement membranes of the inflamed glomeruli become permeable, which accounts for the proteinuria and hematuria. The urine of these patients typically appears murky brown, resembling bouillon soup. Loss of proteins, mostly albumin, in the urine causes hypoalbuminemia which, in turn, results in edema. The hypertension is caused by reduced blood flow through the arterioles leading to the inflamed glomeruli, which elicits a release of renin from the juxtaglomerular apparatus in the afferent arteriole. Reduced blood flow also results in oliguria.

The glomerular inflammation is usually short-lived, and most patients recover completely. In 1 percent to 2 percent of affected patients, however, the disease may cause acute renal failure. Chronic glomerulonephritis and end-stage kidney disease

FIGURE 13-5

Acute glomerulonephritis. (A) Normal glomerulus. (B) This affected glomerulus appears hypercellular. This hypercellularity is mostly attributable to inflammatory cells and, in part, to the proliferation of mesangial cells responding to injury. Deposits of immune complexes on the epithelial side of the basement membrane form "humps."

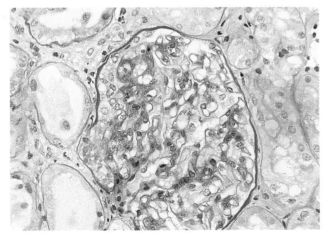

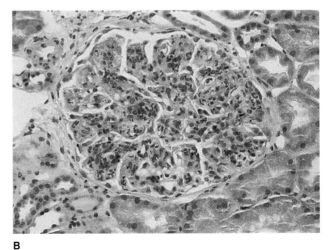

A

B

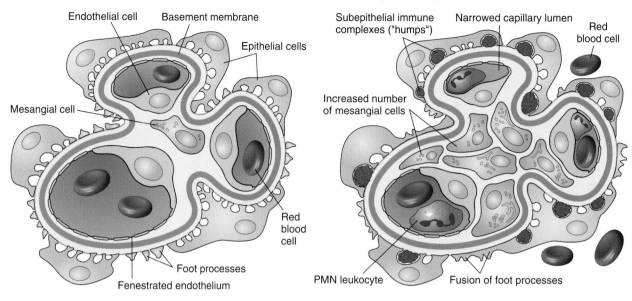

A Normal glomerulus

Endothelial cell Basement membrane

Epithelial cells

Mesangial cell

Red blood cell

Foot processes

Fenestrated endothelium

B Acute glomerulonephritis

Subepithelial immune complexes ("humps") Narrowed capillary lumen Red blood cell

Increased number of mesangial cells

PMN leukocyte Fusion of foot processes

FIGURE 13-6
Histologic appearance of acute glomerulonephritis. (A) Normal glomerulus. (B) Glomerulonephritis. The glomerulus appears hypercellular and the capillaries are narrowed or occluded. PMN, polymorphonuclear neutrophil.

complicate acute glomerulonephritis in less than 10 percent of cases.

Crescentic Glomerulonephritis

Crescentic glomerulonephritis is a term used to describe severe glomerular injury accompanied by the formation of an exudate in the glomerular urinary space. The exudate consists predominantly of macrophages that have crossed through the damaged glomerular capillaries into the urinary space between the capillary tufts and Bowman's capsule (Fig. 13-7). The term derives from the fact that the inflammatory cells surround the compressed capillary loops in the form of a crescent moon.

Crescentic glomerulonephritis usually occurs after focal necrosis of the glomerular capillaries. Such focal necrotizing glomerulonephritis is typically found in *Goodpasture's syndrome,* an autoimmune disease characterized by the formation of antibodies to the body's own basement membrane component: collagen type IV. Injury of collagen type IV in the lungs causes intra-alveolar hemorrhage. In the glomeruli, the antibodies cause rupture of the basement membranes. Macrophages exit through the hole in the basement membrane and accumulate in the urinary space, forming the crescents that compress the capillary loops. Because no blood flows through the compressed capillary loops, glomerular filtration ceases and anuria (i.e., acute renal failure) ensues. Most patients never recover, and their survival depends on continuous dialysis or kidney transplantation.

Crescentic glomerulonephritis is a descriptive diagnosis. In addition to Goodpasture's syndrome, it may be caused by Wegener's granulomatosis, polyarteritis nodosa, or severe poststreptococcal glomerulonephritis.

Membranous Nephropathy

Membranous nephropathy is an immune-mediated glomerulopathy characterized by diffuse ("membranous") thickening of the glomerular basement membranes secondary to massive deposition of immune

FIGURE 13-7
Crescentic glomerulonephritis. The urinary space contains a "crescent" composed of macrophages and some proliferated epithelial cells derived from the lining of Bowman's capsule.

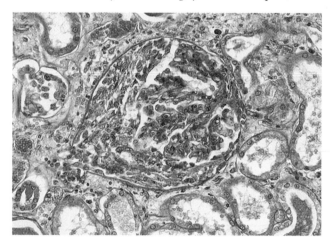

complexes. In contrast to acute glomerulonephritis, which causes nephritic syndrome, membranous nephropathy presents with a typical nephrotic syndrome. There is no evidence of inflammation: the glomeruli do not contain any inflammatory cells, and the urine is devoid of RBCs and inflammatory cells.

Membranous nephropathy is the most common immune nephrotic syndrome of adults. In 85 percent of the cases, its etiology remains unknown. In addition to these idiopathic cases, a "secondary" disease of the same morphology can affect patients who have developed antibodies to tumors, drugs, or infectious agents, such as hepatitis B virus or *Treponema pallidum.*

Light microscopy reveals that the glomeruli have thick basement membranes but are normocellular—that is, they show no proliferative or inflammatory changes (Fig. 13-8A). On electron microscopy, one may see that the thickening of the basement membrane is attributable to the deposition of dense immune complexes (Fig. 13-8B). Immunofluorescence microscopy demonstrates the granularity of these deposits (Fig. 13-8C).

Membranous nephropathy presents with the typical symptoms of nephrotic syndrome and does not respond to therapy. Proteinuria persists in most patients for years, but the disease progresses in only 40 percent of patients. These patients eventually develop chronic renal failure and require dialysis or renal transplantation.

Lipoid Nephrosis

Lipoid nephrosis, also known as *minimal change disease* or *nil disease,* is a disease of unknown etiology that also presents as a nephrotic syndrome. It is the most common cause of nephrotic syndrome in children. The descriptive terms used for this disease reflect our ignorance about its pathogenesis. "Lipoid nephrosis" indicates a nephrotic syndrome with hyperlipidemia and lipiduria. The other terms used as synonyms—*minimal change disease* or *nil disease* (from the Latin term *nihil,* meaning nothing)—indicate that the glomeruli show no changes on light microscopy. On immunofluorescence microscopy, the glomeruli are seen not to contain any deposits of immunoglobulins. The only remarkable findings are seen on electron microscopy, which usually shows

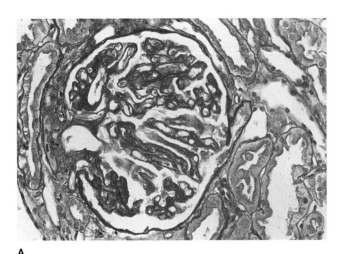

A

B

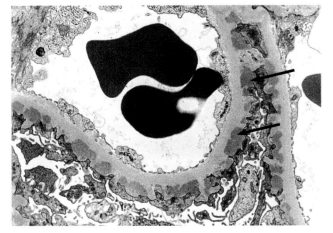

C

FIGURE 13-8
Membranous nephropathy. (A) Light microscopy shows thickening of the basement membranes but no inflammatory cells. (B) Immunofluorescence microscopy shows granular deposits along the basement membrane. (C) Electron microscopy shows immune deposits (arrows) along the basement membrane.

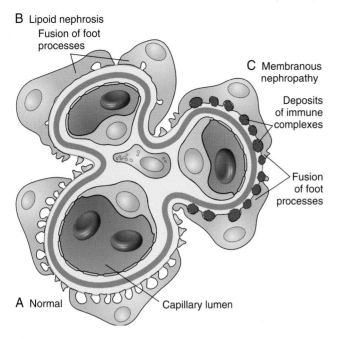

FIGURE 13-9
Schematic drawing of the glomerular changes in two forms of nephrotic syndrome as seen by electron microscopy. (A) Normal appearance. (B) Lipoid nephrosis does not cause any visible basement membrane changes, but fusion of the foot processes of epithelial cells is noted. (C) Membranous nephropathy is characterized by subepithelial dense deposits of immune complexes.

fusion of the foot processes of the podocytes, which are also known as the epithelial cells of the glomerulus. Such changes can readily be distinguished from those of membranous nephropathy (Fig. 13-9). Lipoid nephrosis responds favorably to corticosteroid treatment.

Chronic Proliferative Glomerulonephritis

Kidneys may be affected by several variants of primary immune-mediated glomerulonephropathies. Common to all of these glomerulopathies, which carry names such as IgA nephropathy (Berger's disease), membranoproliferative glomerulonephritis type I and type II, and focal proliferative glomerulonephritis, is that they have a chronic course, they do not respond to treatment, and they slowly, but inexorably, progress to end-stage kidney disease. Kidney biopsies show that these diseases have unique and diagnostic features.

Clinically, these chronic glomerulopathies may present as nephrotic syndrome, or nephritic syndrome with some hematuria, or they may be associated with only mild urinary findings, such as microscopic hematuria and proteinuria, and no clinical symptoms.

Chronic proliferative glomerulonephritis may occur in the course of systemic autoimmune diseases, most notably in *systemic lupus erythematosus* (SLE). Approximately, 60 percent to 70 percent of patients with SLE develop some renal manifestations. The glomerular changes vary from mild to severe, and histologic findings indicate glomerulonephritis or membranous nephropathy with no proliferative changes. The glomerulonephritis of SLE responds well to corticosteroid treatment.

End-Stage Glomerulopathy

Most, if not all, immune-mediated glomerulopathies can progress to end-stage kidney disease. These immune-mediated diseases terminating in uremia have traditionally been called chronic glomerulonephritis. However, by the time chronic renal failure has developed, there has been no evidence of inflammation; hence, the term glomerulonephritis seems unjustified. Furthermore, all chronic glomerulopathies—be they immune, metabolic, or circulatory—appear ultimately identical. As the morphologic study of terminally insufficient kidneys does not indicate the nature of the preexisting disease, it is best to be noncommittal and characterize such kidney diseases as end-stage glomerulopathy.

On gross examination, the kidneys appear to be shrunken symmetrically (Fig. 13-10A). Their surface is finely granular because of the loss of tubules. The fine granules are the remaining tubules surrounded by fibrous tissue. Histologic examination reveals that the glomeruli have undergone hyalinization and appear like solid globules composed of homogenized matrix (Fig. 13-10B).

Metabolic Diseases

Many systemic metabolic diseases affect the kidneys. For example, in gout, which is characterized by hyperuricemia, there are deposits of uric acid crystals in the kidneys. In multiple myeloma, renal failure develops owing to deposits of light chains of immunoglobulins secreted by neoplastic plasma cells. The most important of these diseases is diabetes mellitus.

Diabetes Mellitus

Diabetes mellitus is the most important metabolic disease affecting the kidneys. Diabetic kidney disease is very common; indeed, of the 20 million Americans who have diabetes, 5 percent to 10 percent have some renal problems.

Diabetic nephropathy may present in several forms depending on which portion of the kidney is

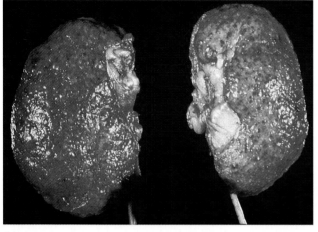

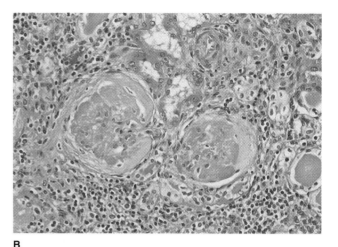

A

B

FIGURE 13-10
End-stage glomerulopathy—chronic glomerulonephritis. (A) The kidneys appear small, are uniformly shrunken, and have a finely granular external surface. (B) Histologic examination of the kidneys shows hyalinization of glomeruli and tubular atrophy. Fibrous tissue in the dilated interstitium surrounds atrophic tubules.

affected. Pathologic changes can be seen in the glomeruli, in the arteries and arterioles, and in the interstitium. The glomerular changes include thickening of the basement membranes and an increased amount of mesangial matrix. This pathologic change is known as *diffuse glomerulosclerosis*. The mesangial matrix expansion may lead to the formation of nodules, which is typical of *nodular glomerulosclerosis* or *Kimmelstiel-Wilson disease* (Fig. 13-11). Regardless of the form of glomerulopathy, the basement membranes of the altered glomeruli show increased permeability, which typically results in proteinuria. Proteinuria usually develops 10 to 20 years after the onset of diabetes. Proteinuria may be massive, and if it exceeds 3 g of protein per day (called nephrotic-

FIGURE 13-11
Nodular glomerulosclerosis of diabetes (Kimmelstiel-Wilson syndrome). The glomerulus shows mesangial nodules, a change associated with the nephrotic syndrome.

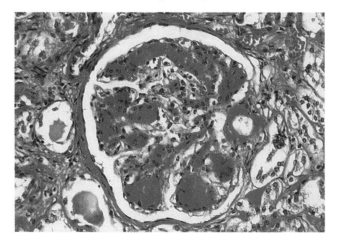

range proteinuria), it causes nephrotic syndrome. Severe proteinuria heralds deterioration of renal function, and chronic renal insufficiency usually develops over a period of 5 years.

The vascular changes caused by diabetes are most prominent in the arterioles, which typically show hyalinosis, accompanied by thickening of the vessel wall and narrowing of the vascular lumen. These changes lead to ischemia and tubular atrophy. The most prominent chronic changes are seen in the papillary part of the medulla. Ischemic papillae may become infected and slough off onto the renal pelvis. This *papillary necrosis* is a serious complication of diabetes, and can cause urinary obstruction and colic as the necrotic papillae detach and occlude the ureter.

The kidneys of diabetic patients are prone to bacterial infections, and pyelonephritis is an important complication. Recurrent bouts of bacterial pyelonephritis may ultimately destroy the kidneys. Such patients develop uremia and require dialysis or renal transplantation.

Urinary Stones

The formation of **urinary stones** or calculi (*urolithiasis*) is quite common. At least 5 percent of all adults in the United States will experience this condition at some point in their lives.

Urinary stones can be classified, on the basis of their chemical structure, into four main groups: calcium, struvite, uric acid, and cystine stones. *Calcium stones,* composed of either calcium oxalate or calcium phosphate, account for 75 percent of all stones. These stones are often associated with hyperexcretion of calcium in patients who have abnormal calcium metabolism (e.g., hyperabsorptive hypercalciuria). Such patients absorb too much calcium in the intestines. The tendency to form calcium stones may be inherited. *Struvite stones,* composed of magnesium ammonia phosphate or sulfate, account for 15 percent of urinary calculi. These stones are typically a complication of UTIs, which lead to formation of ammonia from the urea in the urine. *Uric acid stones* account for about 5 percent of all urinary stones. About 50 percent of the patients with this type of stone have hyperuricemia or gout, whereas others do not have an obvious metabolic disorder predisposing to stone formation. *Cystine stones* account for 1 percent of urinary calculi. These rare stones are found in patients with inborn errors of amino acid metabolism, such as *cystinosis.*

Urinary stones are most often found in the renal pelvis or the urinary bladder. With the exception of struvite stones, which may be relatively large, most other stones are smaller than 3 mm in diameter. The stones may resemble crystals or they may be small, round, or elongated grains or irregular masses. Struvite stones, also known as *staghorn calculi,* are larger and more irregular than the other types of stones. They grow progressively by the apposition of minerals and can fill the entire pelvis (Fig. 13-12).

Urinary stones are more common in men than in women. Most patients experience an attack of urinary stones at the age of 20 to 30 years. Typical symptoms of upper urinary tract stones include hematuria and urinary colics (i.e., spasmodic pain caused by the contraction of an obstructed ureter). Stones in the bladder tend to occur in older patients and are often associated with chronic infection.

Small stones can be voided spontaneously, whereupon the urinary symptoms resolve. The treatment of larger urinary stones, however, requires surgery or mechanical extraction. This is often achieved only after the stones have been broken into smaller pieces by a process called *lithotripsy.* New

FIGURE 13-12
Irregularly shaped struvite stone in the renal pelvis.

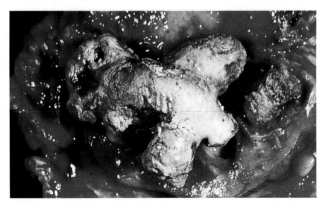

techniques for the removal of urinary stones include ultrasonic targeting, which is used to fragment the stones into small pieces so that they can be voided spontaneously.

Urinary Tract Infections

Among the various infections of the urinary tract, the most important are those caused by bacteria. Viral and fungal infections are less common. Parasitic infections, such as cystitis caused by *Schistosoma haematobium,* reportedly affect 50 million people worldwide but are rare in the United States.

Bacterial infection of the kidney is called **pyelonephritis,** whereas infection of the urinary bladder is called *cystitis.* Both conditions can occur simultaneously or in succession. Clinically and pathologically, both pyelonephritis and cystitis can occur in an acute and a chronic form. Bacteria may reach the urinary tract either from blood (*hematogenous infection*) or, more often, through the urethra and the lower urinary tract (*ascending infection*) (Fig. 13-13).

Hematogenous infection is typically preceded by septicemia. In such cases, the urinary tract is secondarily infected from a primary focus in another organ from which the bacteria spread into the blood. The primary infection may be in the endocardium, lungs, or gastrointestinal tract. Ascending infection, which is more common, may be acquired during sexual intercourse ("honeymoon cystitis"), following urinary bladder catheterization, or following surgical procedures (e.g., removal of urinary bladder tumors). In many instances, there is no obvious cause of UTI. UTI is more common in women than men, partially owing to the shorter urethra in women, which allows easier bacterial colonization of the urinary bladder. Pregnancy also predisposes women to UTI, in part because of the mechanical effects of the enlarged uterus on the urinary bladder and the ureters, and in part because of the relaxing effects of estrogen and progesterone on the smooth muscles of the urethra, urinary bladder, and ureter. Other conditions that predispose individuals to UTI are presented in Fig. 13-13.

UTIs may involve the entire urinary tract or they may present as localized infections, (e.g., pyelonephritis, cystitis). *Acute pyelonephritis* is a suppurative infection of the kidneys. On gross examination, the kidneys contain foci of pus (*abscesses*). In severe cases, the pus may permeate the entire kidney and fill the renal pelvis (*pyonephrosis*).

Chronic pyelonephritis may evolve from acute pyelonephritis, especially if there are recurrent attacks of acute infection. Persistent infection leads to destruction of the renal parenchyma and broad parenchymal scar formation. Ultimately, owing to loss of renal tissue, the affected kidney becomes small and

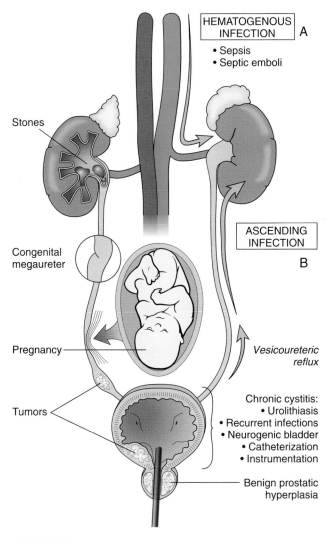

FIGURE 13-13
Routes of urinary tract infection. (A) Hematogenous infection. (B) Ascending infection—causes of urinary tract obstruction that predispose individuals to urinary tract infection.

FIGURE 13-14
Small, shrunken, irregularly scarred kidney of a patient with chronic pyelonephritis. The other kidney is of normal size, but also shows scarring on the upper pole.

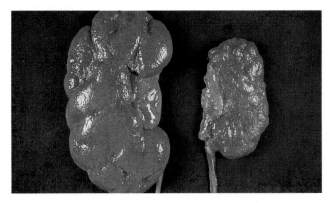

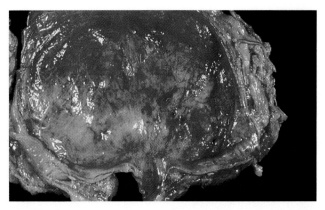

FIGURE 13-15
Acute cystitis. The mucosa of the bladder is red and swollen.

irregularly scarred (Fig. 13-14). As the bacteria do not grow at the same rate in both kidneys, and because the infection is often unilateral, kidneys affected by chronic pyelonephritis are typically asymmetrical. Indeed, it is not uncommon for one kidney to be completely shrunken and the other one to be spared.

Cystitis is an infection of the bladder that may occur in an acute or chronic form. Acute cystitis is characterized by grossly visible congestion and mucosal hemorrhages (Fig. 13-15). These changes are best visualized by cystoscopy, a procedure in which the urologist observes the inside of the bladder with an instrument that has been introduced through the urethra. In severe cases, the mucosa may be covered with pus or be ulcerated. Bladder biopsy specimens usually show the typical histologic features of acute inflammation. In chronic cystitis, the appearance of the mucosa varies considerably and includes foci of hemorrhage, ulceration, or thickening. The wall of the bladder is often thick, especially if cystitis is caused by chronic obstruction, as in urolithiasis or prostatic hyperplasia (Fig. 13-16).

UTIs are treated with antibiotics and/or sulfa drugs. The infections are often resistant, and in many patients, tend to recur. UTIs that are associated with diabetes, calculi, or prostatic hyperplasia are especially resistant to treatment.

Circulatory Disturbances

Circulatory disturbances and vascular diseases affect the kidneys in many forms. Such disturbances may cause acute or chronic renal insufficiency.

Acute Tubular Necrosis

A sudden decrease in arterial pressure will result in acute hypoperfusion of the kidneys with blood. This typically occurs following myocardial infarction, any

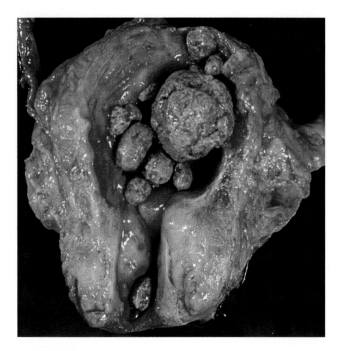

FIGURE 13-16
Chronic cystitis. Note the thickening in the wall of the urinary bladder. The bladder contains stones.

form of cardiac arrest, and all forms of hypotensive shock (e.g., massive bleeding). The reduction of blood flow is more prominent in the cortex than in the medulla. Cortical tubules, especially the highly specialized proximal convoluted tubules, are most affected. However, in severe hypotensive shock, the entire cortex may undergo necrosis ("renal cortical necrosis").

Renal failure that begins as prerenal becomes "renal" once ischemia has destroyed all the tubules. Such failure persists even after cardiac function has been restored or blood volume has been restored following massive blood loss. Patients who have **tubular necrosis** usually require support with an artificial kidney machine (*renal dialysis*) to survive. However, because the renal tubules may regenerate, the disrupted nephrons will heal spontaneously if one gives them time. Renal dialysis is usually continued for 1 to 2 weeks. Usually during that time, enough tubules regenerate to allow the kidneys to become functional again.

Nephroangiosclerosis

Atherosclerosis of the aorta, the renal artery, and its major branches may cause narrowing of the vascular lumen, which will significantly reduce blood flow through the kidneys. This leads to ischemic glomerulosclerosis and a loss of glomeruli, known collectively as nephroangiosclerosis. Loss of glomeruli is accompanied by tubular atrophy. The kidneys become small and show marked scarring. These scars actually represent multiple small infarcts in which the lost tubules have been replaced by fibrosis. Severe glomerulosclerosis may result in chronic renal insufficiency.

Hypertension

Arterial hypertension often affects the intrarenal arteries and arterioles. Hypertension stimulates renal arterial and arteriolar contraction. Sustained arterial and arteriolar contraction ultimately leads to the thickening of the vessel walls. The arterial walls become fibrotic and multilayered, whereas the arterioles undergo hyalinization, similar to that seen in patients with diabetes. In patients who have malignant hypertension, as is typically seen in young black men who experience a sudden onset of high blood pressure, the arterioles do not have time to adjust. Such arterioles may undergo fibrinoid necrosis. Sustained malignant hypertension will cause hyperplasia of the smooth muscle cells in the vessel wall. These smooth muscle cells form crescentic layers around the narrower lumen of the arteriole, forming so-called "onion ring–like" lesions.

Arterial and arteriolar changes induced by hypertension result in ischemia of the renal parenchyma, causing histologic changes that may be similar to those induced by atherosclerosis or diabetes. Clinically, such changes result in reduced renal function and ultimately may cause renal failure.

Hypertension is, in most instances, idiopathic; that is, it has no obvious cause. However, renal ischemia secondary to hypertensive arterial and arteriolar changes stimulates the renal juxtaglomerular apparatus to release renin. Renin may aggravate hypertension. In clinical terms, idiopathic hypertension could, thus, acquire features of secondary renal hypertension. This illustrates the important relationship of the kidneys and arterial hypertension. Clearly, the kidney can be both the "victim," as well as the cause, of hypertension.

Neoplasms

Tumors of the urinary tract are an important cause of morbidity and mortality. These tumors tend to

- be malignant more often than benign
- affect older people
- be more common in men than in women

For practical purposes, tumors of the urinary tract may be divided into four groups: (1) tumors of the kidney and renal pelvis, (2) tumors of the ureter, (3) tumors of the urinary bladder, and (4) tumors of the urethra (Fig. 13-17). The first group comprises renal

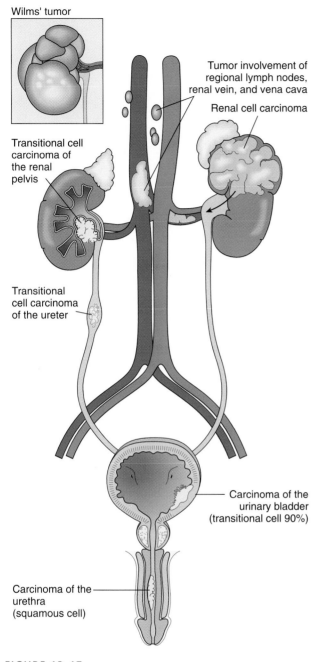

Wilms' tumor

Tumor involvement of
regional lymph nodes,
renal vein, and vena cava

Renal cell carcinoma

Transitional cell
carcinoma of
the renal
pelvis

Transitional
cell carcinoma
of the ureter

Carcinoma of the
urinary bladder
(transitional cell 90%)

Carcinoma of the
urethra
(squamous cell)

FIGURE 13-17
Neoplasms of the urinary tract.

cell carcinomas (85 percent), transitional cell carcinoma of the renal pelvis (8 percent), and Wilms' tumor (5 percent). The remaining 2 percent of the tumors in this group are extremely rare variants that do not warrant mention. Likewise, tumors of the ureter and urethra will not be discussed because of their rarity.

Bladder tumors are the most common neoplasms of the urinary tract. In more than 90 percent of cases, these tumors are transitional cell carcinomas. Benign tumors of transitional epithelium (transitional cell papilloma) are rare and of limited clinical significance.

Renal Cell Carcinoma

Renal cell carcinoma (RCC) is the most common kidney neoplasm, accounting for 85 percent of all tumors involving this organ. Almost 27,000 RCCs are diagnosed every year in the United States, and 11,000 deaths are attributed to this disease annually. RCC occurs in adults, and the median age of patients is 55 years. Males are affected two times more often than females.

The causes of RCC are not known and the risk factors for this tumor have not been defined. Epidemiologic data indicate a link with smoking, but this association is not as strong as that between smoking and lung cancer. Patients with chronic renal disease who receive a kidney transplant are at somewhat increased risk for RCC. These patients tend to develop cystic changes in their original, terminally damaged kidney. RCC develops in approximately 5 percent of such cystic kidneys. The reasons for the increased occurrence of RCC are not known, although it is hypothetically possible that the cystic fluid in these malfunctioning kidneys accumulates carcinogens more readily than normally functioning kidneys.

Pathology. On gross examination, RCCs appear as nodules or masses that are sharply demarcated from the remaining renal parenchyma. On cross section, they tend to be yellow and encapsulated (Fig. 13-18); larger tumors extend through the renal capsule into the peritoneal fat and adjacent organs. It is common for RCC to invade the renal vein. Distant metastases often occur, but their distribution is unpredictable.

Histologic examination reveals that RCC is composed of cuboidal cells reminiscent of the renal tubules. The tumor cells have a clear cytoplasm, which is filled with glycogen and lipids. This accounts for the yellow color of the tumors on gross examination.

Clinical Features. The clinical presentation of RCC is highly variable. The typical triad of symptoms—flank pain, blood in the urine, and a palpable abdominal mass—is found in only 10 percent of patients. About 50 percent of these tumors are discovered accidentally on computed tomography (CT) scans performed for unrelated reasons. Microscopic hematuria, found in one third of all diagnosed cases, is the most common clinical finding. A significant number of tumors present with nonspecific symptoms, such as weight loss, fever, or hypertension. Metabolic "paraneoplastic" findings, such as hypercalcemia, erythrocytosis, and other abnormalities, are found in 20 percent of patients. These variegated clinical and biochemical findings account for the moniker "internist's tumor," as RCC is known colloquially; most of these tumors are diagnosed by in-

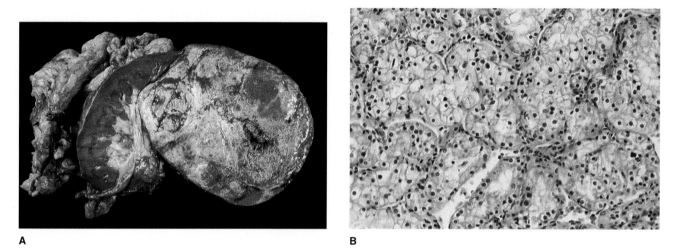

A

B

FIGURE 13-18
Renal cell carcinoma. (A) Gross appearance of the tumor. (B) Histologic examination reveals that the tissue consists of clear cells arranged into tubules.

ternists examining patients for presumably nonrenal complaints. The tumors are treated surgically, but the overall 5-year survival is only 40 percent. In patients with small asymptomatic tumors that have been diagnosed coincidentally by CT scan performed for some other reason, the prognosis is much better, and many of the patients are cured by timely surgery.

Transitional Cell Carcinoma of the Renal Pelvis

These papillary neoplasms resemble transitional carcinoma of the urinary bladder. They are classified as low-grade, intermediate, or high-grade neoplasms or, alternatively, they may be graded I to III, as in the bladder. Most tumors of the renal pelvis present with hematuria or urinary obstruction and colics early in the course of clinical disease. These symptoms provide clues for early diagnosis. Surgical removal yields good results, and the 5-year survival for grade I and II tumors is 70 percent. Grade III tumors have a less favorable prognosis.

Wilms' Tumor

Wilms' tumor or nephroblastoma is the most common of all solid tumors in infants and young children, affecting 1 in 10,000. Many, if not most, Wilms' tumors are present at the time of birth but become clinically apparent only between the second and fourth years of life. At least three distinct genes have been implicated in the pathogenesis of Wilms' tumor. The most important, which is known as Wilms' tumor gene 1 (WT-1), appears to be a transcription factor; the function of WT-1 is not known, but it prob-

ably plays an important role in development. Deletion of WT-1, as a result of chromosomal breaks or mutation of the gene, may result in congenital malformations (e.g., aniridia, or congenital lack of the iris of the eye) or Wilms' tumor formation. These malformations and Wilms' tumor may coexist in the same person.

Pathology. Wilms' tumor typically presents as a renal mass that can be either solitary or multinodular and that replaces the kidney to a large extent. On histologic examination, the tumor is composed of immature cells, similar to those in the developing fetal kidney. These cells may form structures resembling fetal tubules and glomeruli, or they may be arranged into bundles of spindle cells without any evidence of differentiation, resembling renal blastema (fetal primordium of the kidney).

Clinical Features. Most tumors are discovered accidentally by a parent who has palpated the infant's abdominal mass or by a pediatrician during the course of a routine examination. Wilms' tumors are highly malignant neoplasms. Previously, when the only treatment of such tumors was surgery, the mortality was greater than 70 percent. Current therapy, based on surgery and chemotherapy with new cancer drugs, has improved the prognosis for Wilms' tumor such that more than 85 percent of the children with this tumor can now be cured.

Carcinoma of the Urinary Bladder

Urinary bladder cancer represents the most common urinary tract neoplasm. It has a peak incidence in those 60 to 80 years of age, and it is three times more common in males than in females. In the United States, 52,000 new cases are recorded yearly, and 10,000 deaths are attributed to this form of cancer annually. Thus, although bladder cancer is two times more common than renal cell carcinomas, it accounts for approximately the same number of deaths. This discrepancy can be explained in part by the following facts:

- Bladder cancer has a tendency for papillary, exophytic growth into the lumen of the bladder. Bladder cancer is less invasive and less prone to metastasize than renal cell carcinoma. Almost 70 percent of all bladder carcinomas are grade I or II exophytic tumors that have a favorable prognosis.
- Bladder tumors present with symptoms early in the course of their development. Intravesical growth causes urinary irritation and hematuria. Tumor cells may be readily identified in cytologic masses prepared from the urine. All of these factors make early diagnosis feasible.
- Bladder tumors respond better than renal cell carcinomas to combined surgical/chemotherapeutic treatment.

The etiology of bladder carcinomas is, in most instances, unknown. The most important risk factor in the United States is cigarette smoking, which increases the likelihood of bladder cancer proportionate to the total number of cigarettes smoked over the life span. Industrial carcinogens, such as azodies and chemicals used in the rubber industry and textile printing, have been linked to bladder cancer, but with improved industrial hygiene, such chemicals have become less important. In Egypt and other parts of the world in which infection with S. *haematobium* is endemic, the high incidence of bladder cancer is related to the chronic cystitis caused by this parasite.

Pathology. Most bladder cancers (90 percent) are transitional cell carcinomas (Fig. 13-19). The remaining tumors comprise squamous cell carcinoma (7 percent), adenocarcinomas, and sarcomas.

On gross examination, the tumors are either papillary or flat. Papillary tumors are characterized by wart-like protrusions, whereas the flat ones appear as mucosal plaques or thickening. In either case, the tumors may be invasive or noninvasive, which can be determined only by histologic examination of biopsy specimens. Transitional cell carcinomas are graded histologically on a scale from I to III. Grade I tumors are almost never invasive and have an excellent prognosis, with only a 2 percent to 3 percent 10-year mortality. Grade II and III tumors have a 50 percent and 70 percent 5-year mortality, respectively. By contrast, 70 percent of patients with squamous cell carcinomas are dead by the end of the first year.

Carcinoma of the urinary bladder is often multifocal, indicating a "field effect"—that is, the causative agent initiates malignant transformation of the bladder mucosa in several spots. Many grossly visible tumors are thus associated with additional flat lesions which, on histologic examination, appear as carcinoma in situ (i.e., as a full-thickness neoplastic transformation of the bladder epithelium). These superficial lesions tend to become invasive. Such multifocal cancers can be treated only by radical surgery, with removal of the entire bladder.

Progression of bladder cancer leads to the extension of the tumor into the muscle layers of the bladder and into the adjacent pelvic organs. Metastases are initially found in the pelvic lymph nodes, but in

FIGURE 13-19
Bladder cancer. (A) Gross appearance of an intraluminal mass. (B) Histologic examination reveals that the mass is a papillary transitional cell carcinoma.

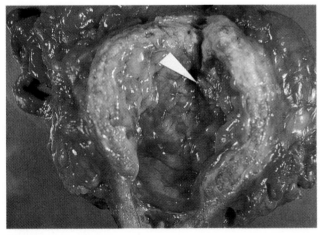

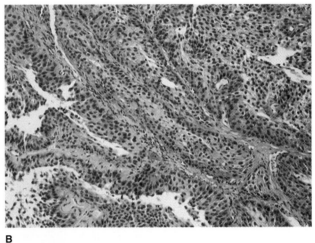

A

B

later stages of disease, the tumor may metastasize to distant sites as well.

Clinical Features. Bladder cancer presents with urinary symptoms, such as hematuria, dysuria, or lower abdominal pain. The diagnosis made by cystoscopy must be confirmed by histologic examination of the tumor biopsy specimen. Cytologic examination of urinary sediment is also useful, especially in the case of early lesions, such as carcinoma in situ or multifocal flat lesions.

Treatment of bladder cancer is based on surgical resection of tumors and chemotherapy. Good results have also been achieved by immunotherapy, specifically by intravesical instillation of adjuvants and immunopotentiators, such as an attenuated *Mycobacterium tuberculosis* known as *bacille Calmette-Guérin* (BCG). BCG stimulates granuloma formation and delayed hypersensitivity, thus destroying tumors locally.

The final prognosis depends on the histologic grade (I to III), histologic type (transitional, squamous, adenocarcinoma), and clinical stage (A to D). Even the low-grade localized tumors tend to recur, so a life-long urologic follow-up is thus mandatory. Recurrent tumors or new lesions can usually be resected with the aid of a cutting device attached to the cystoscope. Large tumors and invasive tumors require complete urinary bladder resection (cystectomy), whereupon a urinary receptacle is formed from the bowel loops and the ureters are implanted into it. Stage A, grade I tumors that are localized to the mucosa have a 98 percent 5-year survival, whereas stage D tumors (i.e., those with metastases) have only a 15 percent 5-year survival.

Review Questions

1. Explain how urine is formed and excreted.
2. Describe the principal portions of the nephron, and explain how they function.
3. What is the functional significance of transitional epithelium?
4. Describe the effects of various hormones on the kidney.
5. Which hormones and growth factors does the kidney produce?
6. List the most important symptoms of kidney disease.
7. How common are renal developmental disorders and which one of them is the most common?
8. Correlate the pathology of autosomal dominant polycystic kidney disease with the clinical features of this disease.
9. Classify glomerular diseases.
10. List the most important immunologic glomerular diseases.
11. List the most important metabolic glomerulopathies.
12. Explain how circulatory disorders affect glomeruli.
13. List the four most important syndromes related to glomerular diseases.
14. Compare nephrotic and nephritic syndrome.
15. Explain the pathogenesis of acute glomerulonephritis and correlate the pathologic and clinical findings in this disease.
16. Explain the pathogenesis of crescentic glomerulonephritis and relate the pathologic and clinical findings in this disease.
17. Explain the pathogenesis of membranous nephropathy and relate the pathologic and clinical findings in this disease.
18. What is lipoid nephrosis and how is it diagnosed?
19. What do most forms of chronic proliferative glomerulonephritis have in common?
20. What is the cause of end-stage kidney disease and how does it present clinically?

21. How does diabetes mellitus affect the kidneys?

22. List the four most common forms of kidney stones.

23. Compare ascending and descending urinary tract infection and list the most common predisposing conditions for these infections.

24. Compare the pathologic and clinical features of acute and chronic pyelonephritis.

25. Compare the causes of cystitis in men and women, and in young and old people.

26. Compare the pathologic and clinical features of acute and chronic cystitis.

27. Explain how circulatory collapse causes renal tubular necrosis.

28. Explain the effects of hypertension on the kidneys.

29. List three common tumors of the urinary tract.

30. Compare renal cell carcinoma and Wilms' tumor.

31. Compare transitional cell carcinoma of the renal pelvis and renal cell carcinoma.

32. How common is carcinoma of the urinary bladder?

33. Correlate the macroscopic and microscopic features of urinary bladder carcinoma with the clinical features of this tumor.

34. What are the typical symptoms of urinary bladder carcinoma?

35. What is the outcome of treatment of urinary bladder carcinoma?

Learning Objectives

After reading this chapter, the student should be able to:

1. Describe the external and internal male reproductive organs.

2. Define cryptorchidism and list two possible consequences of this disorder.

3. Define orchitis, epididymitis, prostatitis, and balanitis and list the most common causes of each of these conditions.

4. List common sexually transmitted diseases and discuss their impact on the society.

5. Describe the macroscopic and microscopic pathology of benign prostatic hyperplasia and relate these findings to clinical symptoms.

6. List in order of highest incidence tumors of the penis, prostate, and testis.

7. Compare the ages of patients with tumors of the prostate and testis.

8. Discuss the importance of histologic diagnosis of testicular tumors in the treatment and prognosis of this neoplastic disease.

9. List three markers of testicular tumors.

10. Discuss the significance of pathologic findings for the diagnosis of prostatic cancer.

11. Describe the spread of prostatic cancer and the course of this neoplastic disease.

12. Describe the gross and microscopic pathologic findings in patients with penile cancer.

Additional Key Terms and Concepts

Benign prostatic hyperplasia

Epididymo-orchitis

Gonorrhea

Infertility

Nonseminomatous germ cell tumors

Prostate-specific antigen

Syphilis

Seminoma

Teratoma

Chapter Outline

The Male Reproductive System

Chapter 14

NORMAL ANATOMY AND PHYSIOLOGY

The male reproductive system comprises the *gonads* (**testes**), *seminal excretory ducts* (**epididymis** and **vas deferens**), the *accessory glands* (**seminal vesicles** and **prostate**), and the *copulatory organ* (**penis**) (Fig. 14-1). The testes are localized in a specialized outpouching of the peritoneum, called the **scrotum**, which is covered on the outside with corrugated skin. The testes are linked with the rest of the reproductive system by the excretory ducts (epididymis and vas deferens). These excretory ducts are confluent with the ducts of the prostate, **seminal vesicles,** and the urethra (i.e., the terminal portion of the lower urinary tract). The **urethra** is located within the shaft of the penis and thus has the double function of conducting and discharging both urine and seminal fluid.

On histologic examination, the testes are composed of **seminiferous tubules** and supporting structures, which include the blood vessels, stromal cells, and connective tissue (Fig. 14-2). The stroma contains hormone-secreting Leydig cells. The seminiferous tubules are lined by germ cells in various stages of maturation and the supporting sex-cord cells, the Sertoli cells. The epididymal ducts are lined by secretory cells that produce a protein- and carbohydrate-rich fluid that bathes the sperm. During ejaculation, the epididymal **sperm** enter the seminal ampule where they are mixed with the **seminal fluid** from the seminal vesicles and the prostatic fluid. This mixture is called the *ejaculate.* Ejaculate, once formed, enters the urethra and is discharged through the tip of the penile urethra outside the body. This fluid provides a vehicle for export of sperm from the testis.

The primary function of the male genital system is the production of sperm. The testes also secrete male hormones, androgens, which are the products of testicular interstitial cells called **Leydig cells.** The most important of the androgenic hormones is **testosterone.** Testosterone secretion is controlled by the pituitary **gonadotropins.**

OVERVIEW OF MAJOR DISEASES

In comparison with the diseases of the female reproductive organs, the diseases affecting the male reproductive organs generally receive less public attention. Note, for instance, that most adult women in civilized societies see their gynecologist at least once a year, whereas most males never consult a urologist during their lifetime. Few people even know that the real counterpart of a gynecologist is technically called an *andrologist* (in Greek, *andros* means man). In practice, "male problems" are treated by urologists, whereas andrologists deal only with male infertility. The pathologists specializing in diseases of the male reproductive organs are called *urogenital pathologists.*

The most important diseases of the male reproductive system are

- infertility
- infections
- tumors

Infertility. As stated in the Bible, God decreed that men should "breed and multiply." Fertility—the ability to produce offspring—is essential for the propagation of all species, including humans. Infertility can

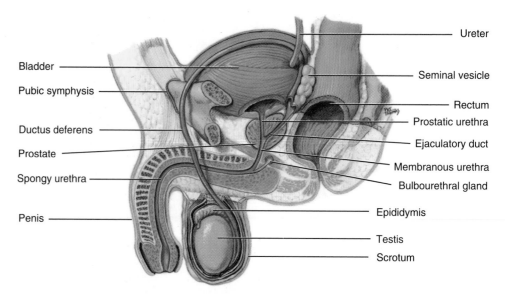

FIGURE 14-1
Male reproductive system (From Applegate EJ: The anatomy and physiology learning system: textbook. Philadelphia: WB Saunders, 1995: 392.)

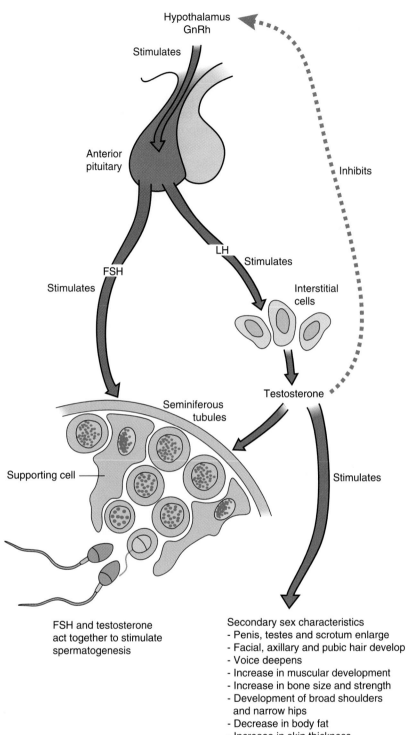

FIGURE 14-2
Histologic features of the testis. GnRh, go-nadotropin-releasing hormone; FSH, folli-cle-stimulating hormone; LH, luteinizing hormone. (From Applegate EJ: The anatomy and physiology learning system: textbook. Philadelphia: WB Saunders, 1995: 399.)

threaten families, tribes, nations, and ultimately, all of humankind with extinction. Problems of fertility have been among the major concerns of humans since time immemorial, and have important medical implications.

Infertility is defined as an inability to have children. Although the cause may lie with either the male or female partner, it is customary to treat the reproductive unit as a whole and thus refer not to infertile individuals, but to *infertile couples*. Statistics show that the causes of infertility are split equally between females and males. It has been estimated that 1 in 6 couples in the United States is infertile, and that the treatment of infertility costs society millions of dollars per year. Considerable advances have been made in the treatment of infertility among women, especially with the introduction of in vitro fertilization. However, no progress has been made in treating male infertility.

Infections. The male reproductive organs are prone to infection for several reasons, two of the most important being the following:

- Sexual intercourse between two persons brings into most intimate contact their genital organs, thus facilitating the transmission of pathogens.
- The ascent of microbial pathogens through the urethra occurs easily because the urethra is an open-ended tube, and even though it is subdivided into several anatomic segments by distinct sphincters, these act more like hurdles than tight valves against ascending bacteria.

Most genital infections are sexually acquired, thus they have the highest prevalence among men in their prime. With age, the pattern of infection changes, so that in older men, most infections are related to urinary retention caused by prostatic enlargement.

Tumors. Among the tumors affecting the male reproductive organs, two deserve special attention: tumors of the prostate and tumors of the testis. Tumors of the prostate are important because they are very common. Malignant tumors of the prostate are incurable. Tumors of the testis are considerably less common. Malignant tumors of the testis are important because they affect men at the height of their productive life (25 to 45 years of age). These tumors can be treated very successfully.

Several facts important for an understanding of diseases of the male reproductive system are presented here, before a discussion of the most common pathologic entities.

1. *Abnormalities of male reproductive organs result from genetic and developmental disorders.* The genetic sex of every individual depends on a normal complement of sex chromosomes. As described in Chapter 5, trisomy of sex chromosomes (47, XXY) results in *Klinefelter's syndrome.* Affected persons have atrophic testes and are infertile. *Cryptorchidism* is a developmental defect that results in incomplete descent of the testis into its normal scrotal position.

2. *Male genital organs are in direct contact with the outside world and, therefore, most infections are acquired through an ascending route (i.e., through the urethra).* Infections in young and middle-aged men are typically acute and are often sexually acquired. Infections in older men tend to be chronic and are often related to urinary tract obstruction secondary to prostatic enlargement.

3. *The testes produce male sex hormones that act on all other reproductive organs.* Abnormalities in testosterone secretion during fetal life result in incomplete development of the reproductive organs, which require testosterone to develop normally. After birth and until puberty, the testes produce little testosterone. However, at **puberty,** under the influence of pituitary gonadotropins, a major surge in testosterone production occurs, determining the maturation of all male sex organs and secondary sexual characteristics. Premature activation of Leydig cells results in *precocious puberty.* The opposite is *delayed puberty.* Both conditions are usually related to hypothalamic and pituitary disturbances. If puberty does not occur, and the testes remain infantile, the condition is called *hypogonadism.* These men are infertile and have eunuchoid body features, without body or pubic hair.

4. *The testis consists of spermatogenic cells, Sertoli cells, and Leydig cells, all of which can give rise to tumors.* Although the testes are small organs, they can give rise to a variety of histologically distinct tumors. This variety of tumors can be accounted for, in part, by the fact that such tumors arise from three distinct cell lineages: germ cells, Sertoli cells, and Leydig cells. Furthermore, neoplastic germ cells can differentiate into embryonic cells, as normally occurs after fertilization (the fusion of male and female germ cells). These embryonic cells can form tumors that are histologically distinct from the normal cells in the testis, and consist of tissues normally found in fetal or adult organs not related to testis. Such tumors are called teratomas, or teratocarcinomas, if malignant.

5. *The prostate is composed of epithelial and stromal cells that express receptors for sex hormones.* The prostate is an organ, the development and function of which depend on male sex hormones. Persons who have accidentally lost testes before puberty, or those that were castrated before puberty, have very small prostates because the prostate does not develop unless properly stimulated by androgens during puberty. Prostatic hyperplasia, commonly found in older men, is a hormonally induced lesion, although its pathogenesis is still unknown. It is thought to be related to an imbalance of male and female hormones that occur as a result of a decrease in testosterone production with advancing age. The role of sex hormones in the pathogenesis of prostatic cancer has been studied extensively, but without any definitive conclusions.

Congenital Abnormalities

The most important abnormality of the male reproductive system is **cryptorchidism.** Other congenital defects of the testes, such as anorchia (absence of

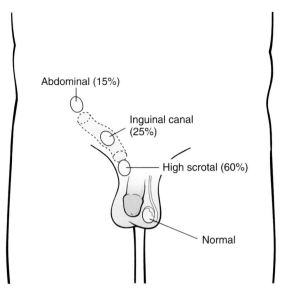

FIGURE 14-3
In cryptorchidism, the testis is not in the scrotum, but may be found in the inguinal canal or the abdominal cavity.

testes) or polyorchidism (3 or more testes), are rare. Abnormalities of the penis are also rare. The most common is **hypospadias,** an abnormal opening of the urethra on the lower side of the shaft of the penis.

Cryptorchidism

Cryptorchidism is a congenital malpositioning of the testes outside of their normal scrotal location (Fig. 14-3).

Pathogenesis. The fetal testes, which develop from the genital ridge, are originally located in the abdominal cavity. During intrauterine life, the testes slowly descend toward the inguinal canal and through it, ultimately reaching the scrotum. The inguinal canal is obliterated, thus preventing the testes from retracting into the abdominal cavity. They remain permanently fixed in the scrotum.

In most boys, the descent of the testes is fully completed by the time of birth. In 3 percent to 4 percent of newborn male infants, however, the inguinal canal remains open, allowing the cremasteric muscle that is attached to the testes to pull them back into the inguinal canal or even into the abdominal cavity. These are called *retractile testes.* In most cases, the inguinal canal nevertheless closes, and by the end of the first year of life, less than 1 percent of all male infants do not have one or both testes in the scrotum. These truly *cryptorchid* testes must be fixed in the scrotum surgically, and the inguinal canal must be closed surgically to prevent formation of a *hernia,* an outpouching of the abdominal organs (usually the intestines) into the scrotum.

The cause of cryptorchidism may be quite evident, as in the case of connective tissue adhesions within the fetal inguinal canal. In most instances, however, the cause remains unknown.

Pathology. Most cryptorchid testes that are surgically repositioned in the scrotum in early infancy develop normally. However, signs of atrophy and hypospermatogenesis are not uncommon. Infertility can result if both testes are cryptorchid, but if only one testis is affected, the other normal one will suffice to maintain fertility.

Cryptorchid testes have a 10-fold greater risk of undergoing malignant transformation than do normal testes. Surgical correction at an early age reduces this risk, but does not eliminate it completely. Apparently, many cryptorchid testes are abnormally developed and, even if repositioned, will retain a predisposition to form tumors.

Infections

Acute and chronic infections may involve the entire male reproductive system, but most often, they are limited to a particular organ or two closely adjacent organs. The most important among these localized infections are *orchitis* (inflammation of the testes), *epididymitis, prostatitis, urethritis,* and *balanitis* (inflammation of the glans penis) (Fig. 14-4). As men-

FIGURE 14-4
Infections of the male reproductive system.

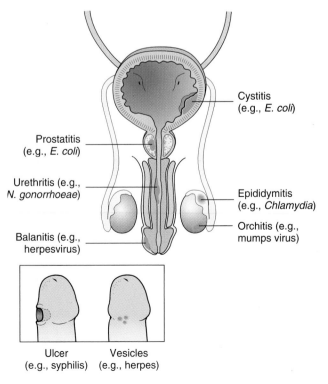

tioned earlier, in adult sexually active males, most infections are sexually acquired.

Balanitis, which may present as localized or diffuse redness, swelling, or ulceration of the mucosa of the glans penis, is usually caused by viruses or bacteria. *Herpesvirus* typically causes vesicles that rupture, giving rise to shallow ulcers. Infection with *Treponema pallidum* causes ulcerations (called syphilitic *chancre*) of the glans or even the skin or the shaft of the penis.

Urethritis with purulent exudate is typical of infection with *Neisseria gonorrhoeae,* diplococci that can be readily demonstrated by microscopic examination of the inflammatory cells expressed from the urethra. If no bacteria are evident and there is no purulent exudate, it is customary to label the condition as *nonbacterial urethritis.* In most cases, it is caused by **chlamydial infection** (*Chlamydia trachomatis*) or *Ureaplasma urealiticum,* a bacteria-like microbe of the Mycoplasma species.

Prostatitis is a disease affecting older men and is usually related to stagnation of urine. The infections are caused by uropathogens, a mixed flora or gram-negative bacteria such as *Escherichia coli* and Proteus.

Epididymitis is caused by ascending infection, usually sexually acquired pathogens, such as *N. gonorrhoeae* and Chlamydia, or uropathogens. A small number of cases are related to hematogenous spread of infection and may be caused by Staphylococcus or Streptococcus species.

Orchitis may occur as an isolated infection or it may accompany epididymitis (*epididymo-orchitis*). Isolated orchitis is a typical complication of hematogenous spread, such as occurs in secondary syphilis or in certain viral diseases. The most important among these is mumps. For unknown reasons, the mumps virus (which typically invades the salivary glands and, occasionally, the pancreas) has a predilection for the testes. One can expect orchitis in one third of all male patients with mumps, and if it is bilateral, infertility may result.

Sexually Transmitted Diseases

The most common **sexually transmitted diseases** are

- genital herpes
- gonorrhea
- nonspecific urethritis caused by Chlamydia or Mycoplasma
- syphilis

Genital Herpes

Genital herpes is caused by herpes simplex virus (HSV) type 2. This virus is closely related to HSV type 1, the cause of cold sores or blisters (*herpes labialis*). Both viruses invade the skin and mucosal cells, disrupting the epithelial layer and producing vesicles filled with clear fluid. The genital lesions are located on the glans or the skin of the shaft of the penis or the scrotum. The vesicles rupture and transform into shallow, painful ulcers that heal without scarring. The vesicles are typical enough to enable one to establish the diagnosis, but it may be confirmed by sampling cells from the vesicles for microscopic examination or virologic culture.

Genital herpes has a tendency to recur. Following the acute disease, the HSV travels along the axons of the peripheral nerves and invades the ganglion cells that enervate the genital area. In the ganglion cells, the virus remains in a balance with the host, causing no clinical symptoms. However, once the balance is disturbed, for example by another infection or in immunosuppressed persons (those with acquired immunodeficiency syndrome [AIDS], for example), the virus is activated and it descends along the nerves into the genital area, producing new vesicular eruptions.

Individuals with active herpetic lesions are contagious, but even asymptomatic carriers or those with atypical nonvesicular lesions may transmit the disease. Permanent cure is not feasible, although antiviral drugs (e.g., acyclovir) provide some relief.

Gonorrhea

Infection with the diplococcus *N. gonorrhoeae* (also known as gonococcus) results in purulent urethritis. Typically, this sexually transmitted disease presents with burning on urination and a yellow urethral discharge 2 to 5 days after exposure.

Gonococcus invades the mucosa of the penile urethra and the adjacent periurethral glands. The inflamed mucosa is red, moist, and covered with purulent exudate which, on histologic examination, consists predominantly of polymorphonuclear neutrophils (PMNs). Gonococcus can be seen in the cytoplasm of inflammatory cells. Penicillin usually cures most infections, although recently, more and more penicillin-resistant strains of bacteria have been reported.

The complications of gonococcal urethritis can be classified as local or distant. Ascending infection may lead to prostatitis and epididymitis. Connective tissue strictures that develop as a consequence of such infection cause narrowing of the urethra and can obliterate the epididymis. Typical consequences of inadequately treated gonorrhea include pain during urination, or infertility secondary to obstructed sperm outflow. Gonococci may also disseminate by blood to distant sites. Gonococcal arthritis is the most common complication of such hematogenous spread.

Nonspecific Urethritis

Nonspecific urethritis, also known as *nongonococcal urethritis,* is caused by Chlamydia and/or Mycoplasma and is the most common sexually transmitted disease. Urethritis caused by these microbes differs from that which accompanies gonorrhea in that it is not accompanied by a purulent discharge. With nonspecific urethritis, the tip of the penis is usually reddened around the meatus of the urethra, and the inflammation typically extends into the urethra itself. Ascending infections may cause prostatitis or epididymitis, but hematogenous dissemination does not occur. Broad-spectrum antibiotics, such as tetracycline, are effective in treating the infection, but the disease may recur.

Syphilis

Syphilis is a sexually acquired disease caused by the spirochete *T. pallidum.* Three stages of the disease—primary, secondary, and tertiary syphilis—are recognized.

Primary Stage. The primary lesion—a painless, indurated ulcer—develops 1 to 12 weeks after exposure. This ulcer, known as the primary *chancre,* develops on the glans penis, on the inner side of the prepuce in uncircumcised men, or on and around the anus in homosexuals. The ulcer is accompanied by local, usually inguinal, lymph node enlargement. Histologic examination reveals that the infected tissue contains numerous spirochetes. *T. pallidum* can be identified by dark-field microscopy of samples obtained by swabbing the ulcer. However, this is rarely done and, in practice, every ulcer of the penis is treated as syphilitic unless proven otherwise. The primary chancre heals spontaneously in about 4 to 6 weeks. With appropriate treatment, it heals in a few days.

Secondary Stage. Symptoms that develop in secondary syphilis are manifestations of systemic spread of spirochetes and an immune reaction to the pathogen. The secondary stage occurs approximately 2 months to 2 years after the primary infection. Clinically, it is marked by systemic symptoms, such as fever, malaise, macular rash, lymph node enlargement, and the appearance of slightly elevated skin lesions (papules) called *condyloma latum.* Many other symptoms and findings also may be present, such as mucosal ulcerations, central nervous system irritation (probably secondary to meningitis), hepatitis, and kidney symptoms. All of these symptoms, however, have a self-limited course and disappear spontaneously.

Tertiary Stage. Following remission of the symptoms of secondary syphilis, the disease may enter a latent phase for an extended period of time. The symptoms of tertiary syphilis occur in a small number of untreated or incompletely treated patients 2 to 20 years after the primary infection. The most important symptoms are related to the pathologic lesions of the cardiovascular and central nervous systems.

Histologic hallmarks of tertiary syphilis include chronic perivasculitis involving the small blood vessels and typical syphilitic granulomas called *gumma.* Lymphocytic and plasma cellular infiltrates around the vasa vasorum of the aorta, the small nutrient arteries in the wall of aorta, cause destruction of the arterial wall with widening of the lumen (*aneurysm*). Gummas of the cardiac valves also cause destruction and insufficiency of the valves, most often at the aortic orifice. Meningovascular syphilis causes destruction of the posterior columns of the spinal cord, evidenced as *tabes dorsalis.* As a result of destruction of sensory nerve axons in the posterior columns, these patients lose proprioception and have difficulty coordinating their movements. In the brain, the loss of neurons secondary to syphilis results in dementia, known as *general paralysis of the insane.* These persons lose all mental faculties and are often paralyzed because of destruction of motor neurons.

In contrast to the effectiveness of antibiotics in the treatment of primary and secondary syphilis, tertiary syphilis is incurable. It is, therefore, most important to diagnose the disease while it is still curable and to treat it appropriately.

Neoplasms

Tumors of the Testis

Testicular tumors account for only 1 percent of all neoplasms in men. These tumors are, nevertheless, clinically important because they occur at a relatively early age; indeed, the peak incidence occurs in men 25 to 45 years of age (Fig. 14-5). The most important aspects of testicular cancer are as follows:

- Most tumors (more than 90 percent) are of germ cell origin.
- The peak incidence of such tumors occurs in adulthood; at an age when most men have few other tumors or potentially lethal diseases. These tumors are rare before puberty and in older men. If a testicular tumor develops in an older man, most likely it represents a disseminated lymphoma or a metastasis from an abdominal primary lesion, and not a primary testicular tumor.
- All malignant testicular tumors follow the same metastatic pathway. Typically, the tumors spread to periaortic lymph nodes in the abdomen. From this site, the tumors metastasize to the upper ab-

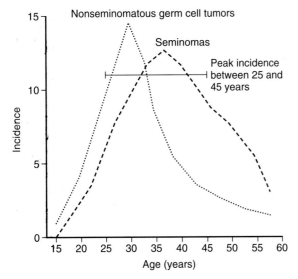

FIGURE 14-5
Incidence of testicular cancer according to age. Testicular tumors have a peak incidence in men aged 25 to 45 years.

domen and may spread hematogenously to the liver, lungs, and the brain.

- Previously, testicular tumors were associated with considerable mortality, but recent advances in chemotherapy have markedly improved the outlook for most patients, and 90 percent can be cured if diagnosed in time.

Etiology and Pathogenesis. More than 90 percent of testicular tumors develop from germ cells. The remaining 5 percent are derived from Sertoli and Leydig cells, and 5 percent represent metastases (Table 14-1). The etiology of testicular tumors is not known. It has been noted that tumors develop more often in developmentally abnormal testes and in cryptorchid testes. Cryptorchidism is the most important predisposing condition. Such testes are at a 10-fold higher risk for neoplastic disease than normal testes.

Malignant transformation of germ cells results in an intratubular tumor known as *carcinoma in situ* (CIS). After a latent period, which can last 5 to 20 years, CIS cells cross the basement membrane and an invasive malignant disease develops. As shown in

Did You Know?

Embryonal carcinoma cells are so called because they resemble normal embryonic cells. Like their normal counterparts, they form embryo-like structures, such as the embryoid body illustrated here. Although it is in a tumor, it resembles almost perfectly an early postimplantation human embryo.

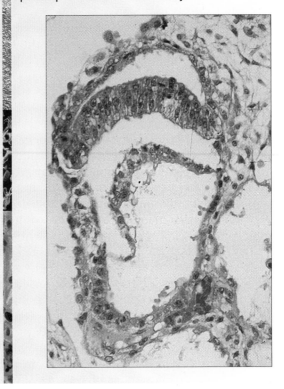

Table 14-1 Testicular Tumors

Germ Cell Tumors	Sex Cord Cell Tumors	Metastases
Seminoma (40%)	Leydig cell tumors (3%)	Lymphoma (2%)
Malignant nonseminomatous germ cell tumors (NSGCTs)	Sertoli cell tumors (2%)	Carcinoma (renal, prostatic, colonic) (3%)
Embryonal carcinoma (10%)		
Teratocarcinomas (20%)		
Choriocarcinoma (<1%)		
Mixed tumors (seminoma + NSGCT) (15%)		
Teratoma (3%)		
Yolk sac tumor (2%)		

Fig. 14-6, the tumors can develop in two directions. If the tumor cells retain the features of primitive gonocytes, forming a neoplasm composed of a single cell type, the resulting malignant lesion is called a *seminoma* (i.e., tumor of seminal epithelium–like cells). However, if the tumor cells acquire the characteristics of embryonic cells, the resulting malignant lesion is called *embryonal carcinoma*. It should be remembered that the germ cells in the testis, like those in the ovary are the precursors of embryonic cells. Embryonic cells are normally formed only from zygotes; that is, they form only following fusion of the male and female gamete. In contrast, embryonal carcinoma (EC) cells are descendants of spontaneously activated male germ cells. It is not known why and how these germ cells give rise to embryonal carcinoma cells. Clearly, they must skip a few developmental steps, as they never mature into sperm or fuse with the female gamete, yet they evolve into embryonic cells. Like normal embryonic cells, EC cells can differentiate into various fetal and adult tissues and even form the components of the extraembryonic membranes (i.e., placenta and yolk sac).

If all the embryonic cells differentiate into mature tissues, a *teratoma* forms. This is a benign tumor composed of somatic tissues (in Greek, *soma* means body) derived from all three embryonic germ layers: ectoderm, endoderm, and mesoderm. In contrast, the malignant tumor that is composed of EC cells and somatic tissues is called a *teratocarcinoma*. Note that both teratomas and teratocarcinomas contain haphazardly arranged and intermixed tissues, such as skin, brain, muscle, and cartilage intestine. Teratocarcinomas also contain malignant stem cells (EC cells), scattered cells of the placental (trophoblastic) and yolk sac epithelium. Trophoblastic cells, like the normal placenta, secrete human chorionic gonadotropin (hCG) into the blood. Because hCG is not normally found in the serum or urine of males (or, for that matter, in females unless they are pregnant), the presence of hCG in a male is strong evidence of a germ cell tumor. Yolk sac cells secrete alpha-fetoprotein (AFP), which is yet another tumor marker of germ cell neoplasia.

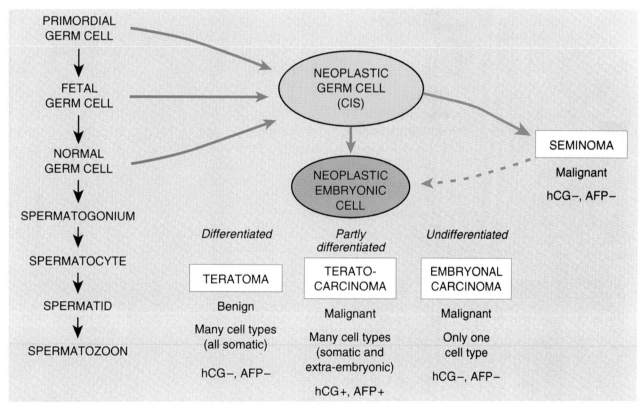

FIGURE 14-6
Histogenesis of malignant testicular germ cell tumors. The tumors originate from intratubular germ cells that form carcinoma in situ (CIS). Tumors derived from CIS are divided into two major groups: seminomas and nonseminomatous germ cell tumors (NSGCTs), the latter of which include several subtypes. hCG, human chorionic gonadotropin; AFP, alpha-fetoprotein. (Reprinted with permission from Scientific American SCIENCE & MEDICINE. Copyright 1995 by Scientific American, Inc. All rights reserved.)

It is important to note that ECs and teratocarcinomas have the same malignant stem cells, the only difference being that, in pure EC (which is rare), these stem cells do not differentiate. Such tumors are composed of monomorphic cell populations. On the other hand, EC cells in teratocarcinomas differentiate and form various tissues. For practical purposes, both ECs and teratocarcinomas are thus considered to be *nonseminomatous germ cell tumors* (NSGCTs), a term that distinguishes them from seminomas, which have a different clinical course and require different treatment. In a small number of NSGCTs, the trophoblastic cells overgrow other tumor components and continue proliferating, forming highly malignant tumors equivalent to placental *choriocarcinomas*. Theoretically, one could predict that, in some NSGCTs, the yolk sac component will also acquire such highly malignant properties, as has been noted in ovarian germ cell tumors. However, pure *yolk sac carcinoma* rarely develops in adults. Tumors composed of yolk sac components are confined to the testes of infants and children younger than 5 years of age. Most appropriately, these are called *yolk sac tumors* (YSTs), not carcinomas, because they can readily be cured by early resection.

For practical purposes, only seminomas and NSGCTs are discussed; other tumors are only briefly mentioned. Classical seminomas constitute 40 percent of all testicular tumors, NSGCTs account for 45 percent, and in 15 percent of the cases, the tumor is mixed seminoma and NSGCT. In the group of malignant NSGCTs, there are pure ECs, teratocarcinomas, and choriocarcinomas, which account for 10 percent, 20 percent, and less than 1 percent of all testicular tumors, respectively. Benign teratomas account for 3 percent, childhood YSTs for 2 percent, and Sertoli and Leydig cell tumors for 5 percent of all testicular tumors.

Seminoma

Seminomas present as firm intratesticular masses which, on cross section, appear yellow and slightly lobulated (Fig. 14-7). Histologic examination reveals that the tumor is composed of large cells with clear, glycogen-rich cytoplasm resembling gonocytes. These cells are arranged into groups separated by connective tissue septa. The septa are infiltrated with lymphocytes and macrophages, probably representing an immune response to the tumor cells.

The peak incidence for seminomas occurs at 40 years of age. Tumors cause enlargement of the testis and few other symptoms. There are no typical serologic tumor markers for seminoma, as the tumor cells do not produce AFP or hCG. Moreover, although most tumors contain a few scattered trophoblastic giant cells that secrete hCG, serum hCG tests yield negative results. Apparently, the tumor does not contain enough hCG-secreting cells to raise the serum levels of hCG above the threshold of detectability.

Seminomas have consistently been associated with a good prognosis, even in the days before the advent of modern chemotherapy. In part, this is because the tumor is radiosensitive. Moreover, the cells evoke a strong immune reaction, manifested by lymphocytic and plasma cellular infiltrates, which retards the growth of the tumor. Survival depends on the extent of tumor spread. Although advanced tumors have a less favorable outcome, the overall cure rate is almost 90 percent.

Nonseminomatous Germ Cell Tumors

NSGCTs are a histologically heterogeneous group of tumors which are composed of malignant stem cells. As a rule, almost all of these tumors contain EC cells, which are their malignant stem cells. The EC cells may

FIGURE 14-7
Seminoma. (A) Cross section of a tumor. The tumor appears lobulated and is uniformly yellow. (B) Histologic examination reveals that the seminoma is composed of groups of clear cells surrounded by fibrous septa infiltrated with lymphocytes.

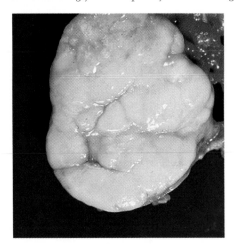

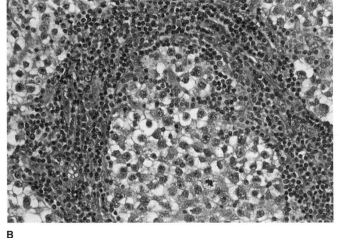

A

B

form monomorphic tumors, as in pure embryonal carcinoma, or they may be admixed with other tissues, as in teratocarcinomas. Approximately 15 percent of testicular germ cell NSGCTs also contain seminoma. Because the seminoma is the less malignant component, all of these tumors should be treated clinically as any other NSGCT.

On gross examination, NSGCTs have a variegated appearance which is partially attributable to their heterogeneous histologic composition; partially to the rapidly proliferating nature of malignant stem cells, which cause necrosis and hemorrhage; and partially to the frequent presence of trophoblastic cells that invade and destroy tissue like their normal equivalents in the placenta (Fig. 14-8). On histologic examination, the tumors may be composed of EC cells only, or EC cells admixed with various other tissues and choriocarcinoma (trophoblastic)– or yolk sac

carcinoma–like cells. Pure choriocarcinoma occurs occasionally, but is extremely rare. Pure yolk sac carcinoma is an almost nonexistent form of NSGCT in adults.

Clinically, NSGCTs present as testicular masses. Affected patients tend to be somewhat younger than those with seminoma (peak incidence occurs at 30 years of age). At the time of diagnosis, many of these tumors will have already metastasized, in contrast to seminomas, most of which are still localized at the time of diagnosis.

Trophoblastic cells and yolk sac cells are found in 75 percent of NSGCTs. These cells produce hCG and AFP, which can be detected in the serum of tumor-bearing patients; thus, these tumors can be monitored by serologic means using AFP and hCG as tumor markers. After removal of the tumor, the elevated serum hCG and AFP levels usually decrease to

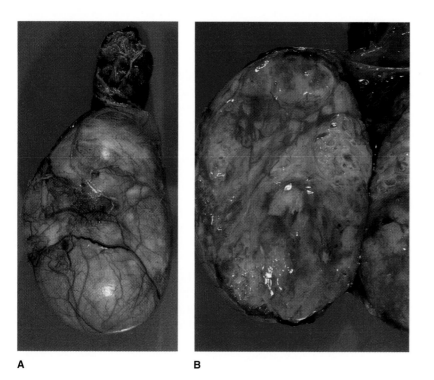

A   **B**

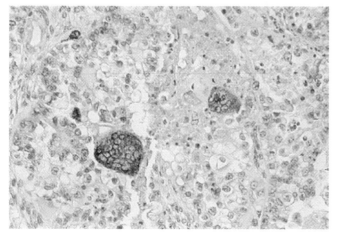

C

FIGURE 14-8

Nonseminomatous germ cell tumor (NSGCT). (A) On gross examination, the tumor is partially cystic and contains heterogeneous portions. (B) On histologic examination, embryonal carcinoma cells are the most important components of this NSGCT. (C) By immunohistochemistry, one can demonstrate human chorionic gonadotropin (dark brown) in trophoblastic giant cells.

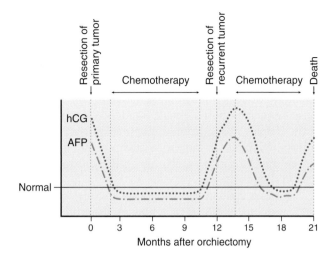

FIGURE 14-9
Alpha-fetoprotein (AFP) and human chorionic gonadotropin (hCG) are good serum markers for testicular nonseminomatous germ cell tumors (NSGCTs). (A) Initial high serum levels of AFP and hCG drop to undetectable levels after resection of the primary tumor. The recurrence of the tumor is marked by rising serum levels of these tumor markers. (B) Inoperable tumor with widespread metastases. Resection of the primary tumor did not significantly reduce the serum levels of these tumor markers. As the tumor load increases, so does the serum concentration of AFP and hCG.

undetectable levels, as one would expect in normal males. However, if the patient has metastases that have not been removed, serum hCG and AFP levels will remain elevated. Similarly, the initial decline in serum AFP and hCG levels will be reversed if there is tumor recurrence (Fig. 14-9).

Until the 1970s, when the new treatment protocols based on platinum salts were introduced into clinical medicine, NSGCTs had a bad prognosis. Today's treatment of NSGCTs includes surgical resection of the primary tumor, resection of lymph nodes involved with metastases, and an intensive course of chemotherapy with several cytotoxic drugs in combination. A second-look operation is sometimes indicated, at which time residual tumor masses may be resected. With this therapeutic course, it is possible to achieve complete tumor eradication and a 5-year survival in excess of 85 percent.

Other Tumors

As indicated in Table 14-1, seminomas and malignant NSGCTs account for 90 percent of all testicular tumors. Other testicular tumors are of lesser importance.

Yolk sac tumors are tumors that occur in infancy and childhood. If resected in time, they have an excellent prognosis.

Leydig cell tumors, like the normal cells from which they originate, are hormonally active. These tumors produce either testosterone or estrogens, can

occur at any age, and although mostly benign, can present as low-grade malignant lesions as well. Excess of testosterone is usually not clinically apparent unless it occurs before puberty. In this age group, Leydig cell tumors may cause precocious puberty. In adult males, estrogen-producing Leydig cell tumors may cause gynecomastia, loss of libido, and feminization.

Sertoli cell tumors are usually benign. Although these tumors may secrete sex hormones, the symptoms are typically related to the testicular mass rather than to the small amounts of hormones produced by the tumor.

Prostatic Hyperplasia and Neoplasms

Enlargement of the prostate may occur as a result of benign prostatic hyperplasia (BPH) or carcinoma of the prostate. BPH is a reactive, benign hyperplastic lesion related to the hormonal changes in the body that occur with aging, whereas carcinoma of the prostate is a truly malignant tumor. It should be noted that prostatic carcinoma does not have a benign neoplastic equivalent; thus, the diagnosis of "adenoma of the prostate" is never made. This does not mean that benign adenomas do not occur in the prostate. Actually, there is no good reason why such benign tumors would not happen in the prostate, but histologically, such benign lesions cannot be distinguished from BPH.

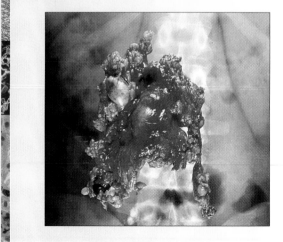

Did You Know?

This is a radiograph of the abdomen of a patient who had a malignant tumor of the testis with metastases. The abdominal lymph nodes are superimposed on the radiograph to indicate the site from which they were resected. The lymph nodes contained metastases.

Self-examination is the best way to diagnose testicular tumors. All men should palpate their own testes every 6 months. Most men who are diagnosed as having testicular cancer present 3 to 6 months after noticing the testicular mass. This delay, to a great extent, reflects self-denial. Most affected persons who are aware of testicular cancer believe that such a disease could never happen to them. In the next stage, they may acknowledge that they have a testicular mass, but they convince themselves that it will disappear on its own. By the time such patients seek medical help, the tumor has had 3 to 6 months to grow. At the time of operation, these tumors measure 5 to 6 cm in diameter (i.e., they have attained the size of a walnut).

Some men have never been taught that the testes can give rise to neoplasms. A survey exploring the reasons for the delay in seeking medical treatment disclosed widespread ignorance about testicular tumors. Some respondents who had a tumor thought that an enlarged testis was a sign of their masculinity—the bigger, the better. Needless to say, they were surprised by the diagnosis of tumor. (Illustration reproduced with permission of Primary Care & Cancer.)

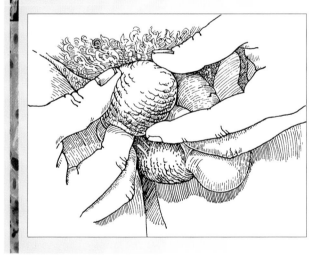

Benign Prostatic Hyperplasia

BPH is a reactive enlargement of the periurethral portion of the prostate and the so-called median bar (median lobe), a part of the prostate located at the neck of the urinary bladder (Fig. 14-10). As the prostate undergoes nodular hyperplasia, it compresses the urethra, and the median lobe may even act as a moving valve impeding urination. The centrally located hyperplastic nodules compress and expand the peripheral tissue. This is called the surgical capsule of the prostate because it loosely envelopes the abnormal tissue. BPH nodules can be surgically "shelled out" from the capsule, which is usually done by inserting a finger between the nodules and the cleavage plane formed underneath the capsule.

Pathogenesis. The pathogenesis of BPH is not fully understood. All theories proposed so far invoke a hormonal mechanism, implying that testosterone plays a crucial role. It is known that the development of the prostate at puberty occurs only in the presence of male sex hormones. Young men who are castrated before the onset of puberty have a small, nonfunctioning prostate. Experimental studies in dogs (which have a human-like prostate and are typically used for prostate cancer research) reveal that the small prostates resulting from prepubertal castration can be made hyperplastic with exogenous testosterone, and even more so with simultaneous administration of estrogen. It is possible that estrogen sensitizes the prostatic cells to the action of testosterone, or that the male and female hormones act synergistically.

A similar interaction of estrogen and testosterone probably accounts for the BPH that occurs in older men; even though older men produce less testosterone than younger men, the relative increase of estrogen that occurs with age probably facilitates and augments the action of testosterone on the periurethral portion of the prostate. This part is apparently most sensitive to estrogens. Metabolic inhibitors of testosterone, which counteract the effects of male sex hormones, are often used instead of surgery to treat prostatic hyperplasia.

Pathology. On gross examination, prostates that are enlarged as a result of BPH appear nodular, distort the urethra, and compress the peripheral portions of the glands into a fibrous capsule ("surgical capsule"). On palpation, the tissue is of uneven consistency, but is generally soft and pliable. On histologic examination, the tissue consists of numerous hyperplastic glands surrounded by an increased amount of fibromuscular stroma. The ratio of glandular to stromal hyperplasia varies from one case to another, and even within a single prostate, there is considerable variation from one area to another. The proliferated glands may dilate cystically and accumulate prostatic secretions (Fig. 14-11). This may predispose the affected individual to infection, which is quite common with BPH.

Clinical Features. The clinical symptoms of BPH are related to urethral compression and retention of urine. It should be noted that the periurethral location of hyperplastic nodules is associated with urinary symptoms early in the course of the disease, in contrast to peripherally located prostatic carcinoma, which produces such symptoms only in later stages

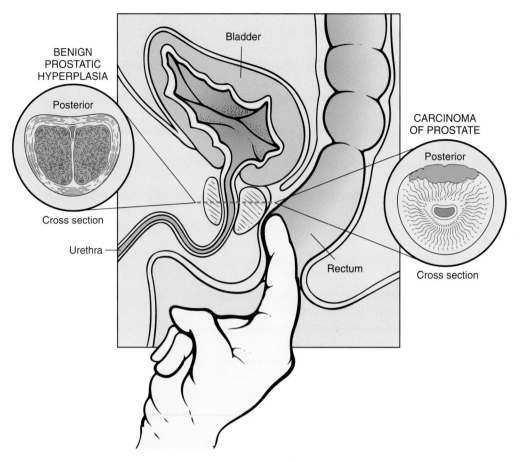
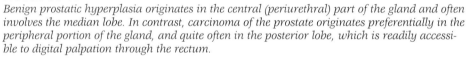

FIGURE 14-10
Benign prostatic hyperplasia originates in the central (periurethral) part of the gland and often involves the median lobe. In contrast, carcinoma of the prostate originates preferentially in the peripheral portion of the gland, and quite often in the posterior lobe, which is readily accessible to digital palpation through the rectum.

of the disease. BPH causes distortion and elongation of the urethra, which also affect the sphincters regulating urination. The patient feels an urgency to void, but cannot begin urinating. The stream of urine is weak and the patient must strain to empty all the

FIGURE 14-11
Cross section of a prostate showing cystic dilation of benign hyperplastic glands.

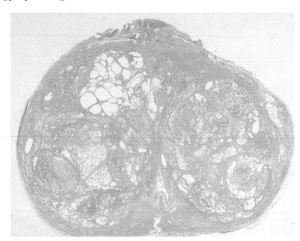

urine. At the end of micturition, the urine keeps dribbling and the patient often experiences loss of control and incontinence. Urinary frequency and dysuria (painful urination) are common, and usually indicate a superseding infection that develops in the residual urine.

Long-standing obstruction of the bladder neck is typically associated with infections of the urinary bladder. Such infection may spread into the upper urinary tract. The increased pressure of urine in the bladder may cause reflux of urine into the ureters, dilatation of ureters (*hydroureters*), and dilatation of the renal collecting system (*hydronephrosis*).

Carcinoma of the Prostate

The significance of prostatic carcinoma can be summarized as follows:

- It is the most common cancer in males.
- It is the third most common cause of cancer-related deaths in males.
- It is a tumor of older men and, as the longevity of the population increases, there is a constant increase in the incidence of prostatic cancer.

- There is still no adequate treatment for tumors that have extended beyond the confines of the prostate. More than 75 percent of all patients are diagnosed with such advanced tumors. The American Cancer Society estimates that 100,000 men will be diagnosed as having prostatic cancer this year, and 30,000 will die of this disease.

The overall incidence of prostatic cancer is 75 per 100,000, but these figures are misleading because such statistics take into consideration men of all ages. If the data are stratified by age, the incidence is more than 500 cases per 100,000 in the group 70 to 75 years of age, and more than 1000 per 100,000 in those older than 80 years of age.

Etiology and Pathogenesis. The etiology and pathogenesis of prostatic carcinoma are poorly understood, and no definitive risk factors have been identified so far. As with BPH, the hormonal theories have the most proponents, and it is widely believed that testosterone stimulates the growth of prostatic cancer. There are several lines of evidence supporting this view, including the following:

- Prostatic carcinoma does not develop in persons who are castrated before puberty.
- Castration of patients with prostatic cancer is thought to retard tumor growth.
- Anti-testosterone drugs retard tumor growth.
- Testosterone receptors have been demonstrated on prostatic carcinoma cells.

Hormonal theories have been refuted by proponents of other explanations. Typically, patients with prostatic carcinoma do not have elevated serum testosterone levels. Actually, most of them show an age-related decrease in testosterone output. Many urologists do not believe that castration improves the survival of such patients. The hormonal theory of prostatic cancer is, thus, far from being proven!

Another puzzling aspect of prostatic cancer relates to the enormous racial differences noted in the incidence of this tumor. For example, the incidence of prostatic cancer in Orientals is more than 10 times lower than that among whites. Some of these differences may be related to environment and lifestyles, as Americans of Oriental origin have a greater incidence of prostatic cancer than do their relatives living in Asia. Epidemiologists hope that these racial and environmental differences may also hold some clues about the causes of prostatic cancer.

Pathology. Carcinoma of the prostate originates in the peripheral (posterior lobe) glands. The initial tumor is limited to the glands, but it gives rise to locally invasive lesions. Cancer spreads through the lymphatics and into the adjacent organs, primarily the rectum, urinary bladder, and other pelvic structures. Perineural invasion is particularly common. Pelvic lymph nodes and, subsequently, retroperitoneal abdominal lymph nodes are involved relatively early in the course of the disease.

Distant metastases occur via the lymphatics or blood. Among the most common distant organs involved are the vertebral bones, lungs, and liver. The lumbosacral vertebral and sacral bones are most often involved, presumably as a result of retrograde spread through the vertebral venous plexus, which drains venous blood from both the prostate and lower vertebrae and sacrum.

Histologic studies reveal that most prostatic malignant lesions are adenocarcinomas. Some tumors are well differentiated, whereas others are less well differentiated. Histologic grading of tumors is clinically important and is, therefore, done routinely by pathologists.

From a diagnostic point of view, it is important to note that prostatic cells produce *prostate-specific antigen* (PSA), a serine protease that is secreted normally into the semen. Its role is to liquefy the coagulum that forms from ejaculated sperm. PSA is normally present in prostatic secretions, and only a small fraction of it enters the blood. In healthy men, blood contains less than 4 ng/mL of PSA. Prostate cancer cells also produce PSA. However, because tumor cells are not arranged normally, considerable amounts of PSA secreted by prostate carcinoma cells will enter the blood. Blood levels of PSA exceeding 10 ng/mL are typically found in cancer patients. Unfortunately, about 30 percent to 40 percent of all patients with prostate cancer have only mild elevation of PSA levels. Furthermore, other prostatic diseases, such as prostatitis or prostatic hyperplasia, can also cause PSA elevations in blood. Clearly, a "positive PSA test" must be interpreted judiciously and in the context of other clinical findings.

Alkaline phosphatase is yet another blood enzyme that deserves to be mentioned in this context. In contrast to prostatic acid phosphatase (PAP) and PSA, alkaline phosphatase is not expressed or produced by prostatic cells. However, it is abundant in osteoblasts. When the prostatic carcinoma cells metastasize to the bone and evoke an osteoblastic reaction, the proliferation of osteoblasts results in an increase of alkaline phosphatase in the blood. Clearly, any tumor that causes osteoblastic metastases will cause elevation of serum alkaline phosphatase levels. However, elevated serum alkaline and acid phosphatase levels in an older man are virtually diagnostic of prostatic carcinoma that has metastasized to the bones.

Clinical Features. The clinical presentation of prostatic cancer has few diagnostic features. This is primarily attributable to two factors:

- The tumor usually occurs in older men who already have some prostatic problems, usually

BPH. Gradual worsening of the symptoms thus may go unnoticed.

- Prostatic carcinoma originates in the peripheral parts of the prostate; therefore, it does not cause compression of the urethra or urinary problems until late in the course of the disease.

Early tumors—i.e., those that are limited to the prostate and that are the only form of prostatic cancer amenable to successful treatment—are typically asymptomatic. Tumor extension into the surrounding organs usually is associated with pain (nerve invasion), dysuria or hematuria (urinary tract invasion), or constipation and intestinal obstruction (rectal invasion). Bone metastases cause dull and persistent pain. Bone fractures are uncommon, but may occur, especially in patients with advanced disease.

Currently, the only feasible approach to combating prostatic cancer is early detection and surgical resection before the tumor has spread beyond the prostate. The good news is that the prostate can readily be palpated using a finger inserted into the rectum. Indeed, no physical examination should be considered to be complete without a rectal examination, which is an absolute must in all men older than 50 years of age. If palpation reveals suspicious areas, those can be further evaluated by ultrasonography. The ultrasound probe is introduced into the rectum, from which location even small tumors can be efficiently localized. This technique is very useful in delineating the extent of tumor spread in patients with more advanced disease. Finally, any suspicious lesions can readily be sampled for cytologic examination by thin needle (or larger) cytologic aspiration or for a "through-cut" tissue biopsy using a thicker needle.

Prostatic cancer is best treated surgically, but extensive tumors usually are also treated with radiation therapy, and occasionally, with chemotherapy. Palliative radiation therapy is used to relieve pain in advanced cases.

The prognosis depends, to some degree, on the histologic grade of the tumor (tumors that are well differentiated have a better prognosis), but the most significant prognostic factor is the extent of tumor (those that are well differentiated grow more slowly). The histologic grade assigned correlates closely with the extent of tumor spread (i.e., the stage of tumor). Nevertheless, wide variations have been reported in the survival of patients, even when they have the same stage of disease, presumably because many of them have clinically inapparent metastases. It has been estimated that one third of all patients with tu-

Did You Know?

Thousands of prostatectomies (surgical removal of the prostate) are performed every year for prostatic carcinoma or benign prostatic hyperplasia. During this rather complicated operation, it is not uncommon for the urologist to sever the nerves innervating the urinary bladder sphincters or the penis, and some patients become either incontinent or impotent or both. To avoid these complications, many modern urologists perform so-called "nerve-sparing" operations. Satisfied patients are a major source of referral of new clients for these highly skilled surgeons.

mors presumed to be confined to the prostate have lymph node metastases. The 5-year survival of patients with tumor limited to the prostate is 75 percent. Patients with tumors that have spread beyond the confines of the prostate have a 35 percent to 50 percent 5-year survival rate, depending on the exact stage of the tumor.

Carcinoma of the Penis

Carcinoma of the penis is rare in the United States, where it affects only 1 to 2 men per 100,000. However, in parts of the world where neonatal circumcision is not practiced and genital hygiene is poor, this form of cancer is much more common. For example, in some countries of South America, such as Paraguay, it accounts for more than 10 percent of all cancers in men. Carcinoma of the penis is, therefore, considered to be an environmentally induced cancer, probably related to poor genital hygiene. Smegma—the product of the penile coronal glands, desquamated cells, and bacteria—is considered to be a possible major carcinogenic influence. Because this material accumulates under the prepuce of uncircumcised men, it is believed to play a role as a contact carcinogen for the mucosal cells of the glans. Indeed, almost all tumors are located on the glans of the penis. Histologic examination reveals the tumors to be squamous cell carcinomas.

Treatment includes surgical amputation combined with radiation therapy. The prognosis depends on the stage of the disease: localized lesions have a good prognosis, whereas advanced lesions are less responsive to treatment.

Review Questions

1. Describe how sperm is formed and excreted.
2. How are the functions of the testis regulated?
3. What is cryptorchidism and how does it present clinically?
4. Explain the pathogenesis of infections, such as balanitis, urethritis, prostatitis, epididymitis, and orchitis.
5. Compare genital herpes simplex infection and gonorrhea with nongonococcal urethritis.
6. What are the pathologic and clinical features of primary, secondary, and tertiary syphilis?
7. How common are testicular tumors, and in which age group are they most often encountered?
8. Classify testicular germ cell tumors.
9. What is the difference between seminoma and nonseminomatous germ cell tumors?
10. What is the difference between teratoma and teratocarcinoma?
11. Which serologic tumor markers are useful for diagnosing testicular tumors?
12. How are testicular germ cell tumors treated, and what is the usual outcome of such treatment?
13. Compare Leydig cell tumors and Sertoli cell tumors.
14. What is benign prostatic hyperplasia and what are its causes?
15. Correlate pathologic and clinical findings in benign prostatic hyperplasia.
16. How common is carcinoma of the prostate?
17. Discuss the possible role of hormones in the pathogenesis of prostatic carcinoma.
18. Correlate the pathologic and clinical findings in prostatic carcinoma.
19. What is the value of prostate-specific antigen in the diagnosis of prostatic carcinoma?
20. What is the outcome of treatment of prostatic carcinoma?
21. On what does the prognosis of prostatic carcinoma depend?
22. Correlate the pathologic and clinical features of carcinoma of the penis.

Learning Objectives

After reading this chapter, the student should be able to:

1. Describe the normal external and internal female organs.

2. Discuss the physiologic events at the time of menarche, during the normal menstrual cycle, and at the time of menopause.

3. Briefly describe the critical events of pregnancy: fertilization, implantation, placentation, and delivery.

4. List the most important causes and consequences of infection of the female genital tract.

5. List the most common causes of vaginal bleeding.

6. List the important causes and consequences of hyperestrinism.

7. List the risk factors for various forms of cancer in the female genital tract.

8. Name the most common tumors of the female genital tract and discuss their symptoms.

9. List and explain the procedures used to diagnose cancers of the cervix, uterus, and ovary.

10. Discuss the symptoms and consequences of endometriosis.

11. List the most common causes of abortion.

12. Explain ectopic pregnancy, including its causes, and list the most common sites where it occurs.

13. Describe gestational trophoblastic disease with special emphasis on hydatidiform mole and choriocarcinoma.

14. Discuss toxemia of pregnancy and eclampsia.

Additional Key Terms and Concepts

Ectopic pregnancy

Germ cell tumors

Infertility

Pelvic inflammatory disease

Sex cord tumors

Sexually transmitted diseases

Chapter Outline

The Female Reproductive System

Chapter 15

NORMAL ANATOMY AND PHYSIOLOGY

The female reproductive system consists of both external and internal genital organs. The external genitalia can be seen on physical examination; in contrast, the internal genitalia, which are located in the pelvis, cannot be seen without special instruments, such as a vaginal speculum or laparoscope.

The principal parts of the female reproductive system are the vulva, vagina, uterus, fallopian tubes, and ovaries (Fig. 15-1). The **vulva** includes the labia majora and minora, the clitoris, and the urethral orifice. In adult women, it is surrounded by the hairy skin of the mons pubis. The vulva is the entrance into the **vagina,** a tube-like organ connecting the external and internal genital organs. The upper end of the vagina is occluded by the **cervix** of the uterus. However, because the cervix has a central canal, the vagina is not sealed shut, and it actually communicates with the cavity of the uterus. The **uterus** extends into two tube-like structures, the **fallopian tubes,** which reach laterally from the top portion of the uterus to the ovaries. The fallopian tubes open freely into the abdominal cavity and are not attached to the ovary.

Histologically, there are several important features of the female genital organs that deserve mention. The vulva, vagina, and external surface of the cervix are covered with *squamous epithelium.* The cervical canal, the uterine cavity, and the fallopian tubes are lined by *glandular tissue.* Squamous epithelium is more resistant to minor trauma and friction during intercourse, and to bacterial invasion, than is the glandular epithelium. As we shall see later, this factor is important to an understanding of infections of the genital tract. It is also worth remembering that the glandular epithelium of the uterus—called the **endometrium**—changes during the menstrual cycle.

The uterus and the fallopian tubes have two additional layers. On the outside, these organs are covered with serosa, which is equivalent to the peritoneum enveloping other abdominal organs. The wall of the uterus and fallopian tubes consists of smooth muscle. The muscle layer of the uterus is called the **myometrium.**

The **ovary** is an almond-shaped organ composed of a connective tissue stroma, sex cord cells, and oocytes. The ovarian surface is covered with peritoneal cells. Below it are oocytes surrounded by specialized sex cord cells: *granulosa* and *theca cells.* Oocytes and sex cords form functional units known as *follicles.*

The functions of the female reproductive organs are regulated by hormones of the hypothalamic-pituitary-ovarian axis (Fig. 15-2). In adult women, the hypothalamus cyclically secretes gonadotropin-releasing hormone (GnRH), which stimulates the pituitary to produce **gonadotropins**—the follicle-stimulating hormone (FSH) and lutenizing hormone (LH). FSH and LH stimulate the ovary to produce **estrogen** or **progesterone** which, in turn, act on the endometrium, promoting either proliferation of glands and stroma or glandular secretion, typical of the proliferative and secretory phase of the **menstrual cycle,** respectively (Fig. 15-3). Ovarian hormones prime the endometrium for the implantation of the fertilized ovum in **pregnancy.** If pregnancy does not occur, the endometrium is shed and menstrual bleeding occurs.

The primary function of the female reproductive system is reproduction. The vagina serves for copulation and a receptacle for ejaculated sperm. *Fertilization* takes place in the fallopian tubes. The fertilized ovum

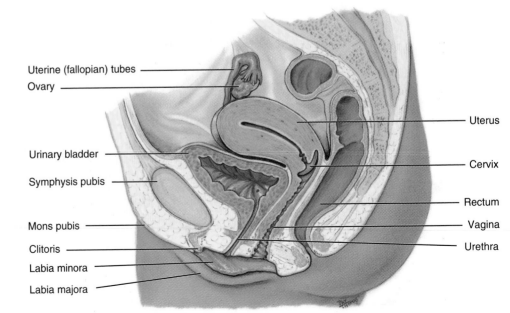

FIGURE 15-1
The female reproductive system consists of both external and internal genital organs, including the vulva, vagina, uterus, fallopian tubes, and ovaries. (From Applegate EJ: The anatomy and physiology learning system: textbook. Philadelphia: WB Saunders, 1995: 400.)

Uterine (fallopian) tubes
Ovary
Urinary bladder
Symphysis pubis
Mons pubis
Clitoris
Labia minora
Labia majora
Uterus
Cervix
Rectum
Vagina
Urethra

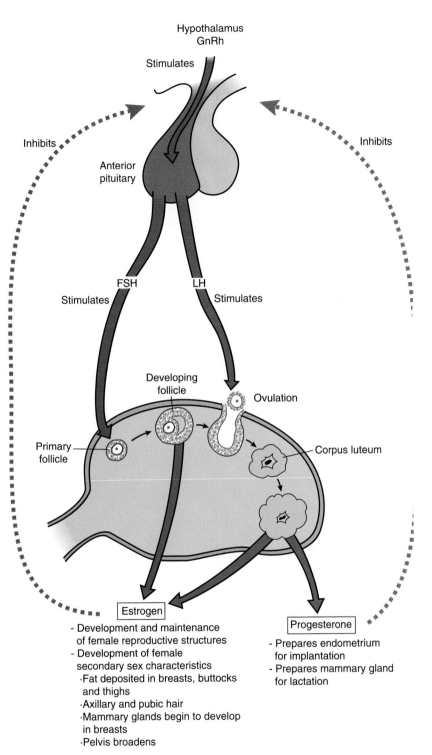

Hypothalamus
GnRh

Stimulates

Inhibits

Anterior
pituitary

Inhibits

FSH   LH

Stimulates   Stimulates

Developing
follicle

Ovulation

Primary
follicle

Corpus luteum

Estrogen

- Development and maintenance
  of female reproductive structures
- Development of female
  secondary sex characteristics
  ·Fat deposited in breasts, buttocks
   and thighs
  ·Axillary and pubic hair
  ·Mammary glands begin to develop
   in breasts
  ·Pelvis broadens

Progesterone

- Prepares endometrium
  for implantation
- Prepares mammary gland
  for lactation

FIGURE 15-2
The hypothalamic-pituitary-ovarian axis controls the functions of the female reproductive system. Cyclic release of gonadotropin-releasing hormone (GnRH) stimulates the secretion of pituitary gonadotropins that act on the ovaries. Ovarian estrogens stimulate the proliferation of endometrium, whereas progesterone stimulates endometrial secretion and prepares the uterus for implantation of the embryo. FSH, follicle-stimulating hormone; LH, luteinizing hormone. (From Applegate EJ: The anatomy and physiology learning system: textbook. Philadelphia: WB Saunders, 1995: 406.)

(*zygote*) travels to the uterus where it implants. Implantation occurs only if the uterus is properly primed by hormones. The implantation is mediated by trophoblastic cells that form the outer layer of the embryo and are the precursors of the **placenta.** These cells, like the placenta, secrete *human chorionic gonadotropin* (hCG), a hormone essential for the maintenance of pregnancy. Serum levels of hCG rise in pregnancy and also spill over into the urine, where hCG can be detected biochemically with a *pregnancy test.*

OVERVIEW OF MAJOR DISEASES

The physicians treating the diseases of female reproductive organs are called gynecologists (derived from the Greek word *gyne,* meaning woman). The most important diseases of the female reproductive system are

- infections
- hormonal disorders

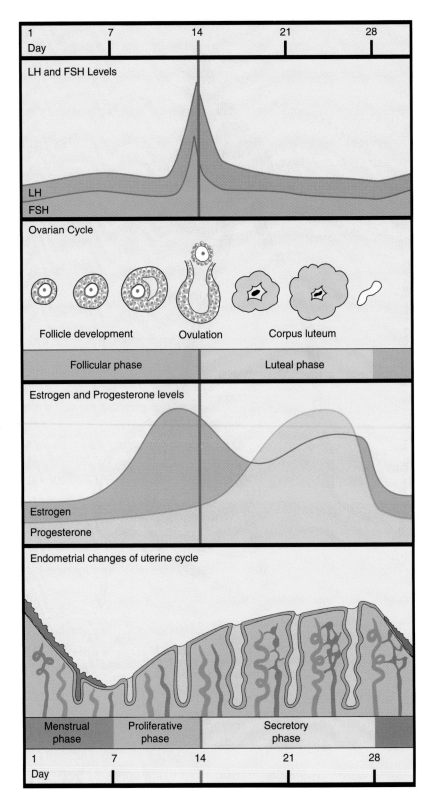

FIGURE 15-3
The normal menstrual cycle consists of a pro-liferative (follicular) and a secretory (luteal) phase. Menstrual bleeding occurs after the luteal phase. LH, luteinizing hormone; FSH, follicle-stimulating hormone. (From Applegate EJ. The anatomy and physiology learning system: textbook. Philadelphia: WB Saunders, 1995: 407.)

- benign or malignant tumors
- disorders related to pregnancy

Several facts important to an understanding of gynecologic pathology are presented here, before a discussion of specific pathologic entities.

1. *The female reproductive system is in direct con-tact with the external world.* Because of this direct con-tact, the female reproductive system is extremely prone to infections. Clinically, these infections range in severity from being asymptomatic to producing only minor irritation and discomfort, to causing major problems, especially if the infection is recur-rent as in chronic pelvic inflammatory disease (PID).

PID is a major cause of pain and suffering. It has been estimated that the treatment of PID and the work days lost owing to the disease cost the U.S. economy more than 2 billion dollars per year!

2. *Many infections of the female reproductive system are venereal in nature.* Venus was the Roman goddess of love, and the term *venereal infections* is a synonym for *sexually transmitted diseases.* The sexually active female, particularly if she has multiple partners, or a single promiscuous partner, is at risk for infection. If infected, she may transmit the disease to her future sexual partners, or the infection may be spread transplacentally or during vaginal delivery of her offspring. Clearly, then, infectious diseases affect not only the health of the infected person, but also other individuals, and thus have major social consequences.

3. *Infections of the female genital system are an important cause of infertility.* It is estimated that 50 percent of infertile women have, or have had in the past, a genital infection. PID is the most common cause of infertility. PID is also an important cause of *extrauterine pregnancies,* most of which are located in the tubes.

4. *Hormonal disorders are another frequent cause of reproductive tract pathology.* Abnormal secretion of estrogen and progesterone from the ovary may cause menstrual abnormalities, such as *oligomenorrhea* (scant bleeding), *amenorrhea* (no bleeding at all), or *menorrhagia* (profuse bleeding). Estrogen may cause endometrial hyperplasia, and it is thought to contribute to the development of endometrial cancer. Hormones have a less pronounced effect on the fallopian tube. Predictably, carcinomas of the fallopian tubes occur much less frequently than carcinoma of the endometrium.

5. *Tumors of the reproductive tract are related to sexually transmitted diseases or hormonal influences.* The causes of gynecologic tumors, like those in other organs, are not fully understood. Nevertheless, carcinoma of the cervix or vulva often contains human papillomavirus. The incidence of this cancer correlates with exposure to other sexually transmitted viruses. Endometrial and ovarian cancer appear to have a hormonal basis.

6. *Screening for gynecologic cancer has reduced the mortality from this disease.* Prior to the midpoint of this century, squamous carcinoma of the cervix was one of the most common fatal cancers of women. It is a tribute to the preventive efforts of the health care system that death secondary to cervical carcinoma is less common today than before. This, in large part, is a result of screening with the Papanicolaou test (Pap smear), which detects premalignant cervical abnormalities and allows efficient treatment. Uterine tumors are also readily detectable because they present as abnormal bleeding. This accounts for the good

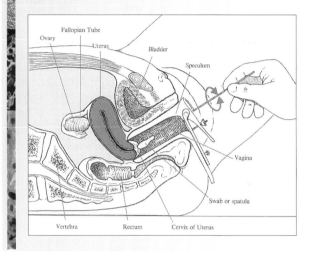

Did You Know?

A Papanicolaou smear is a painless procedure. It is the best and most efficient way of detecting early cervical neoplasia. The procedure is performed during a vaginal gynecologic examination. The examiner inserts a swab or spatula and scrapes the cervix to obtain cells for cytopathologic examination. (Illustration reproduced with permission of Primary Care & Cancer.)

treatment results of both cervical and uterine cancer. Unfortunately, malignant diseases of the ovary are not so easily detected, and these tumors still claim many lives.

7. *Pathology of pregnancy occurs as a result of disturbances in critical events essential for the maintenance of pregnancy.* Considering the complexities of human reproduction, it is a minor miracle that pregnancy occurs at all. The inability to conceive (*infertility*) has been recorded in every sixth marriage. Pregnancy may be abnormal from the beginning. For example, the embryo may implant in the wrong place, such as in a fallopian tube that cannot support embryonic development (*ectopic pregnancy*). The placenta may develop abnormally and give rise to *hydatidiform mole* and *choriocarcinoma.* The adverse effects of pregnancy are best exemplified by *toxemia of pregnancy,* a systemic disease that affects all major organs.

Developmental Abnormalities

Developmental anomalies of the female genital organs are rare, which is surprising considering the complexity of their formation during fetal life. *Agenesis of the vagina or uterus, duplication of the uterus,* and *bicornuate uterus* are mentioned here as possible, albeit rare, causes of sexual dysfunction and infertility.

A discordance between the genetic sex and the phenotypic sex of an individual may result in developmental abnormalities known as hermaphroditism. Such intersexual individuals have both male and female features or something in between. The historic term *hermaphroditism* (derived from the names of two Greek gods, one male [Hermes] and one female [Aphrodite]) has been replaced by three more specific terms:

- *True hermaphroditism* is diagnosed when the gonads are both male and female. For example, one gonad may be a testis and the other an ovary, or they may be fused into an *ovotestis*.
- *Male pseudohermaphroditism* occurs when a person is genetically male, but has female features. For example, in testicular feminization syndrome, the genetic males have a vulva, vagina, and well-developed breasts. The gonad is, however, a testis, usually located inside the abdomen. Testes secrete male hormones, but the tissues have no receptors for testosterone and cannot respond to androgenic stimulation. Hence, the external genitalia become female.
- *Female pseudohermaphroditism* is the correct term when a person is genetically female but has male features. For example, in congenital adrenal hyperplasia, the genetic females show virilization of the vulva. The clitoris enlarges and transforms into a micropenis. *Congenital adrenal hyperplasia,* the most common form of intersexualism, affects 1 in 4000 female neonates.

The most important chromosomal anomaly associated with abnormal genital development is Turner's syndrome or monosomy X (discussed in Chapter 5). This is a congenital disorder that affects one in 3000 newborn babies.

Inflammatory Diseases

Inflammatory diseases of the female genital system may be considered from several points of view and classified accordingly.

Classification

1. *Anatomic classification.* This classification system is based on the clinical or pathologic assessment of inflammation. The inflammation may be *localized,* or it may *diffusely* involve all of the genital organs, or even the adjacent structures, such as the urethra or pelvic organs. Terms such as *vulvitis, vaginitis,* and **cervicitis,** are self-explanatory designations for the inflammation of these organs, although quite often, more than one adjacent anatomic site is involved. It is thus common to diagnose **vulvovaginitis** or cervi-

covaginal infection. Infection of the body of the uterus is usually limited to the endometrium and is thus called **endometritis.** Inflammation of the fallopian tubes is called **salpingitis,** and inflammation of the ovaries is termed **oophoritis.** Inflammation of the entire female reproductive tract is known as **PID.**

2. *Chronologic classification.* With regard to the *duration* of the disease, the inflammations can be classified as *acute, chronic,* or *recurrent.* Recurrent infections may be caused by a new pathogen or represent an exacerbation of latent, clinically dormant infections.

3. *Pathogenetic classification.* On the basis of pathogenesis, genital infections can be classified as ascending or descending, depending on the route by which the pathogens have reached the reproductive system. **Descending infections** typically occur as a result of hematogenous or lymphatic spread of pathogens from some other organ in the body (Fig. 15-4). For example, tuberculosis of the genital organs is always secondary to a focus of primary infection elsewhere, such as the lungs. **Ascending infections** are acquired mostly through sexual contact. The vagina is in direct continuity with the upper genital organs, so any microbe introduced into the vagina can ascend upstream into the uterus and the fallopian tubes. Some ascending infections are complications of pregnancy, whereas others occur following medical procedures, albeit rarely. Previously, illegal abortions were a major cause of infection. Ascending infections are often more common than descending infections.

4. *Etiologic classification.* On the basis of etiology, genital tract infections may be classified as bacterial, viral, chlamydial, fungal, or protozoal. Many cases are caused by more than one pathogen and are classified as *polymicrobial.*

Bacterial infections are extremely common. *Gardnerella vaginalis* causes vaginitis. *Neisseria gonorrhoeae* (the cause of gonorrhea) and *Treponema pallidum* (the cause of syphilis) are among the most common pathogens causing **venereal disease.** Streptococcus and staphylococcus are widespread bacteria that may cause infection of the genital organs by an ascending or descending route. Mixed bacterial infections are commonly found in patients with PID.

Viral infections are also commonly acquired by sexual contact. The most important pathogens are the herpes virus and human papillomavirus (HPV), which typically affect the vulva, vagina, and cervix.

Chlamydial infections are caused by sexually transmitted *Chlamydia trachomatis.* These microbes are obligate intracellular organisms sharing features of viruses and bacteria. Chlamydia organisms cause cervicitis and urethritis, and are important pathogens in PID. Chlamydia is the most common sexually transmitted pathogen in the United States.

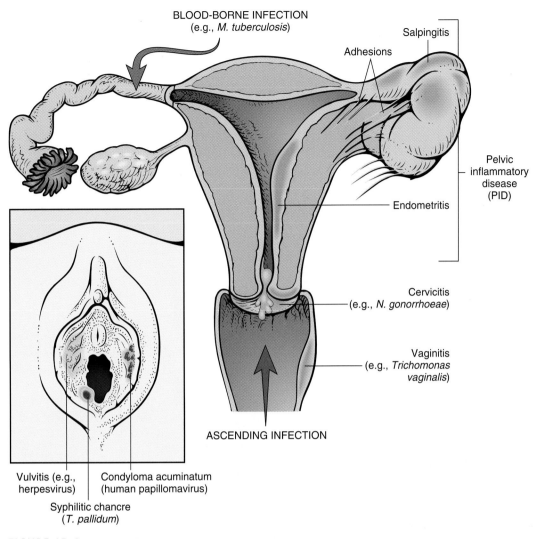

BLOOD-BORNE INFECTION
(e.g., *M. tuberculosis*)

Salpingitis

Adhesions

Pelvic
inflammatory
disease
(PID)

Endometritis

Cervicitis
(e.g., *N. gonorrhoeae*)

Vaginitis
(e.g., *Trichomonas
vaginalis*)

ASCENDING INFECTION

Vulvitis (e.g.,
herpesvirus)

Condyloma acuminatum
(human papillomavirus)

Syphilitic chancre
(*T. pallidum*)

FIGURE 15-4
Pathology and pathogenesis of infections involving the female genital organs. Ascending infections are usually caused by sexual contact, pregnancy, or instrumentation. Descending infections are hematogenous or lymphogenous.

Fungal infections typically cause vulvovaginitis. The most common fungal pathogen is *Candida albicans* (also known as *Monilia*), which lives on moist surfaces (e.g., the vagina) and does not invade deeper into the tissues.

Protozoal infections are typically limited to the vagina. The most important pathogen is *Trichomonas vaginalis,* a common cause of vaginal discharge in women of reproductive age.

The most important genital infections are listed in Table 15-1.

Clinical Features. The incubation period for various genital infections—that is, the time between exposure and the onset of symptoms—varies considerably. Many infected women are asymptomatic or never realize that they are infected. Such persons are a major source of sexually transmitted diseases.

The pathologic changes caused by various pathogens can be classified as local or systemic. *Local symptoms* predominate, but they may also be associated with *systemic symptoms,* such as fever, malaise, and general uneasiness. Entry of pathogens into the circulation may cause *septicemia* and widespread infection of other organs. Entry of bacteria into the peritoneal cavity, usually through the open, fimbriated end of the fallopian tubes, may result in *peritonitis.*

Genital herpesvirus infection, caused by type 2 herpesvirus, typically presents as grouped blisters on the vulva or the perineal skin. Infection with HPV can result in the formation of warts on the vulva, called *condyloma acuminatum.* HPV infection of the cervix or the vagina results in plaques known as *flat condyloma.*

Infectious vaginitis caused by parasites, bacteria, or fungi is associated with a copious discharge. The

Table 15-1 Common Genital Infections

Disease	Organism	Estimated Occurrence (cases per year)	Typical Genital Pathology
Genital herpes	Herpes simplex virus type II	500,000	Painful, recurrent, genital blisters
Human papillomavirus (HPV) infection	HPV	1 million	Labial, vaginal, and cervical warts (condyloma); carcinoma
Infectious vaginitis	*Trichomonas vaginalis, Gardnerella vaginalis,* or *Candida albicans*	7 million (mostly undiagnosed)	Vaginitis with discharge
Chlamydial infection	*Chlamydia trachomatis*	4 million (mostly undiagnosed)	Urethritis or cervicitis with discharge; pelvic inflammatory disease (PID)
Gonorrhea	*Neisseria gonorrhoeae*	1.5 million	Urethritis or cervicitis with discharge; PID
Syphilis	*Treponema pallidum*	>50,000	Vulvar ulcers

discharge may be clear or turbid and yellow, mucinous or frothy, and often has a foul smell. Infectious vaginitis can be treated with drugs: metronidazole is administered for Trichomonas, antibiotics for bacteria, and fungicides for Candida infection.

Chlamydial infections present as nonspecific inflammation of the vulva and internal female genital organs. As urethritis is common, dysuria is an important symptom. A vaginal discharge accompanies vaginitis and cervicitis. The infection may enter the uterus and fallopian tube. Such PID causes lower abdominal pain and tenderness, and is often accompanied by fever and systemic symptoms. Infertility is a common complication.

Gonorrhea affects the lower and the upper genital system. It also causes urethritis (dysuria) and may even cause proctitis (infection of the rectum). PID and infertility are important and common complications. Septicemia and arthritis are found in a significant number of affected patients.

Syphilis presents in females as vulvar ulcers, chancre, or as cervicitis or vaginal lesions. As in men, the primary stage of this disease, if left untreated, may progress to secondary and even tertiary syphilis.

The most important complication of all genital infections is **pelvic inflammatory disease.** The fallopian tubes bear the brunt of the infection, becoming red, swollen, and filled with pus. An abscess involving the fallopian tube and ovary (*tubo-ovarian abscess*) may form. The patient typically has severe lower abdominal pain, fever, nausea, and vaginal discharge or bleeding. Diffuse inflammation of the peritoneum (*peritonitis*), a very serious complication, may result.

As the infection progresses, other bacteria of vaginal origin may invade the fallopian tubes, which accounts for the fact that multiple bacteria can be isolated from older lesions. During the healing phase of inflammation, the fallopian tubes may become scarred and obstructed. If blockage is complete, infertility ensues. PID also predisposes individuals to ectopic pregnancy because the inflamed folds of the fallopian tube may entrap the fertilized ovum and not allow it to pass to the uterus.

Hormonally Induced Lesions

The normal function of the female reproductive system depends on the proper output of ovarian hormones, which in turn, depends on the normal function of the hypothalamic-pituitary-ovarian axis. Lesions can be caused by an excess or a lack of hormones.

Endometrial Hyperplasia
The normal menstrual cycle that typically lasts 28 days is divided into three phases (see Fig. 15-3). The pivotal moment of the normal cycle is the ovulation that occurs on the 14th day. If the ovulation does not occur, the proliferative phase of the menstrual cycle will continue and the secretory phase will never be initiated. This is called an *anovulatory cycle.* The endometrium will continue to proliferate owing to continuous estrogenic stimulation unopposed by progesterone, resulting in marked thickening of the endometrial mucosa (**endometrial hyperplasia**). However, because the endometrium cannot proliferate indefinitely, it finally outgrows its own blood supply. The superficial layers that do not receive enough blood become ischemic and necrotize. The endometrium then begins to shed, resulting in uterine bleeding. This occurs typically 2 to 3 weeks after the expected time of menstruation.

The causes of anovulation may be *organic* or *functional*. The functional disturbances are more common than the organic lesions, which are rare. For example, anovulation is common in pubertal girls in whom the normal cycle of the hypothalamus has not yet been established. Psychological factors, such as anxiety induced by examination or imagined pregnancy, can also cause anovulation. Anorexia nervosa and bulimia are typically associated with anovulation, and it may persist for a long time. Anovulation is also common in athletes. It is important to remember that the ovary contains a finite number of oocytes, and once all the oocytes have been exhausted, menopausal anovulation will ensue. This typically occurs between the ages of 48 and 55 years. Some women, however, enter *early menopause* and stop having menstruation in mid-life.

Endometrial hyperplasia can be caused by an excess of estrogen. Hyperestrinism may be exogenous (e.g., induced by hormone pills or injections). Endogenous hyperestrinism reflects ovarian dysfunction or, less commonly, may be related to estrogen-producing tumors (e.g., thecoma of the ovary).

The hyperplastic endometrium contains an increased number of glands. These glands may be cystic, as in *simple* or *cystic hyperplasia* (colloquially known as "Swiss cheese" hyperplasia) (Fig. 15-5). Alternatively, the glands may be more crowded, producing *complex hyperplasia*. Complex hyperplasia is classified by pathologists into two categories: complex hyperplasia without atypia and complex hyperplasia with atypia.

It is important to note that simple hyperplasia is not a precursor of complex hyperplasia. Complex hyperplasia may, however, progress to atypical hyperplasia, or further to adenocarcinoma. Clearly, simple hyperplasia is an innocuous change, whereas the other forms of hyperplasia should be considered as possible precursors of cancer. Approximately 2 percent to 3 percent of patients with complex hyperpla-

sia without atypia develop cancer. As many as 25 percent to 30 percent of the women who have complex hyperplasia with atypia develop endometrial adenocarcinoma.

Neoplasia and Related Disorders

Tumors of the female tract are common and are an important cause of morbidity in women. Tumors can occur at any age, but are most common in women of reproductive age and are especially common in those that are postmenopausal. The following facts illustrate the magnitude of this problem:

- Gynecologic malignant lesions account for 15 percent of all malignant tumors and for 10 percent of all cancer deaths in women.
- An estimated 70,000 new cases of gynecologic cancer and 23,000 cancer-related deaths are expected each year. The most common malignant tumors are listed, by anatomic site, in Table 15-2.
- For every malignant tumor, there are approximately five benign tumors diagnosed and even more tumor-like conditions, like cysts and endometriosis. It has been estimated that 25 percent of women older than 30 years of age have uterine leiomyomas. Ovarian cysts are found in two thirds of women of reproductive age, although most of these are non-neoplastic, small, and clinically insignificant.

Carcinoma of the Vulva

Carcinoma of the vulva accounts for 3 percent of all gynecologic cancers. The most important facts about vulvar malignant disease are as follows:

- Carcinoma of the vulva is a carcinoma of older women. The median age at diagnosis is 60 years.

FIGURE 15-5

Endometrial hyperplasia. In the presence of estrogens, the menstrual cycle is disrupted and the endometrial cells continue to proliferate.

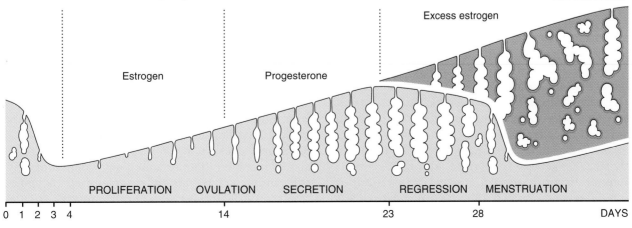

Table 15-2 Estimated New Cases and Number of Deaths Resulting Yearly from Gynecologic Cancer in the United States

Site	New Cases	Death
Cervix uteri	13,000	7,000
Body of the uterus	34,000	3,000
Ovary	19,000	12,000
Other sites	4,000	1,000
TOTAL	70,000	23,000

Data from the American Cancer Society

- The tumor can be recognized by gross inspection of the external genitalia. It presents as a wart-like or slightly raised (macular) mucosal lesion or ulceration. Invasive carcinoma is preceded by carcinoma in situ (CIS), and by preneoplastic lesions that can be diagnosed on the basis of histologic findings following biopsy. Clinically, many of these precursors of cancer present as leukoplakia or erythroplasia (i.e., white or red patches, respectively).
- Clinical symptoms include itching, discomfort, frank pain, and bleeding, but a significant number of patients, at least one in five, are asymptomatic.
- Histologically, the tumor almost always presents as a squamous cell carcinoma.

The tumor grows slowly, and if the diagnosis is made before it has metastasized to the lymph nodes, the patient has a 70 percent chance of surviving 5 years following surgical resection. Patients with tumors that have spread to the lymph nodes have a less favorable prognosis. Treatment includes surgical resection of the tumor and, sometimes, of the entire vulva (*vulvectomy*), supplemented by radiation therapy and chemotherapy in advanced cases.

Carcinoma of the Vagina

Carcinoma of the vagina accounts for 2 percent of all gynecologic cancers. In most aspects, it resembles vulvar cancer, in that it is a disease of older women and it is histologically a squamous cell carcinoma. It can be detected only upon gynecologic examination. Vaginal Pap smears are also useful for diagnosis.

A peculiar form of vaginal cancer, called *clear cell adenocarcinoma,* was identified in the 1970s in young women. It has since been shown that the mothers of these women took diethylstilbestrol (DES) during pregnancy, and that the tumor was related to intrauterine exposure to DES. Today, DES is not used during pregnancy, so vaginal clear cell adenocarcinomas have become rare, as they were before the 1960s.

Carcinoma of the Cervix

Carcinoma of the cervix, once the most common form of gynecologic cancer, accounts for approximately 20 percent of all malignant tumors of the female reproductive tract. Nevertheless, it is still ranked as the eighth major cancer-related cause of death, and it causes more deaths than carcinoma of the body of the uterus, vagina, and vulva together. The reduced mortality achieved over the last 50 years is directly related to early detection of cervical cancer and related preneoplastic conditions by routine use of Pap smears by gynecologists. For each carcinoma reported to the cancer registry, the official statistics still show four CIS or dysplasias, confirming that the incidence of cervical cancer has not decreased, but that detection in early stages has improved.

Etiology. The causes of cervical cancer, like those of most other cancers, are unknown. Nevertheless, clinical, epidemiologic, and virologic studies have identified several risk factors that may play an important role in the pathogenesis of carcinoma of the cervix. Cervical carcinoma is most common in women who

- begin having sexual intercourse at an early age
- have multiple sexual partners (for example, prostitutes are at increased risk)
- have evidence of HPV infection, especially certain subtypes
- have had other venereal diseases, such as herpes or syphilis

All of these facts point to environmental causes of cervical neoplasia. No wonder that many authorities consider carcinoma of the cervix to be an infectious disease transmitted by intercourse and caused by viruses. However, conclusive proof of the viral etiology of cervical cancer is not available and most likely, even if viruses cause it, many other factors play an important role. For example, it has been shown that cigarette smoking represents a significant risk factor, independent of other sexual determinants of cervical neoplasia.

Pathogenesis. Carcinoma of the cervix is a squamous cell carcinoma. As mentioned earlier, the outer surface of the cervix (exocervix) is covered with squamous epithelium, whereas the endocervical canal is lined by columnar epithelium. The point where these two epithelia meet is called the *transformation zone.* Most cervical carcinomas originate in this zone, marked by intense cell proliferation. It should be noted that this zone may widen after cervical trauma, which typically occurs during vaginal delivery of a baby when the cervix ruptures to allow birth. Chronic inflammation of the transformation zone causes its widening. One could assume, then, that women who have had numerous vaginal deliveries or those who are infected because of promiscuity have an altered transformation zone. Because proliferating cells are increasingly susceptible to viral infection, exposure to an oncogenic virus (such as HPV) could induce neoplastic transformation of the transformation zone. The transformed cells do not respond to normal regulatory stimuli operating in the tissue. They do not mature as the normal cervical cells, but remain undifferentiated and proliferate uncontrollably.

The lack of normal maturation of squamous epithelium can be histologically recognized as *dysplasia*. It is customary to grade dysplasia as mild, moderate, or severe (Fig. 15-6). Severe dysplasia may progress to carcinoma that initially is limited to the boundaries of the normal epithelium and is, therefore, called CIS. Carcinoma cells may cross the basal membrane and invade the underlying connective tissue stroma. At this point, the carcinoma is considered to be invasive. Such tumor can further spread locally or by invading the lymphatics and the blood vessels and metastasizing to distant sites.

The preinvasive neoplastic lesions—dysplasia and CIS—are also called *cervical intraepithelial neoplasia* (CIN) and are graded from I to III. Because the abnormal cells are shed into the vagina and can be scraped by the gynecologist, the diagnosis can also be made on the basis of cytologic studies as well. This painless procedure, the Pap smear, has saved many lives and is still the most efficient way for detecting cervical lesions.

Viral studies of cervical biopsy specimens show that more than 50 percent of all CIN lesions contain HPV. In cytologic smears, such lesions present with "koilocytes," vacuolated cells typical of HPV infection. Only types 16 and 18 and, to a lesser extent, types 31, 33, 34, and 35 HPV, are associated with cancer. Other HPV types (e.g., types 6 and 11) are found in benign lesions, such as condyloma acuminatum, and are not related to cancer. Accordingly, it is important not only to identify HPV infection by recognizing the koilocytic cells, but also to type the virus, as it may provide new data for risk assessment and the prognosis of cervical lesions.

Pathology. Carcinoma of the cervix is histologically a squamous cell carcinoma. The earliest lesions are barely recognizable by naked eye examination. Colposcopy may be used to identify the mucosal abnormalities. These changes are typically described as "mosaic" or "punctate." The cervix changes from a normal, smooth pattern to these pathologic patterns as a result of the presence of abnormal cells, irregular maturation of cells, and ingrowth of new blood vessels into the tumor zone.

FIGURE 15-6

Carcinoma of the cervix. The diagram shows the progression from mild to severe dysplasia and invasive cancer. The preinvasive lesions may be graded as mild, moderate, or severe dysplasia, or as carcinoma in situ or cervical intraepithelial neoplasia (CIN I–III). Compare the lack of epithelial maturation in CIN with the normal epithelium that shows distinct basal, suprabasal, and superficial layers. Also note that the basement membrane is intact in all forms of CIN, but is breached in invasive cancer.

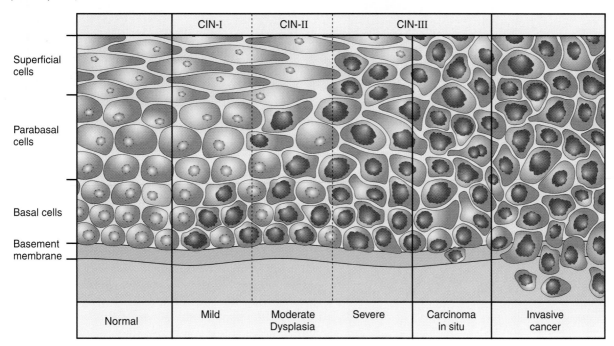

Once an invasive tumor develops, it may take several forms, classified as exophytic or endophytic depending on whether the predominant direction of growth is inside or outside of cervix. Exophytic tumors protrude into the vagina and are cauliflower-like fungating masses. Invasive tumors, called endophytic ("inside growing"), usually present as crater-like ulcerations. A variegated appearance is common in advanced cancers, which do not follow any prescribed mode but grow indiscriminately in all directions.

Because the clinical prognosis of cervical cancer depends primarily on the extent of tumor spread, staging is imperative. This is done according to the following criteria (Fig. 15-7):

Stage 0—no gross lesions; carcinoma limited to the mucosa (CIS or CIN III)

Stage I—invasive carcinoma confined to the cervix

Stage II—carcinoma extending beyond the confines of the cervix, but not reaching the pelvic wall and not extending below the upper part of the vagina

Stage III—tumor reaching the pelvic wall and/or invading the lower third of the vagina

Stage IV—tumor that has spread beyond the pelvis or has infiltrated the adjacent organs. These tumors are also associated with metastases.

FIGURE 15-7
Staging of carcinoma of the cervix. Staging provides the most important data for determining prognosis in patients with cervical carcinoma.

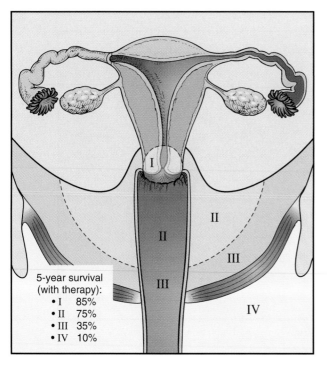

5-year survival (with therapy):
- I   85%
- II   75%
- III 35%
- IV   10%

Did You Know?

Colposcopy is performed with an instrument called a colposcope, which is inserted into the vagina and used to observe the external surface of the cervix. The top figure shows the colposcopic appearance of a normal cervix, whereas the bottom one shows a cervix altered by cervical intraepithelial neoplasia. The normal cervix is smooth, whereas the abnormal cervix shows irregularities that are readily identified. (Photographs courtesy of Dr. Warren Lang.)

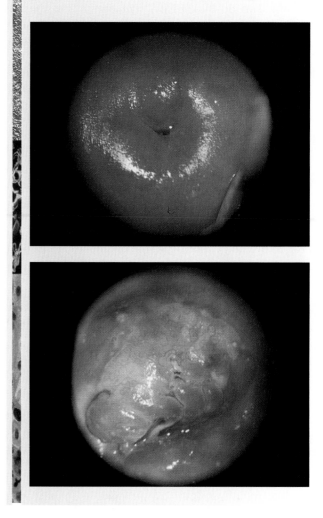

Clinical Features. The median age of patients diagnosed with invasive carcinoma of the cervix is 50 years. In contrast, the median age of women diagnosed with CIN is 35 years. Because we know that CIN precedes invasive carcinoma in almost all cases, it is safe to conclude that it takes approximately 15 years for an invasive tumor to develop. During this period of time, most women have either no symptoms or only nonspecific minor symptoms, such as increased vaginal discharge or bleeding after intercourse. Once the tumor develops, all these symptoms may become more prominent. The discharge ultimately becomes bloody or purulent and foul-smelling. Vaginal bleeding is scant, even in advanced cases, and is not a common finding. Pain is not a feature of cervical cancer, and it occurs only after the tumor has spread extensively beyond the cervix. Note how nonspecific these symptoms are, and how long it takes for them to truly interfere with daily life. Without active surveillance, most women with cervical cancer would probably seek medical treatment only after the tumor had spread well beyond the treatable stages!

Advanced carcinoma invades the adjacent organs, most notably the urinary bladder and the rectum, causing urinary urgency or obstruction. Complete urinary tract obstruction causes slowly progressive renal failure, which is still the most common cause of death in these patients. The metastases tend to follow the lymph drainage of the cervix and typically involve the pelvic lymph nodes. Distant metastases to the abdominal and thoracic organs may occur in terminal stages.

CIS and other forms of CIN can be resected surgically with a scalpel (knife) or with laser ablation, cryotherapy (freezing), or electrocautery. Radiation therapy can be applied as well. Equally good results have been obtained when stage I and II lesions have been treated surgically, or by irradiation. Advanced lesions are treated surgically, in combination with radiation therapy and chemotherapy, but the results are not too encouraging.

The prognosis of carcinoma of the cervix depends primarily on the stage of the tumor. The preinvasive cancer (CIN) is entirely curable, whereas stage IV cancer is almost always lethal and has a 5-year survival rate of 15 percent.

From all that you have learned so far about carcinoma of the cervix, the most important fact to remember is that this cancer can be recognized early and that a simple test (the Pap smear), performed on a regular basis, can save the lives of at least 7000 women annually in the United States. Remember that a few dollars, spent on prevention, can save more lives than thousands spent for the treatment of advanced lesions. The various diagnostic and therapeutic procedures used by gynecologists to treat cervical cancer are listed in Table 15-3.

Tumors of the Uterus

The body of the uterus consists of two tissues—endometrium and myometrium—both of which can give rise to **uterine tumors.** Theoretically, these tumors can be benign or malignant. However, in practice, most tumors originating from the myometrial smooth muscle cells are benign (**leiomyomas**) and the malignant ones, *leiomyosarcomas,* are very rare. In contrast, essentially all tumors originating from

Table 15-3 Diagnostic Tests and Therapeutic Procedures for Carcinoma of Cervix

Test/Procedure	Description	Objective
Pap smear	A wooden spatula is used to scrape cells from the exocervix. A brush is inserted into the endocervical canal to remove the cells.	To detect dysplastic and early neoplastic cells; HPV infection; Trichomonas infection
Colposcopy	The colposcope, a stereoscopic microscope, is used to examine the vagina and cervix in order to magnify and detect lesions invisible to the naked eye. With this instrument, one cannot see beyond the lower endocervical canal.	To detect dysplastic lesions; often used following routine screening with a Pap smear if dysplastic cells are detected
Punch biopsy	A surgical instrument is used to remove small portions of abnormal tissue for microscopic examination.	To provide tissue for pathologic examination; may be curative for small lesions
Cone biopsy	Surgical removal of a cone-shaped portion of exocervical and endocervical tissue. (This technique removes a relatively large segment of tissue and may be associated with complications. Thus, it is generally not used if the previous techniques can adequately characterize the lesion and guide treatment.)	To allow more extensive tissue sampling for pathologic evaluation; may be curative for noninvasive lesions
Hysterectomy	Surgical removal of the uterus	To treat advanced cancer
Pelvic exenteration	Surgical removal of all pelvic organs	Used as a last resort to reduce the tumor burden ("debulking")

the endometrium are malignant. These include *endometrial adenocarcinomas* derived from endometrial glands, endometrial *stromal sarcomas* derived from stromal cells, and *carcinosarcomas* (also called mixed mesodermal tumors or mixed müllerian tumors) derived from both the glands and the stroma. Only the two most common tumors—endometrial adenocarcinomas and leiomyomas—are discussed here because all other neoplasms are rare.

Endometrial Carcinoma

Endometrial carcinoma is the most common malignant tumor of the female genital tract, accounting for approximately 50 percent of all gynecologic malignant disease (see Table 15-2). Histologically, the tumor is an adenocarcinoma, indicating that it arose from the epithelial cells lining the endometrial glands.

Benign endometrial tumors, which in other organs would be called *adenomas,* are not recognized clinically. As mentioned earlier, the endometrium is shed every month; in all likelihood, the benign tumors included in such endometrium are discarded in the menstrual blood. Those benign glandular proliferations that persist are, however, indistinguishable from *endometrial hyperplasia,* a hormonally induced lesion already discussed. Accordingly, even though the endometrium does not have benign tumors, complex adenomatous hyperplasia could be considered to be the benign equivalent of adenocarcinoma. As mentioned before, complex adenomatous hyperplasia may evolve into atypical hyperplasia, and this can then progress to adenocarcinoma in a sequence reminiscent of the progression of cervical dysplasia to CIS and squamous cell carcinoma.

Etiology and Pathogenesis. In view of the fact that endometrial carcinoma originates in a hormonally sensitive tissue, it has traditionally been considered to be a sex hormone–induced malignant lesion. As mentioned earlier, estrogens stimulate endometrial proliferation in the proliferative phase. Several clinical studies have found an association between hyperestrinism and endometrial cancer, regardless of the source of estrogens. Thus, endometrial cancer is more common in women who

- are taking exogenous estrogen in the form of pills or injections
- have estrogen-producing tumors
- are obese and form estrogen at an increased rate by peripheral (fat tissue) conversion of other endogenous steroids. Diabetes mellitus and hypertension are both known to be risk factors, but it is not clear whether these risk factors have a direct or an indirect effect. Because diabetes and hypertension are often associated with obesity, the potentiation of carcinogenic risk may be indirect.
- are nulliparous or have early menarche and late menopause. These women have longer exposure to estrogens than women who have a shorter reproductive life (e.g., those who have late menarche and early menopause).

Because pregnancy is dominated by progesterone rather than estrogen, and because it provides the endometrium a respite from proliferation, multiple pregnancies reduce the risk of endometrial cancer. Thus women who have many children have less endometrial cancer than nulliparous women.

It has been postulated that estrogens stimulate the proliferation of endometrial glands, which ultimately undergo malignant transformation. In experimental animals, it is possible to induce endometrial cancer with prolonged estrogen treatment. Even more tumors can be induced by combining estrogen treatment with chemical carcinogens, which suggests that, in humans, the effects of estrogens may be potentiated by some chemical or viral carcinogens. These natural or man-made carcinogens remain unknown at the present time.

Exogenous estrogens are used extensively in clinical medicine, especially for replacement therapy in postmenopausal women whose ovaries have a reduced capacity for estrogen production. Estrogen has many beneficial effects; most notably, it prevents bone loss that occurs at an accelerated rate after menopause (*postmenopausal osteoporosis*). On the other hand, estrogen increases the risk of endometrial cancer and so the beneficial effects must be counterbalanced with the potentially adverse consequences. In practice, the beneficial effects are considered to outweigh the risk for cancer, primarily because endometrial cancer can be detected early and treated quite successfully. Note that 80 percent of all endometrial cancers are detected while the tumor is confined to the uterus, and affected women have an excellent prognosis. On the other hand, among older women, at least 15,000 deaths per year are related to major bone fractures, most of which are a consequence of osteoporosis caused by estrogen deficiency.

Hyperestrinism has also been implicated in the pathogenesis of tumors originating from other hormone-sensitive organs, such as the breasts and ovaries. Indeed, women with endometrial cancer are also at increased risk of developing carcinoma of the ovaries and breast.

Pathology. Most endometrial adenocarcinomas are exophytic and grow into the endometrial cavity. On gross examination, the fully developed tumor appears as a fungating mass protruding into the uterine lumen (Fig. 15-8). In earlier stages, these tumors

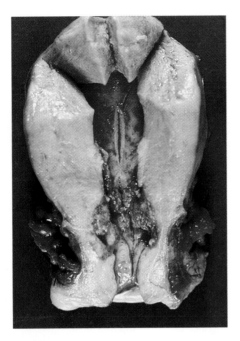

FIGURE 15-8
Endometrial carcinoma. The lower segment of the uterine cavity contains a tumor.

may appear as small polyps or thickened mucosal patches. The tissue is friable and soft because it consists predominantly of atypical glands and very little connective tissue stroma. It is prone to fragmentation and bleeding is common. Histologically, these tumors are classified as adenocarcinomas. Several histologic subtypes of adenocarcinoma are recognized, but these have no clinical relevance. More important for the pathologist is an assessment of the degree of histologic differentiation, as this information is used to grade tumors into three categories:

Grade 1—well-differentiated tumors

Grade 2—moderately well-differentiated tumors

Grade 3—poorly differentiated tumors

Approximately 80 percent of all tumors are well- or moderately well-differentiated.

The most important prognostic feature of endometrial carcinoma is the stage of the tumor (i.e., the size of the lesion and the extent of spread). The stage is determined according to the criteria defined by FIGO (Fedération Internationale de Gynecologie et Obstetrique), as follows (Fig. 15-9):

Stage I—carcinoma confined to the endometrium

Stage II—carcinoma extending into the cervix and invading the myometrium. The depth of myometrial invasion is important for prognosis.

Stage III—carcinoma extending through the wall of the uterus, but not outside the true pelvis

Stage IV—Carcinoma infiltrating the bladder or the rectum, or extending outside the true pelvis

Clinical Features. Endometrial carcinoma is a disease of older women. It is rare before 35 years of age, but its incidence increases steadily thereafter. The most common presenting symptom of endometrial cancer is vaginal bleeding. It may occur as spotting between two menstruations or as prolonged and more pronounced menstrual bleeding (*menorrhagia*). *Metrorrhagia*, massive uterine bleeding, may occur in later stages, but is uncommon initially.

Many tumors remain clinically inapparent for prolonged periods of time, especially in younger premenopausal women. Any abnormal vaginal bleeding should prompt the gynecologist to find its causes, and indeed, that is how most endometrial cancers are diagnosed. Postmenopausal women should be scrutinized even more carefully. Final diagnosis is made by endometrial biopsy, which should be performed in all patients in whom the disease is suspected.

Endometrial biopsy is performed by gynecologists. It is a relatively minor procedure that is done in an office setting. The tissue may be sampled with an aspirator, a plastic tube that is introduced through the cervix into the uterine cavity. Additional tissue can be obtained by dilating the cervix and scraping the endometrium with a curette, a procedure commonly known as *dilatation and curettage* (D & C).

The tissue obtained by these procedures is fixed in formalin and submitted to the pathology laboratory for histologic examination. The pathologist then

FIGURE 15-9
Staging of endometrial carcinoma is important for determining prognosis. Tumors detected in early stages have an excellent prognosis.

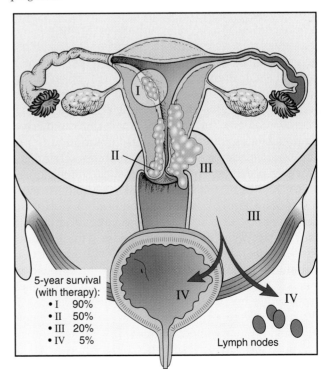

5-year survival (with therapy):
• I   90%
• II   50%
• III 20%
• IV   5%

Lymph nodes

determines whether the tissue is malignant or not, and will also grade the tumor histologically. Staging usually requires additional clinical examinations to determine the extent of tumor spread.

Malignant cells shed from endometrial carcinomas may be found in routine vaginal Pap smears. Although Pap smears are not as efficient for detecting endometrial cancer as they are for cervical cancer, cytology remains an important diagnostic approach. Aspiration cytology provides improved results because the sample is obtained directly from the uterine cavity. However, this procedure is more traumatic than biopsy, and so most gynecologists prefer to obtain tissue by curettage or biopsy instruments.

The treatment of endometrial cancer requires a *hysterectomy*, which is removal of the affected uterus (in Greek, *hysteron* means uterus and *ectomy* means removal). If the tumor has metastasized to the lymph nodes, the gynecologist will resect as many enlarged lymph nodes as can be identified. Such lymph nodes are examined histologically to determine whether they are involved by cancer. Radiation therapy is prescribed for patients with advanced disease, for those in whom the tumor cannot be resected completely, or when it is believed that some lymph node metastases have remained undetected. Chemotherapy is used for inoperable cases.

Two major determinants of prognosis of endometrial cancer are the age of the patient and the stage of the tumor. Younger patients (i.e., those who are premenopausal) fare better than the older ones. Early diagnosis provides the best, and often the only, hope for curing endometrial carcinoma.

Leiomyoma

Leiomyomas are benign tumors originating from the smooth muscle cells of the myometrium. Most myometrial tumors are benign; only 1 percent to 2 percent are malignant. These are called *leiomyosarcomas*. It seems that leiomyosarcomas originate *de novo* and not from pre-existing benign tumors. Thus, leiomyomas are not premalignant lesions and have no predilection to malignant transformation.

Leiomyomas are the most common uterine tumors. Approximately 20 percent of all women of reproductive age have leiomyomas, although in most instances, these are small and clinically inapparent. Leiomyomas are not seen in prepubertal girls, and they do not develop after menopause. Those tumors that originate during the reproductive years but persist after menopause shrink in size owing to a loss of smooth muscle cells. Only the stromal fibroblasts surrounded by collagen fibers remain, imparting to the tumors their firm consistency and whitish color. For such tumors, the term *fibroids* (often used in clinical practice) is truly justified.

The symptoms of leiomyomas vary, depending primarily on their size and location (Fig. 15-10).

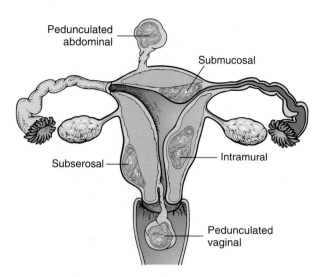

FIGURE 15-10
Leiomyoma of the uterus. The tumors may be subserosal, intramural, or submucosal. Subserosal and submucosal tumors may be pedunculated and may protrude from the uterine surface or into the uterine cavity, respectively. The stalk of pedunculated tumors may also become twisted.

Small tumors are asymptomatic. Large and multiple tumors (especially those that are subserosal) produce a "mass effect" (i.e., symptoms related to the compression of the rectum and urinary bladder). Abdominal heaviness, urinary urgency, and constipation are commonly encountered. On the other hand, tumors located underneath the mucosa tend to grow into the endometrial cavity and cause menstrual irregularities and endometrial bleeding (Fig. 15-11).

Endometriosis

The term **endometriosis** is used for foci of endometrial tissue that form tumor-like nodules outside the uterus. Endometriosis is most often located on the ovary or on the pelvic peritoneum, but occa-

FIGURE 15-11
Leiomyoma of the uterus. The tumor fills the endometrial cavity and distends the uterus. On cross section, the tumor has a whorled appearance.

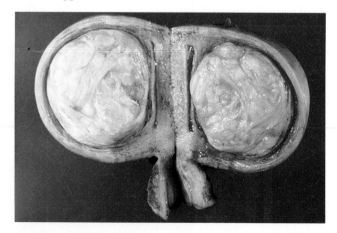

sionally, it may be found outside the pelvis, even on the umbilicus.

The foci of endometriosis are composed of uterine glands and stroma. These glands respond to estrogenic stimulation and proliferate concomitantly with the normal endometrium in the first phase of the menstrual cycle, transforming into secretory glands in the second. At the time of menstruation, the glands degenerate and bleeding occurs. However, the blood cannot be discharged because the endometriotic foci are encased by normal connective tissue and peritoneum. The lesions grow during the proliferative phase, and enlarge even more at the time of menstruation when they become engorged by blood. The foci of endometriosis may persist for a long time, although in many cases, the extravasated blood finally destroys the glands, transforming them into fibrotic scars impregnated with brown blood–derived pigment (hemosiderin).

The pathogenesis of endometriosis is not understood. According to the most popular theory, the endometrial tissue is regurgitated during normal menstruation and, instead of entering the vagina, it is transferred upstream where it enters the abdominal cavity through the fallopian tubes. The endometrial glands implant on the serosa of the ovary or the peritoneum, forming typical red nodules or plaques. The fact that most foci of endometriosis are located close to the orifice of the fallopian tube supports this explanation.

Endometriosis is important for the following reasons:

- It is very common. It has been estimated that 15 percent to 20 percent of all women of reproductive age have endometriosis.
- The lesions expand during the menstrual cycle and are infiltrated with blood at the time of menstruation. This causes peritoneal irritation and pain. Suppression of menstruation (e.g., with contraceptive pills) alleviates the symptoms of endometriosis.
- Endometriosis causes infertility. The exact link between endometriosis and infertility is not understood, but the treatment of endometriosis may cure infertility in many women having both of these problems.
- Endometriosis is a benign, self-limited disorder that does not progress to cancer. It is important to assure patients who have endometriosis that this is not a dangerous condition, although it may cause them considerable pain and discomfort.
- Ovarian endometriosis may present with relatively large cystic lesions measuring 1 to 5 cm in diameter. Typically, cysts are filled with brownish-red viscous fluid derived from decomposed blood. These endometriotic cysts appear like tumors and are called *endometriomas*, or more col-

loquially, "chocolate cysts." Pain and discomfort are the most common reasons for their removal. The larger lesions resemble tumors on gynecologic examination.

Tumors and Tumor-like Conditions of the Ovary

Neoplasms represent the most important pathologic lesions of the ovaries and deserve considerable attention. Nevertheless, we should not forget that there are other, non-neoplastic, conditions that can enlarge the ovaries and that can be mistaken for tumors, such as cysts and endometriosis.

Ovarian Cysts

Cysts of the ovary are common. Remember that the ovarian follicles enlarge during the proliferative stage of the menstrual cycle and transform into graafian follicles. Only one graafian follicle ruptures at ovulation. Those follicles that have not ruptured may remain filled with follicular fluid and may further enlarge into fluid-filled *follicular cysts.* Similarly, if the ovulated follicle transforms into a corpus luteum, but does not involute and transform into a fibrotic corpus albicans, its cavity could fill in with fluid and a *corpus luteum cyst* could form.

Most ovarian cysts are solitary. Ovaries that are bilaterally enlarged and studded with follicular cysts cause a functional disturbance known as *polycystic ovary syndrome* (POS). Originally, it was thought that affected women did not ovulate because the cortical fibrous tissue did not allow the follicles to rupture. A surgical incision ("wedge resection of the ovary") was performed to allow the passage of oocytes. However, today, we know that anovulation is not caused by anatomic abnormalities. Rather, these women have complex hormonal disturbances and do not ovulate, despite high output of gonadotropins from the pituitary. Furthermore, the persistent follicles also contribute to the hormonal imbalance.

Cortical stromal cells secrete androgens, causing masculinization (e.g., facial hair growth, acne, and body hirsutism). Infertility is the most important clinical complaint.

Ovarian Neoplasms

Ovarian tumors form a complex group of benign and malignant lesions that belong to several subtypes. These can be divided on the basis of their cell of origin into four major groups, as follows (Fig. 15-12):

- Tumors of the surface (germinal) epithelium
- Tumors of the germ cells
- Tumors of the sex cord stromal cells

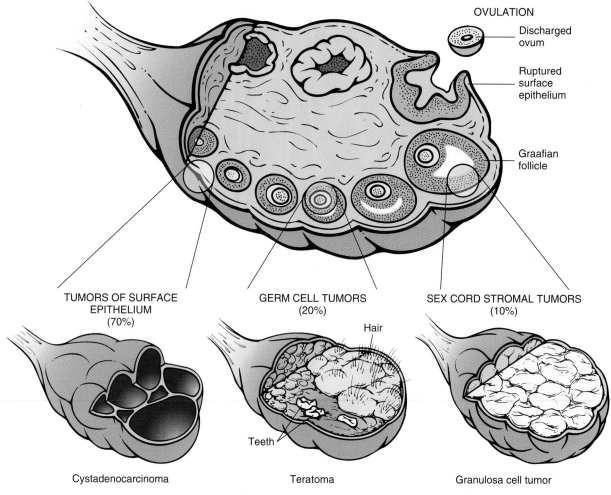

FIGURE 15-12
Histogenesis of ovarian tumors. Tumors may originate from the surface epithelium, germ cells, or sex cord stromal cells.

- Nonspecific tumors of the ovarian stroma or metastases from other organs

The benign tumors are, fortunately, more common than the malignant ones. Nevertheless, a few important facts should be mentioned to understand the magnitude of the problem:

- Ovarian cancer is the second most common gynecologic cancer, but is ranked first for death caused by gynecologic cancer. It causes more deaths than all other tumors of the reproductive female tract.
- Ovarian cancer is the fourth most frequent cause of cancer.
- Approximately 19,000 new cases of ovarian cancer are expected annually, and 12,000 individuals die of ovarian cancer every year.

Etiology and Pathogenesis. Very little is known about the pathogenesis of ovarian tumors, especially the most common variety, which involve the surface epithelium. Nevertheless, from the available clinical data and the experimental models, it is possible to suggest several hypotheses that provide at least partial explanations for these neoplasms.

Surface epithelial cells, the most common progenitors of tumors in the ovary, are akin to the mesothelial cells lining the peritoneal surface of other abdominal organs. Nevertheless, ovarian cells are somewhat specialized and are probably developmentally distinct from other peritoneal lining cells. It is not known how these cells become malignant. However, it is known that the surface epithelium of the ovary is ruptured at each ovulation, and that this little wound heals by the proliferation of epithelial cells adjacent to the site of rupture. Apparently, these proliferating cells are at increased risk of becoming transformed into tumors than are the nonproliferating ones. Women who do not ovulate (such as those who have no oocytes, as in Turner's syndrome) do not develop ovarian cancer. Oral contraceptives suppress ovulation and reduce the risk of ovarian cancer. We should also mention that the best animal models for human ovarian cancer are hens. Egg-laying hens traumatize their ovarian surface epithelium in the same way that ovulating women do. If the hens are not slaughtered for human consumption but are allowed to age, many of them will develop ovarian cancer similar to human epithelial cancer.

Germ cell tumors originate from activated oocytes. There is considerable experimental evidence to show that these cells undergo parthenogenetic activation (in Greek, *parthenos* means virgin and *genesis* means formation). Recalling the information presented in most basic biology courses, you may remember that, in many lower animals, the female germ cell can become parthenogenetically activated without the fertilization that occurs following fusion with the sperm. Activated oocytes give rise to embryonic cells, which further develop, finally producing the entire organism. In mammals, parthenogenetically activated oocytes cannot progress so far, and a fetus cannot be formed without the male gamete. Nevertheless, it has been shown in mice (and this probably occurs in women as well) that the parthenogenetically activated oocytes may form various normal embryonic structures. These structures are arranged in a haphazard manner and form tumors, called *teratomas*. The embryonic cells derived from such eggs—called *embryonic carcinoma cells*—can also proliferate, retaining their embryonic nature.

Sex cord cells (i.e., granulosa and theca cells) of the ovarian follicles are hormone-secreting cells, the function of which is controlled by pituitary gonadotropins. In experimental animals, granulosa and theca cell tumors can be induced by overstimulating the animals with gonadotropins, or by combining the hormonal treatment with some chemical and viral carcinogens.

Ovarian Surface Epithelial Tumors

Ovarian *surface epithelial tumors* are classified on the basis of their biologic features and whether they are benign or malignant. They can be further subclassified, on the basis of their histologic characteristics, into more specific categories (serous, mucinous, endometrioid, etc.). These classifications are rather complex and are usually hotly debated by pathologists and gynecologic oncologists. To simplify these complex issues, only the most salient features of epithelial ovarian tumors are presented here, as follows:

- Essentially, almost all tumors of the surface epithelium of the ovary are adenomas or adenocarcinomas.
- On the basis of cell type and the nature of their secretion, the most common tumors are classified as serous, mucinous, or endometrioid.

Serous tumors secrete clear fluid resembling serum, whereas those that are mucinous secrete mucin. Endometrioid tumors resemble endometrial glands and do not secrete anything. All other forms of ovarian epithelial tumors are rare.

- Serous and mucinous tumors are cystic, whereas endometrioid tumors are solid. From the gross appearance of the tumor and its content, one can tentatively classify most tumors. Histologic examination must be performed to determine whether the tumor is benign or malignant.
- Serous and mucinous tumors are classified as benign, borderline-malignant, or malignant. All endometrioid tumors are malignant.

If these facts are combined, then the tumors can be classified as follows:

Benign Lesions	Intermediate-Malignant Lesions	Malignant Lesions
Serous cystadenoma	Serous tumor of borderline malignancy	Serous cystadenocarcinoma
Mucinous cystadenoma	Mucinous tumor of borderline malignancy	Mucinous cystadenocarcinoma
—	—	Endometrioid adenocarcinoma

Serous tumors are the most common form. They often consist of several cysts lumped together within a common outer capsule. Serous tumors are benign in 60 percent of cases, borderline in 15 percent, and malignant in 25 percent. Approximately 30 percent of benign tumors and 60 percent of malignant tumors are bilateral. The malignant tumors often form papillae, and the cells tend to grow through the capsule of cysts (Fig. 15-13). Malignant cells implant on the mesothelioma of the peritoneal cavity and cause ascites.

Compared to serous tumors, *mucinous tumors* are more often benign and less commonly bilateral (10 percent to 30 percent). Most of these tumors are benign, and the ratio of benign to malignant tumors is 7:1. The cavity of these tumors is filled with thick yellowish or white jelly-like material (Fig. 15-14). If these tumors rupture or the malignant tumors invade the peritoneum, the entire belly is filled with mucus. This is called **pseudomyxoma peritonei** or "jelly-belly."

Endometrioid carcinomas are solid malignant tumors. Histologically, they are composed of glands that resemble endometrial glands. In about 20 percent of cases, the clinical symptoms of ovarian surface epithelial tumors are relatively nonspecific. Because these small tumors do not produce symptoms,

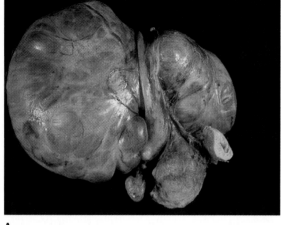

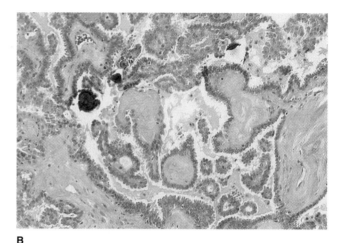

A

B

FIGURE 15-13
Serous cystadenocarcinoma of the ovary. (A) External view of a bosselated tumor. The nodular surface corresponds to cysts filled with fluid. (B) Histologic examination reveals that the cysts are lined by serous cuboidal epithelium. The same cells line the papillae that project into the lumen of the cavity. The dark material represents calcifications, which are common in these tumors.

once they are recognized, it is often too late for treatment. In about 20 percent of cases, there is also a uterine tumor, suggesting that endometrial and ovarian tumors can arise at the same time, or that a tumor involving one organ has metastasized to the other.

The prognosis of these tumors depends on the histologic diagnosis and the stage of disease (i.e., the extent of spread of the tumor). The primary role of the pathologist is to determine whether the tumor is benign, malignant, or of intermediate malignancy. Benign tumors have an excellent prognosis and the 5-year survival is 100 percent. Borderline-malignant tumors also have a good prognosis, although their 5-year survival is somewhat lower than 85 percent.

Surgery and chemotherapy are of limited assistance, and the overall 5-year survival for malignant epithelial ovarian tumor is 10 percent to 40 percent, depending on the stage of the tumor.

Germ Cell Tumors

Germ cell tumors account for 20 percent of all ovarian tumors. There are several histologic types (Table 15-4). As only the most important characteristics of ovarian germ cell tumors are mentioned here, those who are interested in details of histogenesis should refer to the discussion of testicular germ cell tumors.

The most important facts about ovarian tumors are as follows:

FIGURE 15-14
Mucinous cystadenoma of the ovary. (A) The cysts are filled with mucin, a jelly-like substance. (B) Histologic examination reveals that the mucinous cells are filled with clear material (mucin) and have basally located nuclei.

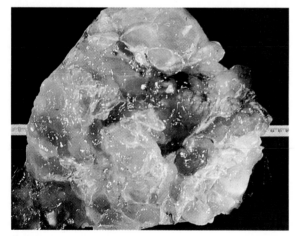

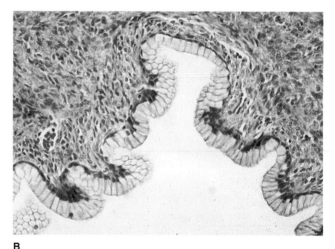

A

B

Table 15-4 Germ Cell Tumors of the Ovary

Tumor Type	Gross Appearance	Histologic Findings	Serologic Markers
Teratoma	Cyst	Skin and other mature tissues; teeth; bones	None
Immature teratoma	Solid, soft mass	Neural tissue, but may contain other fetal tissue as well	None
Teratocarcinoma (mixed germ cell tumor)	Solid	Embryonal carcinoma cells; various embryonic tissues; yolk sac; trophoblastic cells	AFP, hCG
Embryonal carcinoma	Solid	Embryonal carcinoma cells that do not differentiate	None. Possibly, AFP or hCG
Yolk sac carcinoma	Solid	Yolk sac–like structures	AFP
Choriocarcinoma	Solid, hemorrhagic	Cytotrophoblast and syncytiotrophoblast, like placental villi	hCG
Dysgerminoma	Solid	Clear cells surrounded by lymphocytes (like seminoma of testis)	None, although slightly elevated hCG levels may be noted

AFP, alpha-fetoprotein; hCG, human chorionic gonadotropin

- Germ cell tumors occur predominantly in women younger than 25 years of age.
- The most common germ cell tumor of the ovary is benign cystic teratoma, which accounts for 95 percent of all these tumors.
- Overall, teratoma is the most common ovarian tumor in women younger than 25 years of age.
- Teratomas may contain teeth or calcified parts that can be recognized on radiographic studies. However, they do not produce serologic markers. On the other hand, mixed germ cell tumors (teratocarcinomas) secrete alpha-fetoprotein (AFP) and hCG, which serve as serologic markers for these neoplasms and aid in their diagnosis. Pure yolk sac carcinomas secrete only AFP.

Teratoma presents as a cyst that is lined on the inside with hairy skin. The wall of the tumor contains other tissues, most often teeth and cartilage. The skin appendages, such as sebaceous and sweat glands, secrete sebum and sweat into the cavity. This remains there and decomposes into malodorous, mushy material. When the tumor is resected and the cavity is opened, the contents stink, the same way our skin would stink if it were not washed for a few years!

Teratomas are benign tumors that nevertheless should be resected. If they are left in place, the skin, as well as the other tissues of its wall, may gradually undergo malignant transformation. This usually occurs in older women; although it is rare, it should not occur at all if the woman is under appropriate gynecologic supervision.

Sex Cord Stromal Tumors

Sex cord stromal tumors originate from the specialized, ovarian stromal cells forming the follicles. They account for 5 percent of all ovarian tumors. Three tumor types are recognized: granulosa cell tumors, theca cell tumors, and Sertoli-Leydig cell tumors.

Granulosa cell tumors are solid tumors composed of cells resembling the granulosa cells of the ovarian follicles. These tumors may be hormonally inactive or they may produce estrogens, thus causing menstrual irregularities. The small tumors are usually benign, but the larger ones may be malignant. However, even these grow slowly and are not too aggressive.

Thecomas or theca cell tumors, are solid tumors that secrete estrogens. They are always benign and often cause menstrual irregularities and endometrial hyperplasia.

Sertoli-Leydig cell tumors are also solid tumors, and are composed of hormonally active cells that secrete androgens and cause virilization. Typical signs are deepening of the voice, facial hair, male-pattern baldness, hairy chest and abdomen, and hypertrophy of the clitoris. Menstrual irregularities and infertility are signs of smaller tumors and those that are less active hormonally. Sertoli-Leydig cell tumors may be benign or malignant.

Metastases

Metastases involving the ovaries originate most often from carcinomas of the endometrium and breast. These tumors often have estrogen receptors, which could explain their predilection for metastasing to the ovaries. Tumors of the gastrointestinal tract also metastasize to the ovaries. Most notable among these is carcinoma of the stomach, which tends to produce bilateral enlargement of the ovaries. These are called **Krukenberg tumors** in honor of the pathologist who first described this form of metastasis.

Pathology of Pregnancy

Pregnancy may be disrupted or pathologically altered at several points in time. The pathology of pregnancy is discussed here in terms of abnormal fertilization, implantation, placentation, and maternofetal interaction.

Pathology of Fertilization

Fertilization marks the fusion of the sperm and ovum. The oocyte matures into an ovum in the graafian follicle and is expelled from the ovary into the abdominal cavity at the time of ovulation. It then enters the fallopian tube, where it meets the spermatozoa. Normal fertilization occurs in the fallopian tube. The fertilized ovum (the zygote) travels to the uterus and implants into a receptive (i.e., properly hormonally primed) endometrium.

There are four types of factors that can prevent fertilization: ovum-related, sperm-related, and genital organ–related factors, as well as systemic factors affecting the male or female partner.

Ovum-related factors are poorly understood. The ovum may be immature if meiotic division was incomplete. From the experience gained with in vitro fertilization, it is known that some women have "better" ova than others. The ova of older women are generally of inferior quality, but for unknown reasons, even mature, apparently normal ova of young women do not fertilize in 20 percent of cases.

Sperm-related factors are also poorly understood. Sperm quality varies from one man to another. Some men produce no living spermatozoa (*azoospermia*), whereas others do not produce enough sperm (*oligospermia*). Still others have immotile spermatozoa, or spermatozoa that do not swim fast enough and thus have a reduced capacity to penetrate the ovum.

Genital organ factors that prevent fertilization most often occur in women and are related to fallopian tube pathology and PID. It has been estimated that PID accounts for 30 percent of all causes of infertility in women. In such cases, the fallopian tubes are occluded or deformed by chronic inflammation or adhesions, or they contain pus that prevents the normal union of the ovum and the spermatozoa. Even if fertilization does occur, many zygotes are killed by the inflammatory cells that permeate the tissues. Fortunately, women with PID usually have a normal capacity to produce oocytes. If these ova are surgically retrieved, they may be fertilized by the mate's sperm in a test tube. The zygotes thus formed in vitro are then transferred into the uterus, bypassing the abnormal fallopian tube.

Systemic factors causing infertility are poorly understood. The best known are immune mechanisms. Antibodies to spermatozoa or ova may prevent fertilization, implantation, or the development of the placenta.

Pathology of Implantation

Following fertilization in the fallopian tube the ovum travels into the uterus where it implants approximately 6 days after ovulation. For this to happen, the uterus must be receptive—that is, it must be hormonally primed to accept the zygote. In women with hormonal problems, the uterus cannot accept the zygote and cannot provide support for the outgrowth and development of the embryo. Similarly, if there is chronic endometritis or intrauterine adhesions (*Asherman's syndrome*), implantation cannot take place. Endocrine defects are usually treated by hormonal replacement therapy, whereas intrauterine adhesions are generally removed by curettage or by intrauterine surgery with the guidance of a hysteroscope (an instrument used for inspection of the uterine cavity).

Ectopic pregnancy is a term used to denote all forms of extrauterine pregnancies in which implantation occurs outside the uterus. This can occur in many locations, such as the ovary, fallopian tube, and even the abdominal cavity (Fig. 15-15). Most ectopic pregnancies (95 percent) occur in the fallopian tubes; less often, they may involve the ovary or pelvic peritoneum. In most affected women, the fallopian tube has been pathologically altered by PID, previous surgery, or foci of endometriosis. The intratubal adhesions located between the chronically inflamed mucosal folds form a barrier to normal passage of the zygote, and the zygote then implants at the site of obstruction. The trophoblast cells of the placenta that forms at the site of implantation penetrate the thin wall of the tube. It can erode the wall of some of the major vessels, causing bleeding, or it can destroy the muscle layer of the tube and rupture it. Rupture of a fallopian tube containing an ectopic pregnancy sac is a catastrophic event that requires immediate surgical intervention to prevent fatal hemorrhage.

Pathology of Placentation

The human placenta consists of a disk and chorionic amniotic membranes that together form the fetal sac. The fetus, which is attached to the placenta by the umbilical cord, floats within the sac in amniotic fluid.

Placental anomalies include abnormalities in the size, shape, or function of the placenta and membranes, the placental cord, and the amniotic fluid. Most of these represent variations from normal that have no direct consequences on the outcome of pregnancy. For example, the placentae of twins are often multiple or segmented, but these variant forms are

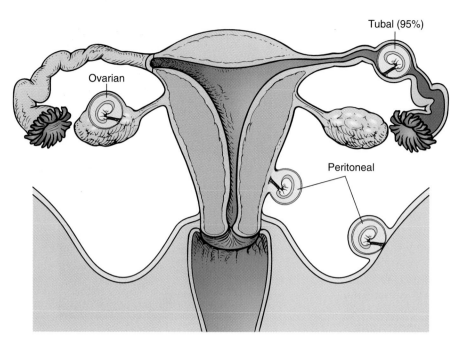

Tubal (95%)

Ovarian

Peritoneal

FIGURE 15-15
Ectopic pregnancy. The fallopian tube is the most common site for ectopic pregnancies, but they can also occur on the ovary or the peritoneal surface of the abdominal cavity.

as efficient in supporting the fetuses as the classic placenta.

Placenta accreta is the result of deep penetration of the placental villi into the wall of the uterus. This usually occurs because the endometrial stroma does not undergo decidual transformation and does not form the so-called decidual membrane. This membrane provides the normal bedding for the placenta and limits the invasion of trophoblast into the uterus. In its absence, the placenta extends into the muscularis. In such cases, the placenta does not shell out spontaneously from the uterus at the time of birth, and this may cause extensive bleeding. Manual extraction of the placenta must be performed to remove it from the uterus after the delivery.

Placenta previa is the result of implantation of the zygote in the lower segment of the uterus, with consequent positioning of the placental disk over the internal orifice of the cervix. Patients with this abnormality are prone to bleeding.

Abortion

Abortion is an interruption of pregnancy prior to the term of fetal viability, which, by convention, means a body weight of 500 g, or 20 weeks' gestation. *Spontaneous abortion* denotes abortions that do not have an identifiable cause; by contrast, *induced abortions* are those performed at the woman's request, usually by a gynecologist.

Spontaneous abortions may be further classified clinically as complete, threatened, incomplete, or missed. *Complete abortion* is when the fetus and placenta are expulsed and the woman resumes normal menstruation without any intervention. *Incomplete*

abortion is one that is marked by cervical dilatation and expulsion of some fetal parts and placenta, with others being retained. A *missed abortion* is characterized by the death of a fetus which nevertheless remains in utero for some time, usually several weeks. The macerated fetus must be evacuated surgically if it is not delivered spontaneously. *Threatened abortion* is a condition in which there is cervical bleeding but the cervix does not dilate, and the pregnancy may continue uneventfully.

It has been estimated that at least one third of all pregnancies end in spontaneous abortion. There are many possible causes of spontaneous abortion, but in most cases, the real cause remains obscure. Developmental anomalies of the embryo and the placenta account for most cases.

Gestational Trophoblastic Disease

Abnormalities of placentation that lead to tumor-like changes in the placenta or placental malignant disease represent a spectrum of changes grouped together under the name of **gestational trophoblastic disease** (GTD). The trophoblast—the epithelium lining the placental villi—consists of two cell types: cytotrophoblastic and syncytiotrophoblastic cells. GTD is a disease that involves this epithelium, and it includes a spectrum of proliferative lesions. The benign form of GTD, marked by limited proliferation of the trophoblastic cells, is called *hydatidiform mole*. The malignant form of GTD is called *choriocarcinoma*.

Hydatidiform Mole

Hydatidiform mole is a placental abnormality that occurs in one of every 2000 pregnancies. It is marked by trophoblastic proliferation and hydropic degeneration of the chorionic villi. In the most common form—so-called *complete mole*—the fetus cannot be identified in the amniotic sac. The *incomplete mole* usually has attached to it fetal parts and even partially preserved normal placental tissue.

It has been shown that complete hydatidiform moles result from abnormal fertilization. Normally, the fetus and the placenta have 46 chromosomes, half of which have been inherited from the mother and the other half from the father. The cells of the complete mole have a 46, XX karyotype. All the chromosomes are, however, of paternal origin. Apparently, at the time of fertilization, the maternal chromosomes are lost from the zygote upon which the paternal 23, X set of chromosomes reduplicates, bringing the number of chromosomes to 46. This process is called *androgenesis*. Without the maternal chromosomes, the embryo proper cannot develop, and the placenta undergoes hydropic degeneration.

The incomplete moles evolve from oocytes fertilized with two spermatozoa; therefore, the cells have 69 chromosomes—one set from the mother and two sets from the father. This chromosomal combination is also lethal, but the embryo does not die immediately, as in androgenesis. Parts of the embryo are found encased among the hydropically altered placental villi and normal placental tissue.

Clinical Features. The diagnosis of hydatidiform mole is based on the observation of an enlarged uterus corresponding to the calculated duration of pregnancy, but without any signs of fetal movement. Ultrasonographic examination is the best method for early detection. High serum and urine levels of hCG are also typically found.

Moles are aborted spontaneously in mid-pregnancy. However, if the diagnosis is made earlier, an abortion is usually performed. It is important to remove all parts of the abnormal placenta because the remaining trophoblastic cells could give rise to malignant tumors, such as choriocarcinoma.

Pathology. On gross examination, the placenta appears to be transformed into numerous vesicles resembling a bunch of grapes (Fig. 15-16). Each of the placental villi is filled with fluid, rounded up, and covered with hyperplastic epithelium. This epithelium produces large quantities of hCG, which appears in serum or urine, usually in amounts that are higher than expected for that stage of pregnancy.

Choriocarcinoma

Choriocarcinoma is a malignant tumor composed of cytotrophoblastic and syncytiotrophoblastic cells. In 50 percent of cases, choriocarcinoma arises from a

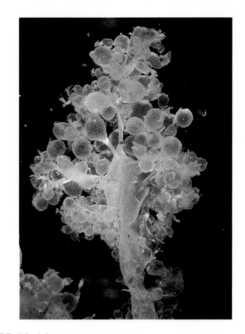

FIGURE 15-16
Hydatidiform mole. The placental villi are transformed into grape-like vesicles.

preexisting complete mole. In 25 percent, it arises from placental cells retained after abortion, and in another 25 percent, it arises from normal placenta after completion of a normal pregnancy. Like the normal trophoblast, choriocarcinoma cells are highly invasive and secrete hCG. This hormone is a convenient serologic marker; it is used for estimating the amount of tumor tissue and for monitoring tumor recurrence after chemotherapy.

Choriocarcinoma forms bulky hemorrhagic nodules in the placental bed. It invades through the wall of the uterus and often implants in the vagina. By invading the veins, it metastasizes to the lung, liver, and, most ominously, to the brain. Fortunately, this tumor responds well to chemotherapy with metothrexate (a folic acid antagonist). Cure rates of 80 percent to 100 percent have been achieved, but only in those patients who do not have brain metastases.

Toxemia of Pregnancy

Toxemia of pregnancy is a disease that occurs as a result of an abnormally functioning placenta or abnormal maternoplacental interaction. The causes and pathogenesis of this condition are unknown. It has been proposed that the symptoms are attributable to hypoperfusion of the placenta by maternal blood. Immune mechanisms have also been postulated, but remain unproven. The possible roles of prostaglandins and intravascular coagulation are currently being studied.

Clinically, two distinct forms of toxemia are recognized: preeclampsia and eclampsia, the latter of which is the more severe form. The triad of hypertension, edema, and proteinuria characterizes both forms of toxemia. In eclampsia, this triad is accompanied by convulsions (seizures) that may be life-threatening.

Some evidence of preeclampsia is found in 6 percent of pregnant women. Primiparae are most often affected. Mild preeclampsia requires no medical treatment, but in severe cases, hypertension is treated and medical support of the failing kidneys must be provided. Eclamptic seizures are life-threatening and must be controlled with appropriate drugs. The overall prognosis is good, and most women recover with no residual problems.

Review Questions

1. Describe the anatomy and function of the vagina, uterus, fallopian tubes, and ovaries.
2. Describe the effects of hormones on the female genital system.
3. What is the difference between hermaphroditism and pseudohermaphroditism?
4. What is PID?
5. List the most common sexually transmitted (venereal) diseases.
6. Discuss the pathogenesis of endometrial hyperplasia.
7. How is endometrial hyperplasia classified, and how does it relate to endometrial cancer?
8. How common is gynecologic neoplasia, and what are the most common tumors in this anatomic location?
9. Correlate the pathologic and clinical features of carcinoma of the vulva.
10. What is the significance of the diagnosis of leukoplakia and erythroplasia?
11. What is the significance of clear cell adenocarcinoma of the vagina?
12. What are the risk factors for carcinoma of the cervix?
13. Explain the evolution of carcinoma of the cervix from cervical intraepithelial neoplasia.
14. Describe the colposcopic features of cervical neoplasia.
15. How is carcinoma of the cervix staged?
16. What is the significance of Pap smears in the diagnosis of cervical cancer?
17. What is the most common tumor of the body of the uterus?
18. What is the most common malignant tumor of the body of the uterus?
19. How is adenocarcinoma of the uterus related to endometrial hyperplasia?
20. What are the risk factors for endometrial adenocarcinoma?
21. Describe the gross and microscopic pathologic features of endometrial adenocarcinoma.
22. How is adenocarcinoma of the endometrium graded and staged, and how are these findings related to the prognosis of this cancer?
23. What are the clinical features of endometrial adenocarcinoma?
24. Compare the features of submucosal, intramural, and subserosal leiomyomas.
25. What is endometriosis?
26. Discuss the pathogenesis and the complications of endometriosis.
27. What is the significance of ovarian cysts, and how are these cysts classified?
28. What is the pathogenesis and clinical significance of polycystic ovary syndrome?
29. How common are ovarian tumors, and how are these tumors classified?
30. Compare the pathogenesis and pathology of ovarian tumors originating from surface epithelium, germ cells, and sex cord cells.
31. What are the most important tumors originating from the ovarian surface epithelium?
32. Compare serous and mucinous cystic tumors of the ovary.
33. How do ovarian malignant tumors spread?
34. What is the most common germ cell tumor of the ovary?
35. Compare benign and malignant ovarian germ cell tumors.
36. List the most common sex cord stromal tumors of the ovary.
37. Compare granulosa cell tumors with thecomas and Sertoli-Leydig cell tumors.
38. What is Krukenberg tumor?

39. Explain the various forms of infertility.

40. What are the most common sites of implantation in ectopic pregnancy?

41. Compare placenta accreta and placenta previa.

42. Compare the placenta of monozygotic and dizygotic twins.

43. What is the difference between spontaneous and induced abortion?

44. What is the difference between complete and incomplete abortion?

45. Describe the pathologic features of gestational trophoblastic disease.

46. Compare complete and incomplete hydatidiform mole.

47. What is choriocarcinoma, and which hormone does it secrete?

48. Describe the pathogenesis and clinical features of toxemia of pregnancy.

Learning Objectives

After reading this chapter, the student should be able to:

1. Describe the normal anatomy of the breast, its development, and how it changes in pregnancy and lactation.

2. Explain the relationship of acute mastitis to lactation.

3. Explain the exaggerated cyclic changes in menstruating women, and relate this to the premenstrual syndrome.

4. Discuss the pathogenesis of fibrocystic changes and describe the three typical histologic changes.

5. Name the most common benign breast tumor and describe its gross appearance, histologic features, and the peak age of incidence.

6. Discuss the incidence of breast cancer and the impact of this disease on the society.

7. List five risk factors of breast cancer.

8. Describe the typical gross and microscopic pathologic changes in breast cancer and list the clinical and pathologic findings that have most significant prognostic value in breast cancer.

9. Discuss various approaches to early diagnosis of breast cancer, with special emphasis on self-examination, mammography, and biopsy.

10. Discuss carcinoma of the male breast and compare it with carcinoma of the female breast.

Additional Key Terms and Concepts

Fibroadenoma

Fibrocystic change

Gynecomastia

Mastitis

Chapter Outline

The Breast
Chapter 16

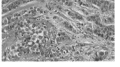

NORMAL ANATOMY AND PHYSIOLOGY

The **breast** is a specialized excretory gland, the primary function of which is to produce milk (*lactation*) for the nourishment of the newborn infant. Breasts attain functional maturity only upon completion of pregnancy. In nonpregnant women, breasts do not mature completely into a milk-producing organ. In males, the breast remains rudimentary.

Breasts develop from modified skin glands located along the so-called *milk line*. This line can best be seen in mammals (like dogs and cats) that have several breasts. Humans develop only two glands on the anterolateral side of the chest. At birth, and until puberty, both the male breast and the female breast consist only of the **nipple** and ducts, and are essentially identical in appearance. At the time of puberty, the female breasts enlarge. This is marked by proliferation of the **ducts** and formation of small epithelial buds, which are precursors of acini. The female sex hormones also stimulate the proliferation of connective tissue and fat cells, which account for the bulk of breast tissue in normally developed female breasts.

The functional units of the female breast are called **lobules** (Fig. 16-1). These consist of a central excretory duct leading toward the nipple on one side and ending blindly in the epithelial buds on the other. The epithelium is surrounded by loose, intralobular, connective tissue. The intralobular spaces contain dense connective tissue and fat tissue. It is important to note that the epithelium and the intralobular connective tissue respond to sex hormones secreted in a cyclic manner during the normal menstrual cycle. Under hormonal stimulation, there is swelling of connective tissue, which accounts for the premenstrual engorgement and enlargement of breast. After the onset of menstrual bleeding, the extraneous water is lost and the breasts detumesce.

Under the influence of the hormones of pregnancy, the terminal buds of the breast ductules develop into functionally fully differentiated **acini.** Acini are lined with secretory cells which produce milk in response to the pituitary hormone *prolactin*. If the child does not suck at the mother's breast, the acini involute and the breast size decreases to prepregnancy dimensions.

The size and shape of the breasts varies from one woman to another. Hereditary and racial differences have been noted, although it is not clear why some women, even those from the same family, have small breasts and others have large breasts. However, it is important to note that the size of breast may vary considerably during the normal life span of a woman. As already mentioned, the breasts enlarge during pregnancy and remain large during lactation. In older women, the breasts gradually atrophy (*involution*) after menopause. The postmenopausal breast contains atrophic ducts, relatively more dense connective tissue, and fewer fat cells.

Breasts have abundant complex **lymphatics** which drain into the axillary and parasternal lymph nodes. Approximately 75 percent of the total lymph flow is directed toward the axilla. If the axillary pathway is blocked, more lymph will drain in the other direction.

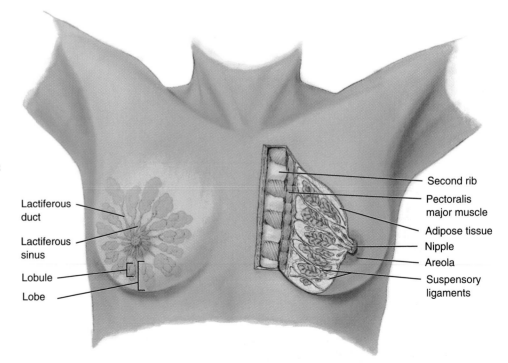

FIGURE 16-1
Normal female breast. (From Jarvis C. Physical examination and health assessment. Philadelphia: WB Saunders, 1992:443.)

Lactiferous duct
Lactiferous sinus
Lobule
Lobe
Second rib
Pectoralis major muscle
Adipose tissue
Nipple
Areola
Suspensory ligaments

OVERVIEW OF MAJOR DISEASES

The most important diseases affecting the breast are

- tumors
- hormonally induced diseases
- inflammatory diseases

Some hormonal and neoplastic diseases may be interrelated.

Several facts pertaining to diseases of the breast should be kept in mind, as follows:

1. *Breast diseases predominantly affect females.* This does not mean that males do not have breast diseases, but in comparison with females, such diseases are relatively unimportant. This point is best illustrated by the fact that, for every breast cancer diagnosed in men, there are 100 such carcinomas diagnosed in women.

2. *The breast consists of cells and tissues that respond to hormones.* Normal female breasts swell and become tense or even painful before the onset of menstruation. Hormonal disturbances of the pituitary and ovary, including the effect of exogenous hormones injected into the body, also affect the breast and may even modify pathologic processes in the breast. Some breast cancers, like normal cells, express hormone receptors and respond to steroid hormones. Blocking the estrogen receptors on cancer cells may slow the growth of tumors.

3. *Each age group of women is affected by different breast diseases* (Fig. 16-2). *Fibroadenomas,* which are benign tumors of the breast, occur mostly in postpubertal girls and young women. Fibrocystic disease is most prevalent in middle-aged women. Breast cancer is most common in older women.

4. *The functional status of the breast predisposes this organ to different diseases.* For example, acute inflammation (*acute mastitis*) is almost exclusively found in lactating women.

5. *Some breast diseases show racial differences.* For example, breast cancer is less common in Japanese women than in caucasian women.

6. *Cancer is the most important disease affecting the breast.* Next to lung cancer, breast cancer is the most common malignant tumor in women. At the present time, 1 woman in 14 in the United States will develop breast cancer during her life span.

Because of the high incidence of breast cancer and the significant mortality of this malignant disease, it is important to take all possible measures to diagnose this tumor. However, one should remember that not all breast masses are cancerous. Malignant lesions must be distinguished from benign ones, which also produce breast lumps. The final distinction between benign and malignant lesions can be made only by cytologic or histologic examination of breast tissue. Many breast nodules turn out to be benign, but that does not mean that the biopsy should not have been performed. Benign lesions, such as fibrocystic disease and fibroadenoma, account for approximately 50 percent of all breast masses that are subjected to surgical biopsy; the remainder are malignant.

Developmental Anomalies

Developmental anomalies of the breast are rare and are usually of minimal clinical significance. *Amastia* refers to congenital absence of the breast. *Polymastia*

FIGURE 16-2
Age-related incidence of various breast diseases. (A) Fibroadenoma is a disease of young women, with a peak incidence in the twenties. (B) Fibrocystic disease affects women of reproductive age, typically increasing in incidence after the age of 30 years. (C) The incidence of breast cancer increases sharply after the age of 45 years and peaks in postmenopausal women.

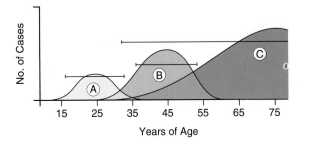

Did You Know?

Despite all the attempts to make women more aware of breast cancer and to encourage them to seek medical assistance as soon as they note any abnormalities on breast self-examination, many women still ignore such advice. As shown in this photograph, some women present with advanced cancer.

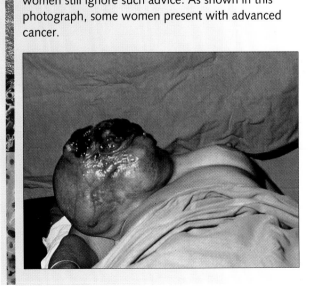

denotes conditions in which more than two breasts have developed. *Supernumerary breasts* can occur, usually along the milk line (as one would find in cats and dogs). *Polythelia* is a condition in which there are supernumerary nipples without glands. *Accessory breast* tissue without a nipple may occasionally be found in the axilla. Such nodules are composed of normal tissue and should not be confused with tumors.

Inflammation of the Breast

Like any other part of the body, breast tissue may be invaded by microbes that can cause **infection,** accompanied with typical signs of **inflammation.** Inflammation of the breast is called *mastitis.* It may be acute or chronic.

Acute mastitis is the most important and the most common inflammatory disease of the breast. Usually, it affects women who are lactating. Typically, it is caused by purulent bacteria, such as staphyloccus or streptococcus. The microbes invade the breast through the dilated milk ducts or through skin lacerations or minor injuries acquired during suckling (Fig. 16-3). Stagnant milk in breasts that have not been fully emptied by suckling provides a good growth medium for the bacteria.

Acute inflammation may spread through the entire breast or cause a localized abscess to form. In either case, the lesion develops quickly and causes localized or diffuse swelling of the breast. The inflamed area appears red, is painful, and is sensitive to palpation.

The entire area is edematous, and histologically, is infiltrated with numerous acute inflammatory cells, mostly polymorphonuclear leukocytes (PMNs). The excretory ducts may contain pus, and if massive suppuration occurs in conjunction with destruction of tissue, an *abscess* will develop. However, this does not usually happen if acute mastitis is recognized early and the lesion is properly treated. In most cases, drainage of the inflammatory exudate can be achieved through the ducts, thereby alleviating the problem. If infection persists, antibiotics may be indicated. Only in the worst cases is a surgical incision required to release pus from an abscess.

Chronic mastitis is a rare disease, the causes of which are unknown. Because it produces small lumps in the breast and may mimic cancer, affected patients occasionally undergo biopsy. In such cases, the biopsy sample is submitted for histologic diagnosis by pathologists. Chronic mastitis does not require any additional treatment.

Hormonally Induced Changes

The epithelial cells lining the ducts and acini of the breast, as well as the intralobular connective tissue, respond to sex hormones during the normal menstrual cycle. After menopause, when the ovaries cease secreting estrogens, the breasts undergo atrophy and shrivel. The fact that atrophy can be prevented by administering estrogen to older women shows that the breasts are sensitive to estrogens and progesterone throughout the life span.

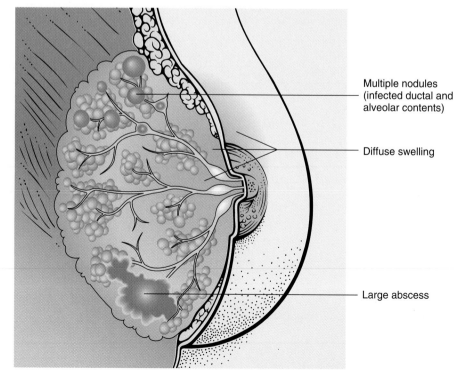

FIGURE 16-3
Acute mastitis typically occurs during lactation. It may present as a diffuse swelling of the breast, as multiple nodules, or as a large abscess.

Multiple nodules (infected ductal and alveolar contents)

Diffuse swelling

Large abscess

Pubertal Changes

At the time of puberty, the breasts enlarge under the influence of sex hormones. Excessive response of the breast tissue to estrogens causes enormous enlargement of the breast in some women. This usually affects only one breast, suggesting an abnormal local tissue response rather than an excess of hormones. This condition is called *juvenile hyperplasia of the breast,* or virginal hyperplasia. Reduction mammoplasty, a procedure designed to remove excess tissue, may be performed for cosmetic purposes to equalize the size of the breasts.

Gynecomastia

Male breasts do not develop and do not enlarge at the time of puberty. However, in some boys, the hormonal changes associated with puberty may cause breast enlargement secondary to an inordinate proliferation of the excretory ducts and the surrounding connective tissue. This is called **gynecomastia,** (derived from the Greek word *gyne,* meaning woman, and *mastos,* meaning breast). Female-like enlargement of the male breast may also occur in adult life, usually owing to an excess of estrogens. Estrogen-secreting tumors are a well-known cause of gynecomastia. The relative excess of estrogen that can accompany cirrhosis of the liver, especially in alcoholics, is another example of a condition that predisposes an individual to gynecomastia.

Fibrocystic Change

Fibrocystic change is a term used to describe fibrosis and cysts—that is, the reactive and degenerative changes that occur in the breasts of some adult women. Previously, these changes were considered to be signs of a specific disease and were collectively referred to as *fibrocystic disease.* This term is no longer used for these changes, which are partially consequences of hormonal stimulation and inappropriate tissue reaction of the breast and partially the results of changes related to aging.

Histologic signs indicative of fibrocystic change are found in approximately 50 percent of all women whose breasts are examined at biopsy or autopsy. Clinical signs of fibrocystic change are less common; indeed, it is estimated that only 10 percent to 15 percent of women between 20 and 50 years of age have symptoms pertaining to fibrocystic change. Fibrocystic change does not occur before puberty, and it is unusual to diagnose the onset of fibrocystic change clinically in postmenopausal women. Women who have symptoms related to fibrocystic disease report gradual improvement after menopause.

Pathogenesis. Sex hormones—estrogen and progesterone—stimulate the proliferation of cells in the excretory ducts of the breast and the intralobular stroma. During the secretory phase of the menstrual cycle, presumably under the influence of progesterone, there is marked accumulation of fluid in the breast, primarily because of the hydration of the loose connective tissue matrix inside the lobules. A decrease of circulating hormones at the time of menstrual bleeding reverses the hydration of connective tissue and leads to cessation of the proliferative activity. At the same time that these cyclic changes are occurring in the epithelium and the *intralobular stroma,* the dense connective tissue forming the *interlobular stroma* is not affected. Hyperplastic reactive and degenerative changes will develop in the breast parenchyma (1) if the hormonal cyclicity is disturbed, (2) if the proliferation of ducts continues unopposed and no involution occurs; or (3) if the hormone-responsive intralobular stroma is replaced by hormone-insensitive dense collagenous tissue. These changes may include dense fibrosis, cystic dilatation of the ducts, and various ductal proliferative changes.

The most constant feature of fibrocystic change is *fibrosis.* In this condition, the loose intralobular connective tissue of the breast is typically replaced by dense connective tissue that is rich in collagen but unresponsive to hormones (Fig. 16-4). The border between the intralobular and interlobular connective tissue becomes blurred and indistinct. The breast consists of dense, broad sheets of collagenous tissue, and the loose connective tissue of the lobules is not visible.

The ductal epithelium, which retains its responsiveness to hormones, continues to proliferate even though the surrounding stroma is hormone-insensitive. These dilated ducts may become entrapped by the connective tissue strands, leading to formation of *cysts.* The cells lining these cysts continue to secrete fluid that cannot be discharged owing to fibrous tissue obstruction. This enlarges the cysts even more. At the same time, the interruption of blood supply caused by fibrous strands will cause degenerative changes, necrosis, and subsequent calcification of the stroma.

The epithelial cells of the breast ducts retain the capacity to respond to hormonal stimuli. Because the epithelium and the surrounding intralobular stroma are in a delicate balance, and because the stroma directly or indirectly regulates the proliferation and maturation of the epithelium, the ducts that are devoid of their normal surroundings may proliferate in an unregulated manner, giving rise to *sclerosing adenosis.*

Pathology. As the name fibrocystic change implies, two constant features of this condition are *fibrosis* and *cysts.* The third component of this change, which is not reflected in the name but is almost always present, is *epithelial proliferation.* This occurs most often

Fibrous tissue "strangles" the ducts

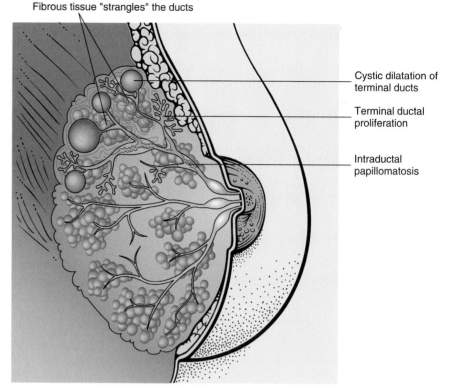

Cystic dilatation of terminal ducts

Terminal ductal proliferation

Intraductal papillomatosis

FIGURE 16-4
Fibrocystic change. Typical features include epithelial proliferation, fibrosis, and cysts. Intraductal papillomatosis occurs in a minority of patients.

in the form of ductal budding and crowding of ductules, known as *sclerosing adenosis*.

In addition to these typical features, 10 percent of those affected show intraductal proliferation of cells that form several layers (*atypical ductal hyperplasia*) and small papillary projections (*papillomatosis*). This intraductal proliferation, especially if associated with atypical nuclear changes, may progress to invasive cancer, and is considered an unfavorable finding.

Clinical Features. Fibrocystic changes usually affect both breasts. Because the changes are asymmetrical, however, patients may complain mostly of one-sided pain, nodularity, and sensitivity on palpation. Careful palpation will usually reveal fine nodularity, which imparts a string-like consistency to both breasts. Small lumps that fluctuate (corresponding to fluid-filled cysts) are also easily palpated. Mammography may reveal condensed areas, cysts, and even areas of calcification. As calcific areas are indistinguishable from those seen in cancer, biopsy examination is the only safe way to establish a definitive diagnosis.

Typical fibrocystic change does not require treatment. However, if premalignant changes such as papillomatosis and atypical ductal hyperplasia, are found in the tissue sample, additional surgical resection is recommended. Most surgeons perform an extended lumpectomy in such cases; that is, they remove the indurated glandular part of the breast parenchyma. The prognosis, even for women so affected, is excellent.

Benign Tumors

Fibroadenoma is the most important and most common of the *benign tumors* of the breast. Typical tumors measure 2 to 5 cm in diameter and are well-encapsulated, round, and lobulated. As the name implies, the tumor is composed of two components: fibrous stroma and glandular epithelium (Fig. 16-5). The fibroblastic component of the tumor corresponds to the hormone-sensitive intralobular connective tissue, whereas the glands represent excretory ducts.

Fibroadenomas are tumors that affect young women (see Fig. 16-2). Because they consist of hormonally sensitive cells, it has been hypothesized that the tumors represent an abnormal exaggerated response of breast tissue to sex hormones. These well-encapsulated and sharply demarcated tumors can be shelled out, and are removed easily by surgeons without serious consequences. Fibroadenomas do not recur and do not undergo malignant transformation; therefore they have an excellent prognosis.

Malignant Tumors

Carcinoma of the breast is the most important breast tumor. The following statistics illustrate the public health impact of breast cancer in the United States:

- Breast cancer is the most common cancer in women, surpassed in lethality only by lung cancer.

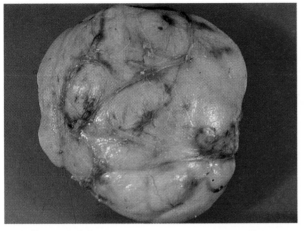

A

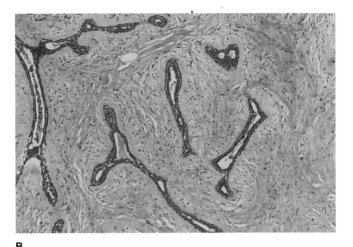

B

FIGURE 16-5
Fibroadenoma. (A) This tumor, which was shelled out from the breast, appears to be well encapsulated and smooth. (B) Histologic features of fibroadenoma include elongated ducts surrounded by connective tissue that is similar to the loose, intralobular, connective tissue in the normal breast.

- Estimates are that 1 woman in 14 will develop breast cancer during her life span (Fig. 16-6).
- At least 180,000 new cases of breast cancer are diagnosed each year. The number of new cases is increasing steadily.
- Approximately 46,000 women die of breast cancer every year.

Etiology and Pathogenesis. The cause of breast cancer is unknown. However, several important risk factors for breast cancer have been identified. The most significant leads point to *hormonal* and *genetic etiologic* influences. The search for these carcinogenic factors has led to discovery of tumor suppressor genes, which play a critical role in breast cancer. These genes, known as BRCA-1 and BRCA-2, account for 80 percent of familial breast cancers and are probably involved in some other cancers, such as those involving the ovary and the prostate. BRCA-1 and BRCA-2 are not involved with nonfamilial breast cancer, the etiology of which remains enigmatic.

Breast cancer has been studied in experimental animals, which have provided important clues to the pathogenesis of human tumors. Breast cancer–inducing *viruses* have been identified in mice, and it is possible that similar viruses exist in humans. Similarly, *chemical carcinogens* are known to induce breast cancer in rats, which makes it plausible that some human breast cancers are related to chemicals. *Hormonal* factors have also been found to be important in laboratory animals. Despite these leads, the causes of human breast cancer are not fully understood.

FIGURE 16-6
Incidence of breast cancer. Breast cancer is the second most common cancer in women. Approximately 180,000 new cases are diagnosed every year in the United States. Approximately 46,000 women die of breast cancer each year. One woman in 14 will develop breast cancer during her lifetime.

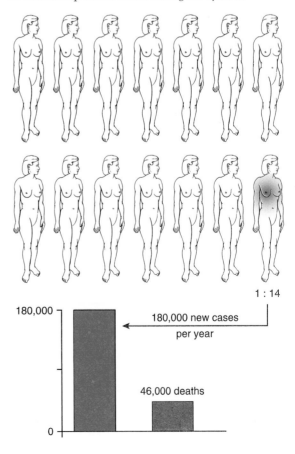

Risk Factors. The most important risk factors of breast cancer identified thus far are as follows:

- *Sex.* Females are affected 100 times more often than males.
- *Genetic predisposition.* Breast cancer occurs more often in some families. If a mother had or has breast cancer, all daughters have an increased risk. The same is true for sisters of a patient with breast cancer. A history of familial cancer increases the risk for relatives by 5- to 10-fold and possibly even higher in some families.
- *Hormonal factors.* Women who are exposed to estrogen for prolonged periods tend to develop breast cancer more frequently than those who are not. Thus, breast cancer is more common in women who have an early menarche and late menopause and are, therefore, under the influence of ovarian sex hormones for a prolonged period. Similarly, nulliparous women are at greater risk for breast cancer than those who have numerous children, presumably because pregnancy interrupts the cyclic secretion of ovarian estrogen. The fact that many breast tumors have estrogen receptors, and that the growth of these cells can be inhibited or slowed down by synthetic antiestrogens, points to an important role of hormones in breast cancer.
- *Presence of other cancer.* The incidence of breast cancer is increased in women who have cancer in the other breast, as well as in those who have *ovarian* or *endometrial* cancer. It is possible that all of these cancers are hormonally induced, occurring in women in whom there is hyperestrinism or dysregulation of the pituitary-ovarian axis.
- *Premalignant fibrocystic changes.* Papillomatosis and *atypical intraductal hyperplasia* are premalignant changes that occur in the breasts of some women with fibrocystic changes. Most of these intraductal lesions will progress to invasive carcinoma during a period of several years if they are not removed in time.
- *Age.* Breast cancer is very rare before puberty and quite unusual in young women. The incidence slowly rises after the age of 35 years and peaks in postmenopausal women who are about 60 years of age.
- *Race.* Breast cancer is uncommon in Japanese, Chinese, and other Oriental people. Of all races, it is most common in Caucasians, and it is especially prevalent among Jews.

The most important risk factors are summarized in Table 16-1.

Pathology. Most malignant breast tumors are of epithelial origin and are, therefore, carcinomas. Histologically, there are several subtypes of breast carcinoma, but more than two thirds are classified as

Table 16-1 Risk Factors for Breast Cancer

Risk Factor	Low Risk	High Risk
Sex	Male	Female
Age (years)	< 30	> 45
Race	Orientals	Caucasians (especially Jews)
Family history	—	Mother or sister with breast cancer
Reproductive history	Multiparity Breast-feeding Pregnancy at an early age	Early menarche Late menopause No children (nulliparity) Late age at first pregnancy
Other cancer	—	Cancer of Breast Ovary Uterus

infiltrating duct carcinomas. Other histologic subtypes of carcinoma, such as *medullary* or *mucinous carcinoma,* are less common. This is unfortunate because these subtypes have a somewhat better prognosis than infiltrating duct carcinomas.

Infiltrating duct carcinoma of the breast—the prototype of this tumor—is an adenocarcinoma that is accompanied by a very strong desmoplastic reaction. Thus, the tumor cells infiltrating the tissue are surrounded by dense connective tissue that is produced by the host in response to the tumor (*desmos* meaning connection in Greek, and *desmoplastic reaction* meaning a connective tissue stromal reaction to the tumor). Because of this dense connective tissue, the tumor appears firm and gritty on sectioning (Fig. 16-7). The dense connective tissue pulls on the adjacent tissue, causing puckering of the skin and retraction of the nipple, which are typical signs of a malignant breast lesion. On palpation, these tumors are firm. They do not have sharp margins, as they infiltrate into the surrounding tissues.

Most breast carcinomas (45 percent) occur in the upper lateral quadrant (Fig. 16-8). Approximately 25 percent of breast cancers are central, underneath the areola.

Breast cancer tends to metastasize via the lymphatics. Because most lymph ducts drain into the axillary lymph nodes, it is to be expected that most metastases are found in the axillary area. Medially or centrally located tumors may spread into the internal mammary lymph nodes. From the lymph nodes, the tumor cells enter the blood circulation and are carried away hematogenously to all major organs. Distant metastases are common in the lungs, liver, bones, brain, and adrenals (see Fig. 16-8).

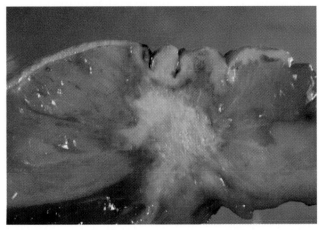

A

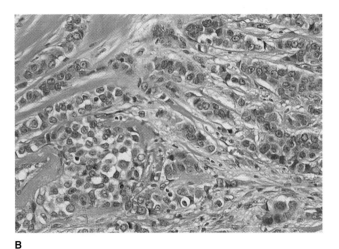

B

FIGURE 16-7

Breast carcinoma. (A) On gross inspection, the tumor appears to be grayish white owing to the abundance of connective tissue between the tumor cells. Such desmoplastic tumors are firm and gritty on sectioning. (B) Histologic appearance of an infiltrating duct carcinoma of the breast. Note the abnormal ducts surrounded by abundant collagenous connective tissue that stains pink.

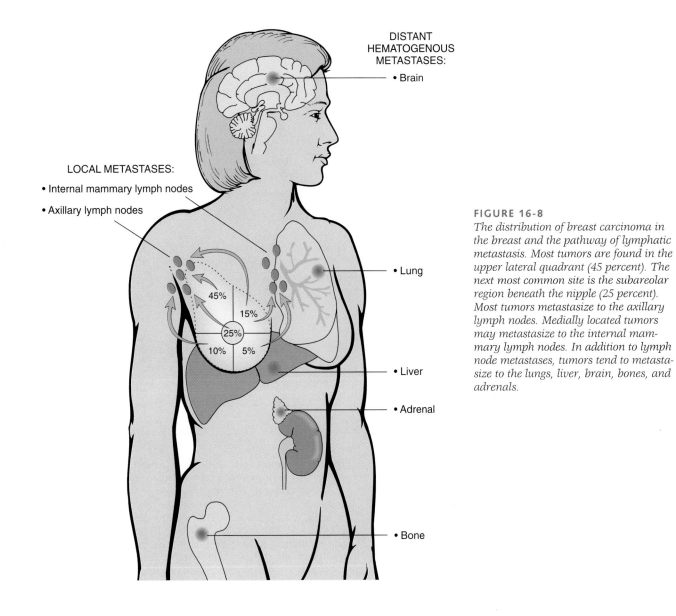

FIGURE 16-8

The distribution of breast carcinoma in the breast and the pathway of lymphatic metastasis. Most tumors are found in the upper lateral quadrant (45 percent). The next most common site is the subareolar region beneath the nipple (25 percent). Most tumors metastasize to the axillary lymph nodes. Medially located tumors may metastasize to the internal mammary lymph nodes. In addition to lymph node metastases, tumors tend to metastasize to the lungs, liver, brain, bones, and adrenals.

Table 16-2 Clinical Presentation of Breast Cancer

Mode of Diagnosis/Presentation	Incidence	
Breast mass discovered by palpation	+ + +	80%–90%
Asymptomatic tumor discovered by mammography	+ +	
Pain (mastodynia, or painful breast mass)	+	10%–20%
Nipple retraction, eczematoid reaction or discharge	+	
Distant metastases	+	

+ + +, very common; + +, common; +, not so common (10% or less).

Clinical Features. Carcinoma of the breast presents as a mass lesion. Typically (in 80 percent to 90 percent of cases), the lump is detected by self-examination, by palpation in the doctor's office, or by mammography. It may be of any size, frequently measuring 1 cm to several centimeters in diameter. Occasionally, it is associated with enlarged axillary lymph nodes. Other modes of presentation are less common (Table 16-2).

Self-examination is very important for breast cancer diagnosis. The American Cancer Society recommends the following procedure of self-examination for all women, as outlined in Fig. 16-9:

1. Stand in front of the mirror and observe the breast for any lumps, swelling, irregularities or marked asymmetry.
2. Raise your arms above your head.
3. Place your hands on your hips.
4. Flex your shoulders forward.
5. Then cradle the left breast and gently feel it with the fingers of the opposite hand.
6. Repeat this palpation on the right side.
7. While lying on your side, with your right hand stretched above your head, palpate the right breast with the fingers of your left hand.
8. Reverse your position and repeat this step, this time palpating the left breast.

A complete physical examination of females must, in all instances, include palpation of the breast. The breasts must be inspected and palpated routinely, with special emphasis on the detection of minor and major irregularities in texture, consistency, and shape. Any patient with suspicious masses or nodules should undergo breast biopsy.

Mammography is a specialized x-ray technique that allows detailed examination of the breast with low-density radiographs. Tumor masses can be de-

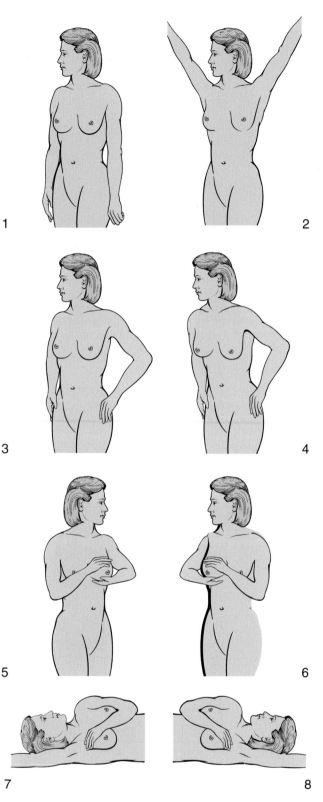

FIGURE 16-9

Breast self-examination. While in an upright position, the woman stands in front of a mirror and inspects her breasts in the normal position. The inspection should be repeated while she assumes three additional positions: raising her arms above her head, placing her hands on her hips, and flexing her shoulders forward. The breasts should then be palpated while in upright position by holding the breast with one hand and by examining it with the fingers of the other hand. Palpation should be repeated while lying down with one hand extended above the head.

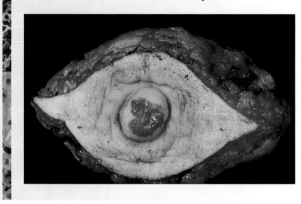

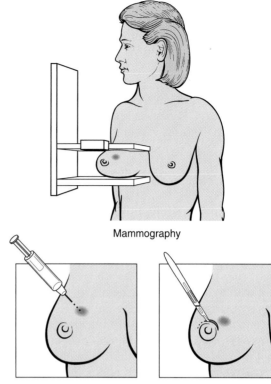

Mammography

Fine-needle aspiration

Incisional biopsy

FIGURE 16-10

Mammography and breast biopsy. Mammography is a noninvasive, usually painless procedure that is easily performed with a special x-ray machine. Fine-needle aspiration biopsy of the breast requires only local anesthesia and is simple to perform. Surgical breast biopsy is performed in the operating room using general anesthesia.

FIGURE 16-11

Survival rates of patients with breast carcinoma. The 5-year survival rate following mastectomy depends on the stage of the disease. Small tumors that are diagnosed before they have metastasized have an excellent prognosis, with a 5-year survival rate exceeding 80 percent. Advanced tumors have a poor prognosis.

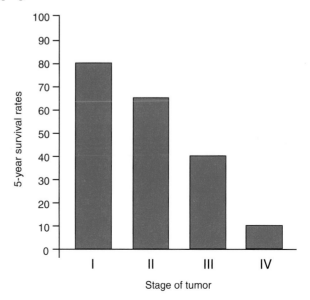

tected in early stages of development, even before they have reached a size that can be palpated (Fig. 16-10). Indeed, the smallest tumors that can be detected by palpation are 2 to 2.5 cm in diameter, whereas by mammography, one can detect lesions measuring less than 0.5 cm. Such lesions are typically recognized as an area of increased density on the radiograph, and frequently, calcifications are detected within them. The American Cancer Society recommends that mammographies be performed at regular intervals in all women older than 45 years. Today, mammography represents the best approach for early diagnosis of breast cancer.

If a lump is detected on self-examination or by a doctor or nurse, or an abnormality is seen on mammography, a breast biopsy should be performed to obtain material for pathologic diagnosis. The biopsy can be performed in an outpatient clinic or doctor's office using *thin-needle aspiration* biopsy and local anesthesia. A *surgical biopsy* requires incision of the skin, and so is performed under general anesthesia in an operating room (Fig. 16-11).

Each of these approaches has its advantages and disadvantages. A fine-needle aspiration biopsy specimen is relatively small and consists of cells that are smeared on a slide for cytologic examination. When these cells are examined by a cytopathologist, this approach has an accuracy rate exceeding 95 percent. Occasionally, the sample may be too small to establish a definitive diagnosis, and the procedure must be repeated. If the cytopathologist cannot establish the diagnosis, a larger specimen, removed by surgical biopsy, should be submitted in all cases in which there is clinical evidence of a possible tumor.

By comparison, surgical biopsy specimens provide more tissue and are therefore more appropriate for final diagnosis. However, this procedure requires general anesthesia and is more traumatic than fine-needle biopsy. Thus, in most cases, the initial screening is done by fine-needle biopsy. If cytologic examination reveals cancer, the diagnosis is confirmed by surgical biopsy.

The treatment of breast cancer includes surgical resection of the primary tumor and any metastases, as well as chemotherapy. Radiation therapy is used for patients with advanced cancer. Tumors composed of cells that express estrogen receptors are also treated with synthetic antiestrogens.

Several surgical procedures are currently in use. *Lumpectomy* is the most conservative surgical procedure, as it is limited to resection of the tumor. *Mastectomy* refers to removal of the entire breast, which is often associated with lymph node dissection.

The prognosis of breast cancer depends on the stage of the disease. Staging is performed on the basis of the gross appearance of the tumor and the extent of its spread to local lymph nodes and distant organs. *Stage I* cancer includes relatively small, localized tumors (less than 2.5 cm in diameter) without any distant metastases. Surgical removal of the tumor is associated with an 80 percent 5-year survival rate. *Stage II* tumors measure more than 2 cm, but less than 5 cm, in diameter. There may be local lymph node metastases, but there is no evidence of distant spread. The 5-year survival rate in these patients is 65 percent. *Stage III* tumors measure more than 5 cm in diameter, with or without regional spread, but without distant metastases. The 5-year survival rate is 40 percent. *Stage IV* tumors may be of any size, and may or may not be associated with local metastases in the lymph nodes, but are associated with distant metastases. The 5-year survival rate is only 10 percent.

Even though the staging of breast tumors provides the most accurate prognostic data, other factors should also be taken into consideration. As mentioned before, the *histologic subtype* of the tumor is important, and there are several variants that have a relatively better prognosis. However, most breast carcinomas are of the infiltrating duct carcinoma type, and the more favorable variants are less common. *Histologic grading* of the tumor is important. Tumors that are relatively more anaplastic and show a more rapid growth rate have a worse prognosis than slower growing, well-differentiated (lower-grade) tumors. *Estrogen* and *progesterone receptors* are expressed on some tumors, but not on others. If receptor-positive, the tumor will respond to antiestrogens and removal of the ovaries.

Breast carcinoma is a tumor that may progress rapidly and cause death within 1 to 2 years. On the other hand, there are numerous, well-documented cases in which the tumor has regressed following treatment, only to recur many years later. Therefore, patients should not be considered cured even if they have survived tumor-free for 5 years after diagnosis. The overall *10-year survival* of patients operated on for breast cancer is in the range of 50 percent.

Lesions of the Male Breast

The male breast is a rudimentary organ, smaller than the average female breast. It has a nipple from which the ducts extend into the subcutaneous tissue. However, lobules are not formed and fibrofatty tissue is scant. The most important pathologic conditions affecting the male breast are *gynecomastia,* which was discussed earlier, and *breast cancer*.

Breast cancer in males is 100 times less common than in females. In most cases, it is diagnosed relatively late—mostly because men do not think that they can develop breast cancer. This delay adversely affects the prognosis, which is generally worse than the prognosis of breast cancer in females. Breast cancer in men has the same histologic features as do cancers of the female breast.

Review Questions

1. Describe the main anatomic parts of the breast, such as the nipple, lactiferous ducts, lobules, and acini.

2. What are the most important breast disease?

3. What is acute mastitis and when does it usually occur?

4. How do hormones affect breasts in women and men?

5. What is gynecomastia?

6. How common is fibrocystic change of the breast and how does it present clinically?

7. What are the pathologic features of fibrocystic change?

8. What is fibroadenoma and how does it present clinically?

9. What are the risk factors for breast cancer?

10. What is the most common microscopic type of breast cancer?

11. Correlate the macroscopic and microscopic pathology of infiltrating duct carcinoma.

12. How does breast cancer metastasize?

13. How should the self-examination of breasts be performed?

14. How is breast cancer usually diagnosed?

15. What are the diagnosis and the survival rates of breast carcinoma diagnosed in various clinical stages of the disease?

Learning Objectives

After reading this chapter, the student should be able to:

1. Describe the normal anatomy and functions of the pituitary, thyroid, parathyroids, and adrenals.

2. Explain the pathogenesis of pituitary hormonal hyperactivity and list at least three syndromes that may develop under these conditions.

3. Describe the symptoms of pituitary insufficiency and explain its causes.

4. Define Graves' disease and explain its pathogenesis and main symptoms.

5. List three causes of hypothyroidism and five principal symptoms of this condition.

6. List the four most important thyroid tumors and their main features.

7. List three causes of hyperparathyroidism and explain the pathologic findings in this disease.

8. Explain the symptoms and laboratory abnormalities caused by hypoparathyroidism.

9. List the three most important syndromes of adrenocortical hyperfunction and explain the symptoms of these disorders.

10. List three causes of Addison's disease and the primary symptoms of this disease.

11. Describe the symptoms of pheochromocytoma and neuroblastoma and the associated laboratory findings.

Additional Key Terms and Concepts

Acromegaly

Addison's disease

Cushing's syndrome

Diabetes insipidus

Goiter

Graves' disease

Panhypopituitarism

Chapter Outline

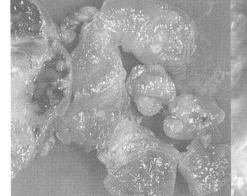

The Endocrine System
Chapter 17

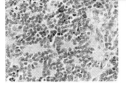

The endocrine system (a term derived from the Greek words *endo,* meaning inside, and *krinein,* meaning to secrete) comprises several glands (pituitary, thyroid, parathyroid, adrenals) and scattered cells in the gonads, pancreas, intestine, and other organs (Fig. 17-1).

The primary function of endocrine cells is to produce hormones. In contrast to exocrine glands, which secrete their products into an external space through excretory ducts, the endocrine organs do not have ducts and so are called the "ductless" glands. Hormones are secreted into the blood or extracellular spaces. Hormones that are released into the circulation act on distant organs (*endocrine effect*), whereas hormones that are released locally into the tissue spaces act on adjacent cells (*paracrine effect*). For example, pituitary hormones exert an endocrine effect on the thyroid, adrenals, or gonads. Glucagon, secreted by the alpha cells of the islets of Langerhans, has a local paracrine effect on insulin-secreting beta cells.

In this chapter, discussion is limited, for practical reasons, to the four major endocrine glands: the pituitary, thyroid, parathyroid, and adrenals. The endocrine functions of the islets of Langerhans have been discussed previously in Chapter 12, and the endocrine functions of the gonads have already been discussed in Chapters 14 and 15. Traditionally, diseases involving these organs are treated by *endocrinologists.* In this context, it is worth noting that dia-

betes mellitus is the most important endocrine disorder. With the exception of diabetes, all other endocrine diseases are uncommon.

NORMAL ANATOMY AND PHYSIOLOGY

The pituitary, thyroid, parathyroids, and adrenals are unrelated to each other and have distinct anatomic locations (see Fig. 17-1). The **pituitary** is located intracranially in an indentation of the base of the cranium called the sella turcica (a Latin term meaning Turkish saddle). The pituitary consists of two parts (anterior and posterior), which are connected to the **hypothalamus** via a stalk that contains extensions of neurons and the vessels of the pituitary portal system. These blood vessels transport—from the hypothalamus into the pituitary—the neuroendocrine releasing factors that regulate the function of the pituitary cells.

The *anterior pituitary,* or adenohypophysis, consists of five distinct cell types, each of which is named according to the hormone it secretes. These hormones are

- growth hormone (GH)
- prolactin (PRL)
- adrenocorticotropic hormone (ACTH)
- the gonadotropins (luteinizing hormone [LH] and follicle-stimulating hormone [FSH])
- thyrotropic hormone (thyroid-stimulating hormone [TSH])

The functions of pituitary hormones are summarized in Figure 17-2.

The secretion of hormones of the anterior pituitary is regulated by positive stimulation exerted by the cells in the hypothalamic centers and by the negative feedback inhibition created by the hormones produced by the target endocrine cells in the thyroid, adrenals, and gonads. Pituitary hormones do not have any influence on the parathyroid or the medulla of the adrenals, which thus are not part of the hypothalamic-pituitary regulatory axis.

The *posterior pituitary,* or neurohypophysis, is composed of cytoplasmic processes of neural cells whose nuclei and perikaryons are located in the hypothalamus. These cells release *oxytocin* (pitressin) and the *antidiuretic hormone* (ADH). In contrast to the hormones of the anterior pituitary, which are trophic and stimulate the functions of other endocrine glands, the hormones of the posterior pituitary have no trophic functions. These hormones act on nonendocrine cells; oxytocin stimulates the contraction of the pregnant uterus and ADH promotes the reabsorption of water from the renal tubules.

The **thyroid** is an endocrine gland located in the neck. It consists of two types of cells: follicular cells

FIGURE 17-1
Endocrine glands (From Applegate EJ: The anatomy and physiology learning system: textbook. Philadelphia: WB Saunders, 1995:208.)

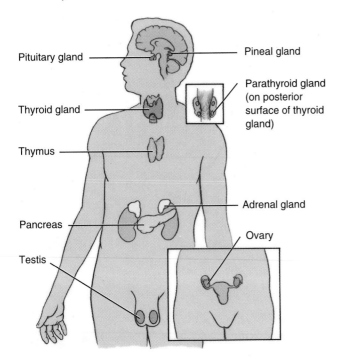

Pituitary gland

Thyroid gland

Thymus

Pancreas

Testis

Pineal gland

Parathyroid gland (on posterior surface of thyroid gland)

Adrenal gland

Ovary

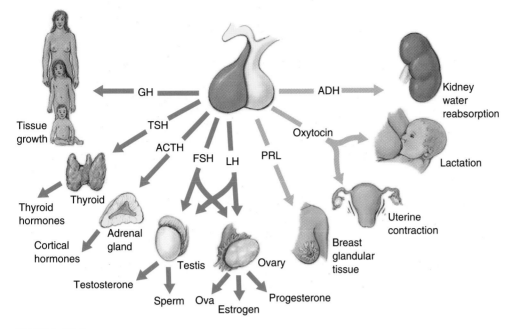

FIGURE 17-2
The effect of pituitary hormones on target tissues. GH, growth hormone; TSH, thyroid-stimulating hormone; ACTH, adrenocorticotropic hormone; FSH, follicle-stimulating hormone; LH, luteinizing hormone; PRL, prolactin; ADH, antidiuretic hormone. (From Applegate EJ: The anatomy and physiology learning system: textbook. Philadelphia: WB Saunders, 1995:211.)

and C cells. *Follicular cells* secrete thyroid hormones (*thyroxine* [T_4] and *triiodothyronine* [T_3]), which are essential for maintaining the intermediate metabolism. The *C cells* secrete *calcitonin,* a polypeptide that is involved in the maintenance of calcium homeostasis. The secretion of T_3 and T_4 is regulated by TSH. The secretion of calcitonin is influenced by the concentration of calcium in serum.

The **parathyroids** are located in the neck, behind the thyroid. There are usually four glands, each of which is the size of a coffee bean. Parathyroid glands secrete the polypeptide parathormone, which is involved in regulating homeostasis of serum calcium and phosphate.

The adrenals are located in the abdomen and are attached to the upper pole of each kidney. Each adrenal consists of a cortex and a medulla. The **adrenal cortex,** which is under the influence of ACTH, consists of three zones

- zona glomerulosa, which secretes mineralocorticoids (e.g., aldosterone)
- zona fasciculata, which secretes glucocorticoids (e.g., cortisone)
- zona reticularis, which secretes sex steroids (e.g., estrogens and androgens)

The steroid hormones of the adrenal cortex regulate the homeostasis of potassium and sodium and the metabolism of carbohydrates, as well as acting on sex hormone–responsive tissues. In addition to these primary functions, the adrenal steroids are involved in

many other metabolic processes. These hormones also modulate inflammation and somatic responses to external stimuli.

The **adrenal medulla** consists of cells that secrete *epinephrine* and *norepinephrine.* These biogenic amines act on smooth muscle cells, heart cells, and many other cells that have adrenergic receptors. In addition to providing sympathetic stimuli, epinephrine and norepinephrine also influence the intermediate metabolism of carbohydrates. Among other effects, epinephrine and norepinephrine cause elevation of blood pressure, tachycardia, and hyperglycemia.

OVERVIEW OF MAJOR DISEASES

The most important diseases involving the endocrine glands present as

- hyperfunction
- hypofunction
- tumors

Several facts important to an understanding of endocrine pathology are presented here, before a discussion of the most important pathologic entities.

1. *The function of the endocrine glands is tightly regulated by positive and negative stimuli.* The function of the thyroid, adrenals, and gonads is regulated by the anterior pituitary, which secretes the trophic hor-

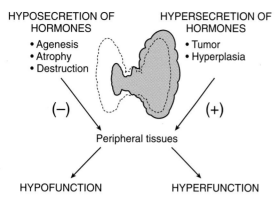

FIGURE 17-3
Hypofunction and hyperfunction of the endocrine glands.

mones TSH, ACTH, LH, and FSH. The function of the pituitary is, in turn, regulated by the hypothalamic *releasing factors* (e.g., gonadotropin-releasing hormone [GnRH]). The hormones of the peripheral target glands released into the blood have a negative inhibitory influence on the hypothalamus and the pituitary (Fig. 17-3). Lack of trophic stimuli leads to incomplete development or atrophy of peripheral endocrine glands. For example, congenital pituitary aplasia is accompanied by incomplete gonadal development and small testes or ovaries. A lack of response of the target peripheral endocrine organ and a decreased feedback inhibition leads to hypersecretion of pituitary trophic hormones. For example, destruction of the adrenals by tuberculosis in Addison's disease is accompanied by hypersecretion of ACTH.

2. *Prolonged hyperstimulation by trophic hormones or metabolic signals leads not only to hyperfunction, but also to physical enlargement of the peripheral endocrine glands.* The thyroid, when overstimulated by TSH, enlarges and becomes nodular. ACTH stimulation leads to adrenocortical hyperplasia.

3. *Hyperfunctioning endocrine glands may be hyperplastic or neoplastic.* Hyperfunctioning endocrine glands are usually enlarged. The enlargement may be attributable to hyperplasia (i.e., a reactive increase in cell number) or to benign or malignant tumors. The distinction between hyperplasia and neoplasia is not always clear-cut. For example, adenoma of the parathyroids is histologically indistinguishable from parathyroid hyperplasia. Because pathologists cannot differentiate between these two processes, they designate symmetrical enlargement of all four parathyroid glands hyperplasia. If only one gland is enlarged and the others are of usual size, the enlarged gland is considered to be involved by an adenoma.

4. *Hypofunction of the endocrine glands is usually attributable to the destruction of secretory cells.* Destruction and loss of endocrine cells or the entire gland may be caused by several mechanisms, the most im-

portant of which are inflammation, tumors, and medical interventions. Inflammation may be caused by infectious organisms or autoimmune processes. Tumors, be they benign or malignant, primary or secondary, may destroy adjacent endocrine cells. For example, adrenal hypofunction (Addison's disease) may be secondary to adrenal destruction by tuberculosis, autoimmune adrenalitis, or metastatic carcinoma. Inadvertent surgical removal of the parathyroid glands during neck surgery for cancer is the most common cause of hypoparathyroidism in adults.

5. *Neoplastic or hyperplastic enlargement of the endocrine glands results in mass lesions that compress adjacent structures.* Local symptoms caused by endocrine gland enlargement are most evident in diseases of the pituitary and the thyroid. Enlargement of the pituitary, which is in close proximity to the optic nerve decussation, produces defects in the visual field (so-called *bitemporal hemianopsia*, or bilateral loss of peripheral [temporal] sight). Thyroid tumors may produce a bulge on the anterior side of the neck or compress the larynx, trachea, and the nerves or blood vessels of the neck. Neoplastic adrenal enlargement rarely presents with signs of compression unless the tumor has reached a considerable size or has invaded adjacent organs. Parathyroid adenomas are so small that they rarely, if ever, produce symptoms of local compression.

6. *Adenomas of the pituitary, parathyroids, and adrenals cannot always be distinguished from carcinomas on the basis of their histologic features.* Benign tumors of the anterior pituitary, parathyroid glands, and the adrenals may have the same histologic features as carcinomas of these organs. The only definitive sign of malignancy of such tumors is the presence of metastases. The histologic diagnosis of thyroid malignant lesions is much easier to establish, as these tumors show clear and readily recognizable signs of malignancy.

7. *Tumors of one endocrine gland may be associated with neoplasia and/or hyperplasia of other glands.* Multiple endocrine neoplasia (MEN) is a hereditary syndrome that occurs in at least three forms: MEN-1, MEN-2A, and MEN-2B. In MEN-1, the tumors originate from the pituitary, parathyroids, and pancreatic islets of Langherhans. In MEN-2A, the tumors include medullary carcinoma originating from C cells of the thyroid, pheochromocytoma originating from the medulla of the adrenal, and parathyroid adenoma or hyperplasia. MEN-2B, which resembles MEN-2A and has the same endocrine lesions, also includes additional multiple skin and mucosal nerve tumors. The occurrence of these familial tumors has been related to defects in tumor suppressor genes. Distinct tumor suppressor genes have been identified for each of these three hereditary syndromes.

8. *Endocrine symptoms may be paraneoplastic; that is, they may be caused by hormones secreted by tumors of nonendocrine glands.* Such symptoms may be indistinguishable from those caused by hyperfunction of the endocrine glands themselves. The best examples are lung tumors. Small cell carcinomas of the lung may produce ACTH, and thus cause Cushing's syndrome, like pituitary tumors. Squamous cell carcinomas of the lung may produce signs of hyperparathyroidism by secreting a parathyroid hormone–related polypeptide.

Pituitary Diseases

Diseases of the pituitary are uncommon, but may present as

- pituitary hyperfunction
- pituitary hypofunction
- a localized mass lesion causing compression of the optic chiasm or the basal portion of the brain

Pituitary Hyperfunction

Pituitary hyperfunction may present in several forms depending on which one of the five cells is hyperfunctioning. The pituitary is usually enlarged (Fig. 17-4). The enlargement may be attributable to macroscopic or microscopic adenomas, which are composed of a single cell type or several cell types. Most common are tumors composed of lactotropic cells (also known as *prolactinomas*). Less common are somatotropic and corticotropic adenomas. Tumors composed of TSH-, LH-, or FSH-secreting cells are extremely rare.

Prolactinomas (lactotropic adenomas) are usually small, benign tumors composed of prolactin-secret-

Did You Know?

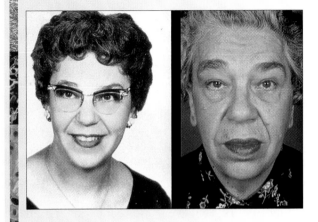

Right: This patient has coarse facial features typical of acromegaly. *Left:* Compare the patient's face several years before she developed the pituitary tumor. (Courtesy of the Group for Research in Pathology Education)

ing cells. The typical symptoms of hyperprolactinemia are easily recognized in women of reproductive age and include amenorrhea (lack of menstruation), galactorrhea (spontaneous milk secretion unrelated to pregnancy), and infertility. Hyperprolactinemia inhibits the pulsatile secretion of LH, which is essential for normal ovulation to occur. In addition, prolactin stimulates milk production in the breast. In males, the symptoms of prolactinomas are usually vague and may include impotence or loss of libido. The function of prolactinomas can be inhibited with bromocriptine, which acts like dopamine, the natural inhibitor of prolactin secretion. Surgery, performed through the nose (transnasal approach to the sella turcica), is reserved for large tumors only.

Somatotropic adenomas are composed of cells synthesizing growth hormone. In contrast to prolactinomas, which are usually microscopic, 75 percent of clinically apparent somatotropic adenomas are visible by the naked eye or modern radiologic techniques (e.g., computed tomography [CT] scanning) and are thus classified as macroadenomas.

The clinical symptoms of hypersecretion of growth hormones depend on the age of the patient. In prepubertal patients—i.e., before closure of the epiphyseal growth plate of the long bones—these tumors stimulate longitudinal skeletal growth, resulting in *gigantism*. Some of these pituitary giants are more than 8 feet tall. In postpubertal patients, somatotropic adenomas cause *acromegaly* (from the Greek words *acros*, meaning end portion, and *megalos*, meaning big), which presents as enlargement of the

FIGURE 17-4
Pituitary adenoma. The enlarged pituitary can be seen bulging from the sella turcica at the base of the skull.

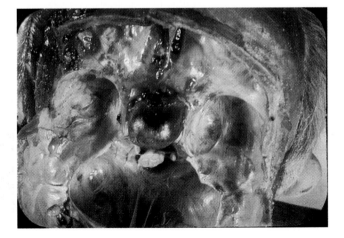

acral parts of the extremities (fingers, hands, toes), the tongue, jaws, and nose. The internal organs are also enlarged (e.g., cardiomegaly). Excess of growth hormone causes metabolic disturbances, such as hyperglycemia and hypercalcemia.

Surgical removal of the tumor is the treatment of choice. The metabolic symptoms improve, but the bone changes do not regress.

Corticotropic adenomas are composed of ACTH-secreting cells. Most tumors are microadenomas and are clinically recognized by the typical signs of *Cushing's disease.* These symptoms are similar to those caused by corticosteroid-producing adrenocortical lesions, and will be described under that heading later. Removal of the pituitary tumor results in an improvement in clinical symptoms.

Tumors of the pituitary are usually benign. Most hormonally active tumors are recognized early in their development and removed. Symptoms related to the extension of tumor into the adjacent intracranial structures or its invasiveness are rare in functioning tumors. However, approximately 25 percent of pituitary tumors are hormonally inactive and are not recognized unless they cause compression of adjacent structures. Such tumors may compress the normal pituitary or the stalk, causing symptoms of hypopituitarism or diabetes insipidus secondary to destruction of the posterior pituitary. Suprasellar growth of pituitary tumors may lead to compression of the optic chiasm and partial blindness.

Pituitary Hypofunction

Endocrine insufficiency of the pituitary causes hypofunction of secondary organs, which depend on trophic stimuli from the pituitary. **Pituitary hypofunction** is rare, but it may be encountered in any age group. It may involve all pituitary cells (*panhypopituitarism*) or it may be selective—i.e., limited to one subset of anterior pituitary cells (e.g., hypogonadism secondary to the deficiency of gonadotropic cells) or posterior pituitary cells (e.g., diabetes insipidus).

The causes of pituitary hypofunction include

- congenital developmental defects, as in *pituitary dwarfism or hypogonadism*
- tumors that destroy the pituitary (e.g., nonfunctioning pituitary adenoma) or the hypothalamus (e.g., craniopharyngioma or glioma)
- ischemia, as in postpartum necrosis (*Sheehan's syndrome*)

The diagnosis of pituitary insufficiency may be suspected clinically but must be confirmed by appropriate biochemical tests, which will show hormone deficiency.

Panhypopituitarism of adults (*Simmonds' disease*) is marked by general weakness, cold intolerance,

poor appetite, weight loss, and hypotension. Women affected by this disease do not menstruate and men suffer from impotence and loss of libido. Pituitary insufficiency of childhood results in dwarfism.

Diabetes insipidus is marked by a lack of ADH secondary to destructive lesions of the hypothalamus, pituitary stalk, or posterior pituitary. It may be caused by tumors, infection of the brain or meninges, intracranial hemorrhage, or trauma involving the bones of the base of the skull. Patients with diabetes insipidus secrete large amounts (5 to 6 L/day) of hypotonic urine.

Pituitary insufficiency requires substitution therapy with appropriate hormones. The most spectacular results have been achieved in the treatment of congenital pituitary dwarfism; affected patients can achieve normal growth if treated appropriately. Substitution therapy with ADH is effective in the treatment of diabetes insipidus.

Thyroid Diseases

Thyroid diseases are common, but fortunately, they can be diagnosed readily and treated with very good results. Thyroid diseases present as functional disturbances (*hyperfunction* or *hypofunction*) or as mass lesions (neoplasms or non-neoplastic enlargement, known as *goiter*).

Hyperthyroidism

Hyperthyroidism (*thyrotoxicosis*) is caused by an excess of thyroid hormones. The most important causes of hyperthyroidism are the following diseases, which account for 85 percent of all cases (Fig. 17-5):

- Autoimmunity, as in Graves' disease
- Idiopathic nodular hyperplasia of thyroid, as in toxic goiter
- Tumors, such as hyperfunctioning thyroid adenoma

Other causes, such as lymphocytic thyroiditis, and Hashimoto's disease are less common. Uncontrolled intake of thyroid hormone pills which are often used for the self-treatment of obesity, may cause self-inflicted hyperthyroidism (Fig. 17-6).

Graves' disease is an autoimmune disorder caused by antibodies to the TSH receptor on the surface of thyroid follicular cells. The disease occurs 10 times more often in women than men and may be associated with other autoimmune disorders. The circulatory antibodies bind to the surface of thyroid cells, exerting a stimulus similar to the effect of TSH itself. Antibodies bound to the TSH receptor stimulate hypersecretion of thyroid hormones (T_3 and T_4). Histologically, the enlarged thyroid is composed of hyper-

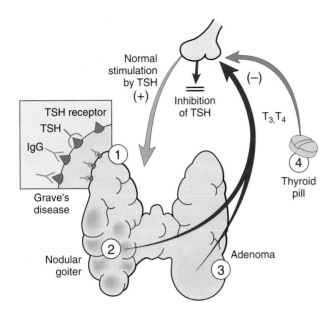

FIGURE 17-5

Hyperthyroidism may have several causes, among them (1) Graves' disease, (2) nodular goiter, (3), toxic adenoma of the thyroid, and (4) exogenous thyroid medication. Triiodothyronine (T_3) and thyroxine (T_4) normally inhibit secretion of thyroid-stimulating hormone (TSH), which accounts for the low concentration of TSH in these forms of hyperthyroidism. IgG, immunoglobulin G.

plastic follicles that are lined by hyperactive, tall, cuboidal cells. The thyroid also contains lymphoid follicles, which are yet another sign that this disease is immune-mediated.

Nodular goiter is a less common, but nevertheless important, cause of hyperthyroidism. The thyroid gland is enlarged and nodular. *Thyroid adenomas* may occasionally be hyperactive and cause hyperthyroidism. Such tumors appear as solitary nodules that concentrate radioactive iodine and are diagnosed as "hot nodules" on radioactive scanning.

Clinical Features. The symptoms of hyperthyroidism result from an excess of thyroid hormones and include restlessness, nervousness, emotional lability, sweating, and tachycardia. Cardiac palpitation, muscular tremor, and diarrhea are common. Weight loss is often seen even though the patient has an increased appetite. Furthermore, most patients with Graves' disease also have *exophthalmos* (bulging eyes). The cause of exophthalmos is not known, but it is thought to be related to the systemic immune disorder that causes thyroid hyperfunction. Hyperthyroidism caused by nodular goiter or thyroid adenoma is not associated with exophthalmos.

The treatment of hyperthyroidism depends on the underlying pathologic process. Best results are achieved in patients with solitary hyperfunctioning nodules that can be removed surgically. Graves' disease and diffuse multinodular goiter are treated with

antithyroid drugs; if these are ineffective, subtotal thyroidectomy is recommended.

Hypothyroidism

Hypothyroidism results from a functional failure of the thyroid gland and its inability to meet the body's demands for T_4 and T_3. The most important causes of hypothyroidism are

- *Developmental defects* (e.g., *congenital thyroid aplasia*). This condition is found in 1 of 4000 newborn children.

FIGURE 17-6

Comparison of hyperthyroidism and hypothyroidism.

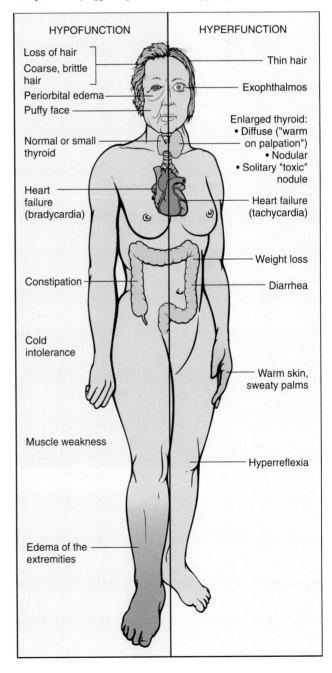

- *Thyroiditis.* Inflammation of the thyroid is most often immune-mediated and includes several disorders known as lymphocytic thyroiditis, Hashimoto's thyroiditis, and related diseases.
- *Thyroidectomy* (surgical removal of the thyroid). Such iatrogenic hypothyroidism typically evolves postoperatively, following resection of a thyroid that has been infiltrated by tumor.
- *Iodine deficiency.* The human body requires iodine, and if the food and water consumed do not contain adequate amounts of iodine, as occurs in some parts of the world (e.g., the Alpine mountains of Switzerland or the Andes of South America), hypothyroidism may ensue. Iodine is preventively added to the salt in most Western countries and, thus, iodine deficiency is rare in the United States.

Pathology. The pathologic basis of hypothyroidism varies depending on its causes. Children born with congenital thyroid aplasia do not have a thyroid. Thyroiditis initially leads to thyroid enlargement, which is usually symmetrical. Histologically, such a gland is infiltrated with lymphocytes, which destroy thyroid follicles. Subsequent healing and fibrosis may actually reduce the size of the thyroid.

Deficiency of iodine in food and water is usually associated with nodular enlargement of the thyroid (*goiter*). Because the thyroid cannot synthesize enough T_3 and T_4, its follicles undergo compensatory hyperplasia in an attempt to increase the production of hormones. Low concentrations of T_3 and T_4 in serum results in inadequate feedback inhibition of the pituitary, which responds to low levels of thyroid hormones by overproducing TSH. TSH stimulation without adequate supplies of iodine further promotes the enlargement of the thyroid, but cannot correct the hormone deficiency.

Clinical Features. The symptoms of hypothyroidism depend on the age of the patient. In children, the deficiency of thyroid hormones affects the growth of the entire body and, most specifically, development of the central nervous system. If the thyroid deficiency is not recognized, the growth of the child is stunted (*thyroid dwarfism*) and mental development is retarded (*cretinism*). These children also have numerous other metabolic disturbances. The hypothyroidism of adults is also known as *myxedema,* named so because the skin of these patients appears edematous, dough-like, and puffy.

Deficiency of thyroid hormones affects essentially all organs in the body, slowing down their function. The patient is sleepy, lacks mental alertness, tires easily, and lacks endurance. The heart beats slowly (*bradycardia*), the intestines lose mobility (*constipation*), and the skeletal muscles are weak, stiff, and aching.

The diagnosis of hypothyroidism is based on biochemical measurements of thyroid hormones in circulation. T_4 and T_3 levels are low, whereas the TSH level is elevated. Treatment with synthetic thyroid hormones yields excellent results in most cases, although such substitution therapy may then be required for the rest of patient's life.

Nodular Goiter

Enlargement of the thyroid is called *goiter* or *struma* (from the Latin term *strumo,* meaning to pile up). The term goiter is noncommittal and includes enlargements caused by a functional disturbance (as in Grave's disease), iodine deficiency, or neoplasia. Most often, the cause of goiter is unknown (*idiopathic goiter*).

Pathology. The nodular goiter consists of nodules that enlarge and deform the thyroid (Fig. 17-7). Histologically, these nodules consist of thyroid follicles that vary in size and shape and are usually filled with colloid. Between the nodules, the struma consists of vessels and collagen fibers infiltrated with lymphocytes and macrophages. Secondary changes, such as calcification, hemorrhage, and atrophy of the compressed follicles in the surrounding parenchyma, are common.

Clinical Features. Most goiters are euthyroid; that is, they do not cause either hyperthyroidism or hypothyroidism. The symptoms are related to the compression of adjacent structures, and include coughing and hoarseness secondary to the pressure of the enlarged thyroid on the larynx or recurrent laryngeal nerve. The treatment of goiter includes resection of the enlarged portions of the thyroid.

FIGURE 17-7
Nodular goiter. The enlarged thyroid consists of multiple colloid nodules.

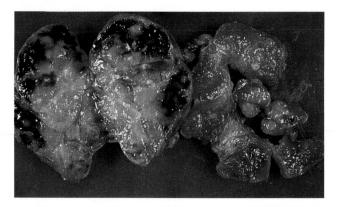

Thyroid Neoplasms

Thyroid tumors may be benign or malignant. Benign thyroid tumors are common. Although they are found in 3 percent to 4 percent of all adults, they are of limited clinical significance, primarily because such tumors are small. Malignant thyroid tumors are rare. Only three to four cases of thyroid cancer are diagnosed yearly per 100,000 people, and less than 1000 people die of thyroid cancer yearly in the United States.

Adenomas. Adenoma of the thyroid is the most common benign tumor. It presents as a nodule, which may vary in size. Most adenomas are small, well encapsulated with fibrous tissue, and composed of thyroid follicles *(follicular adenoma)*. Typically, adenomas comprise cells that do not take up radioactive iodine more avidly than does normal thyroid. On radioscanning with radioactive iodine, therefore, such adenomas cannot be distinguished from normal tissue. Other tumors are composed of afunctional thyroid cells that form so-called "cold nodules," which are unable to concentrate radioactive iodine. In this respect, such cold nodules resemble carcinomas, many of which cannot concentrate iodine either. The final diagnosis can be made only by microscopic examination of biopsy material. Thyroid adenomas are not premalignant, so most small nodules do not require any treatment.

Carcinoma. Carcinoma of the thyroid occurs in several histologic forms, including *papillary, follicular, medullary,* and *anaplastic* carcinoma. All of these tumors except medullary carcinomas originate from follicular cells. No risk factors for developing thyroid tumors are known. Thyroid tumors are, for unknown reasons, more common in females than males.

Papillary carcinoma accounts for 80 percent of all malignant thyroid tumors. It is a low-grade malignant lesion. Papillary carcinoma is a hormonally inactive tumor and usually presents as a cold nodule on radioscans. The tumor tends to metastasize to the local lymph nodes, but distant metastases are not found until late in the disease.

Papillary carcinoma is four times more common in women than in men. It occurs relatively early in life and has a peak incidence in the third to fifth decade. This tumor has a very favorable prognosis; indeed, 80 percent of patients are alive 10 years after diagnosis.

Follicular carcinoma is much less common than papillary carcinoma, accounting for only 15 percent of thyroid malignant diseases. Most patients are older than 40 years of age and 75 percent are female. The tumor grows more aggressively than papillary carcinoma, but it still has a good prognosis. Overall, 65 percent of patients survive 10 years. The tumor cells resemble normal follicular cells of the thyroid and form colloid.

Clinically, follicular carcinoma presents as a slowly growing nodule that may be cold or hot. Many of these tumors concentrate radioactive iodine and produce thyroid hormones. Those tumors that do concentrate iodine can be treated with radioactive iodine, as accumulated radioactive iodine is a strong source of internal radiation and it kills cells. This treatment is especially suitable for patients who have widespread metastases.

Medullary carcinoma differs from other thyroid tumors in that it is derived from C cells. Like the normal C cells, medullary carcinomas produce *calcitonin,* a hormone involved in regulating the homeostasis of calcium. Histologically, medullary carcinoma is composed of round or oval neuroendocrine cells arranged into groups and nests. The stroma of the tumor contains amyloid, which is derived from calcitonin.

Medullary carcinoma may be inherited, and it can occur concomitantly with other endocrine tumors, such as pheochromocytoma in MEN-2. Familial medullary carcinomas are usually discovered early and have a good prognosis if surgically removed. Sporadic tumors, which occur at 60 years of age and older, have a less favorable prognosis.

Anaplastic carcinoma is a rare tumor. It has an extremely unfavorable prognosis, and most patients die within 1 year of diagnosis. Histologically, such tumors are composed of undifferentiated, large or small tumor cells that bear no resemblance to normal thyroid cells.

Diseases of the Parathyroid Glands

Diseases of the parathyroid glands present as either hyperfunction (oversecretion of parathyroid hormone [PTH]) or hypofunction. These diseases cause disturbances in the homeostasis of calcium and phosphate.

Hyperparathyroidism

Hyperparathyroidism is defined as **parathyroid gland hyperfunction** that results in increased levels of PTH in circulating blood. Hyperparathyroidism may be primary (i.e., caused by parathyroid hyperplasia or neoplasia) or secondary, in which case it is usually related to chronic renal failure.

In 80 percent of cases, *primary hyperparathyroidism* is caused by a benign parathyroid adenoma; in 18 percent, it is the result of the hyperplasia of parathyroid glands. In 2 percent of cases, it is caused by parathyroid carcinoma. There are normally four

PARATHYROID HYPERPLASIA   PARATHYROID NEOPLASIA

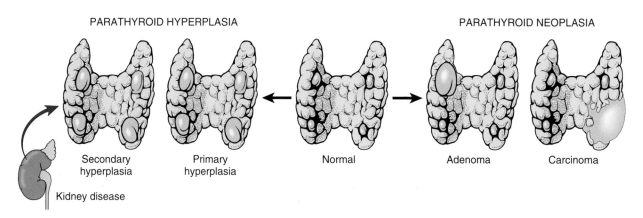

Secondary   Primary   Normal   Adenoma   Carcinoma
hyperplasia   hyperplasia

Kidney disease

FIGURE 17-8
Parathyroid hyperplasia and neoplasia.

parathyroid glands. *Parathyroid adenomas* or *carcinomas* are characterized by enlargement of one gland, with the other glands being normal (Fig. 17-8). In *parathyroid hyperplasia,* all four glands are enlarged (Fig. 17-9). Because the diagnosis of adenoma or hyperplasia cannot be made preoperatively, it is essential for the surgeon to explore all four glands. If adenomatous enlargement of one gland is identified, that gland is usually removed, whereas the others are left intact. If all four glands are enlarged, the surgeon will usually remove three glands and leave behind only one, which should suffice to maintain normal calcium-phosphate homeostasis.

Secondary parathyroid hyperplasia is indistinguishable from primary hyperplasia, as all four glands are symmetrically enlarged. Enlargement of the parathyroid glands and their hyperfunction is a compensatory mechanism triggered by hyperphos-

phatemia caused by chronic renal disease. Osteomalacia caused by hypovitaminosis D, as in rickets, may have the same results.

Pathologic Findings. The histologic changes in the parathyroid glands are identical, regardless of the cause of hyperparathyroidism. Parathyroid adenomas or carcinomas, as well as hyperplastic glands, are composed of parathyroid cells arranged into dense sheets. These cells replace the fat cells that are normally found inside the gland. In parathyroid adenomas, one may occasionally see remnants of the compressed preexisting gland, but this is not always evident. In hyperplastic glands, there is no evidence of normal parathyroid tissue. Parathyroid carcinomas may consist of invasive cells extending beyond the normal confines of the gland.

Hyperparathyroidism is characterized by an ex-

FIGURE 17-9
(A) Parathyroid hyperplasia. All four glands are symmetrically enlarged. (B) Parathyroid adenoma presents as a solitary nodule involving one parathyroid.

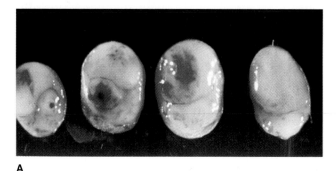

A

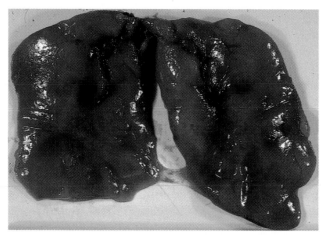

B

cess of PTH in the circulation. PTH acts primarily on the bones and kidneys. In the bones, it promotes bone resorption and the release of calcium into the circulation. In the kidneys, PTH promotes resorption of calcium from the tubular lumen, thus diminishing excretion of calcium in urine. PTH also promotes the formation of the active form of vitamin D_3 in the kidney which, in turn, facilitates the uptake of calcium from food in the intestine (Fig. 17-10). Hypercalcemia and compensatory hypophosphatemia are thus the primary biochemical abnormalities detected by blood analysis. PTH serum concentrations are also elevated.

Clinical Features. The clinical symptoms of hyperparathyroidism are related to increased PTH activity. The bones show signs of decalcification and are prone to fractures. Hypercalcemia leads to deposition of calcium salts in the kidney (*nephrocalcinosis*) and formation of renal stones (*nephrolithiasis*). Ocular and skin calcifications may be present. An excess of calcium produces lethargy, muscle weakness, and conduction defects in the heart.

The treatment of primary hyperparathyroidism includes surgical exploration of the neck and resection of the hyperfunctioning glands or the tumor. Secondary hyperparathyroidism can also be surgically treated, but at the same time, it is important to correct the basic metabolic defect that has caused PTH

hypersecretion. There is no need to rush with parathyroid surgery, however. Following renal transplantation, the glands may regress to normal size and the metabolic disturbances disappear. If renal transplantation does not normalize calcium and phosphate balance, one can assume that the hyperfunction of parathyroids has apparently taken an autonomous course. Such cases, which are called *tertiary hyperparathyroidism,* are rare. Surprisingly, chromosomal analysis of the enlarged parathyroids of patients with tertiary hyperparathyroidism has revealed chromosomal changes identical to those seen in parathyroid adenomas. This suggests that prolonged metabolic stimulation can cause irreversible neoplastic changes in the parathyroid cells. Because tertiary hyperparathyroidism represents a form of metabolically induced neoplasia, like any other tumor, it can be cured only by surgery.

Hypoparathyroidism

Hypoparathyroidism results from **parathyroid hypofunction** or a complete loss of function of the parathyroid glands. Overall, it is a rare condition that most commonly occurs following inadvertent removal of all four parathyroid glands during cancer surgery of the neck. Congenital, genetic, or autoimmune causes of hypoparathyroidism are extremely rare.

The clinical symptoms of hypoparathyroidism reflect metabolic disturbances caused by a deficiency of PTH. The most important of these is hypocalcemia, which results in changes in neuromuscular excitability and muscular contraction. The skeletal muscles tend to become spastic (*hypocalcemic tetany*). The heart action becomes irregular, and in severe cases, even cardiac arrest may occur. The activity of the nerves is also altered, fluctuating between hyperexcitability and depression. All the symptoms can be ameliorated by substitutional hormonal therapy with synthetic PTH.

Diseases of the Adrenal Cortex

Diseases of the adrenal cortex cause metabolic disturbances that reflect an excess or a deficiency of adrenal steroids. Each of the three zones of the adrenal cortex—zona glomerulosa, zona fasciculata, and zona reticularis—may be affected, either separately or jointly. The secretion of mineralocorticoids, glucocorticoids, or sex steroids may be altered; the excess or deficiency of these hormones will produce either disturbances in the metabolism of minerals (sodium, potassium, and chloride), carbohydrate metabolism, or sexual problems.

FIGURE 17-10
Metabolic consequences of hyperparathyroidism. PTH, *parathyroid hormone.*

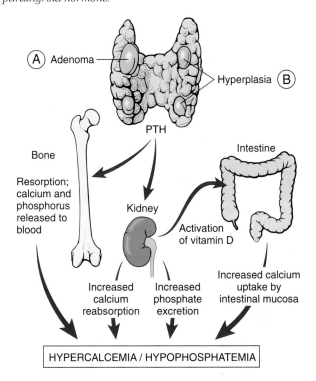

Adrenocortical Hyperfunction

Adrenocortical hyperfunction results in three partially overlapping syndromes:

- hyperaldosteronism (or Conn's syndrome), which is caused by hypersecretion of mineralocorticoids (aldosterone)
- hypercortisolism (or Cushing's syndrome), which is caused by hypersecretion of glucocorticoids (cortisol)
- adrenogenital syndrome, which is caused by hypersecretion of the adrenal sex steroids (androgens)

Cushing's syndrome is the most common of these three syndromes. Hypercortisolism is caused either by adrenal hyperplasia or neoplasia. In about 70 percent of cases, hypercortisolism occurs as a result of hypersecretion of ACTH from pituitary adenomas. This association was originally described by the Canadian neurosurgeon, Harvey Cushing, and is, therefore, called *Cushing's disease.* Subsequently, it was noticed that the same symptoms could occur as a result of hypersecretion of corticosteroids from adrenocortical tumors, a clinical entity that was called *Cushing's syndrome* to distinguish it from the disease caused by corticotropic adenomas of the pituitary. Adrenocortical tumors account for about 20 percent of the cases of hypercortisolism. Approximately 10 percent of cases are caused by extrapituitary tumors, like small cell carcinoma of the lung, which is the most common source of ectopically secreted ACTH (Fig. 17-11). Hypercortisolism may also be found in patients treated with synthetic steroids for rheumatoid arthritis, systemic lupus erythematosus, and other autoimmune diseases.

Pathology. Hyperplasia of the adrenals leads to bilateral thickening of the adrenal cortex. Tumors of the adrenal appear as discrete nodules or marked irregular enlargement of the entire gland. These tumors may be benign adenomas or malignant lesions (carcinomas). Typically, adrenocortical tumors are yellow because of their high lipid content (Fig. 17-12). Adenomas are usually well circumscribed, whereas carcinomas tend to extend into the adjacent tissues. Histologically, adenomas and well-differentiated carcinomas cannot always be distinguished from one another. Invasive carcinomas, however, show marked cellular pleomorphism.

Clinical Features. Symptoms of hypercortisolism include a peculiar "central" obesity that is most prominent on the face and trunk, resulting in a so-called "moon face" and "buffalo hump" (Fig. 17-13). The patients appear red in the face because of a plethora of blood, hypertension, and thinning of the skin. Glucose intolerance and overt diabetes are the most common biochemical disturbances. Typically, affected patients experience fatigue and weakness, and are mentally unstable. They also have numerous

FIGURE 17-11
Hypercortisolism in Cushing's disease and Cushing's syndrome. Excessive production of cortisol is related to the overstimulation of adrenals by ACTH. Cushing's syndrome can be caused by hormone-producing adrenocortical tumors or primary adrenocortical hyperplasia or exogenous corticosteroids.

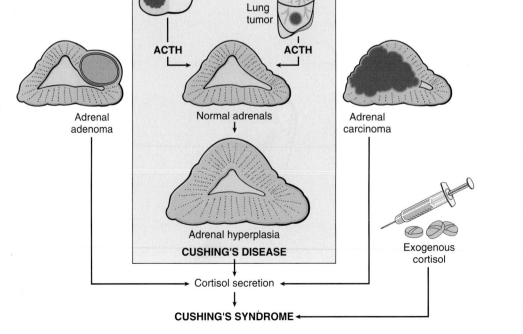

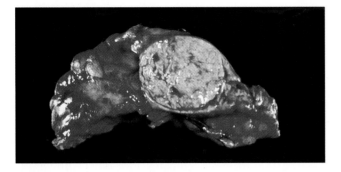

FIGURE 17-12
Adrenocortical adenoma. The neoplastic nodule is yellow owing to increased lipid content.

FIGURE 17-13
Comparison of adrenocortical hyperfunction and hypofunction.

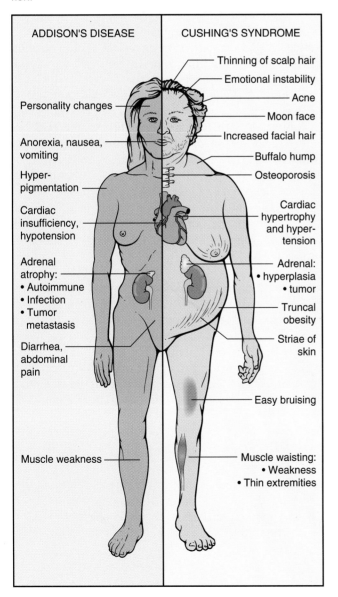

ADDISON'S DISEASE | CUSHING'S SYNDROME

Thinning of scalp hair
Emotional instability
Acne
Personality changes
Moon face
Increased facial hair
Anorexia, nausea, vomiting
Buffalo hump
Hyper-pigmentation
Osteoporosis
Cardiac insufficiency, hypotension
Cardiac hypertrophy and hypertension
Adrenal atrophy:
• Autoimmune
• Infection
• Tumor metastasis
Adrenal:
• hyperplasia
• tumor
Truncal obesity
Diarrhea, abdominal pain
Striae of skin
Easy bruising
Muscle weakness
Muscle waisting:
• Weakness
• Thin extremities

other minor problems, reflecting abnormal intermediate metabolism of carbohydrates.

Endogenous Cushing's syndrome and Cushing's disease are rare. In clinical practice, the most common cause of Cushing's syndrome is the administration of exogenous steroid hormones, which are commonly used for the treatment of various immune disorders, such as rheumatoid arthritis or asthma, renal diseases (e.g., nephrotic syndrome), and many skin diseases. Exogenously induced Cushing's syndrome responds well to gradual tapering off and cessation of steroid treatment.

Hyperaldosteronism is a rare disease that is typically caused by an adenoma of the zona glomerulosa. Adenoma is found in 70 percent of cases, whereas the remaining 30 percent have cortical hyperplasia. Clinically, hyperaldosteronism presents with retention of sodium and loss of potassium. Changes in the concentration of minerals, accompanied by a retention of water, result in hypertension (hypernatremic hypokalemic hypertension). Although this adrenal disease is rare, occurring in less than 0.1 percent of hypertensive patients, it is important to bear in mind that it is surgically treatable. Removal of the patho-

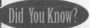

Did You Know?

Patients treated with corticosteroids develop the clinical features of Cushing's syndrome. As shown in the photograph, they have cushingoid features—"moon face," obesity, and cutaneous striae.

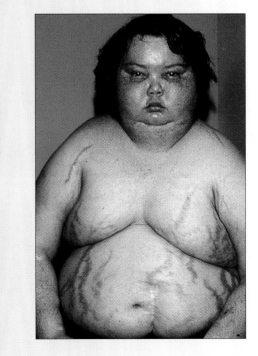

logically altered adrenal gland will result in complete cure of the hypertension.

Primary hyperaldosteronism must be clinically distinguished from *secondary hyperaldosteronism,* a much more common disease. The secretion of aldosterone is physiologically stimulated by angiotensin, which is formed from angiotensinogen under the influence of renin. Renin is secreted from the juxtaglomerular apparatus of the kidney, and elevated levels of renin are typically found in various renal diseases. Hence, secondary hyperaldosteronism is associated with hyperreninemia, in contrast to primary hyperaldosteronism, which is renin-independent and associated with normal levels of renin in circulation. Measurements of renin and aldosterone in blood are important in determining whether hyperaldosteronism is caused by a renal or adrenal disease.

Adrenogenital syndrome, which is also known as *adrenal virilism,* is a rare disease that can affect neonates or adults. As the name implies, the disease is typically found in females who experience virilization owing to an excess of androgenic hormones.

Adrenogenital syndrome may be congenital (i.e., present at birth), or it may develop in adulthood. In neonates, this disease is related to one of several inborn errors of steroid metabolism (e.g., 21-hydroxylase deficiency). An excess of androgens results in partial virilization of the external female genitalia. The vulva in these patients shows partial fusion of the labioscrotal folds, and the clitoris may be enlarged (*clitoromegaly*). Some of these female children are assigned the wrong sex. Although genetically female, they are reared as males. In adult women, the adrenogenital syndrome is usually related to androgen-producing tumors, which cause virilization with hirsutism, deepening of the voice, and loss of menstruation.

The treatment of adrenocortical hyperfunction depends on the cause of the disease and usually involves either surgical resection of hyperfunctioning tumors or medical suppression of the abnormal endocrine stimulatory pathway. For example, in congenital deficiency of 21-hydroxylase, virilization of the female external genitalia can be reversed by treating the child with cortisol. Cortisol is not produced in these children. Exogenous cortisol will provide the negative feedback impulse to the pituitary, inhibiting the excessive release of ACTH that occurs because of the lack of a natural inhibitor (endogenous cortisol). By reducing ACTH secretion, the exogenous cortisol reduces the overproduction of androgen in the adrenal. Without androgenic stimulation, the external female genitalia lose their male features and resume normal development comparable to that of normal female children.

Adrenocortical Hypofunction

Adrenocortical hypofunction is usually a consequence of adrenal destruction. This can occur suddenly in an acute form, as in meningococcal septicemia (so-called *Waterhouse-Friderichsen syndrome*), or slowly owing to the destruction of the adrenocortex by autoimmune disease (*autoimmune adrenalitis*). Infections, such as tuberculosis or histoplasmosis, or a primary or metastatic malignant tumor may also destroy the adrenals, causing adrenal insufficiency. Carcinomas of the breast and lungs are the most common tumors that metastasize to the adrenals, and if the metastases are bilateral, such tumors cause adrenal insufficiency.

Adrenal insufficiency results in a clinical syndrome known as *Addison's disease.* Today, 70 percent of the cases of Addison's disease are caused by an autoimmune adrenalitis, in contrast to previous times, when the disease was mostly caused by tuberculosis. However, infections, such as tuberculosis and fungal diseases, still account for 25 percent of cases and are most common in immunosuppressed patients with cancer or acquired immunodeficiency syndrome (AIDS). Malignant tumors are a rare cause of Addison's disease.

The pathologic basis of Addison's disease varies. In early stages of autoimmune adrenalitis, the cortex is infiltrated with lymphocytes and plasma cells. In later stages of the disease, the entire cortex is destroyed and may be replaced with fibrous tissue or fat cells. At autopsy, it is almost impossible to identify the adrenals, which have been destroyed by granulomas and pathogen-induced necrosis. Tumoral destruction of the adrenals is marked by an overgrowth of metastatic malignant cells and a loss of adrenocortical tissue.

Clinical Features. Addison's disease presents insidiously with fatigue, weight loss, and nausea. Affected patients are hypotensive and have frequent syncope. They are extremely susceptible to infections. They do not tolerate any stress, and cannot work or maintain many of the usual daily routines. Numerous metabolic disturbances may be detected.

> ### Did You Know?
>
> President John F. Kennedy had adrenal insufficiency (Addison's disease), most likely owing to an autoimmune disease that destroyed his adrenals. The President's disease was a well-kept secret during his lifetime.

The serum typically exhibits low levels of sodium and chloride, elevated potassium levels, and low glucose levels. If untreated, these mineral disorders lead to cardiac conduction problems, which can be lethal. Steroid levels in the blood are low.

The final diagnosis is made on the basis of an ACTH test. Normally, ACTH stimulates secretion of corticosteroids. In Addison's disease, such stimulation has no effect, proving that the adrenal has been destroyed and cannot respond to physiologic stimuli. Treatment with steroids results in fast recovery. However, exogenous steroids must be administered at regular intervals for the remainder of the patient's life.

The comparative features of Cushing's syndrome and Addison's disease are shown in Figure 17-13.

Diseases of the Adrenal Medulla

The most important diseases of the **adrenal medulla** are two **tumors:** *neuroblastoma* and *pheochromocytoma.*

Neuroblastoma

Neuroblastoma is a tumor composed of neuroblasts—i.e., undifferentiated precursors of neural cells that are also precursors of normal adrenal medullary cells. The adrenal medulla is derived from cells of the neural crest that migrate during fetal development and invade the primordium of the adrenal. Normally, these migrating neuroblasts differentiate into chromaffin cells of the adrenal medulla. Differentiation is recognized by the appearance of epinephrine- and norepinephrine-rich granules, visible in the cytoplasm of these cells by electron microscopy. If the migratory neuroblasts do not differentiate, but instead retain their embryonic-fetal undifferentiated phenotype, they undergo malignant transformation and form a malignant tumor. Such tumors, composed of undifferentiated neuroblasts, are called neuroblastomas. Similar tumors can occur in the brain or at the site of extraspinal and sympathetic ganglia, which are also derived from the neural tube and neural crest. Nevertheless, the adrenal is the most common site of neuroblastomas.

Neuroblastomas are developmental malignant lesions that predominately occur in neonates and young children. These tumors grow fast, forming large abdominal masses that may be palpated by the child's mother or by an examining physician. Neuroblastomas are highly malignant tumors, evidenced by the fact that most tumors have already metastasized by the time of diagnosis. Histologically, the tumor is composed of neuroblasts, undifferentiated small cells that have very little cytoplasm (Fig. 17-14).

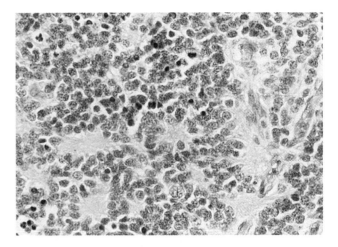

FIGURE 17-14
Neuroblastoma. Histologically, the tumor is composed of "small blue cells" corresponding to neuroblasts. These cells are arranged focally into "neural rosettes" (arrow), similar to those found in fetal neural tubes.

The few cells that differentiate usually evolve into neurons. Such cells release neurogenic amines, which may be detected in the urine as catecholamines or their degradation products, such as vanillylmandelic acid (VMA).

Neuroblastomas are rapidly growing and metastasizing tumors that previously were invariably lethal. With modern chemotherapy, however, these tumors have become more treatable; indeed, more than 90 percent of patients diagnosed today are cured completely with a combined regimen of surgical, medical, and radiation therapy.

Pheochromocytoma

Pheochromocytoma is the most common tumor involving the adrenal medulla of adults. It occurs only rarely, having an incidence of 1:10,000 per year. This tumor is important because it is a cause of surgically treatable hypertension. If the tumor is diagnosed and removed, the hypertension caused by it is cured instantaneously.

Pheochromocytoma is, in most instances, a benign, solitary tumor originating from the medulla of the adrenal (Fig. 17-15). Approximately 10 percent of all tumors originate in extra-adrenal locations and are derived from sympathetic paraganglia. Also, 10 percent of all pheochromocytomas are multiple, and 10 percent are malignant. Histologically, the tumor is composed of polygonal cells resembling those of the normal adrenal medulla.

Clinical Features. Pheochromocytomas are, in most instances, functionally active tumors that se-

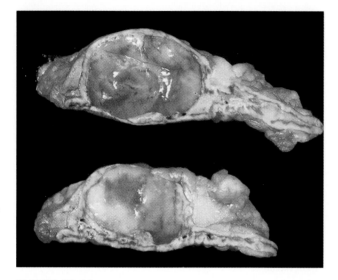

FIGURE 17-15
Pheochromocytoma. The adrenal contains a grayish-white nodule that is sharply demarcated from the normal tissue.

crete epinephrine and norepinephrine. The release of these catecholamines into the circulation causes hypertension. Patients usually have attacks of paroxysmal hypertension corresponding to a sudden release of catecholamines from the tumor. Prolonged exposure to epinephrine or norepinephrine may cause heart lesions (*catecholamine cardiomyopathy*).

The diagnosis of pheochromocytoma is made clinically and is confirmed biochemically by demonstrating elevated levels of epinephrine or norepinephrine, or both, in blood. Levels of VMA, the primary degradation product of these biogenic amines, are elevated in urine. In complex cases, it is necessary to perform functional studies that are based on the inhibition or stimulation of catecholamine release from the tumor cells.

Pheochromocytomas are treated surgically. The prognosis is excellent, as most of these tumors (90 percent) are benign, well encapsulated, and readily removable.

Review Questions

1. Which hormones are secreted by the pituitary?
2. Describe the anatomic components and cells of the thyroid, parathyroid, and adrenals, and list the hormones they secrete.
3. Compare the signs of pituitary hyperfunction in children and adults.
4. What are the signs of pituitary hypofunction?
5. List the most important pituitary tumors and their clinical manifestations.
6. What are the causes of hyperthyroidism?
7. What are the clinical features of hyperthyroidism?
8. What are the causes of hypothyroidism?
9. What are the clinical features of hypothyroidism?
10. Correlate the pathologic and clinical features of nodular goiter.
11. List the most important thyroid neoplasms and discuss their prognosis.
12. What are the causes of hyperparathyroidism?
13. What are the clinical features of hyperparathyroidism?
14. What are the metabolic consequences of hyperparathyroidism?
15. Compare the clinical features of hyperparathyroidism and hypoparathyroidism.
16. What are the causes of adrenocortical hyperfunction?
17. Describe the clinical features of the three most important syndromes caused by adrenocortical hyperfunction.
18. What are the causes of adrenocortical hypofunction?
19. What are the clinical features of adrenocortical hypofunction?
20. Compare neuroblastoma and pheochromocytoma.

Learning Objectives

After reading this chapter, the student should be able to:

1. Describe the normal skin and list its functions.

2. Describe and define the principal skin lesions, such as macule, papule, vesicle, pustule, ulcer, and scar.

3. Describe skin lesions caused by mechanical trauma.

4. Explain the short-term and long-term effects of ultraviolet light on the skin.

5. Describe skin infections caused by bacteria, viruses, fungi, and parasites, and give an example of each.

6. Describe the typical lesions of acne vulgaris and explain their pathogenesis.

7. Discuss various causes of eczema.

8. Define bullous lesions and explain their possible pathogenesis.

9. Describe two manifestations of seborrheic dermatitis.

10. Compare the clinical and pathologic features of seborrheic keratosis, basal cell carcinoma, and squamous cell carcinoma.

11. Compare freckles, nevi, and malignant melanoma.

12. List the most important neoplastic skin lesions involving the dermis.

Additional Key Terms and Concepts

Albinism

Folliculitis

Hirsutism

Melanoma

Nevus

Chapter Outline

The Skin
Chapter 18

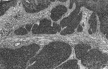

NORMAL ANATOMY AND PHYSIOLOGY

The skin is the external covering of the body, and its primary function is to protect the body from undue outside influences. The Greek term for skin is *derma;* accordingly, the subspecialty of medicine concerned with skin diseases is called *dermatology.* Dermatopathology is the synonym for pathology of the skin.

The skin is an organ that consists of three layers: **epidermis, dermis,** and **subcutis** (Fig. 18-1). The outer epidermal layer is predominantly composed of **keratinocytes** and scattered melanocytes (see Fig. 18-1). The dermis consist of **connective tissue.** It also contains blood vessels, nerves, hair follicles, and skin **adnexal glands.** The hypodermis or subcutis is predominantly composed of fat tissue.

The surface of the skin is constantly abraded, and the epidermis is constantly regenerated from the proliferating cells in the basal layer. This is essential for maintaining the integrity of the skin and its primary function—**protection** against external injury. Intact skin represents a formidable barrier; therefore, it is imperative for the body to keep its "armor" intact.

The epidermis undergoes keratinization, which is the second most important protective mechanism. Epidermal cells have the capacity to produce *keratins,* which are cytoskeletal proteins that are highly resistant to mechanical and chemical injury. The keratin layer thus represents the final stage of epidermal cell differentiation. It varies in thickness from one anatomic site to another, and is most prominent on the palms and soles.

Keratin provides limited protection against sunlight by preventing the penetration of light through the skin. In this function, the keratinocytes are abetted by **melanocytes,** the pigment-producing cells. Melanocytes are located in the basal layer. However, these cells have branching cytoplasmic processes that extend to several adjacent cells and link them with keratinocytes. Melanocytes produce melanin, a brown pigment, which is packaged into membrane-bound cytoplasmic bodies (melanosomes) and transferred through the cytoplasmic processes into keratinocytes. This transfer of pigment accounts for the browning of the skin upon exposure to sunlight. Keratinocytes injected with melanin are more resistant to ultraviolet light, and therefore, protect the body against the adverse influences of sunlight more efficiently than do nonpigmented keratinocytes. Over time, the suntan fades and the skin pigmentation disappears as the pigmented keratinocytes are lost and replaced with new cells that do not contain melanin.

The epithelial components of the dermis, often referred to as *skin appendages,* are anatomically distributed in an uneven manner. *Hair follicles,* with the sebaceous glands attached to them, are prominent on the scalp but are not evident on the palms or plantar side of the foot. *Eccrine sweat glands* are present all over the body except for some sites, such as the margins of the lips and nipples. The primary function of these sweat glands is perspiration and thus, indirectly, **thermoregulation.** *Apocrine* or *odoriferous sweat glands* are located in some areas, such as the axilla and pubic areas. Under the control of sex hormones, these glands produce a clear, sweat-like fluid

FIGURE 18-1
The skin consists of three layers: epidermis, dermis, and subcutaneous tissue. (From Jarvis C. Physical examination and health assessment. Philadelphia: WB Saunders, 1992: 225.)

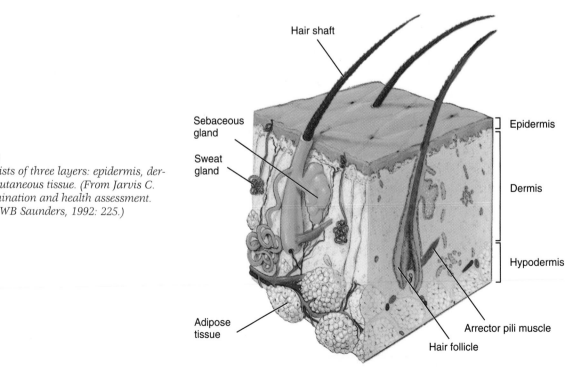

Hair shaft

Sebaceous gland

Sweat gland

Epidermis

Dermis

Hypodermis

Adipose tissue

Arrector pili muscle

Hair follicle

that is rich in organic substances. The organic components of sweat decompose under the influence of skin bacteria, resulting in distinct odors.

The hypodermis or subcutis is the third layer of the skin. It is predominantly composed of fat cells and connective tissue. The thickness of this layer, which is poorly demarcated from the overlying dermis, varies. Its primary function is to provide thermal and mechanical protection to the body by its fat pad (*panniculus adiposus*). It also allows us to sit comfortably in one place and study for exams!

OVERVIEW OF MAJOR DISEASES

The most important diseases involving the skin are as follows:

- Traumatic lesions caused by mechanical, chemical, or thermal injury
- Infectious disease
- Immune diseases and diseases of presumptive immune etiology
- Metabolic diseases and those secondary to diseases of internal organs
- Tumors

It is also important to remember that the causes of many skin diseases remain unknown. The treatment of skin diseases is still, in many cases, empirical and symptomatic, and not fully understood or scientifically justified. Thus, dermatologists still have a reputation for assigning each skin disease a long Greek or Latin name and then treating them all with the same creams!

Several facts important to an understanding of skin diseases are presented here, before a discussion of specific pathologic entities.

1. *The skin protects the body primarily by maintaining its own integrity.* Intact dry skin is the best barrier against infection. Wounds caused by mechanical trauma or minor cuts provide entry sites for bacteria. Moist skin, caused by sweating (as during a hot, wet summer), also facilitates the entry of bacteria. This explains why skin infections are more common among manual laborers whose skin is easily traumatized, and especially those working in tropical climates.

2. *Skin can be traumatized mechanically, thermally, chemically, or by various forms of radiation.* Various forms of mechanical skin trauma induce different lesions. Just compare a knife wound and a penetrating bullet wound. Likewise, many of us have been burned or had frostbite, rarely stopping to consider these as forms of thermal trauma. Blisters produced by exposure to early summer sun are prime examples of radiation-induced skin trauma. The sunlight is a mixture of ultraviolet, visible light and in-frared rays, all of which can damage the skin under appropriate conditions.

3. *The effects of acute injury are distinct from those caused by chronic or repeated injuries.* For example, gradual exposure to sunlight allows gradual pigmentation of the skin. However, if the skin were exposed to the same amount of radiation in one long day on the beach, it would not tan but would burn, blister, and finally undergo acute scaling. Long-term exposure to sunlight causes chronic skin injury and accelerates aging of the skin.

4. *Skin is covered normally with bacteria* that do not affect it adversely. Our skin is not sterile, but is covered with a myriad of saprophytic bacteria. That is why surgeons must wash their hands before operations so that they do not infect the operating field if the gloves rupture. Saprophytic bacteria are innocuous as long as they remain on the intact skin. However, they may infect wounds and cause overwhelming infections in weak or immunosuppressed persons.

Bacteria, viruses, fungi, and parasites that are transferred onto the skin may cause diseases. Bacteria, such as staphylococci, may invade hair follicles or sebaceous glands, as occurs in acne. Viruses, such as herpesvirus, may invade the epidermis and cause vesicles. Fungi tend to grow in the keratin layer, causing dermatophytic infections, such as "athlete's foot." Lice tend to grow on hair shafts. Subcutaneous infections with worms occur frequently in the tropics, but are not usually seen in the United States.

5. *Skin participates in an* **immune reaction** *to foreign substances.* The skin is constantly exposed to foreign substances, many of which are immunogenic and act on the immune system of the body. For example, many people are allergic to nylon underwear, cats, or house dust. Such substances may induce allergic contact dermatitis and even systemic symptoms. Childhood *atopic dermatitis* and *eczema* are the most common immune-mediated skin diseases.

6. *Skin may be affected by systemic, metabolic, and immune diseases.* The etiology of many such diseases is still unknown. For example, systemic sclerosis, a multiorgan disease of the connective tissue, produces hidebound skin known as *scleroderma*. Diabetes mellitus is a systemic disease affecting the metabolism of carbohydrates and lipids, which often manifests as skin lesions. Diabetes also predisposes individuals to bacterial infections and causes microcirculatory disturbances.

7. *Skin diseases may present with hypopigmentation or hyperpigmentation. Albinism* represents generalized genetic hypopigmentation. Localized hypopigmentation is called *vitiligo.* Hyperpigmentation may be a consequence of suntanning, but also may be hormonally induced.

8. *The skin is the most common site of tumors in the human body.* This can be explained, in part, by the fact that such tumors are more easily diagnosed than small tumors of the same size in internal organs. However, one should also remember that the skin is constantly exposed to various carcinogens: chemicals, radiation, viruses, and probably many other influences of unknown carcinogenic potential. Contact with known carcinogens should be avoided. The most important skin carcinogen—the *ultraviolet light* in sunshine—can be avoided to some extent, but never entirely.

9. *The skin has a limited way of responding to injury.* Morphologically, identical skin lesions can be induced by different means. For example, blisters (*bullae*) can result from sunbathing; an allergic reaction to poison ivy; a systemic disease, such as porphyria; or a primary skin disease of unknown etiology, such as bullous pemphigoid.

Pathology of Basic Skin Lesions

In view of the fact that the skin has a limited reaction pattern and that many diseases produce the same symptoms, it is important to learn and understand the terms used for skin lesions in dermatologic practice. The most important of these are presented in Fig. 18-2.

Macule—flat lesion measuring less than 2 cm in diameter; not raised or depressed; primarily representing a change in skin color. The best example is the freckle: a brown, pigmented spot.

Patch—similar to a macule, but larger than 2 cm in diameter. The best example is the skin rash that occurs in measles, a childhood viral disease.

Papule—slightly elevated, small induration of the skin with a diameter of less than 1 cm. Papules are the hallmark of eczema, which is usually caused by allergy.

Nodule—similar to a papule but larger (1 to 5 cm in diameter). Nevi or moles, which are pigmented, slightly raised skin lesions, are the best examples of this lesion.

Tumor—nodule with a diameter exceeding 5 cm. Squamous cell carcinoma and a variety of other skin neoplasms are examples of skin tumors.

Vesicle—fluid-filled elevation of the epidermis measuring less than 1 cm in diameter. Herpesvirus infections produce vesicles on the border of lips.

Bulla—Vesicles measuring more than 1 cm in diameter. Burns can cause bullae, some of which are confluent and may cover large surfaces of the skin.

Pustule—vesicle filled with pus. Impetigo, a bacterial infection of the skin that usually affects children, is a typical example.

Ulcer—defect of the epidermis. Syphilitic chancre, which most often appears on the skin or mucosa of the genitals, is a good example.

Crust—a skin defect that is covered with coagulated plasma or blood. Healed wounds are covered with crusts.

Scales—keratin layers that cover the skin in flakes or sheets and that can easily be scraped away. Pemphigus and seborrheic dermatitis are relatively common skin diseases of unknown etiology which cause scaling of the skin.

Squames—large scales. Ichthyosis, a congenital thickening of the skin, forms numerous squames.

Excoriation—superficial skin defect caused by scratching. Any chronic skin disease accompanied by an itch will ultimately result in excoriations, mostly self-induced by the patient.

Fissure—sharp-edged defect of the epidermis that extends into deeper layers of the skin. Athlete's foot, a fungal disease, typically produces fissures.

FIGURE 18-2
The appearance of various skin lesions.

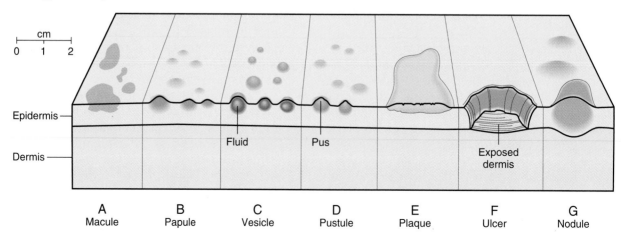

Congenital Disorders

Congenital diseases of the skin may present at birth, early in life, or later on. These include minor cosmetic imperfections (so-called "birthmarks") and/or diffuse afflictions affecting the entire body integument. The **nevus** or birthmark is the most common congenital skin anomaly (in Latin, *naevus* means "birthmark"). Nevi represent congenital developmental defects or hamartomas (in Greek, *hamartion* means "body defect") whereby normal skin elements are arranged in an abnormal manner. Brown birthmarks (*melanocytic nevi*) are composed of melanocytes. *Nevus flammeus,* also known as port-wine mark, is a congenital aggregate of small blood vessels, usually found on the face. Congenital nevi are innocuous lesions that require no treatment.

Many skin diseases have a significant hereditary component; some are even inherited as mendelian traits. For example, **ichthyosis congenita** is inherited as an autosomal dominant trait. In this disease, the child is born covered with thick squames resembling fish skin (in Greek, *ichthys* means "fish").

Albinism (*albinus* meaning "white" in Latin) is a generalized hypopigmentation caused by an inborn error of metabolism. Affected persons lack one of the enzymes essential for the synthesis of melanin from the amino acids tyrosine and phenylalanine. These individuals appear strikingly pale and never tan. They have white hair and red eyes because their hair and retina also lack pigment. Albinos are at increased risk for developing sunburns and skin cancer, and they should avoid exposure to the sun altogether. There is no treatment for this pigmentary defect.

Epidermolysis bullosa is a term used to denote several congenital skin disorders, all of which are characterized by the formation of blisters upon rubbing of the skin or minor trauma. The most severe form, which is fortunately rare, may present during intrauterine life. The milder forms present with blisters that form spontaneously, usually on the palms and soles. There is no effective treatment for this disease.

External Injury

Skin can be injured by a variety of **external injuries.** These can be classified as

- mechanical trauma
- thermal injury
- electrical injury
- radiation injury

Mechanical Trauma

Humans are exposed to mechanical trauma throughout their lives. Minor trauma does not even register. Major trauma, however, may have serious consequences, and because it is usually not limited to the skin alone but involves other organs as well, it may be even lethal.

It is customary to categorize mechanical trauma according to the means by which it is inflicted. *Blunt trauma* is caused by objects, such as a club or hammer. It usually results in *contusion* (*contusio* meaning "bruise" in Latin). Bleeding into the skin and soft tissue occurs from mechanically disrupted blood vessels. *Laceration* involves disruption of the skin and the underlying soft tissue. It usually requires surgical treatment and does not heal easily. *Sharp trauma* (wound) is caused by sharp objects, such as a knife or bullet.

Thermal Injury

Skin can be injured by relatively short exposure to very high or very low temperatures, or by prolonged exposure to moderately high or low temperatures. The most important forms of injury are *burns,* caused by heat, and cold injuries, such as *frostbite* and *immersion foot injury.*

Burns. The extent of skin burns depends on the mode of exposure (e.g., sunburn, hot metal, hot air, fumes), the duration of exposure, the temperature, and the anatomic site of injury. For example, the palms and soles have a thicker keratin layer and are more resistant to burns than the skin of the face. Thermal injury may be localized (e.g., sunburn on the face) or widespread (e.g., total body burns, as might be incurred in a house fire). The final clinical outcome of burns depends on the depth of skin injury and the extent of the body surface affected.

Burns are graded clinically by establishing the depth of skin injury. First degree burns are the mildest form, producing only erythema and swelling. Histologically, the epidermis shows spotty, single cell necrosis, as well as edema. Such lesions are transitory, reversible, and heal spontaneously without any consequences.

Second degree burns are characterized by blisters involving the epidermis. The hair follicles and skin adnexa in the dermis are spared. The epidermis heals from the edges of the blisters and from the epithelium of the hair follicles without scarring.

Third degree burns, also known as full-thickness burns, cause massive necrosis of the entire epidermis and dermis and extending, to a variable degree, into the subcutaneous tissue and underlying soft tissue. Localized third degree burns take a long time to heal, usually with prominent scarring. Large surface areas affected by third degree burns cannot heal spontaneously and require specialized treatment, including skin transplantation.

In order to estimate the chances for survival and to determine appropriate treatment modalities, it is important to estimate the total surface of the body that has been burned. For this purpose, it is customary to apply the "rule of nines," which assigns 9 percent of the total body surface area to burns affecting the head and to each of the upper extremities; and 2 times 9 percent to each lower extremity, and to the frontal and posterior surface of the trunk (Fig. 18-3). Any burn exceeding 9 percent of the total body surface is serious and must be treated intensively in a specialized burn unit. With modern treatment, most patients can be saved, even if they have extensive burns, but the scarring that follows may have crippling consequences. Mortality usually results from uncontrolled fluid loss and infection of the denuded body surfaces.

Cold Injuries. Cold injuries are usually less severe and less life-threatening than burns, although prolonged exposure to cold can cause death by freezing. Death in snow blizzards has befallen many a mountaineer and polar explorer, but immersion foot and frostbite are more common injuries seen in daily medical practice.

Immersion foot is the term used to describe tissue injury caused by exposure to nonfreezing cold and a moist environment. It typically affects the legs and was first recognized in soldiers who had to stand for hours in trenches—hence the synonym "trench foot." The principal damage occurs at the level of the small blood vessels which, stunned by cold, become permanently dilated and unable to regulate local blood flow. Venous stagnation occurs, contributing to gradual cooling of tissues and accounting for the bluish color of the skin. Skin necrosis develops, with formation of blisters and ulcers.

FIGURE 18-3
Schematic depiction of the "rule of nines," which subdivides the body into 9-percent areas to allow estimates of the extent of burns (From Applegate EJ: The anatomy and physiology learning system: textbook. Philadelphia: WB Saunders, 1955: 92.)

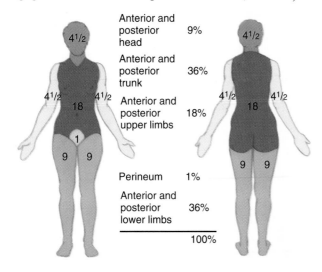

Frostbite or *congelation* (a Latin term meaning freezing) is an injury caused by exposure to subfreezing point temperature. The tissue changes resemble those induced by immersion foot injury, but they develop more rapidly and are usually more pronounced. Any part of the body may be injured. The fingers, toes, and face are most often involved. On reheating, the tissue becomes blotchy red and swollen. Recovery may occur, but necrotic tissue (gangrene) may impede healing. Surgical resection of nonviable tissue may be indicated, but only after spontaneous recovery is deemed impossible.

Electrical Injury

Contact with unprotected and inadequately isolated electrical wires can cause skin wounds. Similar wounds result from lightning, which is electricity that is generated by nature. The passage of electricity through the skin generates heat, which burns the tissues, leaving linear marks along its path. At the point of entry of high-voltage electricity into the body—typically at the site of contact with an unprotected high-voltage wire—the tissue is burned and an "electric mark" of blackened skin forms. However, electrical injury also affects the deeper tissues and possibly even internal organs, and it may cause death by interfering with the electrical conduction system of the heart. In the dermis, electricity damages the blood vessels, provoking thrombosis and subsequent infarctions in the areas to which the thrombosed blood vessels were providing blood before the injury.

Radiation Injury

We are constantly exposed to numerous sources of natural radiation, the most important source of which is the sun. In addition, we are exposed to various forms of artificial, man-made radiation, such as radio waves, television waves, microwaves, and ultrasound. The two most important forms of **radiation injury** are caused by sunshine and ionizing radiation.

Sunlight Injury. *Acute exposure to the sun* over a short period of time leads to hyperemia. Prolonged exposure causes sunburn, accompanied by blisters and peeling of the skin (Fig. 18-4). Acute sunburn represents a first or second degree thermal injury.

Chronic exposure to the sun has cosmetically pleasing beneficial effects, but it also damages the skin. Most of the long-term consequences are related to ultraviolet light. Controlled sunbathing over a relatively short period, such as 2 weeks, stimulates the transfer of melanin pigment from melanocytes to keratinocytes in the epidermis, producing a suntan. Suntan is usually short-lived, however, and the skin

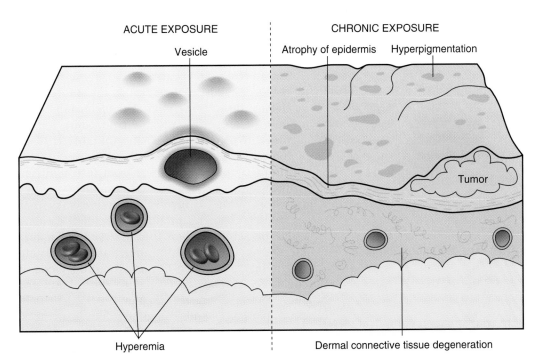

FIGURE 18-4

Short-term and long-term effects of sunbathing. Acute injury results in hyperemia of the dermis and blister formation. Long-term exposure may stimulate pigmentation, but may also promote carcinogenesis and aging of the epidermis and dermis.

color returns to normal after the pigmented keratocytes have been shed (i.e., within about 30 days). The adverse affects of long-term exposure to sun outweigh the short-term cosmetic effects. Two major consequences of prolonged suntanning are

- accelerated aging of the skin
- development of tumors

Aging affects all layers of the skin. The skin becomes more brittle and less elastic, develops wrinkles, and tends to resist injury less efficiently than that of younger people. Wounds also tend to heal more slowly.

Ultraviolet light is carcinogenic for the skin. Skin tumors develop more often on sun-exposed surfaces, such as the face or arms. Furthermore, skin tumors are more common in persons who work in the fields than those who work in offices. Sailors and farmers are at increased risk, for obvious reasons. Moreover, fair-skinned persons are at a greater risk than dark-skinned persons, who are partially protected by the pigment in their skin.

Ionizing Radiation. Short-term exposure to x-rays or other forms of ionizing radiation (e.g., in a laboratory during handling of radioactive isotopes) is not dangerous, and usually produces no obvious pathologic changes. However, prolonged or repeated exposure, or exposure to high doses of ionizing radiation, can produce significant lesions. Whereas alpha particles are large and do not penetrate the skin, beta particles can penetrate up to 1 cm and can cause epidermal changes. Gamma rays and x-rays penetrate tissues easily, causing little damage while passing through the tissue themselves. On the other hand, all of these radiation particles induce secondary ionization of the molecules in tissues; thus, all ionizing particles should be considered potentially damaging.

Short-term exposure to high levels of radiation may induce necrosis because radiation kills cells. Long-term exposure to small doses of radiation stimulates pigmentation, but also may be carcinogenic. Thus, it is no wonder that many old-time radiologists who were inadequately protected while working have developed skin cancer of the hands. Today, it is

Did You Know?

Not everybody can acquire a suntan. Indeed, dermatologists recognize six distinct groups: those who

1. Always burn, never tan
2. Burn readily, tan poorly
3. Burn occasionally, tan well
4. Almost never burn, tan easily
5. Are pigmented all of the time (e.g., Asians)
6. Are black-skinned (e.g., blacks)

unusual to see x-ray–induced cancer in health professionals.

Infectious Diseases

Infectious diseases of the skin are common. In most instances, these infections are localized and do not produce serious systemic symptoms. However, skin infections can have systemic consequences, as well.

Bacterial Infections

Bacterial infections of the skin are classified into three major groups:

- primary bacterial infections, which occur on apparently normal skin
- secondary bacterial infections, which complicate preexisting skin diseases or wounds and ulcers
- systemic bacterial infections, in which the skin involvement is only one of many manifestations of systemic, blood-borne infection.

Primary bacterial infections are typically caused by pus-forming bacteria and, therefore, are called *pyodermas*. Most often, these infections are caused by coagulase-positive staphylococci and beta-hemolytic streptococci, which may produce either superficial or deep lesions.

Impetigo (in Latin, *impeto* means "to attack") is a common superficial infection caused by streptococci or *Staphylococcus aureus*. It is characterized by superficial pustules that rupture, leaving behind honey-colored scabs. Impetigo is most often found on the face of small children. Because these skin lesions are itchy, affected children often spread the infection to other sites on their body, and can infect their playmates as well. Impetigo is highly contagious, but responds well to systemic antibiotic therapy. It heals without any scars.

Folliculitis is a common form of infection limited to hair follicles (Fig. 18-5). It is usually caused by *S. aureus*. Typically, it involves hairy areas, such as the beard. The bacteria produce a purulent exudate that fills the lumen of hair follicles. As the bacteria invade the hair shaft and the infection extends into the perifollicular tissue, a *furuncle* (boil) develops. If the infection spreads to adjacent follicles and the original abscess enlarges to include several hair follicles, a much larger boil, called a *carbuncle,* evolves. Such large abscesses are most often located on the neck and are more common in males than in females. Adequate antibiotic treatment may prevent further spread and recurrence of infection, which is otherwise quite common.

Secondary bacterial infections develop at the site of another disease or in wounds. Bacterial infections impede the healing of primary skin disease. The skin affected by chronic dermatitis, known clinically as eczema, is almost always contaminated with bacteria. Hence, the treatment of most chronic skin diseases must include some antibiotic therapy to eradicate the bacterial contamination.

Systemic infections may spread to the skin through the blood or the lymphatics, or by direct extension of the infection from the underlying tissue to the skin. Such infections are more common in debilitated or immunosuppressed patients. Any case of septicemia or bacteremia—that is, entry of bacteria into the blood—may cause skin abscesses.

Fungal Infections

Fungal infections of the skin are extremely common. Luckily, fungal pathogens—called *dermatophytes*—tend to live in "dead tissues," such as the surface keratin layer, hair, or nails, and cause almost no inflammation in the underlying skin. Nevertheless, such infections cause itching and discomfort, and predispose the individual to secondary bacterial infection, which may lead to the formation of fissures and scaling.

The most common sites of superficial **dermatophytoses** are the feet, head, and nails, and the intertriginous parts of the body, such as the axilla and groin. These lesions are called *tinea* or *ringworm*. *Tinea pedis,* or athlete's foot, typically begins between the toes and spreads locally. *Tinea unguium* is

---

Did You Know?

Skin infections are often caused by bacteria that are normally present on the skin but are in a healthy equilibrium with the human body. In this respect, various parts of the body surface have been compared with geographic ecosystems that sustain life on earth in vastly different forms. The hairy scalp, for instance, has been compared to moutain woods with tall trees that provide the shady grounds for low-lying bacteria and fungi. Similarly, the moist armpits have been likened to a tropical rain forest ideally suited to sustain all sorts of exotic flora; the face has been compared to arid, sun-exposed prairies that harbor bacteria in pit-like follicles; the nails have been said to resemble a desert that does not allow any growth at all, thereby resisting bacterial growth (except in the oasis that corresponds to the paronychium). Clearly, then, different parts of the skin are variously predisposed to distinct infections.

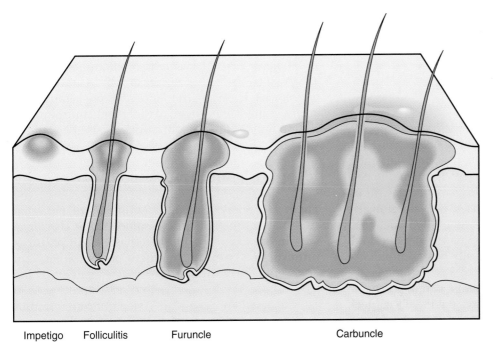

Impetigo   Folliculitis   Furuncle   Carbuncle

FIGURE 18-5
The appearance of various bacterial skin infections.

a chronic nail infection. *Tinea corporis* presents as circular or irregularly shaped patches on the skin that have a pale center and spreading margins. *Tinea cruris* (jock itch) affects the groin region. *Tinea capitis,* or scalp ringworm, typically affects children, causing local hair loss.

The diagnosis of fungal infections is usually made on the basis of clinical findings. To confirm the fungal nature of the disease, one may scrape the squames and examine them under the microscope.

Other fungi besides dermatophytes may affect the skin. The most important of these pathogens is the ubiquitous *Candida albicans,* the cause of common *thrush* in children. Infections caused by Blastomyces, coccidioidomycosis, and similar fungal infections are uncommon in temperate climates but are endemic in the tropics. These invasive, **deep fungal infections** cause large destructive lesions and tumorlike lesions called *mycetomas.* Mycetomas may produce major skin defects and deformities and are resistant to therapy.

Viral Diseases

Viral infections of the skin may be acute and self-limited or chronic. Acute systemic viral diseases are common in childhood and present with either a maculopapullar rash (*exanthem*), as in **measles,** or vesicles, as in **chickenpox. Herpes labialis** and **herpes zoster,** or shingles, are localized, blistering, viral skin diseases affecting adults.

Viral skin diseases may also have a chronic course. The best example of a chronic viral disease of the skin is the common *wart* (*verruca vulgaris*), which is caused by human papillomavirus (HPV). Warts are innocuous lesions that disappear spontaneously after some time, with or without treatment.

Insect Infestations and Bites

Insect bites cause itchy, papulomacular skin lesions that usually have a red dot in the center. Blood-sucking insects that feed on human blood, like fleas, mosquitoes, bed bugs, and lice, are the most common culprits. The skin lesions are caused by substances injected by the insect. Such substances are biologically active and cause edema, itching, or pain. These lesions are usually temporary and do not require treatment.

Many insects, like wasps, use their sting in self-defense. The poison injected by such a sting contains vasoactive substances, which may cause edema, hemorrhage, and even systemic effects. Persons allergic to bee stings may develop a profound local reaction or a systemic anaphylactic reaction which, if untreated, may result in death. It is important to remember that insect bites may cause not only local irritation, but also may transmit serious systemic diseases, as in the case of fleas (typhus), ticks (Lyme disease), and mosquitoes (malaria).

Scabies is a contagious skin disease caused by the mite *Sarcoptes scabiei* (in Greek, meaning "flesh cutter"). This tiny organism, which is barely visible with the naked eye, burrows itself into the superficial layers of the epidermis. The burrows appear like irregular lines on the skin and are most prominent between the fingers and on the dorsal side of the wrist. Typical maculopapullar eruptions evolve, in part induced by scratching and in part caused by a reaction to the bite, to the mites' feces, or to the ova deposited by the female. Treatment with specific anti-scabies ointments is usually effective.

Acne

Acne vulgaris, as the adjective in its official Latin name indicates, is a very common disease (in Latin, *vulgus* means "crowd"). Although **acne** is an infectious disease, it is best to consider it under a special heading, as other factors besides bacteria play an important role in the pathogenesis of typical lesions.

The pathogenesis of acne is not fully understood. Hereditary, hormonal factors, and general cleanliness are important. Acne typically begins at puberty, probably under the influence of sex hormones. Sex hormones, particularly androgens, stimulate the development of sebaceous glands on the face, neck, chest, and back (Fig. 18-6). The secretion of sebum is increased, as evidenced by greasy skin. At the same time, the sex hormones promote hyperkeratosis at the orifice of hair follicles, which blocks the discharge of sebum. The stagnant sebum is colonized by anaerobic bacteria (*Propionibacterium acnes*). This results in formation of *comedos,* which can occur in two forms: open (blackheads) and closed (whiteheads). Through the action of bacterial lipases, the fat of the sebum is broken down to glycerin and free fatty acids, which, upon being released into the tissue, cause inflammation. The entire obstructed follicle and the surrounding connective tissue are transformed into pustules or larger abscesses. These may persist, become confluent (*acne conglobata*), transform into dermal cysts, or heal with scarring (*keloid acne*). Scratching, picking, or pressing of these lesions predisposes the individual to secondary infections.

Acne is a major cosmetic problem in teenagers. Treatment is aimed at decreasing the keratinization of follicles by using retinoic acid or keratinolytic agents, such as benzoyl peroxide, and controlling infection with local antibiotics, such as clindamycin.

Idiopathic and Immune Disorders

There are many skin diseases that have either no identifiable cause or are presumed to be caused by immune mechanisms. Most often, such **idiopathic** or **immune-mediated dermatoses** present as **eczema** or chronic **dermatitis,** or as papulosquamous or bullous disorders. Clinically, such diseases present as localized or widespread skin lesions of variable morphology. Itching is the most common symptom.

Eczema or Dermatitis

Eczema (in Greek, meaning to "boil out") is a term used to denote many forms of inflammatory skin diseases that

- present with nonspecific lesions, such as localized edema, papules, and vesicles
- are uniformly accompanied by *pruritus* (the Latin term for "itching")

Because of the itching, the primary lesions become infected, which causes secondary changes, such as scales, crusts, and oozing. Histologically, eczema is characterized by chronic inflammatory

FIGURE 18-6
Pathogenesis of acne.

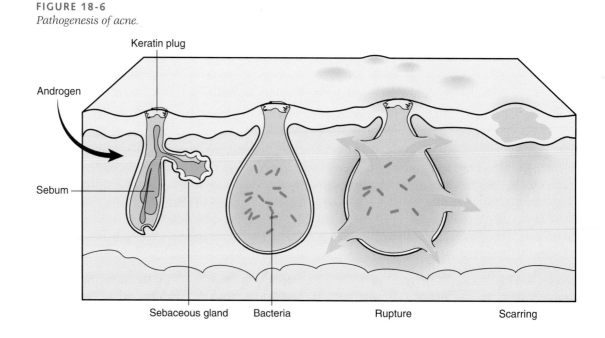

cell infiltrates in the dermis, blood vessel dilatation, and edema. The epidermis shows edema and hyperkeratosis.

It is convenient to classify eczema into two major forms:

- exogenous eczema
- endogenous eczema

Exogenous eczema can usually be traced to a specific cause in the environment; that is, it may be caused by irritants or allergens. Many exogenous chemicals may act as irritants. For example, detergents in soap may cause eczema in housewives, and cement powder may cause hand lesions in construction workers. Skin allergy can also develop in hypersensitive persons. For instance, some people are allergic to plastic, rubber gloves, or even gold rings. Allergies to systemic drugs may also cause eczema. Drug-induced skin eruptions, as may occur in those who are allergic to penicillin, may present as systemic rash.

Endogenous eczema may occasionally have an identifiable cause, but most often, its etiology is unknown. Many systemic autoimmune disorders, such as systemic lupus erythematosus, present with skin lesions. *Atopic dermatitis,* a common disease affecting approximately 10 percent of all children, also is thought to have an immunologic basis. It tends to affect families with other immune disorders, such as hay fever, but its pathogenesis is still unknown.

Seborrheic Dermatitis

Seborrheic dermatitis, a widespread chronic disease that affects 10 percent to 20 percent of the population in the United States, is a multifactorial disorder. It presents with reddening, scaling, and itching of the skin, especially on the nasolabial folds and eyebrows and the upper chest. It leads to the formation of abundant dandruff. Topical steroids provide some relief, but that does not prove the allergic nature of this disease. Special shampoos and soaps containing sulfur also can be used.

Psoriasis

Psoriasis is the most important generalized papulosquamous disease because it affects 1 percent to 2 percent of the entire world population and currently is incurable. It is more common in some families, but its mode of inheritance is not mendelian.

The disease presents with slightly elevated papules and patches. These are covered with silvery scales, reflecting the parakeratotic surface layer. The lesions most often appear on the extensor surface of the extremities, such as the knees and elbows. The scalp and the nails are also often affected. In most patients, the lesions are not itchy, even though the Greek word *psora,* from which the name of the disease is derived, means "to itch."

The papules erupt in crops, symmetrically involving various parts of the body; they then slowly fade away. Exacerbations seem to be related to trauma and emotional stress. The treatment is symptomatic but not too effective. Symptoms relating to internal organs may develop occasionally, most often in the form of psoriatic arthritis.

Neoplasms

Neoplasms of the skin are divided into four groups:

- tumors of epithelial cells
- tumors of pigmentary cells
- tumors of the dermal connective tissue
- tumors of blood-borne "immigrant" cells

All of these tumors may be benign or malignant. The most important tumors are listed in Table 18-1.

Epithelial Tumors

Epithelial skin tumors originate from the surface epidermis, the hair shafts, sebaceous glands, and various eccrine and apocrine sweat glands. Most common are tumors originating from the epidermis itself. Sweat gland and sebaceous gland tumors are much less common. **Seborrheic keratosis** is the most common benign epidermal tumor, presenting in the form of a brownish, solitary or multiple, mulberry-shaped, wart-like exophytic, flat-topped lesion with a corrugated, furrowed surface. The wart-like lesions (also called *senile warts*!) seem to be loosely attached to the skin and can be shaved away with ease. Histologically, the lesion consists of papillae lined with a uniform population of basaloid cells.

Seborrheic keratosis is innocuous and should not be considered premalignant. Some lesions that are very pigmented may be mistaken for malignant melanoma. In contrast to melanoma, senile warts are friable and easily removed.

Basal cell carcinoma is the most common malignant skin tumor of epithelial origin. Fortunately, this low-grade malignant tumor does not metastasize and rarely, if ever, causes death.

Lesions are typically located on sun-exposed skin and thus are probably related etiologically to overexposure to sunlight. The tumor presents as a slightly elevated nodule with a central depression that becomes more and more prominent as the tumor grows (Fig. 18-7). Histologically, the tumor is composed of islands and strands of invasive neoplastic cells resembling those in the basal layer of the epidermis. The treatment, be it surgical resection, cauterization, or radiotherapy, yields excellent results,

Table 18-1 Neoplasms of the Skin

Tumor Category	Benign	Malignant	Cell of Origin
Epithelial cells	Seborrheic keratosis	Basal cell carcinoma	Keratinocyte
		Squamous cell carcinoma	
	Eccrine adenoma	Eccrine carcinoma	Sweat gland
	Sebaceous adenoma	Sebaceous carcinoma	Sebaceous glands
Pigmentary cells	Nevus	Melanoma	Melanocyte
Connective tissue	Dermatofibroma	Fibrosarcoma	Fibroblast
	Hemangioma	Angiosarcoma	Blood vessel
		Kaposi's sarcoma	
Blood-borne cells	Pseudolymphoma	Lymphoma	Lymphocyte
		Mycosis fungoides	
	Urticaria pigmentosa	Malignant mastocytosis	Mast cell
—	—	Metastatic carcinoma	Malignant disease of an internal organ

although some of the flat and multifocal lesions may recur if not removed completely.

Squamous cell carcinoma is a truly malignant tumor of the surface epithelium. Like the basal cell carcinoma, it occurs most often on sun-exposed skin. The lesion presents as a flat plaque; a small, persistent ulcer; or a slightly elevated, keratotic plaque (Fig. 18-8). Histologically, the tumor is a squamous cell carcinoma that is indistinguishable from squamous cell carcinoma in other organs.

On sun-exposed skin, squamous cell carcinoma is often preceded by a malignant, preinvasive stage of disease known as **actinic keratosis.** Colloquially, actinic keratosis is also known as squamous cell carcinoma "one half," so named because it shows many of the cytologic characteristics of cancer but no invasion of the underlying tissue. Actinic keratosis typically progresses into an even more atypical lesion, carcinoma in situ, which, if left untreated, will ultimately become a truly infiltrating malignant process.

Typical squamous cell carcinomas are locally invasive, but less than 2 percent of all tumors metastasize. The prognosis depends primarily on the stage of the disease; therefore, it is imperative that the tumor be diagnosed early. Since none of the clinical signs are diagnostic, it is important to maintain a high degree of suspicion and to perform a biopsy of all suspicious lesions for histologic examination.

The most important tell-tale signs of cancer are as follows:

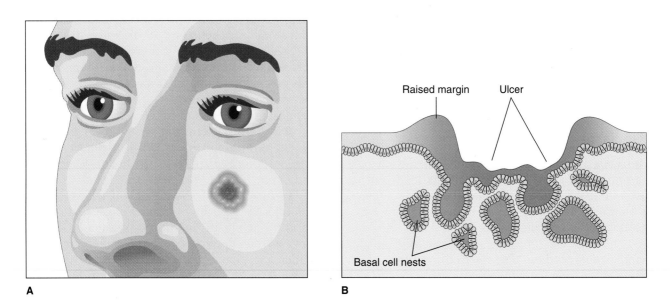

A   **B**

FIGURE 18-7

Basal cell carcinoma. (A) Tumor appears as a nodule with central depression. (B) This crater-like tumor is composed of invasive basaloid cells arranged into nests.

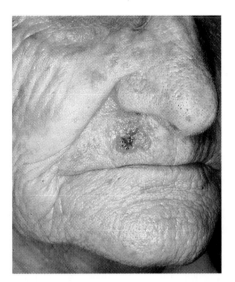

FIGURE 18-8
Squamous cell carcinoma.

- Persistent, nonhealing ulcer
- Ulcer or nodule of irregular shape and indistinct margins
- Friable, bleeding tissue in an ulcer
- Induration of the tissue around an ulcer
- Irregularly textured, multicolored tissue at the bottom of an ulcer
- Indurated skin surrounded by the atrophic and keratotic skin typical of sunlight injury (actinic keratosis)

Pigmented Lesions

The normal skin contains numerous brownish pigmentary lesions (Fig. 18-9), the most common of which are freckles, lentigos, and nevi. A freckle (or **ephelis**) is a patch of skin in which the melanocytes show a hyperreactivity to ultraviolet stimulation. If exposed to sunlight, such spots become darker brown. A **lentigo** is an area of skin occupied by an increased number of melanocytes. Lentigines do not respond to sunlight. A **nevus** or *mole*, as explained previously, is a developmental abnormality of the skin characterized by an accumulation of melanocytes. Nevi may be located in the dermis (*dermal nevus*) or at the dermoepidermal junction (*junctional nevus*), or they may be both junctional and dermal (*compound nevus*). Finally, there are the so-called *blue nevi*, which are composed of deep dermal melanocytes. Because of their deep location, such nevi have a bluish color like the paint of warships.

Nevi are divided into two groups: *congenital nevi*, which are present at the time of birth, and *acquired nevi*. Congenital nevi are birthmarks with no special significance. In Japan, a congenital nevus on the right earlobe portends good luck and is evidence that the person was born under a lucky star. Acquired nevi appear at puberty, become more prominent during adult life, and then involute. Acquired nevi are usually innocuous skin lesions that are typically removed in crops before the sunbathing season for cosmetic reasons. However, some nevi—so-called **dysplastic nevi**—are not so innocuous and may progress to malignant melanoma. Dysplastic nevi occur at a high rate in some cancer-prone families and, if untreated, undergo malignant transformation in more than 50 percent of cases. As a result, some authorities call such lesions malignant melanoma in situ. The malignant potential of ordinary acquired nevi is very low.

Malignant Melanoma

Malignant melanoma is a tumor originating from melanocytes (Fig. 18-10). Approximately one half of malignant melanomas originate from intact skin; the

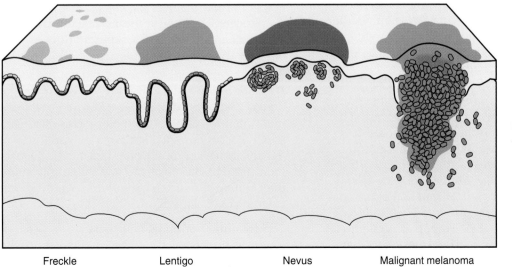

FIGURE 18-9
Pigmented lesions.

| Freckle | Lentigo | Nevus | Malignant melanoma |

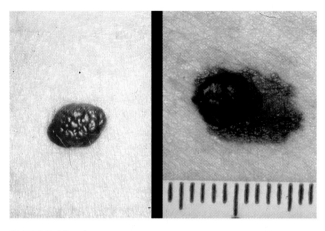

FIGURE 18-10
*Pigmented skin lesions. Left: Benign pigmented nevus (mole).
Right: Malignant melanoma. Note the differences in size and
shape and the irregular borders of the melanoma. (Courtesy of
the National Cancer Institute, Bethesda, Maryland.)*

other half arise from freckles and preexisting nevi.
As melanoma is the most malignant of the skin tumors, it is important to diagnose it as early as possible. Several clinical histologic types of melanoma are
recognized.

Lentigo maligna (melanotic freckle of Hutchin-
son) is a flat, macular lesion that typically originates
in a preexisting freckle, usually in the elderly. It remains localized for up to 10 to 15 years, and if not removed, acquires invasive properties and transforms
into a superficially spreading or invasive nodular
melanoma.

Superficial spreading melanoma accounts for 70
percent of all malignant pigmentary tumors and is
the most common form of clinically recognized
melanomas. These lesions present as irregularly pigmented macules with irregular edges. The lesions
are pruritic, and are most often located on the legs in
women and the back in men. Histologically, these lesions are composed of malignant melanocytes that
grow radially in the epidermis, showing, for a considerable time, no tendency for dermal invasion. As the
tumor progresses, the cells tend to invade superficial
layers of the epidermis and invade the dermis, thus
giving rise to nodular melanoma.

Nodular melanoma is the rapidly growing, infiltrating variant of malignant melanoma. It is marked
by vertical growth and invasion of the dermis. The
extent of dermal invasion is the most important prognostic sign. Pathologists estimate the depths of tumor
invasion by histologic means and then use these
measurements to stage the tumor. For example, if
the tumor invades less than 0.75 mm and is limited
to the papillary dermis, it is considered to be a level I
lesion, and is entirely curable. Tumors invading to a
depth of more than 1.5 mm (i.e., those that have
spread to the reticular dermis) are classified as level

IV and have a 5-year survival of 40 percent. Invasion
of the subcutaneous tissue by tumor (level V lesion)
portends a poor prognosis (a 5-year survival of 25
percent).

Acral-lentiginous melanomas develop on the palms
and plantar surfaces or underneath the nails. This is
the most common variant of melanoma in blacks and
Orientals.

Clinical Features. Malignant melanomas are related to sun exposure and are thus more common in
patients living in tropical areas than in northern climates. The races that have little pigment are more
susceptible than pigmented races. Accordingly, melanomas are quite rare in blacks (except for acral-
lentiginous melanomas). A familial predisposition to
melanomas has been registered in individuals with
multiple dysplastic nevi.

At least one third to one half of all malignant
melanomas originate in preexisting lentigines or acquired and dysplastic nevi. Therefore, it is important
to recognize the transition of these benign or premalignant pigmentary lesions into overt malignant
melanoma. Clinical experience has taught us the "A-
B-C-D of diagnosis," as follows:

A—*Asymmetry of the pigmented lesion.* Any pigmented lesion that has flat as well as elevated
parts intermixed in a haphazard manner should
be considered potentially malignant and warrants careful monitoring.

B—*Borders.* Lesions that have irregular margins,
with notching and leakage of brown pigment
across the borders, are suspect.

C—*Color.* Marked variations in color (ranging
from dark black to dark brown to red), when in-
terspersed with areas that appear bleached, are
signs of "restlessness" of the melanocytes and
their potential for invasiveness. Malignant melanoma cells are not as efficient melanin produc-
ers as normal pigmentary cells. Melanomas are
immunogenic and an immune reaction may destroy some cells. All these aspects of tumor biology account for the paler areas noted in the tumors.

D—*Diameter of the lesion.* Most malignant melanomas that are diagnosed clinically measure
more than 6 mm in diameter. This does not
mean that lesions smaller than 6 mm are not malignant. However, any lesion that has the above-
mentioned A-B-C features and measures more
than 6 mm in diameter should be removed and
examined histologically.

The treatment of malignant melanomas is surgical. Tumors that have distant metastases must be
treated by radiation therapy and chemotherapy. The

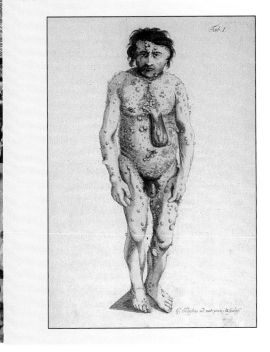

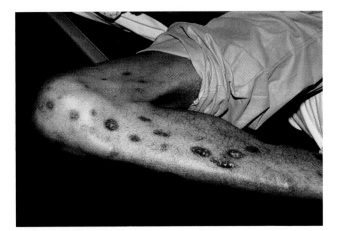

FIGURE 18-11
Kaposi's sarcoma.

overall 5-year survival for all forms of melanoma is 60 percent.

Dermal Connective Tissue Tumors

Dermal tumors may originate from fibroblasts, blood vessels, and many other structures. These are mostly benign lesions or low-grade malignant tumors that are curable by surgical excision. Among these, the most common is the **dermatofibroma.** Dermatofibromas are benign tumors composed of fibroblasts. Surgical excision is the treatment of choice.

Kaposi's Sarcoma

Kaposi's sarcoma is a dermal tumor composed of blood vessels and perivascular connective tissue cells (Fig. 18-11). These red tumors present as hemorrhagic nodules, which are often multiple and confluent. Previously, Kaposi's sarcoma of the skin was extremely rare. However, with the recent epidemic of

acquired immunodeficiency syndrome (AIDS), the incidence of Kaposi's sarcoma has increased dramatically to the point where this tumor has become the most prevalent malignant lesion in patients with AIDS. The relationship of Kaposi's sarcoma to AIDS is not fully understood, but it seems that the state of immunosuppression associated with AIDS somehow facilitates the proliferation of blood vessel–forming cells in the dermis, as well as in other sites.

Herpesvirus type 8 has been isolated from Kaposi's sarcoma cells recently. It has been proposed that the virus may cause tumors in immunosuppressed hosts.

Kaposi's sarcoma is a tumor of low malignant potential which, nevertheless, tends to spread in immunosuppressed patients with AIDS. It may spread widely and cause death. There is no adequate treatment available for this tumor.

Dermal Tumors Derived from Blood-Borne Cells

The skin may be affected by malignant cells that reach it from the blood circulation. It is thus fairly common to see dermal infiltrates of malignant lymphoma or other visceral malignant lesions. T-cell lymphomas have a special predilection for the skin, one form of which is called **mycosis fungoides.** Typically, this disease presents as skin macules and papules that progress to nodules and ulcerating large masses. Histologically, these skin lesions are composed of infiltrates of malignant T lymphocytes.

Urticaria pigmentosa is a peculiar skin disease characterized by dermal infiltrates of mast cells. This disease, typically found in children and young adults, presents with pigmented, brownish-red macules or slightly elevated papules that flare upon touching or stroking. Histologically, these lesions consist of dermal infiltrates of mast cells. These mast cells release histamine and other vasoactive amines, causing

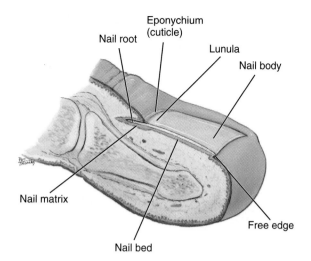

Eponychium
(cuticle)

Nail root

Lunula

Nail body

Nail matrix

Free edge

Nail bed

FIGURE 18-12
Structure of the nail. (From Jarvis C. Physical examination and health assessment. Philadelphia: WB Saunders, 1992: 226.)

swelling and reddened skin patches. The disease usually does not require any special treatment, and it disappears spontaneously with time, usually after puberty.

Diseases of Nails

Nails are specialized coverings on the toes and fingers, which can be considered as modified skin. The nails are derived from the constantly dividing cells of the matrix at the base of the nail, which is partially covered with the cuticle of the nail fold (Fig. 18-12).

Diseases of the nails are manifold; some of them are caused by local conditions, whereas others reflect various systemic disorders. Deformities, such as *onychogryphosis* (from the Greek *onychos,* meaning nail, and *gryphosis,* meaning curvature), are usually without a known cause. Spoon-shaped nails (*koilonychia*) are usually a sign of iron deficiency anemia, whereas nail clubbing is a sign of chronic pulmonary disease. Psoriasis is associated with nail disease in about 50 percent of all patients.

Nails are resistant to infection except for the base and the cuticle. Bacterial infections of the cuticle, which are common, are called *paronychia*. This is most common in individuals who work with their hands immersed in water, such as kitchen personnel. The only clinically significant nail infections are caused by fungi. These *onychomycoses* are typically chronic, quite resistant to treatment, and cause nail deformities, defects, and brittleness.

Hair Diseases

The body is covered with several types of hair that differ with regard to their structure, growth cycle, and many other properties. Compare, for instance, the hair of the pubic skin, the scalp, and the beard. Clearly, each of these forms of hair may react in a different manner to various adverse influences and will show different pathologic changes. Some of these diseases have been mentioned already, such as fungal and bacterial infections. Acne is, in essence, a disease of the hair follicle–sebaceous unit.

An excess of hair is called *hirsutism* (in Latin, *hirsutus* means shaggy). The hair growth on the chin and the chest is stimulated by male sex hormones; thus, normal males have a beard and chest hair. Hirsutism in these areas in the females is usually a sign of hormonal disturbances, such as those caused by androgen-producing ovarian or adrenal tumors or complex hormonal disturbances caused by polycystic ovary syndrome.

Loss of hair from the scalp is called baldness, or *alopecia* (from the Greek *alopex,* meaning fox; thus, alopecia is loss of hair, as in fox mange). Alopecia may be focal (*alopecia areata*) or diffuse. Alopecia areata is usually a sign of an infection caused by fungi (*tinea capitis*) or bacteria, such as that seen in syphilis. Hair pulling (*trichotillomania*) is usually a manifestation of nervousness, and may cause focal hair loss.

Diffuse alopecia involves large portions of the scalp and typically occurs in aging males. Male pattern baldness is marked by recession of the frontotemporal hairline with progressive loss of hair over the convexity of the head. Such baldness is considered to be idiopathic, but has a strong hereditary component. It usually occurs after the age of 30 years and is resistant to treatment. Alopecia in women is usually a sign of hormonal disorders, such as hypothyroidism or some nutritional deficiency (e.g., iron deficiency and protein malnutrition). Alopecia may also be induced by cytotoxic drugs. Drugs used to treat cancer kill the dividing cells, including those in the hair matrix, thus preventing hair growth. Drug-induced alopecia is diffuse and involves not only the scalp, but the eyebrows and body hair as well. After the completion of the therapy, hair growth resumes.

Review Questions

1. What are the main histologic components of epidermis, dermis, and subcutis?
2. What are the main functions of skin?
3. Give clinical examples of a macule, patch, papule, vesicle, pustule, plaque ulcer and nodule.
4. What is ichthyosis?
5. What is albinism?
6. What is epidermolysis bullosa?
7. Explain the effects of mechanical trauma on the skin and subcutaneous tissues.
8. What are the differences between first degree, second degree, and third degree burns?
9. Compare immersion foot and frostbite.
10. Describe an "electric mark" on the skin.
11. Compare the effects of acute and chronic sun exposure.
12. Describe and explain the pathogenesis of impetigo, folliculitis, furuncle, and carbuncle.
13. Compare superficial dermatophytosis with deep fungal infections.
14. List viruses that infect skin.
15. Describe insect bites.
16. What is scabies?
17. Describe the pathology of acne and explain its pathogenesis.
18. What is eczema?
19. What is seborrheic dermatitis?
20. Describe the pathologic and clinical features of psoriasis.
21. Classify skin neoplasms.
22. What is seborrheic keratosis?
23. Compare basal cell and squamous cell carcinoma.
24. What is actinic keratosis?
25. What are the most important tell-tale signs of skin cancer?
26. Comapre freckle with lentigo and nevus.
27. Classify malignant melanomas.
28. List the A-B-C-D of diagnosis of malignant melanoma.
29. What is Kaposi's sarcoma and how is it related to the AIDS epidemic?
30. Compare mycosis fungoides and urticaria pigmentosa.
31. Describe the main features of nail infections.
32. Compare hirsutism and alopecia.

Learning Objectives

After studying this chapter, the student should be able to:

1. Define the portions of a typical long bone: epiphysis, metaphysis, diaphysis, and growth plate.

2. Define and describe the bone cells: osteocyte, osteoblast, osteoclast, and chondrocyte.

3. Describe the anatomy of joints.

4. Discuss achondroplastic dwarfism, osteogenesis imperfecta, and osteopetrosis.

5. Describe the most common forms of osteomyelitis.

6. Describe aseptic necrosis and list at least two anatomic sites affected.

7. Define osteoporosis and discuss its clinical features.

8. Explain the pathogenesis of osteomalacia and rickets and relate the bone changes to clinical symptoms.

9. Describe the healing of simple bone fractures, define callus, and explain the reasons for delayed healing of fractures.

10. List the typical age and the most common anatomic sites of osteosarcoma, chondrosarcoma, and Ewing's sarcoma and describe typical features of these tumors.

11. Define osteoarthritis, explain the pathogenesis of degenerative joint disease, and describe its pathology.

12. Define rheumatoid arthritis and explain its pathogenesis and pathology.

13. List three most important facts about ankylosing spondylitis.

14. Give two examples of infectious arthritis.

15. Define gout and describe the pathology of gout arthropathy.

Additional Key Terms and Concepts

Chondrosarcoma

Ewing's sarcoma

Osteomyelitis

Osteosarcoma

Chapter Outline

Bones and Joints
Chapter 19

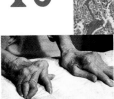

The skeleton is composed of **bones** connected to one another by joints. The diseases affecting the skeleton are classified under the headings of orthopedic pathology and rheumatology.

NORMAL ANATOMY AND PHYSIOLOGY

The human body contains more than 200 bones which can be classified as either long or short and flat. The long bones, also known as tubular bones, form the shaft of the extremities, whereas the short and flat bones form the skeleton of the trunk, the skull, and the terminal portions of the extremities (Fig. 19-1).

All bones are composed of cells (**osteocytes**) and extracellular matrix (**osteoid**) that is impregnated with calcium phosphate salts in the form of hydroxyapatite. In the cortex of long bones, the cells and matrix are arranged into elementary units called **osteons,** which form the *compact* bone. The medullary portion of long, most short, and flat bones is composed of *trabeculae,* forming the cancellous or *spongious* bone. The inside surface of the compact bone and the trabeculae are covered with bone-forming cells (**osteoblasts**) and bone-resorbing cells (**osteoclasts**). The external surface of bones is covered with the *periosteum,* which also contains osteoblasts, fibroblasts, blood vessels, and nerves.

Long bones have a central part, called the *diaphysis,* (Fig. 19-2) and two ends, each of which is covered with a cup of articular cartilage. These terminal portions of bone are called *epiphysis* because they are above the growth plate, which is called the *physis* (in Greek, *physis* means growth). The growth plate and the adjacent terminal diaphysis represent the metabolically most active segment of the long bones. Because it changes dramatically during development, it is, therefore, called the *metaphysis. (*In Greek, the prefix *meta* denotes changes; thus, *metaphysis* means the growth-related, changing part of the bone).

Bone formation during fetal life and until the end of puberty occurs through two mechanisms. The longitudinal growth of long bones is based on osseous transformation of the **cartilage** in the growth plate, called *endochondral ossification.* Most flat bones form through *intramembranous ossification,* whereby bone formation results from direct transformation of fibrous matrix into osteoid, followed by mineralization (i.e., deposition of calcium phosphate salts, predominantly in the form of hydroxyapatite). Intramembranous ossification also accounts for the subperiosteal bone formation of long bones, which is the basis of the appositional growth and widening of long bones. Endochondral ossification ceases by the end of puberty and appears later only exceptionally and under pathologic conditions, as during healing of bone frac-

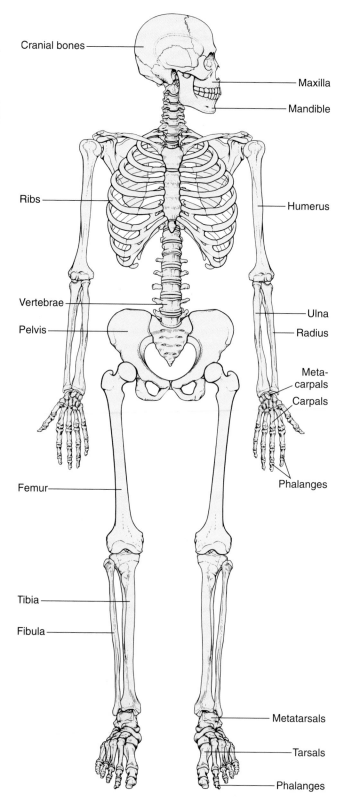

FIGURE 19-1

The human skeleton consists of long bones (e.g., femur and radius), short bones (e.g., tarsal bones and vertebrae), and flat bones (e.g., pelvic bone, scapula, and calvaria).

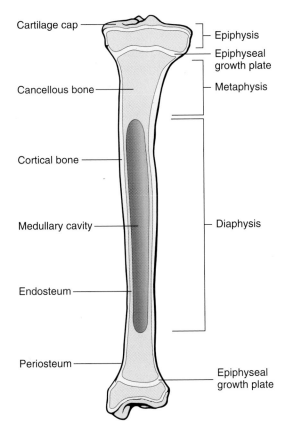

FIGURE 19-2

The long bone has a central part (diaphysis) and two terminal parts (epiphysis). The shaft of the bone is composed of cancellous bone on the outside and trabecular bone on the inside. The marrow contains fat tissue except in the short and flat bones of the trunk, where it is composed of hematopoietic cells. The external surface of the bone is covered with periosteum. The articular surface is covered with a cartilage cap. (From Applegate ED: The anatomy and physiology learning system: textbook. Philadelphia: WB Saunders, 1995:98.)

tures. The intramembranous appositional growth of long bones continues, albeit at a slower rate, throughout the normal life span.

The bone formed by either endochondral or intramembranous ossification is composed of a meshwork of collagen fibers that calcify in a haphazard manner and appear under polarized light as *woven bone*. The woven bone is restructured so that the collagen fibers become arranged into parallel arrays which, under polarized light, appear as *lamellar bone*. Adult bones are composed of lamellar bone except in the case of fractures undergoing repair and pathologically altered bones.

The most important functions of the bone are the following:

- Mechanical support for the muscles, which makes possible the movement of limbs
- Protection of internal organs, such as the ribs forming the thorax or the skull protecting the brain
- Support of hematopoiesis
- Storage of calcium and phosphate salts

The normal structure of bones and their shape depend on two extraosseous influences: their interaction with the muscles and the hormonal regulation of calcium and phosphate metabolism. The normal structure of bones also depends on the proper balance between bone formation and bone resorption. The muscles insert onto the periosteum and, by exerting tension, modulate the shape of bones according to the elementary laws of physics.

Osteoblasts form new bone, whereas osteoclasts remove and remodel old bone under the influence of hormones (e.g., parathyroid hormone), vitamins (e.g., vitamins D and C) and various other biologically active substances (e.g., prostaglandins and interleukins). The calcium and phosphate released from the bone enter the circulation and are in balance with ionized calcium and phosphate in the serum. As discussed in greater detail in the chapter on endocrine pathology, this balance is tightly regulated by parathyroid hormone and vitamin D.

A **joint** (in Latin, called *articulatio*) is the junction between two or more bones, designed to provide support and structural firmness, as well as to allow movement. There are two types of joints: (1) moveable diarthrodial or *synovial* joints, and (2) joints that allow limited or no movement at all, termed *synarthroses*. We shall limit our discussion predominantly to synovial joints, which account for most of the joints of the extremities. Synarthroses interconnect the bones of the head and trunk.

The typical synovial joint is enclosed in a connective tissue capsule composed of **ligaments** (Fig. 19-3). On the inside, the space is lined with synovial cells secreting a viscous fluid that lubricates the joint surface. The joint surfaces are covered with cartilaginous caps covering the epiphyseal bone. Between the two adjacent cartilaginous surfaces of two adjacent bones, some joints, such as the knee, have a similunar disk called the *meniscus;* in other joints, the cartilage caps of opposing bones are in close contact with each other, separated only by a thin film of synovial fluid. Some joints, like the knee, are reinforced by ligaments that hold the bones within the joint in close contact with one another. Joints are richly supplied with blood vessels and nerves.

OVERVIEW OF MAJOR DISEASES

The most important diseases of the bones are

- metabolic diseases affecting the growth, formation, and removal of bone
- fractures and deformities

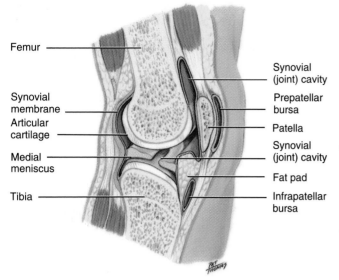

FIGURE 19-3
Schematic drawing of a typical diarthrodial (synovial) joint. (From Applegate EJ: The anatomy and physiology learning system: textbook. Philadelphia: WB Saunders, 1995:119.)

- bacterial infections
- tumors

The most important diseases of the joints are

- inflammatory diseases
- degenerative joint diseases

Several facts important to an understanding of bone pathology are presented here, before a discussion of specific pathologic entities.

1. *Bones have two major functions: mechanical and metabolic.* Although we tend to view the bones only as support structures, one should not forget that bones are the major storage site of calcium and phosphate salts. Bones actively participate in the body's response to vitamin deficiency (e.g., rickets secondary to vitamin D deficiency). Many hormones, such as parathyroid hormone, corticosteroids, and sex hormones have an effect on bones. The joints have only a mechanical function: to stabilize the skeleton and enable movement of bones.

2. *Bones and joints are composed of living tissues that undergo constant changes.* Bones are in an active equilibrium with other parts of the body. For example, the muscles exert constant pressure and tension, influencing the shape of bones and maintaining their normal structure. Loss of muscle strength in people who are paralyzed or confined to bed as a result of chronic illness weakens bones. Exercise has been recommended for delaying age-related bone loss. Prolonged immobilization stiffens the joints and may cause *ankylosis* (in Greek, *ankylos* means stiff).

3. *The extracellular matrix of bones is constantly formed, remodeled, and resorbed.* Bone consists of metabolically active cells (osteocytes) that form and maintain it. Osteoblasts form the bone, whereas osteoclasts resorb it. The structure of bones depends on a balance between osteoblastic and osteoclastic activity. Excessive resorption of minerals from the extracellular bone matrix results in softening of bones (*osteomalacia*). Excessive bone formation without commensurate resorption occurs only rarely (as in a congenital disorder called *osteopetrosis*, or marble bone disease).

4. *The extracellular matrix of the bone consists of osteoid and minerals; cartilage, which is not mineralized, lines the joint surfaces.* Minerals—mostly calcium and phosphate—account for 60 percent of the bone weight, and the osteoid, which is mostly composed of collagen type I, accounts for the remaining 40 percent. Cartilage is made up of collagen type II.

The synthesis of bone collagen and the deposition of hydroxyapatite are two distinct functions of osteoblasts that are under the control of different regulators. Either one of these functions could be deranged. In *osteogenesis imperfecta*, a genetic defect, collagen synthesis is defective. In osteomalacia, mineralization of osteoid is affected. Both conditions lead to weakening of bones caused by a loss of bone substance (*osteopenia*) and an increased incidence of fractures.

5. *Calcium and phosphate stores in the bones are in equilibrium with ionized calcium and phosphate in the blood.* The ratio of ionized calcium and phosphate in the blood is tightly regulated and normally oscillates only within a narrow range. Calcium and phosphate can be mobilized quickly from the bones to compensate for low levels of these minerals in the blood. An excess of calcium or phosphate in blood is counterbalanced by an increased deposition of these minerals in bones or their excretion in the urine or feces.

6. *Bone cells respond to stimuli by hormones, cytokines, and prostaglandins.* Bone cells respond to a variety of hormones: parathyroid hormone, vitamin D (which is actually also a hormone!), calcitonin, estrogens, androgens, growth hormone, corticosteroids, and probably many others. An excess or deficiency of these hormones adversely affects the skeleton. For example, a deficiency of vitamin D in children results in rickets and deformities of the long bones. Bone cells respond to interleukins, transforming growth factor, prostaglandins, and other bioactive substances. In response to activated oncogenes, bone cells may undergo neoplastic transformation and give rise to benign and malignant tumors. Osteoblasts, the most proliferative cells, are the most common sources of these tumors, known as osteoblastomas or osteosarcomas.

7. *Bone diseases are age-specific.* Normal bones change considerably during the human life span.

There are major differences between the growing bones of prepubertal youngsters and those of older adults. Likewise, the diseases that affect the bones in each age group are also distinct. For example, each bone tumor has a typical peak age incidence. Some bone diseases that are common in old people, like osteoporosis, are unusual in children. The same pathogenetic agent or mechanism can produce one set of changes in growing bones and another in nongrowing adult bones. For example, growth hormone stimulates the epiphyseal growth plate in growing bones, promoting longitudinal growth (*gigantism*). In adults, growth hormone stimulates the appositional bone growth of adult bones, resulting in acromegaly. Vitamin D deficiency in childhood causes rickets, whereas in adults, it causes osteomalacia.

Growing bones need more nutrients and are, therefore, more vascularized and receive more blood than the bones of adults. Accordingly, the bones of adolescents are more likely to be infected by bloodborne bacteria than the bones of adults.

8. *Joints are moving structures that may be traumatized easily.* Long-term trauma causes degenerative changes known as *osteoarthritis.* Because the joints are constantly under pressure, they can be easily injured. Such injury can cause joint dislocation (*luxation*).

9. *Unlike bones, joints may be affected by autoimmune diseases. Rheumatoid arthritis* and *systemic lupus erythematosus* are autoimmune diseases commonly affecting the joints. The inflammation typically involves the synovial membranes, the internal lining of the joint capsule.

Developmental and Genetic Disorders

Developmental and genetic bone diseases are rare, occurring in the general population at a rate ranging from 1:20,000 to 1:60,000. Despite great advances in the understanding of these diseases, they remain incurable.

Achondroplasia

Achondroplasia is a genetic defect of endochondral ossification, inherited as an autosomal dominant trait and causing dwarfism. Achondroplastic dwarfs can be easily recognized because they typically have short legs and arms and a body of relatively normal size. As mentioned earlier, long bones grow through endochondral ossification; if this process is faulty, the bones of the extremities will be short. On the other hand, intramembranous ossification is not affected; therefore, the bones of the trunk develop normally. The calvarium of the skull and the bones of

the hands develop normally, but the base of the head, which is of endochondral origin, is thwarted in its growth. The face appears disproportionately small in comparison to the upper part of the head; a typical saddle nose and small jaws are usually present.

Osteogenesis Imperfecta

There are several diseases known as **osteogenesis imperfecta,** a term which, in Latin, means defective bone formation. Recently, it has been shown that the basic defects in these diseases are various mutations involving genes encoding collagen I. These defects are inherited as either autosomal recessive or dominant traits.

Collagen type I is the principal component of the osteoid; therefore, gene mutation results in abnormal osteoid formation. Depending on the extent and the form of the gene defect, the disease may begin in childhood or at puberty, and even later in life. In the most severe form of congenital osteogenesis imperfecta, the affected infant is born with numerous bone fractures. These fractures can be seen on x-ray examination while the baby is still in utero. Affected children have problems with their growth, and are frequently hospitalized for surgical repair of fractures and concomitant deformities. Conversely, the mild forms of osteogenesis imperfecta may appear late in life and cause only minor problems, such as increased susceptibility to bone fracturing.

Collagen type I has widespread distribution in the body. Thus, the symptoms of osteogenesis imperfecta are not limited solely to the bones. Many patients have thin skin, thin dental enamel (*dentinogenesis imperfecta*), and defective heart valves ("*floppy mitral valve*"). Defective collagen formation in the eye imparts a bluish hue to the sclera.

Osteopetrosis

Osteopetrosis, also known as marble bone disease, derives its name from the stone-like, thickened appearance of the bones (in Latin, *petrus* means stone). There are several forms of the disease, which may be inherited either as a dominant or recessive trait. It is thought that the primary defect is in the osteoclasts, which cannot adequately remove the bone matrix. The bones are, therefore, thick but brittle. Fractures are common because the osteons are not modeled properly and cannot withstand pressure. Expansion of the bone matrix into the medulla compresses the hematopoietic bone marrow and causes anemia. Compression of the nerves causes pain and various neurologic symptoms. Compression of the acoustic nerves may cause deafness. There is no efficacious treatment for osteopetrosis. However, newer approaches based on bone marrow transplantation may improve the symptoms of anemia. Also, the transplantation of precursors of osteoclasts may restore a balance between excessive bone formation and inadequate bone resorption.

Infectious Diseases

Bones are relatively resistant to infections, but once infections develop, it may be difficult to eradicate them. An infection located inside the bone is called *osteomyelitis,* whereas an infection of subperiosteal bone and periosteum is called *periostitis*.

Osteomyelitis

Osteomyelitis is a bacterial infection of bones. It may present as an acute infection that progresses to chronic osteomyelitis; less commonly, it takes the form of a slowly evolving, chronic disease.

Etiology. The most common causes of osteomyelitis are pyogenic cocci—most notably, *Staphylococcus aureus.* Drug addicts may develop mixed-flora hematogenous infections. Patients with sickle cell anemia are predisposed to infections caused by Salmonella. Previously, *Mycobacterium tuberculosis* was a common cause of chronic osteomyelitis of the spine (*Pott's disease*), but it is rare today. This disease produces deformities of the back (*hunchback*). In congenitally acquired syphilis, *Treponema pallidum* passes across the placenta from the infected mother to the fetus and tends to colonize the bones.

Syphilitic osteochondritis and periostitis with prominent bone deformities (e.g., "saddle nose" and "saber shins") are well-known features of tardive congenital syphilis. Although congenital syphilis is a rare disease, it still occurs in underprivileged populations.

Pathogenesis and Pathology. *Staphylococcal osteomyelitis* is the best prototype of bone infection. The infection, which usually originates in the metaphysis, typically occurs in growing children. It affects boys more often than girls, presumably because bone trauma is more common in boys.

The metaphysis is the most vascularized portion of the bone, receiving copious blood through one or more arteries. These vessels, known as nutrient arteries, penetrate the cortical bone and deliver the blood into the zone of the epiphyseal growth plate. This "direct access" facilitates the entry of bacteria into the bone during bacteremia. Once the bacteria have reached the "fertile soil" of the metaphysis, which is well supplied with nutrients and oxygen, they multiply rapidly, forming a nidus of infection. Polymorphonuclear leukocytes are soon attracted from the blood, and these cells form pus, which spreads into the adjacent portions of the epiphysis, through the medullary cavity, and through the haversian canals of the compact bone (Fig. 19-4). The pus draining from the cavity is rich in enzymes, which can lyse the bone and cartilage. The devitalized bone fragments remain in the newly formed cavities filled with pus and are called *sequestra* (because they are detached or sequestered from the rest of the bone). Reactive bone forms around the zone of inflammation as an attempt by the body to wall off the infec-

FIGURE 19-4
Osteomyelitis. The bacteria reach the metaphysis through the nutrient artery. Bacterial growth results in bone destruction and formation of an abscess. From the abscess cavity, the pus spreads between the trabeculae into the medulla, through the cartilage into the joint, or through the haversian canals of the compact bones to the outside. These sinuses traversing the bone persist for a long time and heal slowly. The pus destroys the bone and sequesters parts of it in the abscess cavity. Reactive new bone is formed around the focus of inflammation.

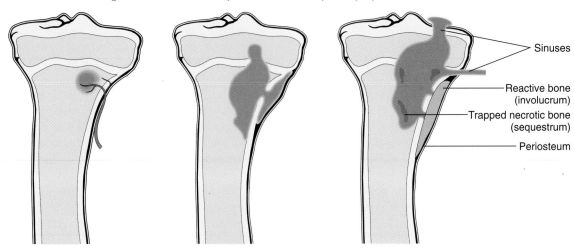

Sinuses

Reactive bone (involucrum)

Trapped necrotic bone (sequestrum)

Periosteum

tion and prevent its spread. This outer shell of new bone is called *involucrum* (in Latin, meaning "wrapper"). These changes result in deformities of the bone, predisposing the bone to fractures that heal poorly as long as there is pus in the area.

In adults, bacterial osteomyelitis occurs as a complication of bone fractures or bone surgery, or as a result of the spread of infection to the bones from the joints and adjacent soft tissues. Gangrene of the toes that is caused by diabetes is also often complicated by osteomyelitis.

Suppurative osteomyelitis must be treated with high doses of antibiotics. However, surgical drainage of the pus and repair of the defect may be unavoidable.

Circulatory Disturbances

A sudden onset of ischemia caused by disruption or complete interruption of blood flow results in bone infarcts. Traditionally, these are called **aseptic bone necrosis**. This term, coined in the last century, when most bone necroses were caused by bacteria (i.e., were "septic"), is still used for historic reasons. Moreover, various forms of aseptic infarcts of growing bones are still called by the names of the physicians who first described them. This list of more than 50 names provides some satisfaction and pleasure to name-droppers with a photographic memory, but would cause desperation among the rest of us if we tried to memorize all these eponyms. These diseases occur mostly in children and adolescents. For example, *Legg-Calvé-Perthes* disease of the femoral head, *Köhler's* disease of the lunate bone, and *Scheuermann's* disease of the vertebrae have the same pathologic substrate and are all caused by an infarction of the ossification centers of various growing bones.

Etiology and Pathogenesis. Bone infarcts may be caused by trauma, emboli, or drug-induced injury of the endothelial cells. Often, the cause of these infarcts is unknown. Traumatic fractures may disrupt the arterial and venous circulation and, thus, cause infarcts.

Nutrient arteries, and especially their smaller branches, may be obstructed by emboli of tumor cells, air emboli in caisson (decompression) disease, or microthrombi and sludges of sickle cells in sickle cell anemia.

Endarteritic occlusion may be induced by radiation therapy or cytotoxic chemotherapy of cancer.

Clinical Features. Aseptic bone necrosis is a disease of growing children and adolescents, but it also occurs at a high rate in the elderly. Certain portions of the growing skeleton are at increased risk and undergo infarction more often than others. The carpal bones are especially vulnerable because of their complex blood supply. In the elderly, the most important site of aseptic necrosis is the head of the femur. Ischemic fractures of the neck of femur, which are especially common in conjunction with osteoporosis of old age, are often incapacitating. The hip joint, which may become afunctional, usually must be replaced, as the chances of spontaneous repair are minimal.

Metabolic Disorders

Osteoporosis

Osteoporosis is a multifactorial disease characterized by an absolute reduction of the total bone mass. It is probably the most prevalent bone disease in our society. Osteoporosis, with all its complications, costs society around $10 billion per year. It has been estimated that one third of women older than 65 years of age have some minor fractures related to osteoporosis. In those older than 85 years of age, one third of all American women and every sixth man is temporarily or permanently confined to bed because of hip fractures, the most incapacitating complication of osteoporosis.

Etiology. It is customary to divide this disease into two basic forms: primary and secondary osteoporo-

Did You Know?

Spontaneous osteomyelitis that occurs without a predisposing cause has become a relatively rare disease. Most cases of osteomyelitis reported today occur after trauma or surgery on the bones. The site of open trauma, caused by severe injury or a bullet wound, typically becomes infected. Such exogenous bacteria may spread through the bone and cause osteomyelitis, which will typically delay healing of a fracture. Likewise, infectious agents may be introduced into the bone during bone surgery. Although surgery is performed under sterile conditions, 1% to 3% of orthopedic operations are associated with subsequent infection at the site of surgery. To reduce this complication, orthopedic surgeons operate in specially designed operating rooms that contain almost no bacteria in the air. The surgeons also use special dress and masks to prevent infection of their patients. Using such precautions, the best centers of orthopedic surgery have reduced the number of cases of postoperative osteomyelitis to less than 0.5%.

sis. For the time being, there are no definitive clues about the etiology of primary osteoporosis, which accounts for most cases. Primary osteoporosis is a disease of the elderly. Secondary osteoporosis may occur at any age and is related to identifiable causes (Fig. 19-5) that include

- hormonal disturbances, which are marked by an excess (e.g., hyperadrenocorticism) or deficiency (e.g., hypogonadism or diabetes) of some hormones
- dietary insufficiency caused by inadequate intake (e.g., calcium or vitamin C deficiency), or malabsorption of nutrients (e.g., intestinal disease or liver disease)
- immobilization, as in chronic diseases or following trauma
- drugs, such as anticonvulsants for the treatment of epilepsy or anticoagulants (e.g., heparin)
- tumors, such as hormonally active lesions of the endocrine glands, or metastases that destroy bone directly. (Breast carcinoma may cause osteoporosis through its hormonal effects and by metastatic spread.)

Osteoporosis often has multiple causes. For example, a postmenopausal chronic alcoholic could develop osteoporosis owing to a lack of estrogen, or excessive alcohol intake could have a direct toxic effect on bones. It also causes cirrhosis, which affects vitamin D metabolism. Moreover, alcoholics often suffer from nutritional deficiencies as well.

Pathogenesis. Osteoporosis is characterized by the simultaneous loss of the organic bone matrix (osteoid) and minerals. Although the pathogenesis of primary osteoporosis remains unknown, several determinants of bone loss have been identified. These include

- initial bone mass
- diet and life style
- hormones
- age-related changes in metabolism

Normal bones are remodeled during the entire lifespan. During the growth phase and up to approximately 30 years of age, bone formation exceeds bone resorption. However, after this, bone resorption outpaces bone formation, resulting in a net bone loss of

FIGURE 19-5

Osteoporosis. Causes of osteoporosis include genetic and hormonal factors, inactivity, and aging. Clinically, loss of bone substance results in postural changes ("widow's hump" or "dowager's hump") and fracture. The bone trabeculae are thin.

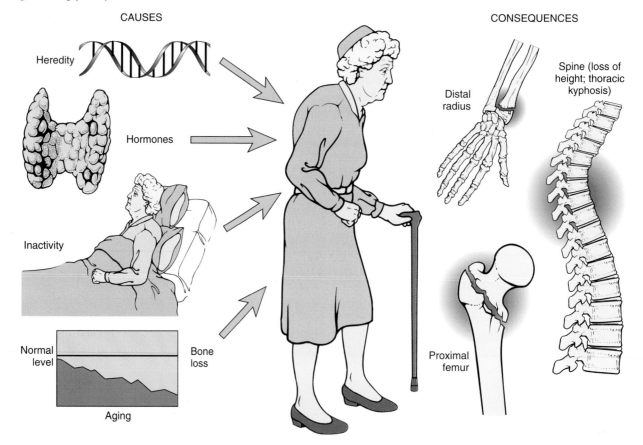

CAUSES

Heredity

Hormones

Inactivity

Normal level

Bone loss

Aging

CONSEQUENCES

Distal radius

Proximal femur

Spine (loss of height; thoracic kyphosis)

0.5 percent of the total bone mass per year. Following menopause, the bone resorption is accelerated in women three- to five-fold, resulting in a bone loss in the range of 1 percent to 3 percent. The reasons for this accelerated bone loss, which occurs over a period of 8 to 10 years, are not known, but they are believed to be related to estrogen. Estrogen replacement therapy can prevent or slow down the development of postmenopausal osteoporosis. Bone loss is less prominent in men, who do not go through menopause; however, even they develop some osteoporosis with advancing age.

Osteoporosis develops more often in gracile white women of small frame, who have a smaller initial bone mass, than in women with large frames ("heavy bones"). Men have denser bones, so their bones take longer to become osteoporotic, even if bone resorption occurs at the same pace in both sexes. Blacks generally have denser bones than whites. Bone density is greater in athletes and muscular persons, and the beneficial effects of exercise in maintaining the bone mass have been amply documented.

Dietary calcium and vitamin D are also important, and thus are added to many items included in the typical American diet to meet the minimum daily requirements. However, if the absorption of vitamin D, a fat-soluble vitamin, and calcium is impaired owing to liver or intestinal disease, deficiencies may develop.

Pathology. Osteoporotic bones are thin and brittle, and are prone to fracture. The bone loss involves both cortical and spongious bone. In type I osteoporosis, which occurs typically in postmenopausal women, trabecular bone loss predominates, occurring most prominently in the vertebrae and distal radius. Major complications of type I osteoporosis are, therefore, *crush fractures* of the vertebral bodies and of the distal end of the radius. Type II or old-age osteoporosis is characterized by a proportional loss of cortical and trabecular bone of the long bones. The most serious fractures of old age are those of the head of femur. However, none of the bones is spared. The vertebrae are common sites of microfractures, which produce wedge-shaped deformities that are most pronounced anteriorly. Multiple wedge-shaped fractures of the vertebral bodies make old people appear smaller and bent forward.

Clinical Features. The symptoms of osteoporosis are extremely variable and are often nonspecific. Vertebral fractures can cause back pain or kyphosis of the spine ("dowager's hump"). Extensive osteoporosis may reduce a person's height up to 15 cm, or 10 percent. Fractures of the long bones, such as the femur, may be incapacitating. More than 1 million

hip fractures occur yearly in the United States, and at least 25 percent of these never heal. Other bones may be affected as well. Despite a marked loss of bone substance, patients with osteoporosis show no biochemical abnormalities. Calcium, phosphate, and alkaline phosphatase levels are normal.

Osteoporosis is best diagnosed by radiographic studies. However, routine x-ray studies detect signs of osteoporosis only after a 30 percent to 50 percent reduction of bone mass has occurred. Additionally, more sensitive techniques for measuring bone density are currently available in specialized centers.

Osteomalacia

Osteomalacia (in Latin, meaning "softening of bones") is a consequence of inadequate mineralization of the organic bone matrix, caused by disturbances of either vitamin D or phosphate metabolism. Osteomalacia of growing bones is called **rickets**.

Etiology. Vitamin D and phosphates are essential nutrients. Vitamin D is derived from diet but is also synthesized in the skin under the influence of ultraviolet light. Meat and dairy products are the primary sources of dietary phosphates.

Vitamin D deficiency may result from the following (Fig. 19-6):

- *Inadequate intake,* as occurs in malnourished children in Africa. In the U.S., many foods are fortified with vitamin D, and the dietary deficiency occurs only in vegetarians or food faddists who do not drink milk supplemented with vitamin D.
- *Inadequate exposure to sunlight,* as occurs in people living above the Arctic Circle.

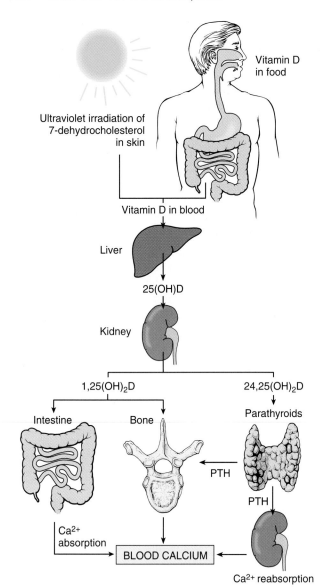

FIGURE 19-6
Vitamin D metabolism and the various pathologic processes that can interfere with it. PTH, parathyroid hormone.

- *Abnormal intestinal malabsorption,* as may occur in primary diseases of the small intestines in which vitamin D is absorbed or in biliary and pancreatic diseases associated with fat malabsorption. Because vitamin D is fat-soluble, any disturbance in fat absorption can cause vitamin D deficiencies.

Hypophosphatemia as the cause of osteomalacia may be related to abnormal absorption or excessive loss of phosphates. Malabsorption may result from intestinal diseases and is an important complication of intestinal resection. The aluminum that is present in some antacids (e.g., Maalox) may bind to phosphorus in the intestinal lumen and prevent its absorption. Parathyroid hormone (PTH) also prevents tubular reabsorption of phosphates; thus, phosphate

wasting in urine is a constant feature of *hyperparathyoidism.*

Pathogenesis. Vitamin D deficiency affects the metabolism in a complex manner, but the most important of all these changes is the reduced absorption of calcium and phosphates in the intestines. Compensatory hyperparathyroidism ensues, which leads to increased bone resorption and increased urinary phosphate loss. Loss of minerals from the bones leads to softening of bones. Loss of bone spicules provokes compensatory new bone formation. However, no calcification occurs and the unmineralized osteoid remains the primary component of the bones. Loss of calcified bone and an excess of osteoid account for the lucency of bones on x-ray examination ("osteopenia"). Clinically, the bones are soft and pliable. Fractures and deformities are typical complications.

Rickets, the osteomalacia of growing bones in children, affects bone formation. Endochondral ossification in the growth plates is most severely disturbed. This results in growth retardation, bone deformities, and fractures of long bones.

Pathology. Osteomalacia is characterized by an excess of osteoid around the calcified core of the trabeculae of spongious bone and on the endocavitary side of compact bones. Fractures are common and heal by exuberant osteoid formation. Softening of the bones may also produce deformities. These are common in children affected by rickets but are rare in adults.

Rickets causes growth retardation, softening of growing bones, and deformities. Typical *bowlegs* result from the inability of soft leg bones to carry the weight of the body. A widened junction between the rib bone and the cartilage—the costochondral junction—appears nodular and can be palpated as beads on the thorax (called "*rachitic rosary*"). Softening of the cranial bones is called *craniotabes. Dentition* is delayed and the teeth may be speckled owing to incomplete mineralization.

Clinical Features. Osteomalacia of adults is often asymptomatic, or it may cause nonspecific bone pain. Muscle weakness is common. Skeletal deformities develop slowly and are not prominent.

Rickets produces typical deformities of the legs, ribs, and head. However, many other bones are affected and the consequences may become clinically important many years later. For example, childhood deformities of the pelvis may persist and may be severe enough to narrow the birth canal and impede normal vaginal delivery of the baby.

The diagnosis of osteomalacia is based on clinical symptoms, radiographic evidence of osteopenia, and typical laboratory findings. In vitamin D–related osteomalacia, calcium and phosphate levels are low in serum, but the PTH level is elevated owing to compensatory parathyroid hyperplasia. In typical osteomalacia due to phosphate deficiency, the serum phosphate level is low, but serum calcium and PTH levels are normal.

Renal Osteodystrophy

Chronic renal failure is associated with complex bone changes (**renal osteodystrophy**), the most important of which are *osteitis fibrosa* and *osteomalacia*. These bone changes are directly or indirectly related to the altered homeostasis of calcium and phosphates in the body.

Because the kidneys cannot excrete phosphorus, the phosphate level in the blood rises. This is accompanied by compensatory hyperparathyroidism. PTH stimulates bone resorption and a release of calcium and phosphate into the blood, resulting in hyperphosphatemia and hypercalcemia.

Damaged kidneys cannot hydroxylate vitamin D and, without the active form of vitamin D, calcium absorption in the intestines is decreased.

The pathologic changes in the bones are highly variable. The total bone mass is reduced. The bone trabeculae are predominantly composed of osteoid and are poorly mineralized (*osteomalacia*). PTH stimulates osteoblasts and fibroblasts, which occupy the bone marrow (*osteofibrosis*). Increased osteoclastic activity may cause cystic changes (*osteitis cystica*). Aggregates of osteoclasts may even form small nodules, which are indistinguishable from the so-called *"brown tumors"* of hyperparathyroidism. Renal osteodystrophy may improve with kidney transplantation or following dialysis.

Paget's Disease

Paget's disease, or *osteitis deformans,* is a chronic disease of unknown origin characterized by irregular restructuring of bone that leads to thickening and deformities of bone. Turnover of bone is increased up to 20-fold over normal. It has been estimated that 3 percent of all men and women older than 40 years have radiologic signs of Paget's disease. Because the disease occurs more commonly in some families than in others and is more common in persons with certain histocompatibility antigens, known as human leukocyte antigens (HLAs), it is possible that it has a genetic basis. The highest prevalence is seen among the British and their descendants in the United States and Australia; the lowest incidence of this disease is in Orientals.

Paget's disease typically has three phases. The first *destructive phase* is marked by bone resorption. In the second *mixed phase,* bone resorption is coun-

terbalanced by new bone formation. In the third *osteosclerotic phase,* the trabeculae appear irregularly thickened and the normal compact bone is replaced by wide, sclerotic, dense bone. This bone is crisscrossed with calcified cement lines demarcating irregularly shaped osteons and the borders between the bone and incompletely calcified osteoid. This gives the bones a typical mosaic pattern that can easily be recognized on histologic examination.

The clinical features of Paget's disease vary. Many patients are asymptomatic or have only minor skeletal pain. The most commonly affected sites are the cranium, and the long bones of the lower extremities. The thickened cranial bones may compress the cranial nerves and cause headaches, hearing loss, or dizziness. The tibia and fibula are thickened and deformed ("bow-legs") (Fig. 19-7). Osteosarcoma develops as a late complication in some patients. Because osteosarcomas are rare in adults, all tumors that develop in patients older than 50 years of age presumably arise in bones affected by Paget's disease.

The diagnosis of Paget's disease is based on x-ray studies. The thickened bones show a "honeycomb" or "cotton-wool" appearance owing to irregular bone structure. Deformities and fractures are common.

Fractures

A **fracture** (in Latin, meaning "break") denotes a disruption of bone continuity caused by mechanical factors, most often by trauma. Fractures are clinically classified as *simple* if there is a single fracture line, or *comminuted* if there are multiple lines and fragments (Fig. 19-8). Simple fractures extending through the entire thickness of the bones are called *complete; incomplete* fractures are those that do not extend from one side to another. If the overlying skin is intact, the fracture is considered to be *closed,* whereas if the skin is disrupted, it is termed *open* or *compound.*

Infected fractures are also called *complicated.* Clinicians also distinguish between *traumatic* fractures, which are related to obvious mechanical injury, and *spontaneous* fractures, which occur without major external trauma. These are also called *pathological* fractures because they occur in structurally abnormal bone that cannot withstand normal outside pressure and tension (e.g., osteoporosis) or bone that has been destroyed by a pathologic process (e.g., bone tumor). Depending on the clinical situation, there are also other clinical terms for specific fractures characteristic of various diseases. *Compression* fracture of the vertebral bones is a complication of osteoporosis; linear *stress* fractures of the tibia are common in sportsmen. *Greenstick* fractures occur in children's bones, which tend to bend rather than break.

Healing of simple fractures occurs in a pre-

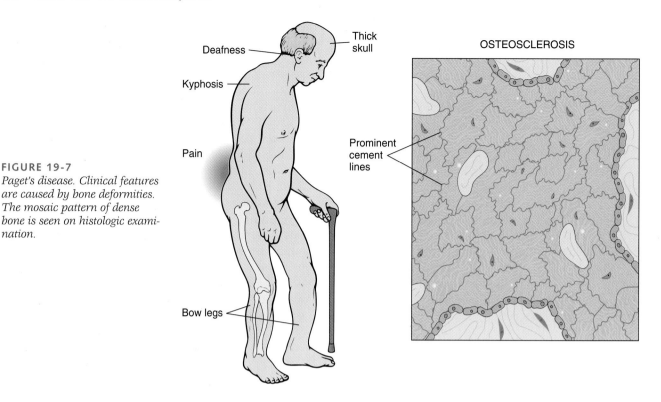

FIGURE 19-7
Paget's disease. Clinical features are caused by bone deformities. The mosaic pattern of dense bone is seen on histologic examination.

dictable manner (Fig. 19-9). Cellular events of healing of fractures have been discussed in Chapter 2.

The initial phases of wound healing require complete immobilization of the fracture site. Any movement that could disrupt the provisional scaffolds and cause additional bleeding into the site of fracture will delay the healing. Therefore, the extremity must be immobilized with casts. However, if the defect is too big, the bone must be reconstructed surgically. This usually includes the removal of necrotic tissue, which cannot be removed readily by granulation tissue, and the insertion of nails and mesh wire to hold the pieces together. Compression of two sides of the fracture promotes healing. Once the fracture heals, the final restructuring of the new bone will occur only after normal movement is reestablished. Reha-

FIGURE 19-8
Types of fractures: simple incomplete, simple complete, compound, comminuted.

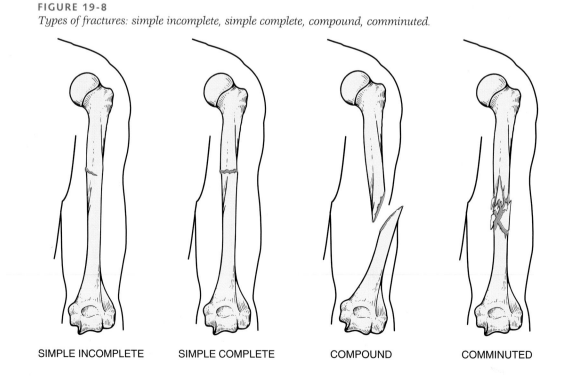

SIMPLE INCOMPLETE   SIMPLE COMPLETE   COMPOUND   COMMINUTED

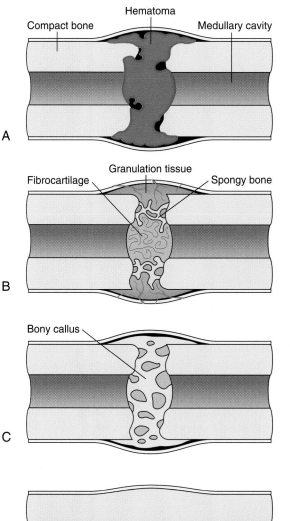

Compact bone   Hematoma   Medullary cavity

A

Fibrocartilage   Granulation tissue   Spongy bone

B

Bony callus

C

D

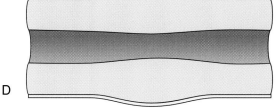

FIGURE 19-9
Fracture healing occurs in four stages: (A) hematoma;
(B) granulation tissue; (C) bony callus; and (D) remodeling.

bilitation exercises are occasionally needed to complete the recovery.

Healing of fractures depends also on the proper influx of nutrients. In malnourished persons, fractures heal poorly. Vitamins, especially C and D, and calcium and phosphorus are important for new bone formation. Infection and foreign bodies introduced by trauma impede fracture healing.

If the fracture site is not immobilized, bone formation may never occur; instead of a callus, the bone defect will be replaced by a fibrous scar (*fibrous nonunion*). The two fragments of bone may even move as in a joint (*pseudoarthrosis*). Also, if the two fragments of bone are not properly aligned, a *mal-*

union, characterized by a remarkable deformity, occurs. Such complications may be purely cosmetic, but they may also cause serious functional disturbances that usually require surgical repair.

Bone Tumors

Primary **bone tumors** form less than 1 percent of all tumors in the human body. Approximately 50 percent of these are derived from blood-forming cells of the bone marrow. These neoplasms, such as multiple myeloma and leukemia, are discussed in Chapter 9. Tumors of bone-forming cells (osteoma and osteosarcoma), cartilage cells (chondroma and chondrosarcoma), osteoclasts (giant cell tumor of bones), and primitive mesenchymal bone marrow cells (Ewing's sarcoma) account for the other 50 percent and will be discussed here. However, before these tumors are presented, it is worth repeating that the most common malignant tumors of bone are not derived from bone cells, but represent metastases of neoplasms of other organs. The most common primary sites of such malignant lesions are the breast, prostate, lung, kidneys, and thyroid. Metastases, which may involve any bone in the body, outnumber primary bone tumors by a ratio of 10:1.

Benign Bone Tumors

Benign bone tumors are composed of bone cells (**osteoma**), cartilage cells (**chondroma**), or fibroblasts (**fibroma**). Typically, these tumors appear as bumps on the outer surface of bones, or small nodules on the inside of the bone that are discovered on routine x-ray examination or because of the pain that they produce owing to expansive growth. The growing tumors are removed only if they cause pain (e.g., those on the nose or the face). Benign bone tumors do not tend to undergo malignant transformation. The only exceptions are chondromas, which occasionally give rise to chondrosarcomas.

Malignant Bone Tumors

The essential data on the four most common malignant bone tumors are summarized in Table 19-1. It should be noted that bone tumors occur more often in males than in females, and that each of them is characterized by a typical peak age incidence and anatomic location (Fig. 19-10).

Osteosarcoma is the most common primary malignant tumor involving bone (Fig. 19-11). The most important facts about this tumor are as follows:

- This bone-forming tumor most often involves the metaphysis of the long bones of the extremities.

Table 19-1 Malignant Bone Tumors

Tumor	Age (years)	Sex Ratio (M:F)	Bones Commonly Involved	Location	Treatment (5-year survival)
Osteosarcoma	10–25	2:1	Long bones of extremities (knee joint), jaws	Metaphysis	S + C (30%)
Chondrosarcoma	35–60	2:1	Pelvis, ribs, vertebrae, long bones (proximal part)	Diaphysis or metaphysis	S (variable, 20%–80%)
Ewing's sarcoma	5–20	2:1	Long bones; may be multiple	Diaphysis	C (30%)
Giant cell tumor	20–40	1:1	Long bones (knee joint)	Epiphysis	S (90%)

S, surgery; C, chemotherapy.

Approximately 50 percent of these tumors are located in the knee joint. The jaw bone is the most common short bone involved.

- Osteosarcoma is a tumor of young persons. Osteosarcomas in adults are rare, and most develop as a result of preexisting Paget's disease.
- Treatment is based on surgical resection and adjuvant chemotherapy. Without chemotherapy, less than 10 percent of affected patients survive 5 years. However, with chemotherapy, 30 percent of these patients can be completely cured, and probably many more will be successfully treated in the future.

Chondrosarcoma is a malignant tumor composed of neoplastic cartilage cells (Fig. 19-12). The most important facts about this tumor are as follows:

- Tumors originate in the axial skeleton (i.e., the bones of the trunk [pelvis, ribs, and vertebrae]) and the adjacent portion of long bones (e.g., the proximal femur and humerus).
- On the basis of the maturity and the level of differentiation of cells, these tumors can be graded (I to III). Tumors composed of well-differentiated cartilage cells have a better prognosis than those composed of undifferentiated cells (80 percent versus 20 percent 5-year survival, respectively). The grading is thus clinically important.
- These tumors usually affect adults, and have a peak incidence in those 35 to 60 years of age.
- Treatment is based on surgical resection, as the tumor cells are insensitive to chemotherapy.
- The prognosis depends on the size of the tumor and its location (i.e., whether it can be resected). Histologic grade is an important prognostic determinant. The 5-year survival varies, but is in the range of 20 percent to 80 percent.

Ewing's sarcoma is a malignant tumor composed of undifferentiated cells, the nature and origin of which have not yet been determined (Fig. 19-13).

The most important facts about Ewing's sarcoma are as follows:

- The tumor is composed of small cells that have hyperchromatic bluish nuclei and very little cytoplasm.
- The cell of origin is not known. Presumably, the tumors arise from undifferentiated stem cells of the medulla. Thus, the tumor is typically located in the diaphysis of long bones.
- Tumor cells invade the cortical bone and spread into the soft tissues of the extremities. The cortical bone reacts and new bone is formed beneath the periosteum. This imparts a "sunburst" or "onion-skin" appearance to the bones on x-ray examination.
- These tumors occur mostly in young persons (5 to 20 years of age) and are more common in males. Ewing's sarcoma is a very malignant tumor and, without chemotherapy, it is invariably lethal. With chemotherapy, 30 percent of affected patients survive 5 years.
- The tumor may metastasize via the blood. Some multiple tumors may represent multifocal primary tumors originating in distant bones at the same time.

Joint Diseases

The most important diseases affecting the joints are *osteoarthritis*, also known as degenerative joint disease, and *rheumatoid arthritis*, which together account for more than 90 percent of all cases in rheumatology practice. *Luxations* are typically treated by orthopedic surgeons and are important traumatic joint lesions. Some luxations and joint deformities are congenital. For the sake of completeness, infectious arthritis shall be mentioned, as well as gout, an important metabolic cause of arthritis. Note that tumors of the joints are rare. The only proliferative joint disease that deserves mention is *pigmented villonodular synovitis.*

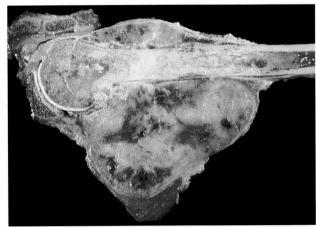

A

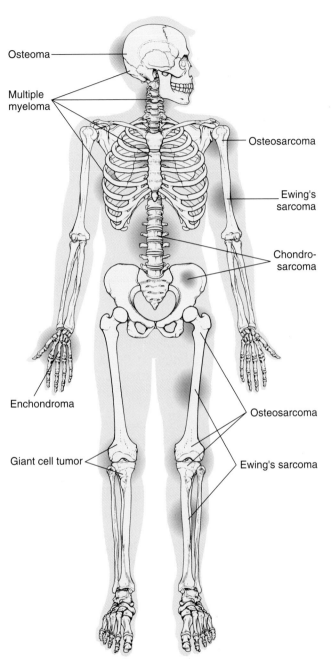

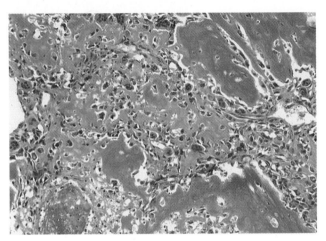

B

FIGURE 19-11
(A) Gross appearance of osteosarcoma. (B) Histologically, the tumor consists of osteoblasts and osteoid or bone.

FIGURE 19-10
Schematic presentation of the most common sites of origin of bone tumors. Most often, osteosarcomas originate in the metaphyses of long bones, chondrosarcomas arise in the axial skeleton, Ewing's sarcomas develop in the diaphyses of long bones, and giant cell tumors originate in the epiphyses of long bones. Osteomas occur most often in the skull, and enchondromas in the small bones of the hand. Multiple myelomas involve the calvaria, vertebrae, and ribs, but also other bones that contain hematopoietic bone marrow.

FIGURE 19-12
Chondrosarcoma is composed of cartilage cells.

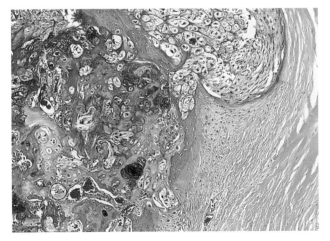

Osteoma

Multiple myeloma

Osteosarcoma

Ewing's sarcoma

Chondro-sarcoma

Enchondroma

Osteosarcoma

Giant cell tumor

Ewing's sarcoma

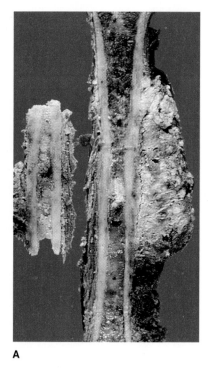

A

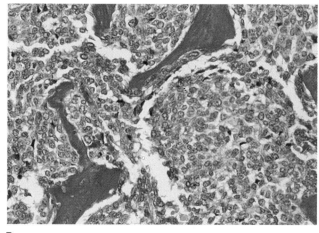

B

FIGURE 19-13
(A) Ewing's sarcoma originates in the diaphysis of long bones.
(B) Histologically, the tumor is composed of a uniform popula-
tion of small blue cells.

However, it is not clear whether this is a benign tumor or a traumatic reactive lesion of the synovium. It should be noted that the tumor known as *synovial sarcoma* is actually a soft tissue sarcoma that does not involve the joints and that, despite its name, is not derived from or related to synovial cells.

Osteoarthritis

Osteoarthritis, or degenerative joint disease (DJD), is the most common joint disease. Osteoarthritis is classified as primary or secondary. The causes of primary osteoarthritis are not known. Secondary osteoarthritis develops under conditions that stress the joint surfaces, such as repeated trauma; in congenitally abnormal joints, such as the hip or knee joints of achondroplastic dwarfs; in structurally abnormal joint structures, such as those affected by various hormonal and metabolic diseases; or in joints that are functionally damaged, as in the neuropathic joints called *Charcot's joints.* Charcot's joints are the result of a loss of sensory nerve function and abnormal gait, as in syphilitic peripheral neuropathy. Loss of sensation interferes with normal gait and exposes the joint surfaces to undue pressure, tear, and wear.

Pathogenesis. The pathogenesis of primary DJD is unknown, but most authorities favor a *"wear-and-tear"* explanation and consider the articular cartilage to be the primary site of injury. Empirical facts in support of the wear-and-tear hypothesis are as follows:

• DJD affects preferentially the weight-bearing joints, such as the knee, hip, and vertebral joints.
• The prevalence of the disease increases with age.

Almost all persons older than 65 years of age have some x-ray findings indicative of DJD.
• Mechanical instability, stress of the joint, or increased stress of the joint surface accelerates the disease.
• Abnormal connective tissue degenerates quickly, and because many of the properties of connective tissue are inherited, the disease has a tendency for familial preponderance. DJD is more common among native Americans than in other ethnic groups.

Proponents of opposing views assert that DJD is either a *metabolic* disorder or is caused by *inflammation.* The joint fluid and the cartilage removed from DJD joints have disclosed many biochemical abnormalities, but the interpretation of these findings is controversial. Abnormalities of collagen and glycosaminoglycans, the main components of the cartilage, are common, but it is not possible to state whether these are the cause or the consequence of joint changes. Inflammation of the periarticular connective tissue is prominent in many cases, especially in the fingers. Because finger joints are not weight bearing, the common involvement of these joints is taken as evidence against the wear-and-tear hypothesis and in support of the primary inflammatory nature of the disease. The beneficial effects of anti-inflammatory drugs is another argument in favor of this hypothesis. However, because these drugs also act as analgesics, the beneficial effect could reflect more a reduction of pain than an effect on the basic process that has caused joint pathology.

Pathology. Pathologic changes in the joints are not specific (Fig. 19-14). Initial changes are seen in the

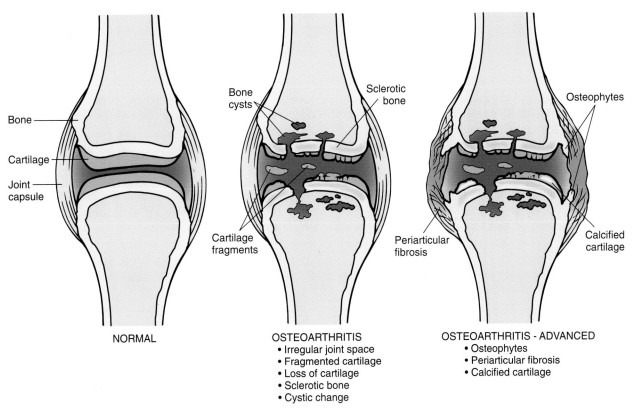

FIGURE 19-14

Schematic presentation of the pathologic changes in osteoarthritis. Fragmentation and loss of cartilage denude the subchondral bone, which undergoes sclerosis and cystic change. Osteophytes form on the lateral sides and protrude into the adjacent soft tissues, causing irritation, inflammation, and fibrosis.

articular cartilage, which shows softening, surface defects, and irregular thinning. Very early in the disease, the cartilage undergoes fibrillation, with formation of vertical clefts. The cartilage fragments are shed into the cavity, leaving behind the denuded surface of the subchondral bone. Continued pressure will induce sclerosis of the subchondral plate, which is called *eburnation* because the bone appears dense, like ivory. Bone degeneration under stress leads to the formation of cysts, which are filled with fluid, and a bone defect that communicates with the joint cavity. At the margins of the joint, spurs of new bone (*osteophytes*) form, projecting into the adjacent connective tissue. The traumatized soft tissue undergoes swelling and inflammation.

Clinical Features. Symptoms of osteoarthritis are nonspecific, and many individuals with prominent x-ray signs of disease and even gross deformities commonly have only minor disability. A list of common symptoms related to pathologic changes is presented in Table 19-2.

The most common symptom is pain, which is relieved by rest. Stiffness typically lasts 15 to 20 minutes and then disappears; this is in contrast to rheumatoid arthritis, in which it persists an hour or more after joint immobility (as during sleep or sit-

ting). All joints show reduced mobility and tend to be deformed as a result of intra-articular changes and superimposed lesions caused by faulty movement, as well as periarticular inflammation. Joint movement is often associated with *crepitus*, a grating of rough articular surfaces. Muscle spasm and contractures tend to develop with progression of the disease as the body attempts to reduce movement in the painful joint.

Table 19-2 Clinicopathologic Correlations in Osteoarthritis (Degenerative Joint Disease)

Symptom	Pathologic Findings
Pain	Osteophytes, periarticular inflammation, bone cysts, destruction, and microfractures
Crepitus	Degeneration of cartilage
Swelling and warmth	Periarticular inflammation
Joint deformation	Osteophytes, periarticular fibrosis, degeneration of cartilage, reactive bone lesions
Loss of normal mobility	Degeneration of cartilage, loose intra-articular bodies, muscle spasm

The disease may be monoarticular or polyarticular. Weight-bearing joints are most often affected, including the hips, knee joints, and cervical and lumbar spine. On the hands, the disease typically involves the distal interphalangeal, proximal interphalangeal, and first carpometacarpal joints. On the foot, the first metatarsophalangeal joints are most often affected. Symptoms depend on the duration of the disease and the anatomic distribution of the joints involved.

Hip involvement, known as *coxarthrosis,* presents with pain in the buttocks and upper thigh, and limited mobility resulting in a so-called *antalgic gait* (from *ante,* meaning "against" in Latin, and *algos,* meaning pain, in Greek). The patient walks hesitantly, trying to avoid pain.

Knee joint involvement may present with pain or crepitus as the joint surfaces erode and roughen. Deformities of the joint result in bowlegs or knock-knee deformities.

The *spine* is most often affected in the cervical or lumbar area. DJD involves primarily the interverbral apophyseal joint, which causes stiffening of the vertebral column. Radicular pain from the compression of spinal nerves is common. In many cases, it is difficult to determine what caused the symptoms—DJD or spondylosis, a degeneration of the intervertebral disks that often coexists with DJD in older people.

The *hands* are often involved. The nodular deformities of the distal interphalangeal joints are called Heberden's nodules, whereas those of the proximal interphalangeal joints are termed *Bouchard's* nodules. The former are the most common manifestations of DJD.

Feet that are affected by DJD show deformities of the toes. The most common is DJD of the first metatarsophalangeal joint, which leads to the formation of a deformity called a *bunion.*

The diagnosis of osteoarthritis is based on clinical symptoms and radiologic findings. Typical x-ray findings include narrowing of the joint space, sclerosis of the subchondral bone, cystic bone changes, and osteophytes. It is important to note that DJD produces no diagnostic laboratory findings. Joint fluid analysis may occasionally be useful. Typically, it shows no signs of joint inflammation, no bacteria, and no evidence of urate crystals. This helps to exclude inflammatory arthropathies and gout, but does not prove that the patient has osteoarthritis.

Rheumatoid Arthritis

Rheumatoid arthritis (RA) is a chronic systemic disease of unknown etiology characterized by:

- chronic, symmetric inflammation of the joints
- significant but not diagnostic laboratory findings, usually with positive serologic data suggestive of an immune disorder
- variable extra-articular manifestations

Etiology. The cause of RA is unknown. The disease affects approximately 1 percent of the world population, but is approximately four times more common among women than men. This could reflect the more common occurrence of autoimmune diseases in women, but could also be related to sex hormones; with advancing age, the sex differences become less prominent. Life style seems to have a role, as it has been shown that the disease is more common and symptoms are more severe in urban than in rural areas, and in cold climates as opposed to warm ones.

Genetic factors are important, and a familial predisposition has been noted. If one identical twin has RA, the other has a 30 percent chance for developing symptoms as well, in contrast to fraternal twins, in whom there is only 5 percent concordance. The genetic basis of the disease is supported by the fact that more than 70 percent of patients have the same human major histocompatibility locus (HLA). HLA loci are inherited as a cluster, together with several other genes located on the immune response region of chromosome 6. Certain HLA genotypes (haplotypes) are associated with autoimmune disorders, but this still does not prove that RA is an autoimmune disease.

Pathogenesis and Pathology. Rheumatoid arthritis is a systemic autoimmune disease that primarily involves the synovial joints. The inflammation begins as synovitis and leads to exudation of fluid and inflammatory cells into the joint cavity (Fig. 19-15). The infiltrates consist of lymphocytes and plasma cells, but the joint fluid contains polymorphonuclear leukocytes (PMNs) as well, albeit in variable quantities. The inflammation stimulates the ingrowth of vessels and proliferation of synovial cells. Ultimately, the exuberant synovial fronds transform into granulation tissue. This is called *pannus* because it covers the articular surfaces like a sheet (in Latin, *pannus* means cloth cover). Like any other granulation tissue, the pannus is rich in inflammatory cells that secrete lytic enzymes and various mediators of inflammation. These biologically active substances destroy cartilage and erode the underlying bone. The joints become immobilized and the intra-articular space may even become completely obliterated as the granulation tissue transforms, in subsequent stages, into collagenous scar, causing *ankylosis.* The immobilized bone on both sides of the joint undergoes osteoporosis that is readily visible on x-ray studies.

Extensive research into the pathogenesis of RA has not yet provided any definitive answers about the pathogenesis of joint inflammation. Major em-

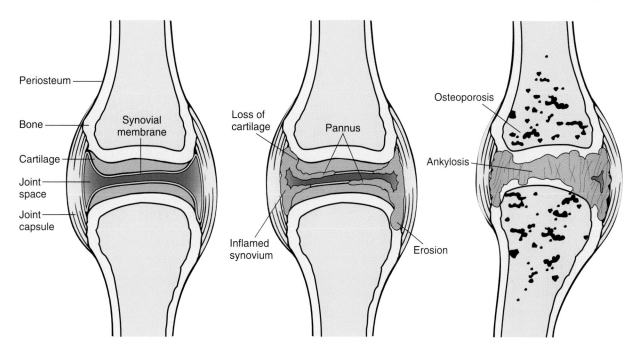

FIGURE 19-15
Schematic presentation of the pathologic changes in rheumatoid arthritis. The inflammation (synovitis) leads to pannus formation, obliteration of the articular space, and finally, ankylosis. The periarticular bone shows disuse atrophy in the form of osteoporosis.

phasis has been placed on elucidating the role of immunoglobulins, prostaglandins, and various interleukins, which promote inflammation and also exert metabolic influences on the adjacent bone and connective tissue. Drugs that inhibit prostaglandin synthesis, like aspirin and indomethacin, are known to improve clinical symptoms.

Clinical Features. The onset of RA is usually insidious, although in some patients the disease presents with an acute onset of joint pain, swelling, and redness. Symmetrical involvement of small joints is typical, but the symptoms may appear in any joint. The most commonly affected joints are the proximal interphalangeal joints of the fingers, the metacarpophalangeal joints, and the joints of the wrist (Fig. 19-16). The elbow and the ankle are also common sites of inflammation, and the large joints of the extremities can be involved as well.

RA has an unpredictable course. In some patients, it heals spontaneously after a single episode; in most people, however, it will recur or persist. In about 10 percent of patients, it will progress and cause severe disability. The onset of disease at an early age has a poor prognosis. At least 50 percent of the patients with juvenile RA develop severe deformities and systemic complications.

The most serious complications are joint deformities and contractures, which cause a loss of full-range mobility. Radial deviation of the wrist, with deviation of the fingers in the opposite direction and anterior slippage of the proximal phalanges, is known as a *Z deformity*. Other terms—like *hourglass, opera glass, swan-neck,* or *boutonnière deformity*—are used to describe the various hand deformities.

RA is a systemic disease that can cause low-grade fever, loss of appetite, malaise, and fatigue. Anemia is common. Pathologic lesions occur in many anatomic sites besides the joints, the most common of which are subcutaneous nodules (*rheumatoid nodules*) composed of central fibrinoid necrosis surrounded by macrophages and lymphocytes. These nodules are painless, small (less than 2 cm in diameter), and cause no symptoms. Rheumatoid nodules do not occur in other forms of arthritis and are, therefore, useful in the diagnosis of RA.

Internal organs often show nonspecific signs of chronic inflammation. In the lungs, this presents as interstitial fibrosis or subpleural fibrosis. Rheumatoid lung disease is commonly associated with pleuritis and pleural effusion. The eyes show scleritis. Pericarditis can develop on the surface of the heart. Rheumatoid vasculitis, provoked by the deposition of immune complexes in the walls of arteries, can occur in all organs and can cause widespread infarcts.

RA that develops in children and adolescents is called *juvenile RA,* also known as *Still's disease.* In contrast to typical RA, juvenile RA most commonly involves the large joints. It has an acute onset and more prominent extra-articular manifestations than typical RA. It also has a worse prognosis than classical RA.

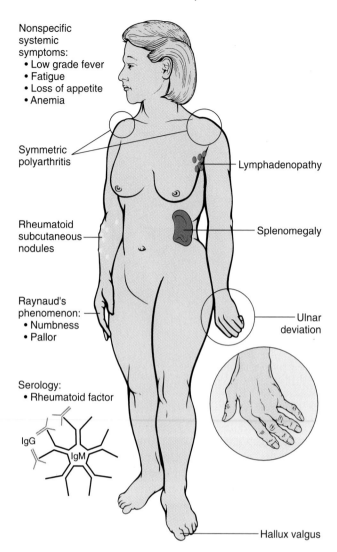

Nonspecific systemic symptoms:
- Low grade fever
- Fatigue
- Loss of appetite
- Anemia

Symmetric polyarthritis

Lymphadenopathy

Rheumatoid subcutaneous nodules

Splenomegaly

Raynaud's phenomenon:
- Numbness
- Pallor

Ulnar deviation

Serology:
- Rheumatoid factor

IgG

IgM

Hallux valgus

FIGURE 19-16

Signs and symptoms of rheumatoid arthritis. IgG, immunoglobulin G; IgM, immunoglobulin M.

The laboratory findings include a variety of abnormalities that accompany systemic inflammation and some immune disturbances, but none of these is diagnostic of RA. Rheumatic factor, an immune complex formed between a patient's own IgM and IgG, is present in 80 percent of patients. Unfortunately, these immune complexes are not diagnostic of RA, as they may be found in other autoimmune disorders, and even in normal persons. Joint fluid analysis is helpful for demonstrating intra-articular inflammation, but is most useful for excluding bacterial arthritis (in RA, there are no bacteria!) and gout (in RA, there are no urate crystals!). Other autoimmune diseases, such as systemic lupus erythematosus, must be excluded on clinical grounds because these diseases may produce the same symptoms and often cause arthritis.

There is no specific therapy for RA. However, treatment with anti-inflammatory drugs may provide relief and slow the progression of the disease.

Infectious Arthritis

Infectious arthritis results from hematogenous spread of pathogens during sepsis or from the spread of infection from adjacent bones, or from direct inoculation of bacteria by trauma or surgical procedures, or from joint fluid removal (*arthrocentesis*). Pyogenic arthritis caused by staphylococci or streptococci is rare. Tuberculous arthritis was common in past years, but is rare today. Gonococcal arthritis, a well-known complication of this sexually transmitted disease, affects less than 5 percent of infected persons who have not been treated properly.

The most common bacterial arthritis is the migratory arthritis of *Lyme disease.* Lyme disease is caused by the spirochete *Borrelia burgdorferi,* transmitted by ticks (*Ixodes dammini*). Arthritis, often in a migratory form, occurs a few weeks or even months after the tick bite, in concert with fleeting skin rash (*migrating erythema*), and nonspecific systemic symptoms. The knee joint is most involved, but other weight-carrying joints, and even smaller joints, may show signs of inflammation as the bacteremia spreads the disease, causing transient exudation of fluid into the joint cavity. Histologically, there is evidence of synovitis marked by infiltrates of lymphocytes and plasma cells. Antibiotic treatment usually eradicates the infection and cures the arthritis.

Did You Know?

Clinicians have been using a variety of terms to describe hand deformities in rheumatoid arthritis. Some of these carry the names of the physicians who first described these changes (e.g., Bouchard's nodes). Other terms are more colorful and less precise, and serve only to help one remember that hand deformities occur often in rheumatoid arthritis. This photograph shows "opera glass deformities." Even people who have never used opera glasses will remember such a term, and some patients may be elated that a fancy term was used to describe their deformity.

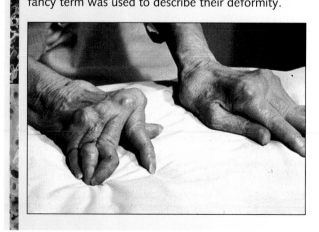

Many viral diseases cause vague pain in the muscles and joints. Such viral infections typically produce a transient, self-limited synovitis. The inflammation is usually mild, heals spontaneously, and leaves no consequences.

Gout

Gout denotes a group of diseases characterized by hyperuricemia and the deposition of uric acid crystals in various tissues, primarily the joints, subcutaneous tissue, and kidneys. Hyperuricemia is a prerequisite for gout, but not all persons who have hyperuricemia will have symptoms of gout. It should be remembered that hyperuricemia is arbitrarily defined as blood levels exceeding 7 mg/dL (415 μmol/L). By this standard, approximately 5 percent to 15 percent of the normal population has hyperuricemia. In the elderly and those who are hospitalized for various reasons, hyperuricemia may be found even more often. It is, thus, comforting to know that only a minority of people who have hyperuricemia develop clinical signs of gout.

The prevalence of gout is 15 to 35 persons per 1000; that is, only 5 percent of those that have hyperuricemia develop gout. It is not known what predisposes patients to hyperuricemia, but genetic hormonal background and environmental factors play a significant role. A significant number of patients have a family history of gout. Almost 95 percent of all patients with gout are males.

Etiology and Pathogenesis. Gout may be classified as primary or secondary. *Primary* or *idiopathic gout* may be classified as *metabolic* (i.e., caused by hyperproduction of uric acid) or *renal* (i.e., caused by underexcretion of uric acid). Most affected patients are overproducers, but the kidney's handling of uric acid is also important. *Secondary gout* is related to another disease or identifiable causes of hyperproduction of uric acid or its underexcretion in the kidneys. The main forms of gout are listed in Table 19-3.

Uric acid is the end-product of purine metabolism. The purines guanine and adenine are nucleic acids essential for the synthesis of DNA and RNA in the cell nuclei and cytoplasm. Purines are derived from ribose through several intermediate steps, the pivotal one of which is the formation of inosinic acid, which is degraded to hypoxanthine and xanthine, and finally to uric acid, to be excreted in the urine or feces. Part of hypoxanthine is salvaged by the enzyme hypoxanthine guanine phosphoribosyl transferase (HGPRT). This enzyme is missing in the inborn error of metabolism known as the Lesch-Nyhan syndrome. Children born without HGPRT develop gout early in their life. Genetic deficiency of other enzymes involved in the intermediary metabolism of purines can also cause hyperuricemia and gout.

Table 19-3 Classification of Gout and Hyperuricemia

Primary metabolic
  Idiopathic overproduction
  Lesch-Nyhan syndrome
Secondary metabolic
  Hematopoietic malignant disease
  Chronic hemolysis
  Obesity
  Alcoholism
Primary renal
  Underexcretion of uric acid
Secondary renal
  Kidney disease
  Drugs (diuretics)
  Lead poisoning

However, these defined enzyme deficiencies are rare, and in practice, most cases of gout do not have an obvious explanation (i.e., they are idiopathic).

Surplus uric acid that is produced in the body is excreted in the urine. However, many patients with gout show decreased clearance of urates in the proximal tubules. Renal excretion of urates includes filtration in the glomeruli, reabsorption in the proximal tubule, and secretion in the proximal tubules, followed by partial reabsorption in the loop of Henle and the collecting tubules. Although the exact mechanisms of renal malfunction in gout are not known, it is well established that the kidneys of most patients underexcrete urates.

Hyperuricemia leads to deposition of uric acid crystals in tissues. Most deposits are in the form of rather insoluble monosodium urate. The disease typically develops after many years of asymptomatic hyperuricemia, usually 15 to 30 years. The most common sites of uric acid deposition are the joints and periarticular connective tissue. In more than 90 percent of cases, the first symptoms occur in the tarsometatarsal joint of the big toe, which is clinically known as *podagra* (meaning foot "seizure" in Greek). Uric acid is probably released from the deposits in the joint capsule by minor trauma. It enters the joint cavity and hypersaturates the fluid. Since the feet are usually colder than the rest of the body and since the low temperature reduces uric acid solubility and promotes crystallization inside the joint, deposition of crystals occurs along the joint surfaces and the periarticular connective tissue. Uric acid crystals are chemotactic and provoke an acute inflammation within the joint (Fig. 19-17). Uric acid also activates the complement system and kallikrein, which promote inflammation, cause pain, and recruit more leukocytes into the joint. Uric acid crystals are phagocytosed by the leukocytes. However, because

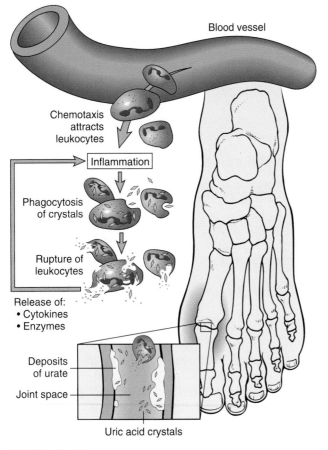

Blood vessel

Chemotaxis attracts leukocytes

Inflammation

Phagocytosis of crystals

Rupture of leukocytes

Release of:
• Cytokines
• Enzymes

Deposits of urate

Joint space

Uric acid crystals

FIGURE 19-17
Gouty arthritis. Deposits of uric acid crystals in the connective tissue have a chemotactic effect and cause exudation of leukocytes into the joint. The inflammation most often affects the metatarsophalangeal joint of the big toe.

these crystals are sharp, they pierce the lysosomes, and a release of acid hydrolases ensues. Such an attack of gout is apparently not only painful, but has all the features of acute inflammation.

Clinical Features. Gout can be classified as acute or chronic. In *acute gout,* the joint is swollen, hyperemic, and warm, and the patient cannot walk because of the excruciating pain. Systemic symptoms include fever, leukocytosis, tachycardia, and general exhaustion. The attack may last 2 to 3 days or longer, and usually subsides spontaneously. Recurrences can occur within weeks, but often occur after a prolonged period of time. Asymptomatic periods tend to become shorter and shorter as the disease progresses. *Chronic gout* is marked by less inflammation but more pronounced bone deformities. In addition to joint involvement, gout often presents with subcutaneous deposits of uric acid known as *tophi.* These are most common on the ears, the extensor sites of the arms, over the olecranon, and over the patella. Tophi are usually not painful. Histologically, they are encapsulated, contain urate crystals, and are surrounded by macrophages, lymphocytes, and giant cells. The crystals of uric acid are birefringent and can be seen in properly fixed tissue under polarized light.

Deposits of urates can be found in many internal organs, but most of these are small or inconsequential. The most significant are uric acid deposits in the kidneys. Renal failure is seen in 25 percent of patients with gout. However, not all of them have "pure" uric acid nephropathy, but a mixture of ischemic, toxic, and infectious renal lesions. Hypertension is common in gout, and it may also damage the kidneys.

Hypersaturation of urine with uric acid may lead to the formation of uric acid stones. Approximately 20 percent of all patients with gout have uric acid stones. This may cause obstructive nephropathy or predispose these individuals to chronic pyelonephritis. Gout also predisposes patients to the formation of calcium stones.

The diagnosis of gout is based on the recognition of typical clinical symptoms, and on laboratory proof of hyperuricemia. Monoarthritic joint pain involving the great toe is highly characteristic of gout. However, if there are doubts, x-ray studies may be useful in demonstrating bone erosion with tophi. Analysis of joint fluid will typically disclose signs of inflammation (i.e., numerous leukocytes and evidence of uric acid crystals).

Review Questions

1. What are the functions of bone cells?
2. Define epiphysis, metaphysis, and diaphysis, and explain why a knowledge of these anatomic term is important for pathology.
3. Compare endochondral and intramembranous ossification.

4. What are the main functions of bones?

5. What is the basic structure and function of joints?

6. What is achondroplasia?

7. What is osteoporosis imperfecta?

8. What is osteoporosis?

9. What are the main causes of osteomyelitis?

10. Describe the principal pathologic feature of osteomyelitis.

11. What are the possible causes of aseptic bone necrosis?

12. Describe typical clinical features of aseptic bone necrosis.

13. What are the causes of osteoporosis?

14. Discuss the pathogenesis of osteoporosis.

15. What are the complications of osteoporosis?

16. What is osteomalacia?

17. Explain the role of vitamin D in calcium homeostasis.

18. Compare rickets and osteomalacia.

19. How is osteomalacia diagnosed?

20. What are the main pathologic features of renal osteodystrophy?

21. Describe the three phases of Paget's disease.

22. Describe various forms of fracture of long bones.

23. Describe the healing of fractures.

24. Classify bone tumors.

25. Describe the main pathologic and clinical features of osteosarcoma.

26. Describe the main pathologic and clinical features of chondrosarcoma.

27. Describe the main pathologic and clinical features of Ewing's sarcoma.

28. What are the main pathologic and clinical features of giant cell bone tumor?

29. What is osteoarthritis?

30. Compare the facts favoring the "wear-and-tear" hypothesis of osteoarthritis with those favoring a metabolic or inflammatory origin for this disease.

31. Describe the pathology of osteoarthritis.

32. What are the main clinical signs and symptoms of osteoarthritis?

33. What is rheumatoid arthritis?

34. What is the role of hormones, genes, and autoimmunity in the pathogenesis of rheumatoid arthritis?

35. What is pannus and how does it evolve?

36. Describe the pathology of rheumatoid arthritis.

37. What are the clinical features of rheumatoid arthritis?

38. What are the main causes of infectious arthritis?

39. What is gout?

40. How common is gout in men and women?

41. Compare primary and secondary gout.

42. How does hyperuricemia lead to podagra?

43. Compare the clinical features of acute and chronic gout.

44. What are tophi?

45. What kind of urinary stones are found in persons who have gout?

Learning Objectives

After studying this chapter, the student should be able to:

1. Describe the histology of skeletal muscle.

2. Describe the neuromuscular junction and explain how the neural impulses are transmitted to the muscle.

3. Classify muscle diseases by their etiology and pathogenesis.

4. Describe the muscle changes that occur following the transection of peripheral nerve and nerve regeneration.

5. List three diseases that cause neurogenic atrophy of the muscle.

6. Explain the pathogenesis of myasthenia gravis.

7. Describe the clinical symptoms of myasthenia gravis and how these can be treated.

8. Define Duchenne type muscular dystrophy and explain the inheritance of this disease.

9. Describe the pathologic changes in the muscles of patients with Duchenne type dystrophy and relate these to the diagnostic laboratory and clinical findings.

10. List two additional muscular dystrophies and compare these with Duchenne type dystrophy.

11. List and briefly explain two metabolic myopathies.

12. Describe the histologic features of polymyositis and relate these to the clinical presentation of the disease and the laboratory findings.

13. Explain the relationship of polymyositis to autoimmune disorders.

14. List three malignant tumors of skeletal muscle and adjacent soft tissues.

Additional Key Terms and Concepts

Cerebral palsy

Myotonic dystrophy

Polymyositis

Rhabdomyosarcoma

Wallerian degeneration

Chapter Outline

Muscles
Chapter 20

NORMAL ANATOMY AND PHYSIOLOGY

Skeletal muscle is composed of striated **muscle fibers.** Each of the anatomically distinct muscles, which vary in size from the very large muscles (such as quadriceps) to exquisitely small muscles (like the ocular muscles), is enclosed in a connective tissue fascia called the perimysium. Thinner connective tissue septa branch from the epimysium, forming strands of perimysium that enclose groups of muscle fibers, separating them from one another into fascicles. Septa within each fascicle, called endomysium, are composed of basement membrane–like material that envelopes each muscle fiber individually (Fig. 20-1). This framework of stromal tissue provides support to muscle cells, blood vessels, and nerves.

The **muscle cells** are postmitotic, terminally differentiated cells that cannot divide. The regeneration of muscle proceeds from the less-differentiated reserve cells. Such regeneration is very inefficient and quite limited.

The muscle cells are specialized cells that are rich in contractile proteins (actin and myosin). In order to perform their primary function (**contractibility**), these cells have a high ratio of cytoplasm to nuclei. The muscle cells are long and extensible; that is, many return to normal length after contraction. To maintain their viability, they have many nuclei, typically located beneath the cell membrane along the entire length of the fiber. The nuclei are positioned so that they do not interfere with the contraction of the fibers that occupy the rest of the cytoplasm.

Each muscle fiber is individually innervated by a branch of the motor neuron axon. The site of contact between the axon and the muscle fiber is called the **neuromuscular junction** (Fig. 20-2). The nerve and muscle are separated from one another by a very narrow space. The nerve ending releases into this space **acetylcholine** (ACh), which acts as a neurotransmitter and binds to receptors on the surface of the muscle cell, causing membrane depolarization and thereby initiating contraction. The enzyme cholinesterase removes the neurotransmitter from the muscle receptors. This is associated with repolarization of the muscle cell membrane and relaxation.

Skeletal muscles are composed of two types of fibers: type I or *slow fibers,* and type II or *fast fibers.* In chickens, these fibers are separated from one another. The red fibers that maintain protracted contraction are found in chicken legs, whereas the white fibers designed for rapid but short movements of the wings are found in chicken breast. In humans, the red and white fibers are intermixed at random in a checkerboard pattern that is easily recognized using special histochemical techniques. Histochemistry makes it possible to distinguish between type I fibers, which are rich in oxidative enzymes, and type II fibers, which contain fewer of these enzymes (Fig. 20-3).

It is important to remember that muscle fibers are not inherently fast or slow; rather, their properties depend on nerve impulses. If a fast white muscle fiber loses its original innervation and is later reinnervated by a "slow" nerve, it will change and become slow. Such changes are commonly seen in

FIGURE 20-1
The normal muscle consists of fibers arranged into fascicles.

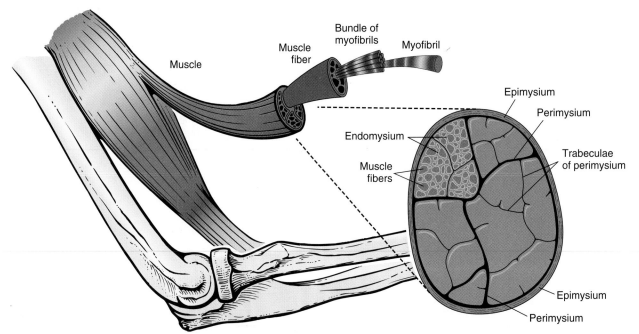

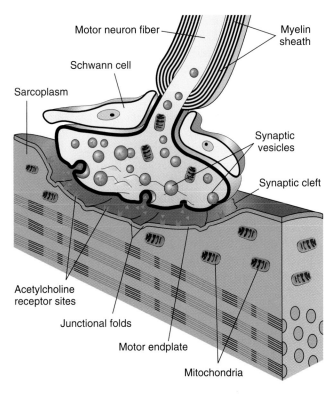

FIGURE 20-2
The neuromuscular junction consists of the nerve ending and the neuromuscular plate on the surface of the muscle cell. Synaptic vesicles loaded with acetylcholine (ACh) are released into the space between the nerve and muscle, and the ACh binds to the receptors on the neuromuscular plate.

reinnervated muscle following regeneration of transected axons.

The muscles are composed of highly specialized cells, the primary function of which is contraction. The contraction of muscles enables the body to move. Muscles are needed to breath and to maintain posture. Muscle contraction also generates heat. On

FIGURE 20-3
Checkerboard appearance of type I and type II muscle fibers in normal muscle.

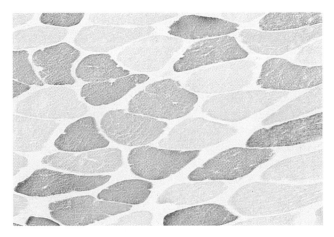

the other hand, muscles are also a **storage site** for metabolites, such as glycogen and fat. Proteins of the muscle cells can be used, under adverse conditions, as sources of energy. (Inmates of concentration camps all appeared wasted because they used muscle proteins to compensate for an inadequate diet!)

OVERVIEW OF MAJOR DISEASES

The skeletal muscles have a limited capacity to respond to injury, and the range of morphologic and functional changes in diseased muscles is quite narrow. Morphologically recognizable changes include

- adaptations, such as atrophy and hypertrophy
- cell injury, referred to in this context as degeneration
- limited regeneration
- inflammation
- neoplastic proliferation

Functionally, muscle diseases are characterized by an inability to contract adequately (*weakness*); an inability to sustain action (*fatigability*); continuous spasm (*myotonus*); or irregular and uncoordinated contraction of groups of fibers (*fibrillation*). However, the most prominent symptom of muscle disease is pain (*myalgia*).

The most important muscle diseases are:

- neuromuscular disorders
- muscular dystrophies
- myositis

Metabolic myopathies, inborn errors of metabolism, muscle diseases secondary to systemic diseases, and trauma will not be discussed. These diseases are very rare, and it is enough to know that they exist. For the sake of completeness, however, examples of such diseases are listed in Table 20-1. Tumors of striated muscles and soft tissues are also uncommon, but are described briefly.

First, let us review some important facts about normal muscles and muscle diseases.

1. *Muscle and peripheral nerves are a single unit.* Without proper nerve stimulation, the muscle undergoes atrophy. The muscle can, however, be reinnervated from the regenerative nerve. Loss of motor neurons—for example, after stroke or spinal cord injury—causes *paralysis* of skeletal muscles.

2. *Transmission of nerve stimuli from nerve to muscle is chemically mediated and depends on the binding of the neurotransmitter to the receptors on the muscular side of the neuromuscular junction.* Chemical destruction of *acetylcholine* (ACh) ((the neurotransmitter) or the blockade of receptors can impede or completely block the transmission of stimuli. Muscle paralysis in

Table 20-1 Classification of Muscle Diseases (with examples of important entities)

Neuromuscular disorders
    Neurogenic muscle cell atrophy
    Myasthenia gravis

Muscular dystrophy
    Duchenne type dystrophy
    Myotonic dystrophy

Congenital myopathy
    Carnitine deficiency
    Nemaline myopathy

Endocrine/metabolic myopathy
    Thyrotoxicosis
    Diabetes

Paraneoplastic myopathy
    Dermatomyositis

Autoimmune and infectious myositis
    Polymyositis/dermatomyositis
    Infectious myositis
    Trichinosis

Traumatic myositis (overexertion)
    Rhabdomyolysis

Tumors
    Rhabdomyosarcoma

myasthenia gravis, an immune-mediated disease, is mediated by antibodies to ACh receptor that impair the transmission of neural impulses.

3. *The function of muscle cells depends on the integrity of its primary cytoplasmic components.* A deficiency of normal structural components is best noted in hereditary muscle disease. A genetic defect involving the plasma membrane protein *dystrophin* causes muscle cell degeneration in Duchenne type dystrophy. Aggregation of tropomyosin in cytoplasmic bodies—so-called *nemaline bodies*—impairs the function of muscle cells in nemaline myopathy.

4. *Muscle cell function depends on the maintenance of transmembrane gradients in the concentration of minerals in the muscle cell and the pericellular fluids.* The hypocalcemia of hypoparathyroidism causes muscle spasms (*tetany*). A disease known as *hypokalemic periodic paralysis* is characterized by attacks of weakness caused by low serum potassium levels, which perturb the normal transmembrane mineral gradient.

5. *Muscle function depends on adequate generation of energy.* Carnitine deficiency, an inborn error of lipid metabolism, and various congenital mitochondrial myopathies are characterized by muscle weakness that can be explained in terms of insufficient energy production. No machine can function without fuel, and muscles that are inadequately supplied by energy are no exception.

6. *Many hormones affect muscle function.* Hormones regulate the intermediary metabolism and influence mineral gradients in the muscle. Thyroid, adrenal, or insulin excess or deficiency may cause muscle weakness. Lack of parathyroid hormone causes spastic contractions.

7. *Many toxins and drugs may affect the muscle.* The effect may be exerted directly on the muscle cell or indirectly through the nerve. Bacterial toxins may cause paralysis or muscle spasm. Botulism, a disease caused by a toxin from *Clostridium botulinum,* is marked by muscle paralysis. Tetanus, a disease marked by muscle spasm (tetany), is caused by toxin from *C. tetani.* Curare, a natural poison used by Indians of South America for their arrows, may cause muscle paralysis. Curare also has a medicinal use as an agent used to induce muscle relaxation during surgery.

8. *Muscle is often affected by autoimmune disorders.* Systemic lupus erythematosus, rheumatic arthritis, and dermatomyositis present with inflammatory muscle lesions. Myasthenia gravis is an autoimmune disorder affecting the neuromuscular junction.

9. *Destruction of muscle fibers is characterized by a release of muscle-specific enzymes, such as creatine kinase (CK).* This enzyme is released into the circulation and is a useful marker of muscle cell injury. Traumatic injury of the muscle, and even exercise-induced rhabdomyolysis (i.e., rupture of striated muscles), as occurs in most marathon runners, causes elevation of CK in blood.

10. *Muscle cells are relatively resistant to infections.* Bacterial infections of the muscles are rare in persons who have intact skin. Infected wounds may, however, cause the spread of bacteria into muscle. Viral infections are probably more common. Most viral infections are mild (but clinically undiagnosed) and have no residual consequences. Aches and pains of muscles during a bout of flu are the best examples of viral myositis. *Trichinella spiralis,* a worm acquired from eating inadequately cooked pork meat, may infest the muscle and cause chronic myositis.

11. *Muscle cells cannot regenerate properly.* Muscle cell loss cannot adequately be compensated for because the regeneration from the reserve cells is limited. Thus, muscle cell loss is, for all practical purposes, irreversible. On the positive side, the nonproliferating muscle cells rarely, if ever, undergo malignant transformation. The most common malignant muscle cell tumor—rhabdomyosarcoma—is very rare in adults. Rhabdomyosarcoma is more common in young persons in whom it is probably derived from fetal or growing muscle cells. Most tumors in the muscles of adults are derived from connective tissue cells. Such tumors are also rare. In medical practice, they are known as *soft tissue sarcomas.*

Neurogenic Atrophy

Neurogenic atrophy is a form of muscle cell atrophy caused by injury of the nerves, classified as follows:

- Upper motor neuron
- Lower motor neuron

The upper motor neuron is located in the central cortex. The lower motor neuron is in the anterior horn of the spinal cord. The axons of the upper neuron connect the cerebral cortical neurons with the spinal neurons. These axons run through the spinal cord. The axons of the lower motor neurons are assembled into fascicles, which form peripheral nerves, extending from the spinal cord to the skeletal muscles (Fig. 20-4).

The most important causes of neurogenic atrophy of muscle are listed in Table 20-2. For example, the lower motor neuron may be damaged in the spinal cord. Poliomyelitis, a viral disease that has been eradicated by successful immunization, destroys the anterior horn neurons and causes paralysis.

The axons are extensions of motor neurons that form peripheral nerves. Nerves are long structures

Table 20-2 Causes of Neurogenic Atrophy

Lower Neuron Injury

Spinal nerve disease
   Poliomyelitis
Nerve root compression
   Intervertebral disk rupture
   Ankylosing spondylitis
Axonal injury
   Knife wound
   Autoimmune neuritis
   Toxic injury (e.g., drug- or alcohol-induced)
Axonal branch injury
   Ischemia (e.g., diabetes, atherosclerosis)

Upper Neuron Injury

Cortical neuron injury
   Stroke
   Amyotrophic lateral sclerosis
Cortical tract injury
   Stroke
Spinal tract injury
   Trauma

and can be injured easily because they are not protected adequately by surrounding soft tissues. For example, nerves can be severed by knife stabbing. The axon can also be damaged by a toxin or by antibodies (*autoimmune neuritis*). Ischemia, most often caused by small blood vessel disease in persons with diabetes, may also damage the nerves or their axons. Overall, diabetic neuropathy is probably the most common cause of neurogenic atrophy of the skeletal muscles.

Upper neuron injury may be related to transection of the spinal cord and the damage of descending cerebrospinal tracts. This is a common consequence of car accidents or sport injuries (e.g., football injuries).

Cerebral bleeding and infarcts ("strokes") that destroy cerebral neurons are the most important causes of upper motor injury. Stroke is typically associated with a massive loss of motor neurons in the cortex. Bleeding into the midbrain and the internal capsule of the basal ganglia may damage axons crossing these parts of the brain. Paralysis of both legs is called *paraplegia. Hemiplegia* is a paralysis of the muscles on one side of the body. All of these conditions are characterized by neurogenic atrophy of skeletal muscles.

Histologic signs of neurogenic atrophy vary depending on the extent of nerve loss. This condition may present as single muscle cell atrophy or fascicular atrophy. Loss of branches of axons, as is commonly seen in diabetic neuropathy or various toxic neuropathies, is accompanied by single muscle cell atrophy. Such fibers are scattered at random throughout the muscle fascicle. They appear *angulated* and

FIGURE 20-4
Upper and lower motor neurons.

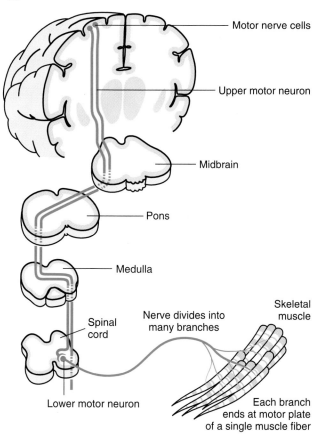

Motor nerve cells

Upper motor neuron

Midbrain

Pons

Medulla

Spinal cord

Nerve divides into many branches

Skeletal muscle

Lower motor neuron

Each branch ends at motor plate of a single muscle fiber

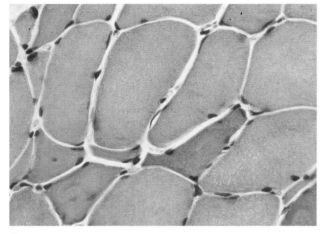

A

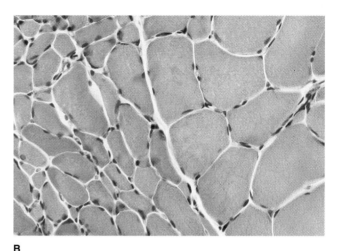

B

FIGURE 20-5

Histologic appearance of atrophic fibers. (A) Single cell muscle atrophy comprises individual, small, angulated fibers (arrows) surrounded by fibers of normal size. This is usually a conse-quence of the loss of axonal branches, as in ischemia secondary to diabetes. (B) Fascicular at-rophy involves the entire muscle fascicle (left side of the figure). It is usually related to transec-tion of a larger nerve or injury of the motor neurons in the brain and spinal cord.

are surrounded and compressed by adjacent normal muscle fibers, many of which actually undergo com-pensatory hypertrophy (Fig. 20-5). Transection of the entire nerve or its parts causes atrophy of larger groups of muscle fibers or the entire fascicle (*fascicu-lar atrophy*).

Spinal cord or cerebral injury leads to atrophy of entire muscles, as is commonly seen in paraplegic persons. Such atrophy is permanent and irreparable. Single cell atrophy may be reversed, and each mus-cle can theoretically regain its size and normal shape if it is reinnervated. In practice, this rarely occurs be-cause the underlying cause of muscle disease is usu-ally incurable.

Transection of the larger nerves also can be re-paired if the proximal part of the axon is preserved (Fig. 20-6). The nerve distal to the transection injury degenerates, together with its myelin sheath. This de-generation, called *wallerian degeneration,* progresses toward the nucleus of the nerve but stops at the first node of Ranvier proximal to the injury. From this area, the Schwann cells proliferate and lay down the path for axonal regrowth. Axonal growth typically progresses at a speed of 1 to 2 cm per week until the terminal branches again reach the denervated mus-cle. The axonal branches reinnervate the muscle, reestablishing functional neuromuscular junctions. We have all heard of "surgical miracles"—operations in which skillful surgeons have reconnected to the body severed arms, fingers, or a penis. In all these cases of reconstructive surgery, the transected nerves were sutured together and axons were allowed to re-generate.

FIGURE 20-6

Wallerian degeneration and regeneration of peripheral nerve. The nerve degenerates distal to the transection and proximally, up to the first node of Ranvier. Schwann cells regenerate and form a new sheath through which the axon will find its way to reinnervate the muscle.

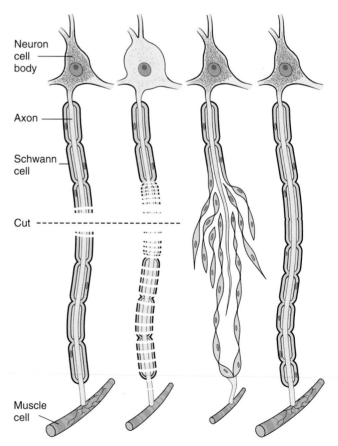

Reinnervated muscles resume normal function and appear normal on histologic examination. The only difference from the preexisting normal state is that groups of muscle fibers are innervated by a single axon. Because the axon determines the muscle type, the fibers in the reinnervated area will all be of the same type—either type I or type II—and will not be intermixed in a checkerboard pattern as before. This is called *fiber type grouping* and is typical of reinnervated muscles.

Myasthenia Gravis

Myasthenia gravis (MG) is an autoimmune disease involving the neuromuscular junction. It is characterized by impaired neural impulse transmission. MG is a rare disease with a prevalence of 1:10,000. It is more common in women than in men (ratio of 3:2). Most affected women are 20 to 35 years of age, whereas affected men are generally older (50 to 60 years of age). In 75 percent of patients with MG, especially those in the younger age group, the disease is associated with enlargement of the thymus.

Etiology and Pathogenesis. The cause of MG is not known. However, almost all patients have antibodies to ACh receptors. The reasons for the formation of such autoantibodies are not known. These antibodies bind to the receptor on the neuromuscular plate, preventing the binding of neurotransmitters and the normal transmission of nerve impulses to the muscle (Fig. 20-7).

Pathology. The striated muscles examined during muscle biopsy are histologically normal or, occasionally, contain aggregates of lymphocytes. By electron microscopy, one observes a decreased number of invaginations of the motor neural plate. It is not known how the antibodies produce these morphologic changes. The loss of invaginations correlates with biochemical and immunohistochemical data, which indicate a reduced number of surface receptor sites for ACh at the motor neural plate. Antibodies bound to the receptor can be demonstrated by immunohistochemical techniques during muscle biopsy. Antibodies are also found circulating in the blood.

Many patients with MG have enlargement of the thymus. Histologically, the enlarged thymus shows

FIGURE 20-7

Schematic drawing of the normal neuromuscular junction (A) and its simplification in myasthenia gravis (B). The antibodies bind to the acetylcholine (ACh) receptor, preventing binding of the neurotransmitter (ACh).

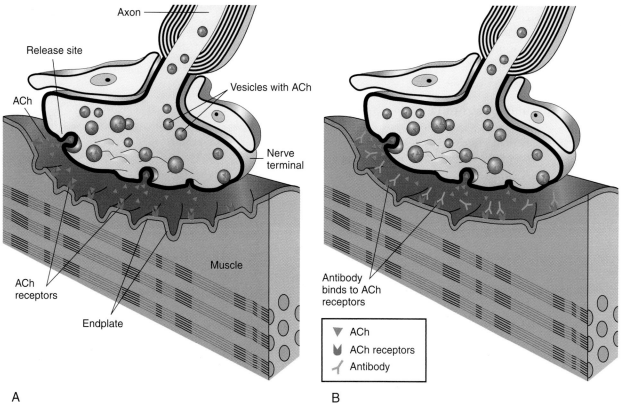

either hyperplasia or neoplasia. Tumors of the thymus are called thymomas. Most thymomas are benign, but some may be malignant.

Clinical Symptoms. MG is characterized by easy fatigability and muscular weakness. Small extraocular muscles and facial muscles are most often involved. In 20 percent of affected patients, the disease remains limited to the eye muscles. The eyelids show drooping (*ptosis*), and the patients typically complain of double vision (*diplopia*) and easy fatigability on reading. Facial muscle weakness produces a bland expression, and these patients often complain of an inability to chew. The disease spreads to the upper extremities, usually involving the proximal muscles. Finally, all the muscles may become affected, and the patient will not be able to move around. Death occurs owing to the paralysis of the thoracic intercostal respiratory muscles and the diaphragm.

The diagnosis of MG is made on the basis of clinical findings and is confirmed with specific tests, including anticholinesterase test, electromyography, and serologic testing for antibodies to ACh receptors. The anticholinesterase test is performed with antagonists of cholinesterase, like edrophonium. This drug may momentarily improve symptoms because the inhibition of the enzyme that normally destroys ACh allows the "flooding" of the neuromuscular junction with ACh to occur. Such an excess of ACh temporarily facilitates the transmission of impulses from the nerve to the muscle. Electromyographic testing, which involves inserting a needle into the muscle and connecting it with a generator of electric current, shows increased fatigability of muscles. Normal muscle fibers contract when stimulated. As the affected muscles are stimulated with consecutive electric impulses, they respond less and less to the stimulation. Antibodies to ACh receptors are, however, the most reliable sign that the patient has an autoimmune disorder that causes the symptoms of MG. Such antibodies are easily detectable in patients' blood.

The treatment of MG is symptomatic because, for the time being, this disease is incurable. Best results are obtained with drugs that inhibit the action of acetylcholinesterase. As in the cholinesterase test, this treatment increases the concentration of ACh at the neuromuscular junction. Plasmapheresis, a procedure whereby antibodies are removed from the blood, provides temporary relief, but cannot stop the progression of the disease (as reported in more than 80 percent of cases). Patients with thymic enlargement should undergo thymectomy, which is usually beneficial, especially in young women. The prognosis is less favorable for older patients and those who cannot be helped by thymectomy; 40 percent of them are dead within the first 5 years after diagnosis.

Muscular Dystrophies

The term **muscular dystrophy** encompasses a group of muscle diseases, all of which show

- genetic defects inherited as mendelian traits
- primary muscle cell pathology
- a progressive course and symptoms related to muscle wasting

The most important diseases of this group are listed in Table 20-3.

Table 20-3 Muscular Dystrophies

Type of Dystrophy	Inheritance/Incidence per 10,000	Age at Onset (years)	Muscles Involved Initially	Symptoms/Course	Associated Findings
Duchenne's	XR/2 (males only)	3–5	Girdle	Severe (death by 25 years of age)	Mental retardation
Becker's	XR/0.2 (males only)	5–10	Girdle	Mild but progressive (death at 40 + years of age)	—
Limb-girdle	AR/0.01	Variable (5–30)	Shoulder, girdle	Moderate weakness	Cardiomyopathy
Facioscapulo-humeral	AD/0.01	Variable (5–30)	Face, shoulder	Mild weakness	Hypertension
Myotonic	AD/1	Variable (10–30)	Eyelids, face, distal limbs	Variably progressive myotonia (death at 50 to 60 years of age)	Mental retardation Frontal baldness Gonadal atrophy Heart disease Diabetes

AD, autosomal dominant; AR, autosomal recessive; XR, X-linked recessive.

Clinically, muscular dystrophies are a heterogeneous group. They differ from one another with regard to

- mode of inheritance
- age of onset
- muscle groups that are initially affected
- severity of the disease
- associated findings

Muscular dystrophies may be inherited as autosomal (dominant or recessive) or sex-linked traits. The diseases may have their onset in childhood, adolescence, or adulthood. Each disease initially involves different muscle groups, and some diseases are named accordingly (e.g., facioscapulohumeral dystrophy). The diseases may be severe or mild, and some of them are associated with other organic lesions.

Because all of these diseases show essentially similar pathologic changes, histologic examination of muscle biopsy specimens is of limited diagnostic value. In all patients with muscular dystrophy, the muscle cells fall apart (degenerate), releasing typical muscle enzymes, such as CK, into the circulation. An elevated CK level in the blood is a reliable sign of muscle injury, but is not useful for distinguishing between the various types of muscular dystrophy. However, recent advances in molecular biology, which have already identified the genes for some muscular dystrophies, offer the most promising means for precise diagnosis.

Duchenne's Muscular Dystrophy

This is the most common muscular dystrophy, caused by a deficiency of *dystrophin,* an integral plasma membrane protein. Dystrophin holds together other structural proteins, linking them to the cell membrane (Fig. 20-8). This abnormality affects muscle fibers and many other cells in the body. Skeletal muscle cells degenerate and muscle weakness ensues.

The gene encoding dystrophin is located on the X chromosome. It is a very long gene. Larger or smaller parts of this gene may be mutated or deleted in muscular dystrophy. Depending on the extent of the mutation or deletion, the symptoms may vary. The milder form is called *Becker's dystrophy.* It is 10 times less common than Duchenne type dystrophy, which indicates that the disease most often presents in a severe form.

Duchenne's muscular dystrophy is a sex-linked recessive disease; thus, it occurs only in boys. The mothers, who are the carriers of the gene, are asymptomatic. In one third of the cases, however, the mother is not the carrier, indicating that a new mutation occurred in the affected male.

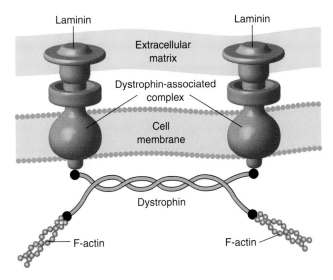

FIGURE 20-8
Duchenne's muscular dystrophy. The disease is caused by an abnormality in the protein dystrophin, which is responsible for the functional integrity of the muscle cells. It binds on one side with actin fibers (F-actin), and on the other with cell membrane glycoproteins. The gene encoding dystrophin is on the X chromosome.

Pathology. Skeletal muscles affected by Duchenne's dystrophy show typical alterations that are not, however, distinct from similar changes in other dystrophies. The histologic picture varies, and as the disease progresses, the changes become more and more prominent. Early stages of dystrophy are marked by individual muscle cell degeneration and loss. The abnormal muscle cells have an irregular shape, and their cytoplasm shows granularity, inhomogeneous staining, or vacuolization and centrally located nuclei. There is progressive muscle cell loss associated with compensatory hypertrophy of viable fibers, and an ingrowth of fibrous tissue and fat cells, which replace the lost fibers. Scavenger macrophages involved in the removal of dead muscle cells may be present. Scattered regenerating muscle fibers may be seen as well, but regeneration is inefficient. With progression of the disease, the entire muscle fascicles are gradually lost and replaced by fibrous tissue and fat cells. Severe wasting of skeletal muscles leads to skeletal deformities. The loss of respiratory muscles is accompanied by difficulties with breathing and recurrent pneumonias. Respiratory insufficiency is the main cause of death in affected individuals.

Clinical Features. Symptoms of Duchenne's dystrophy appear in preschool children, and are caused by a weakness of the weight-carrying muscles of the pelvic girdle and lower extremities. Affected boys have difficulty getting up from a squatting position and must use their arms to lift the body (Fig. 20-9). During this effort, they are typically moving their

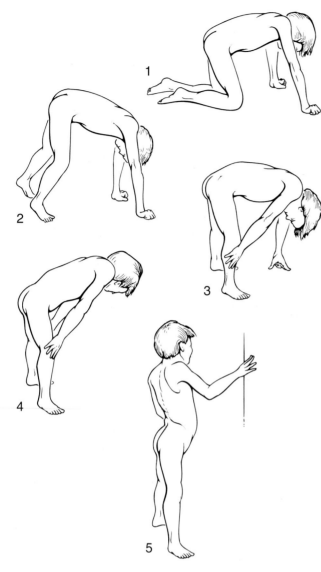

FIGURE 20-9
The clinical diagnosis of Duchenne's dystrophy is made on the basis of a neurologic examination. If a boy with this disease is in a squatting or "all-fours" position and is asked to rise, he will not be able to get up because of the weakness of the pelvic girdle muscles. He will use his arms to raise his body.

hands up their legs, as if climbing a tree. The gait is first waddling, and very soon becomes completely uncontrollable. The disease rapidly progresses, causing deterioration of all muscle functions.

The weakened legs become deformed and cannot be kept straight. By school age, most of these children need braces and often cannot walk on their own. Contractures and deformities of the extremities and the trunk inevitably develop, and by the age of 10 to 12 years, these boys are confined to a wheelchair. Their general health deteriorates because of frequent pulmonary infections that follow aspiration of food during feeding. Symptoms pertaining to other organ systems gradually appear as well. Myocardial weakness may produce signs of heart failure. Ane-

mia reflects red blood cell abnormalities. All affected children have reduced intelligence, and one third of them are severely mentally impaired. Even with the best health care, early death cannot be prevented, and it usually occurs in late teens or early 20s.

The diagnosis of Duchenne's dystrophy is made on the basis of typical clinical findings, the hereditary nature of the disease, and supporting laboratory evidence. CK is released from degenerating muscle, so CK blood levels are elevated. The deficiency of *dystrophin,* the protein encoded by the defective gene, can be demonstrated by molecular biologic techniques. This test can also be performed on fetal cells obtained by chorionic villus biopsy or amniocentesis before birth.

Other Dystrophies

Other dystrophies are less common than Duchenne's dystrophy (see Table 20-3). Note that these dystrophies are generally milder and present later in life than Duchenne's dystrophy. *Becker's dystrophy,* a mild form of Duchenne's dystrophy, is related to the same gene and protein defect. These two dystrophies, however, do not occur in the same families. The symptoms of Becker's dystrophy appear later in life and are generally milder. Nevertheless, the disease has a progressive course and all patients die in their late 40s or 50s.

The symptoms of *limb-girdle* and *facioscapulohumeral dystrophy* are variable. The former is inherited as an autosomal recessive trait, whereas the latter is an autosomal dominant trait. Clearly, these diseases are caused by different gene defects, unrelated to one another or to the dystrophin gene. The proteins encoded by these defective genes have not yet been isolated.

Myotonic dystrophy is the second most common genetic muscle disease, being almost as common as Duchenne's dystrophy. It is inherited as an autosomal dominant gene; thus, it affects males and females at the same rate. The symptoms appear in adulthood. Muscle wasting is relentless and is typically associated with mental deterioration and diabetes. Frontal baldness and testicular atrophy are seen in men.

In contrast to other dystrophies, which show only muscle weakness, myotonic dystrophy is characterized by myotonia. Myotonic muscles can contract, but they remain contracted for some time—that is, they cannot relax immediately. For instance, when such a patient shakes hands with somebody, the hand is held tightly in position, even after the other person has withdrawn the hand. Because of the weakness of the ocular muscles in these patients, the eyelids droop. Facial muscle weakness accounts for the typical "hatchet face" appearance of those affected. Myotonic dystrophy is a multisystemic disease, and premature death (usually in the 50s) is attributable either to complications of diabetes or to heart disease.

Congenital Myopathies

This group of diseases comprises a slew of rare disorders, including inborn errors of lipid metabolism (e.g., carnitine deficiency) and glycogen metabolism (e.g., glycogenosis type II, so-called Pompe disease), characterized by multisystemic involvement. It also includes diseases limited to the muscles, such as nemaline myopathy or central core myopathy. Although these are rare diseases, from time to time, the practitioner may see a child who cannot move and has flaccid limbs. It is important to remember that this *floppy child syndrome* may have a genetic basis. The mother needs to understand that the baby's disease is not related to some mishap in pregnancy, and that genetic counseling may be indicated. Furthermore, such diseases must be distinguished from *cerebral palsy.*

Cerebral palsy is the most common form of muscle weakness in children. Pathologically, it is an

Myotonic dystrophy affects the muscles of the entire body. Atrophy of the face produces a peculiar look, referred to as the "hatchet face." (Photo courtesy of MEDCOM.)

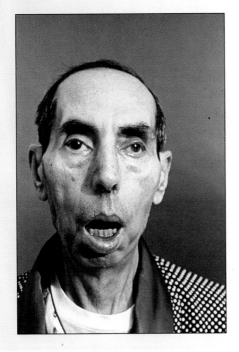

Congenital myopathies cause generalized muscle weakness. If lifted, affected infants cannot hold up their heads. Colloquially, these diseases are known under the name of "floppy infant syndrome." (Photo courtesy of MEDCOM.)

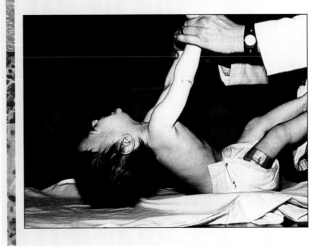

upper neuron disease; it is mentioned here because, in its severe form, it may present as floppy child syndrome. The muscular atrophy, which varies in extent, is related to developmental defects of the motor cortex in the central nervous system. The cause of cerebral changes is not known. It seems that they are caused by prenatal brain injury, rather than birth-related cerebral trauma, as previously held. The nature of the intrauterine brain injury is poorly understood. Neurogenic atrophy of muscles impairs the ability of the child to move. Many children are confined to a life in a wheelchair and develop secondary deformities. In the worst cases, they are unable to walk at all. However, there are also many children, born with a milder form of disease, who can be rehabilitated and function almost normally.

Acquired Myopathies

This term is used to denote nonspecific muscle weakness secondary to some identifiable disease. The term myopathy—which in translation from the Greek means muscle ailment—is in itself noncommittal. Many metabolic and hormonal diseases (e.g., diabetes or thyroid disease) and autoimmune diseases (e.g., rheumatoid arthritis) can cause muscle weakness.

The pathogenesis of acquired myopathies and their course are highly heterogeneous. In thyrotoxicosis, the high metabolic rate reduces the muscle stores of nutrients, whereas in hypothyroidism, the entire metabolism, including the energy-generating metabolism of muscles, is sluggish. *Myopathia rheumatica,* a common diagnosis in persons with rheumatoid arthritis, is probably secondary to rheumatic joint disease. Muscle biopsy reveals only minor and nonspecific changes in all of these diseases. Electromyography is not diagnostic either.

Diabetic Myopathy

Diabetes, a disease of the small blood vessels (microangiopathy), is associated with chronic hypoperfusion of muscles with blood. Diabetes also affects the peripheral nerves and causes neurogenic muscle atrophy and weakness. The disturbances of the intermediary metabolism of carbohydrates and lipids, caused by insulin deficiency or resistance, also adversely influence muscle function. Diabetic myopathy has at least three causes, including a vascular, neurogenic, and metabolic component. Muscle biopsy is rarely performed, as it usually contributes little to the diagnosis. Histologically, the muscle may show focal atrophy. The small blood vessels have thickened walls. The nerves may show some loss of axons.

Cancer Myopathy

Acquired myopathy is a common *paraneoplastic syndrome.* Tumors may produce muscle weakness through several mechanisms. For example, antibodies to tumor antigens may incite an immune-mediated inflammation. Some tumors share common antigens with muscle and skin, and the antibodies to these antigens may cause dermatomyositis or polymyositis. Muscle weakness without any inflammation may be found in other patients. In practice, paraneoplastic myopathy is treated symptomatically with analgesics and muscle relaxants. Muscle biopsy is rarely performed in these patients, and the pathologic basis of paraneoplastic myopathy often remains undetermined.

Myositis

Myositis is a term used to describe inflammatory muscle diseases, which are divided into two major groups: infectious myositis and myositis caused by immune mechanisms. Inflammation usually involves more than one muscle; therefore, the disease is called **polymyositis.** The most important forms of myositis are listed in Table 20-4.

Infectious Myositis

Infectious myositis may be caused by bacteria, viruses, protozoa, or worms. Isolated infectious myositis is rare except in patients with complicated

Table 20-4 Classification of Myositis (with examples of common forms)

Infectious Myositis
Pyogenic bacteria (e.g., staphylococcal sepsis)
Anaerobic bacteria (e.g., gas gangrene secondary to *Clostridium perfringens*)
Virus (e.g., Coxsackie virus myopathy)
Protozoa (e.g., *Toxoplasma gondii* acquired from cats)
Worms (e.g., Trichinella from raw pork meat)
Immune Disorders
Polymyositis
Dermatomyositis
Systemic lupus erythematosus
Sarcoidosis

wounds. Systemic diseases affect the muscles, but the symptoms of myositis are usually overshadowed by other, more serious clinical findings. Pyogenic cocci may be blood-borne and may form an abscess in the muscle. Infected emboli detached from cardiac valves in endocarditis may lodge in the muscle, also causing an *abscess.* Local extension of bacterial infection of the pharynx into the muscles of the neck causes a suppurative myositis and soft tissue gangrene known as *Ludwig's angina.* Ludwig's angina is a very serious disease that still has a high mortality. *Gas gangrene,* caused by *C. perfringens,* is an important complication of wound infections marked by necrosis of muscles and formation of air bubbles in the tissues. Infected wounds are also a source of tetanus infection. Tetanus toxin causes spastic contractions of all muscles, even those at a distance from the site of infection. Tetanus is invariably lethal. Because there is no treatment for tetanus, it is essential that everyone be immunized against tetanus toxin early in life. A booster dose of vaccine is given every 10 to 20 years.

Viral infections are often associated with muscle pain (*myalgia*). It is not known whether myalgia is attributable to invasion of muscle cells by viruses or to inflammation in the interstitial spaces or the connective tissue. Coxsackie virus has a propensity for invading muscle cells and is the best known cause of viral myalgia. Both cardiac and skeletal muscles are affected. One can assume that the chest wall pain in patients presenting with Coxsackie virus myocarditis is caused by invasion of striated muscles with the same virus.

Trichinella spiralis is a worm that may be ingested in raw or inadequately cooked pork meat. The worm has a tendency to invade striated muscles and cause localized myositis (Fig. 20-10).

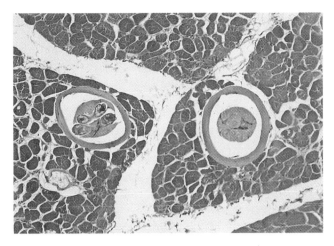

FIGURE 20-10
Trichinosis of the muscle. The encysted parasite is seen surrounded by normal muscle fibers.

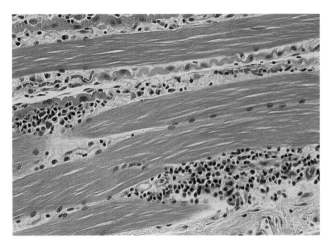

FIGURE 20-11
Polymyositis. The necrotic muscle cells are surrounded by an inflammatory infiltrate of macrophages and lymphocytes.

Immune Myositis

Immune myositis occurs in several forms, including the following:

- *Polymyositis,* which is limited to muscles
- *Dermatomyositis,* in which the inflammation is not limited to the muscles, but may involve other organs as well. Skin changes are prominent.
- *Myositis of systemic lupus erythematosus.* This form of myositis is usually overshadowed by other more serious symptoms of this disease, which is a systemic disease caused by a type III hypersensitivity reaction. The muscle disease, like the other symptoms, is caused by the deposition of immune complexes in vessel walls.
- *Sarcoidosis,* which is a systemic disease caused by a cell-mediated immunity type IV hypersensitivity reaction and characterized by granuloma formation

Pathology. Polymyositis or dermatomyositis is marked by chronic inflammation of the muscles. Histologically, the fascicles are infiltrated with lymphocytes, macrophages, and occasionally, plasma cells (Fig. 20-11). The infiltrated muscle shows reactive changes and focal loss of muscle fibers. Destruction of muscle fibers is associated with attempts of regeneration, hypertrophy of unaffected fibers, and intrafascicular fibrosis.

In systemic lupus erythematosus, the inflammation of the muscles is most prominent around the vessels. Narrowing of the small arteries causes atrophy of muscle cells, typically at the periphery of muscle fascicles (*perifascicular atrophy*). In sarcoidosis, the muscles are infiltrated with epithelioid histiocytes, giant cells, and lymphocytes arranged into noncaseating granulomas.

Clinical Features. The clinical diagnosis of polymyositis is not always easily established because most symptoms are nonspecific. Symptoms typically begin insidiously, and include pain, some muscle weakness, and difficulty moving. The proximal parts of the extremities are more often involved than the distal parts. In general, this helps to distinguish polymyositis from neurogenic muscle diseases, which are more prominent distally. Symptoms of systemic diseases and internal organ involvement, such as problems with swallowing (owing to neck muscle weakness!), may be helpful hints. The lilac blue rash ("heliotropic rash") of the upper lids is a helpful diagnostic finding typical of dermatomyositis.

The laboratory findings may be nonspecific. However, elevation of CK levels is invariably present, and represents the best evidence of muscle disease. Abnormal laboratory findings indicative of immune disorders are also common. For example, many patients have antinuclear antibodies (ANAs). A search for cancer that could be the cause of polymyositis should be included in the evaluation of older patients. Electromyography is useful. In typical cases, it shows so-called "myopathic" changes, which are distinctly different from those in neurogenic muscular atrophy or myasthenia gravis. Muscle biopsy provides the definitive diagnosis.

The treatment of polymositis and dermatomyositis includes corticosteroids and immunosuppressive drugs that are used for similar immune disorders. The response to therapy and the prognosis cannot be predicted, but in many cases, the disease has a prolonged course.

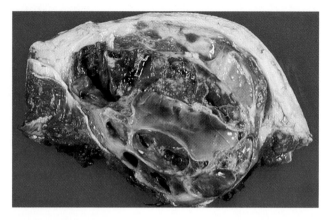

FIGURE 20-12
Soft tissue sarcoma. The tumor is located in the soft tissue of the extremity.

Tumors of Muscles and Soft Tissues

Neoplasms of skeletal muscles and soft tissues may be benign or malignant. These tumors are rare. Nevertheless, every year, approximately 6000 malignant tumors of striated muscle and the soft tissues are diagnosed in the United States.

Benign tumors, such as fibromas, lipomas, or hemangiomas, are of limited clinical significance. Malignant tumors, classified as *sarcomas,* are more important. These tumors invade local tissues (Fig. 20-12) and metastasize to distant sites, most notably, the lungs.

Overall, the most common tumor is *rhabdomyosarcoma,* which originates from striated muscle cells. It has a peak incidence in childhood. Tumors often occur on the arms and legs, but may develop in the trunk muscles as well. In adults, rhabdomyosarcomas tend to originate more often from small muscles, like retro-orbital eye muscles, than from the large muscles of the extremities.

Other soft tissue sarcomas are less common (Table 20-5). *Malignant fibrous histiocytoma* (MFH) is a tumor of undifferentiated connective tissue cells. These cells are pleomorphic and resemble fibroblasts and histiocytes. MFH occurs in middle-aged and older persons, and is actually the predominant soft tissue sarcoma in adults. *Synovial cell sarcoma* is a tumor affecting older teenagers and young adults. Its name was coined under the wrong assumption that the tumor originated from synovial cells in the joints. The cell of origin of synovial cell sarcomas is not known. The tumor cells appear undifferentiated, but may differentiate into epithelial gland–like cells. *Liposarcoma,* the second most common sarcoma of adulthood, is composed of malignant fat cells. *Leiomyosarcoma* is composed of smooth muscle cells, and probably originates from smooth muscle cells of the blood vessels.

There are many other histologic forms of soft tissue sarcoma. It is important to remember that the prognosis of these tumors depends to some extent on their histologic type, but primarily on their size and location. Small tumors close to the skin have a good prognosis and are curable by surgical resection. Tumors that are large and deeply seated have a less favorable prognosis, and surgical treatment usually requires follow-up radiation therapy and chemotherapy. Even so, only 40 percent of affected patients survive 5 years.

Table 20-5 Malignant Tumors of Soft Tissues

Tumor	Cell of Origin	Most Common Sites	Age (years)
Rhabdomyosarcoma	Striated muscle	Various sites	5–10
Malignant fibrous histiocytoma	Mesenchymal stem cell*	Leg, arm, retroperitoneum	40–60
Synovial sarcoma	Mesenchymal stem cell*	Leg	10–40
Liposarcoma	Fat cell	Leg, retroperitoneum	40–60
Leiomyosarcoma	Smooth muscle	Retroperitoneum	40–60
Angiosarcoma	Blood vessel cells	Head and neck	30–50

*The hypothetical mesenchymal stem cell has not been fully characterized, and the origin of synovial sarcoma remains controversial. The names for these tumors are also misleading. Malignant fibrous histiocytoma is not derived from histiocytes. Synovial sarcoma does not originate from the synovial lining of joints.

Review Questions

1. Compare muscle fibers with myofibrils, and fast muscle fibers with slow fibers.
2. How are nerves connected with striated muscle cells?
3. Classify muscle diseases.
4. What are the most important causes of neurogenic muscle atrophy?
5. Compare neurogenic atrophy caused by upper and lower motor neuron disease.
6. Compare paraplegia and hemiplegia.
7. Compare the histologic features of single cell and fascicular atrophy of muscle.
8. Explain wallerian degeneration.
9. What is myasthenia gravis?
10. What is the role of antibodies in the pathogenesis of myasthenia gravis?
11. Which diseases are classified as muscular dystrophies and how do they differ one from another?
12. How are Duchenne's and Becker's dystrophy related to the gene encoding dystrophin?
13. What are the differences between Duchenne's and Becker's dystrophy?
14. Correlate the pathologic and clinical features of Duchenne's dystrophy.
15. What are the clinical features of myotonic dystrophy?
16. What are the possible causes of congenital myopathies?
17. What is cerebral palsy?
18. Give examples of acquired myopathies.
19. What is myositis?
20. Compare infectious myositis with immune myositis.
21. Correlate the pathologic features of polymyositis with the clinical and laboratory findings in this disease.
22. List the most important malignant tumors of soft tissues.

Learning Objectives

After reading this chapter, the student should be able to:

1. Describe the basic anatomy of the nervous system.

2. Describe the morphology and function of the principal cells of the nervous system: neurons, astroglia, oligodendroglia, microglia, and ependymal cells.

3. List the principal functions of the cerebral cortex, basal ganglia, pons, medulla oblongata, cerebellum, and spinal cord.

4. Describe the pathogenesis of dysraphic malformations of the central nervous system and list three typical lesions.

5. Describe the main cerebrospinal lesions caused by trauma.

6. Compare epidural, subarachnoid, and subdural hematoma.

7. Discuss the causes and pathology of cerebrovascular accidents (strokes).

8. Describe the circulation of the cerebrospinal fluid and the pathogenesis of hydrocephalus.

9. Describe the route of infections of the central nervous system and the pathology of meningitis, encephalitis, and cerebral abscess.

10. Describe the main neuropathologic features of AIDS-related encephalopathy.

11. Define multiple sclerosis, discuss its pathogenesis, and describe the principal neuropathologic findings of this disease.

12. Describe the neuropathology of alcoholism.

13. Define Alzheimer's disease, describe the main pathologic findings in the brain, and correlate these with the clinical symptoms of this disease.

14. Describe the pathology of Parkinson's disease and Huntington's disease and correlate the pathologic findings with typical symptoms.

15. List the five most common brain tumors and describe their pathologic and clinical features.

Additional Key Terms and Concepts

Creutzfeldt-Jakob disease

Encephalitis

Epilepsy

Huntington's disease

Meningitis

Psychosis

Stroke

Wernicke-Korsakoff syndrome

Chapter Outline

The Nervous System
Chapter 21

NORMAL ANATOMY AND PHYSIOLOGY

The nervous system consists of two interrelated parts: the **central nervous system** (CNS), which comprises the brain and the spinal cord, and the **peripheral nervous system,** which includes the peripheral nerves and autonomic ganglia. The nervous system is closely interrelated with the endocrine system with which it regulates and integrates numerous body functions. The nervous system is also closely interlinked with the skeletal muscles, the function of which depends critically on proper innervation.

The CNS consists of the brain and the spinal cord (Fig. 21-1). The **brain** comprises the cerebrum, cerebellum (the "little brain"), and brain stem, which can be further subdivided into the midbrain, pons, and the medulla oblongata. The cerebrum, which represents the largest part of the brain, is organized into two hemispheres which, morphologically, appear identical; nevertheless, one of them is dominant over the other. The hemispheres are connected through a number of commissures, the most prominent of which is the corpus callosum.

The external surface of the brain is arranged into gyri which are separated from one another by invaginations called the sulci. On cross section, the brain forming the gyri is seen to be composed predominantly of gray matter, also known as cortex. The brain tissue beneath the cortex appears white and is called the white matter. The deep parts of the brain also contain gray areas, which form the basal ganglia, thalamus, and hypothalamus. The cortex and subcortical gray matter are composed of numerous neurons

and support cells. The axons emanating from the nerve cell bodies extend into the white matter, where they become myelinated. Myelinated axons extend from the white matter into other parts of the brain and into the spinal cord.

The **cerebrum** has four major lobes, known as the frontal, parietal, temporal, and occipital lobes. Each of these lobes has a special function. The frontal lobe primarily controls motor functions, but it also regulates behavior, emotions, and higher intellectual functions. The parietal lobe has primarily sensory functions. The occipital lobe is the seat of the visual center. The temporal lobe has an important role in hearing and smelling. The basal ganglia supply inhibitory stimuli to skeletal muscles, coordinate skeletal muscle contractions, and block unwanted muscle contractions. The thalamus is an important center for integrating sensory stimuli and is an important determinant of consciousness. The hypothalamus serves as a crossroad that connects various parts of the brain; it also regulates many body functions. The centers for regulation of temperature, heart rate, blood pressure, thirst, appetite, and many others are located in the hypothalamus. Moreover, the hypothalamic centers are the source of the neurosecretory substances that stimulate the pituitary to produce various trophic hormones regulating the function of other endocrine glands.

The **midbrain, pons,** and **medulla oblongata** are parts of the brain that contain numerous myelinated nerve bundles connecting the brain with the spinal cord. These structures also contain important centers that regulate elementary body functions. For

FIGURE 21-1

Normal central nervous system. (From Applegate EJ: The anatomy and physiology learning system: textbook. Philadelphia: WB Saunders, 1995:168.)

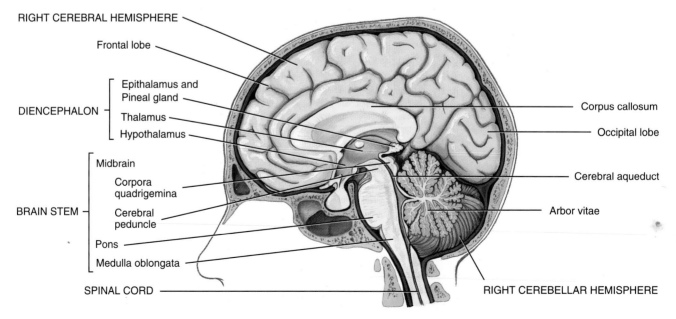

RIGHT CEREBRAL HEMISPHERE

Frontal lobe

DIENCEPHALON
- Epithalamus and Pineal gland
- Thalamus
- Hypothalamus

BRAIN STEM
- Midbrain
- Corpora quadrigemina
- Cerebral peduncle
- Pons
- Medulla oblongata

SPINAL CORD

Corpus callosum

Occipital lobe

Cerebral aqueduct

Arbor vitae

RIGHT CEREBELLAR HEMISPHERE

example, the midbrain contains the visual and auditory reflex centers, whereas the medulla oblongata contains vital centers, such as the cardiac, vasomotor, and respiratory centers.

The **cerebellum** is the major regulator of motor activities. It controls the maintenance of balance, regulates the tone of muscles, and coordinates voluntary movement. The cerebellum receives sensory input from the spinal cord and vestibular organ of the inner ear, as well as motor impulses from the cerebral cortex. These neural signals are integrated in the cerebellum and transmitted to the skeletal muscles to coordinate their function. Damage of the cerebellum affects the coordination of limb and eye movements.

The **spinal cord** consists of gray matter and white matter. In contrast to the brain, the gray matter of the spinal cord is located internal to the white matter around the central canal. The gray matter has a butterfly-like shape on cross section, with anterior and posterior horns that consist of neurons and unmyelinated nerve fibers. The neurons of the anterior horn give rise to peripheral nerves, which extend to the muscles and carry motor impulses. The white matter of the spinal cord consists of myelinated nerve fibers representing the descending motor tracts or ascending sensory tracts. The motor tracts, such as the corticospinal tracts, are located in the anterior and lateral white matter. These myelinated nerves represent axonal extensions of cortical and subcortical neurons of the brain known as the upper motor neurons. Axons of the cerebral nerves connect with distal neurons in the anterior horn of the spinal cord called the lower motor neurons. The sensory spinal tracts, which are located predominantly in the posterior columns, represent the axonal extension of neurons located in the spinal ganglia. Spinal ganglia are located external to the spinal cord, to which they are connected by the dorsal roots.

The *peripheral nervous system* consists of nerves emanating from the CNS and the autonomic nervous system. Each spinal nerve has an anterior root and a posterior root. The ventral root consists of the axons of the lower motor neuron, whereas the dorsal root is composed of spinal ganglia and their cytoplasmic extensions. The sensory and motor neurons form a circuit that is important for reflex movements.

The *autonomous nervous system* regulates involuntary (autonomic) body functions. It consists of a sympathetic and a parasympathetic part. The nerve cells of the autonomic nervous system are located in the peripheral ganglia, which may be paravertebral or located at a distance from the CNS (collateral ganglia). Like the neurons in the CNS, autonomic nerve cells have axons that innervate various internal organs. The autonomic nervous system regulates movement within the intestines, the tonus of blood vessels, urination, ejaculation, and many other automatic or reflux functions. For example, sympathetic stimulation causes vasoconstriction and hypertension, whereas parasympathetic stimuli have just the opposite effects.

The brain is enveloped by specialized connective tissue called *meninges.* The outer layer, called the *dura,* is composed of dense collagenous tissue. The middle layer, called the *arachnoid* (derived from the Greek word for spider web), is loosely structured and consists of loose connective tissue strands and blood vessels. The innermost layer, called the *pia,* is contiguous with the brain and actually represents the external surface of the brain.

The brain is separated from the arachnoid by a thin space filled with cerebrospinal fluid (CSF). CSF is produced by the choroid plexus in the third ventricles. The fluid flows (under relatively low pressure) from the lateral ventricles into the third ventricle and then into the fourth ventricle. From the fourth ventricle, the CSF may enter the central canal of the spinal cord or exit through the lateral openings (foramina of Luschka) and a median opening (foramen of Magendi) into the subarachnoid space. From the subarachnoid space, the CSF is resorbed through the arachnoid granulations of the meninges into the venous system.

The CSF serves as a cushion that protects the brain from injury. At the same time, it allows an exchange of substances between the brain and the blood. In normal adults, the volume of CSF is approximately 150 mL, and it circulates at a constant rate. Children have less CSF. The circulation of CSF depends on a constant rate of production and resorption (approximately 500 mL/day).

Histology of the Brain

The brain consists of neurons and support cells (Fig. 21-2). The neurons are large, very complex cells that have highly specialized functions. Each neuron has three basic components: a cell body, also known as a perikaryon; one or several dendrites; and a single axon. The perikaryon contains the nucleus, which is typically surrounded by a well-developed cytoplasm full of organelles. Dendrites and axons are extensions of the cytoplasm that contain less organelles, and are specialized for the transmission of neural impulses. Axons and dendrites form the cerebral and spinal tracts and the cranial and spinal nerves.

The support cells of the central nervous system are called glia (neuroglia). Glial cells are classified as astrocytes, oligodendroglia, microglia, and ependymal cells. Astrocytes are star-shaped, relatively large cells with cytoplasmic processes that attach to nerves and blood vessels. Oligodendroglial cells are small

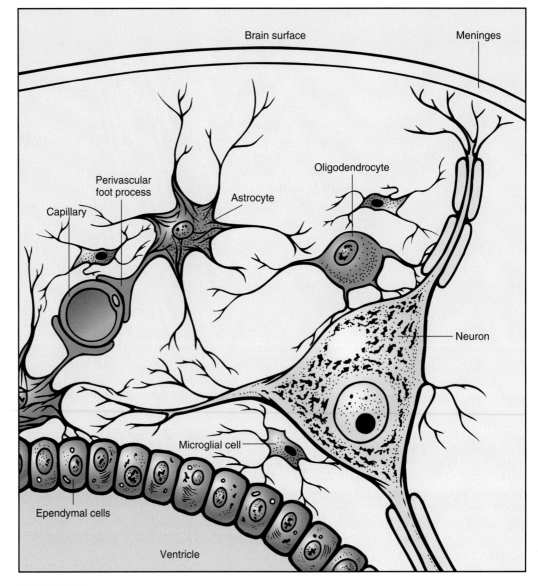

Brain surface

Meninges

Perivascular foot process

Oligodendrocyte

Capillary

Astrocyte

Neuron

Microglial cell

Ependymal cells

Ventricle

FIGURE 21-2
Normal cells of the nervous system.

cells that form long cytoplasmic processes that wrap around the axons. Schwann cells are the peripheral nerve equivalents of oligodendroglia. They form myelin sheaths of peripheral nerves. Microglia are small cells with short cytoplasmic processes. Microglial cells are mobile and phagocytic cells that are derived from bone marrow precursors that have colonized the brain. Ependymal cells line the inside of ventricles of the brain and the central canal of the spinal cord. The cilia on the apical surface of the ependymal cells contribute to the flow of CSF.

OVERVIEW OF MAJOR DISEASES

Diseases of the nervous system are very common, and essentially all health workers must deal with them in their daily practice. The symptoms of neural diseases may be mundane, such as headache or back pain; dramatic, such as an epileptic seizure; or deep seated and unrecognized, such as depression, which may lead to suicide attempts. Common, mild neurologic diseases may be treated by family physicians, nurses, or even local pharmacists, who can often recommend a good and efficient treatment for such ailments. Long-standing headache or severe recurrent headache, known as migraine, may require a more detailed examination, usually performed by a neurologist. In some cases, headache is the first symptom of a brain tumor; in such instances, the patient is referred to a neurosurgeon. Many headaches are "psychogenic," or related to the stresses of daily life. In such cases, the patient may require the assistance of a psychiatrist.

The nervous system may be affected by numerous diseases, the most important of which are

- developmental and genetic diseases
- diseases caused by trauma
- circulatory disorders
- infectious diseases
- autoimmune diseases
- metabolic and nutritional diseases
- neurodegenerative diseases of unknown etiology
- brain tumors

Several facts important to an understanding of CNS pathology are presented here in summary form, before a discussion of specific pathologic entities.

1. *The nervous system consists of highly specialized functional units.* A loss of certain parts of the CNS results in typical functional defects that can be recognized on neurologic examination. The damage is typically irreversible because neurons cannot regenerate. For example, an injury of the Broca area of the frontal cortex results in a loss of speech. A loss of the visual center in the occipital lobe leads to central blindness. Lesions of the respiratory centers, which are located in the medulla oblongata, cause death.

2. *The CNS is protected from mechanical injury by the bones of the skull and vertebrae.* The skull is composed of bones that enclose the brain and shield it from external insults. The bones of the vertebrae protect the spinal cord. The joints between the bones of the skull ossify during childhood, making the entire skull a compact unit. Brain wounds occur only if the integrity of the skull is disrupted. The vertebrae, which protect the spinal cord, are linked to one another by intervertebral disks and tendons that allow them a certain degree of mobility. The spinal cord is, thus, more susceptible than the skull to external trauma. Any rapid body movement that is forceful enough to cause anterior, posterior, or lateral movement of the vertebrae can damage the spinal cord. If the vertebral bodies become detached from one another or severely dislocated, the spinal cord may be completely severed. This typically occurs in traffic accidents.

3. *The CNS is separated from the remainder of the body by meninges and by a blood–brain barrier.* The CNS has an abundant blood supply which assures a constant supply of energy (i.e., oxygen and nutrients). However, the brain must remain relatively isolated from metabolic changes in the body that could adversely affect the functions of the neurons. To this end, the CNS is protected and separated from the rest of the body by the meninges and an anatomic and functional barrier known as the *blood–brain barrier.* The blood–brain barrier acts like a filter, allowing the passage of some substances from the blood into the CSF while preventing the passage of others. For example, bilirubin does not enter the CNS compartment, even in the most severe forms of jaundice. Glucose concentration in the CSF is at a level that is one-half that of the blood concentration. If the concentration of glucose in blood is 100 mg/dL, the concentration in the CSF will be 50 mg/dL. In hyperglycemia, with a blood glucose level of 400 mg/dL, the concentration in the CSF is 200 mg/dL. The protein concentration of normal CSF does not exceed 45 mg/dL, which is just a fraction of the concentration of proteins in serum, which is in the range of 7 mg/dL.

When the blood–brain barrier breaks down, the brain is affected by many substances that cross the blood–brain barrier and enter the neural tissue. The blood–brain barrier of newborn children is not fully functional; therefore, the jaundice of newborn children, especially those affected by maternal-fetal Rh incompatibility (*icterus neonatorum*), is accompanied by impregnation of the basal ganglia by bilirubin (kernicterus), which may be accompanied by irreparable brain injury.

4. *The brain and the spinal cord are surrounded by CSF.* The space between the brain and the meninges is filled with clear CSF. CSF has several functions, the most important of which are to separate the brain from the meninges and to serve as a mechanical buffer between the brain and the bones of the skull. Without the CSF, the brain would be much more vulnerable to trauma.

CSF also serves as a venue for the disposition of metabolites and waste products from the brain. Normally, it has a defined biochemical composition that fluctuates very little. In patients with neurologic diseases, the CSF changes, and these changes can be detected by laboratory tests. For example, bacterial infection of the meninges (meningitis) is accompanied by the appearance of neutrophils in the CSF. Multiple sclerosis is associated with the appearance of gamma globulins (so-called "oligoclonal bands"), which are important for the diagnosis of this disease.

The rate of production, flow, and resorption of CSF remains constant under normal circumstances. Obstruction of CSF flow or blockage of CSF resorption leads to the accumulation of fluid in the brain (*hydrocephalus*). If the obstruction is at the level of the midbrain, preventing communication between the lateral ventricles and the subarachnoid space, the resulting hydrocephalus is designated as noncommunicating. In contrast, communicating hydrocephalus develops if there is an obstruction in the meninges that prevents the resorption of CSF into the venous system.

5. *Neurons, the principal cells of the CNS, are nondividing, postmitotic, permanent cells, whereas the supporting cells, such as the glial cells, are facultative, mitotic (labile) cells that are capable of dividing.* The brain contains billions of neurons, all of which are formed during prenatal, intrauterine life. Neurons are long-lived cells. Nevertheless, every hour of our lives, we lose thousands of neurons owing to programmed natural death. Lost neurons cannot be replaced because the remaining neurons cannot divide and the brain does not contain neuronal reserve cells. Because neural tissue cannot regenerate, every loss of brain substance results in permanent defects.

In contrast to neurons, the glial cells retain a capacity for multiplication and are capable of multiplying in response to certain forms of injury. *Gliosis* (i.e., an increased number of glial cells) is a typical sign of brain injury. Gliosis is found around tumors, brain infarcts, and foci of intracerebral hemorrhages.

The dichotomy between the neurons and glia is important for understanding the histogenesis of brain tumors. Because the adult neurons are incapable of dividing, these cells never give rise to tumors. The malignant tumors of neural cell origin are found only in children, in whom they presumably originate from undifferentiated precursors of neural cells, such as neuroblasts. The primary tumors of the brain in adults are derived from glial cells and are classified as *gliomas*. Other support structures of the brain, such as the meninges and the blood vessels, also contain cells that are capable of proliferation and/or malignant transformation. These tumors are known as *meningiomas* or *hemangioblastomas*.

6. *The CNS may be affected by diseases that involve other organs, but also by diseases that are unique to the CNS.* The CNS is affected by many multisystemic diseases, especially those classified as circulatory, metabolic, or infectious. For example, atherosclerosis of the coronary arteries and aorta is often accompanied by cerebrovascular accidents (CVAs). End-stage kidney disease (uremia) or liver disease is accompanied by metabolic disturbances that typically cause numerous neurologic symptoms. Uremia typically terminates in progressive somnolence and coma. Hepatic encephalopathy is characterized by mental confusion, flap-like movements of the hands (asterixis), and coma. Systemic infections caused by various bacteria or viruses may spread to the brain, usually by a hematogenous route.

Diseases restricted to the brain may be caused by neurotropic pathogens, or they may be a consequence of metabolic changes unique to neural cells. For example, neurotropic viruses, like rabies, infect only nerve cells. Prions—minute infectious particles composed only of proteins—which are smaller than viruses, survive only in nerve cells and are, therefore, selectively harmful to CNS. Prions cause spongiform degeneration of the brain that is typical of such diseases as kuru and Creutzfeldt-Jakob disease. Neurodegenerative diseases, like Alzheimer's disease or Parkinson's disease, are characterized by neuronal degeneration and loss of neurons. The etiology and pathogenesis of these neurodegenerative diseases are unknown.

7. *The symptoms of CNS diseases result from dys-function of or loss of function of neurons.* Overall, symptoms of diseases of the CNS can be *local*, like the headaches that accompany brain tumors, or *systemic*, like the generalized paralysis and coma that ensue following massive intracerebral bleeding.

Local symptoms of intracranial lesions result from direct compression of a nerve center by a mass (e.g., a tumor) or increased intracranial pressure caused by mass effect or cerebral edema. Intracranial tumors and all inflammations of the brain and meninges cause brain edema. Brain edema develops also in shock and in many metabolic diseases, as well as in cases of drug overdose and poisoning.

Increased intracranial pressure is a life-threatening condition. The symptoms depend on the pace at which it develops. A sudden, explosive increase in intracranial pressure, such as that caused by a bullet wound to the head, will cause death instantaneously. By contrast, a rapid but gradual increase of intracranial pressure will present as a severe headache that is usually accompanied by vomiting, blurry vision, and loss of consciousness. Such patients lapse into coma and usually die of apnea (absence of breathing) or develop pulmonary edema secondary to inhibition of the medullary vital centers. Patients with chronic elevation of intracranial pressure—for example, those with brain tumors—generally present with headaches, personality changes, intellectual decline, or emotional lability. As the pressure gradually increases, symptoms of acute intracranial hypertension supersede the nonspecific chronic symptoms.

Death caused by increased intracranial pressure usually results from the compression of vital centers in the brain stem. Most often, the centers of the medulla oblongata are compressed by the edematous tonsils of the cerebellum, which herniates through the foramen magnum (Fig. 21-3). Herniation of the medial portion of the cerebral hemisphere beneath the tentorium cerebelli (uncal or transtentorial herniation) may compress the pons and can also cause death. Other forms of herniation of the brain, such as herniation of the cingulate gyrus of the cerebral hemisphere beneath the falx cerebri or herniation through an opening of a broken skull, are less important.

Symptoms of CNS dysfunction may result from a loss of neurons (e.g., the loss of memory that accompanies Alzheimer's disease), from abnormal function of neurons (e.g., the rigidity of muscles in Parkinson's disease), or abnormal excitation of neurons, such as that which can be recorded by electroencephalography (EEG) during the convulsions typical of epilepsy. Many psychiatric diseases, such as schizophrenia or manic-depressive psychosis, are caused by abnormal function of brain cells, but the nature of these neural cell dysfunctions remains unknown. The underlying defect of psychiatric diseases has not been defined in pathologic terms.

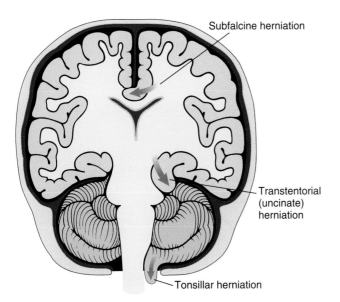

Subfalcine herniation

Transentorial (uncinate) herniation

Tonsillar herniation

FIGURE 21-3
Herniations of the brain. (A) Subfalcine herniation involves the cingulate gyrus protruding beneath the falx cerebri. (B) Transentorial (uncinate) herniation involves the uncus protruding below the tentorium cerebelli. (C) Tonsillar herniation involves the cerebellar tonsils protruding into the foramen magnum.

Developmental Disorders

The cause of most **developmental disorders** is unknown. Some developmental disorders of the brain can be related to genetic and chromosomal abnormalities and abnormal morphogenesis of the brain and spinal cord during early stages of fetal life.

Genetic diseases, such as Tay-Sachs disease, a gangliosidosis caused by a deficiency of hexosaminidase, produce histologic changes but no obvious gross malformations of the CNS. Trisomy of chromosome 21 results in Down syndrome, which invariably presents with mental deficiency, but no distinct gross malformations of the brain. Developmental malformations of the CNS caused by intrauterine infection with toxoplasma, rubella virus, cytomegalovirus, or herpesvirus (well-known causes of the neonatal TORCH syndrome) produce visible changes in the brain, such as calcifications and hydrocephalus.

Anencephaly and Dysraphic Disorders

The CNS develops from the neural plate, which folds and ultimately closes into a neural tube extending along the dorsal side of the body axis (see Fig. 21-4). As the neural tube forms, it becomes internalized and is protected by the overlying skin. The mesenchyme between the neural tube and the skin is induced to form bone, which gives rise to the skull and the vertebral bodies. Each of these bones originates

from separate and often multiple ossification centers. The products of ossification centers must fuse to provide a continuous external envelope to the CNS.

Incomplete fusion of the neural tube gives rise to **dysraphic malformations** (derived from the Greek word *raphe,* meaning suture). Dysraphic malformations occur in several forms (Fig. 21-4). If the calvaria is not formed and the unprotected brain is destroyed in utero, the malformation is called *anencephaly* (see also Fig. 5-23). Milder dysraphic malformations, such as *meningocele, myelomeningocele,* and *spina bifida,* are characterized by a lack of fusion of the posterior bone coverings. If the meninges protrude through the bony defect, the malformation is called meningocele. In myelomeningocele, the protrusion contains not only the meninges but also a portion of the spinal cord. Spina bifida is characterized by an absence of vertebral arches, resulting in exposure of the meninges or the spinal cord to the outer world. Spina bifida may be evident at birth as a deep defect on the lower back, or it may be covered with skin and be inapparent (*spina bifida occulta*).

Anencephaly is incompatible with life. Spinal dysraphic disorders are typically associated with major neurologic deficits, such as paralysis. Although spina bifida cannot be repaired entirely and the neurologic defects are permanent, these children may be rehabilitated to a certain degree by physical therapy.

Intracranial Hemorrhages

Intracranial hemorrhages can be classified, according to their location, into four groups: epidural, subdural, subarachnoid, and intracerebral (Fig. 21-5). These hemorrhages may be caused by trauma (as may occur in boxers) or brain contusions owing to a vehicular accident; rupture of blood vessels that are congenitally abnormal (as in aneurysms) or that are damaged by hypertension; or abnormalities of coagulation, as occurs in various congenital and acquired bleeding disorders.

Epidural hematomas are typically located between the skull and the dura in a space that, under normal circumstances, is almost nonexistent because of the close apposition of the dura to the skull bones. Epidural hematoma develops from a ruptured middle meningeal artery that lies in this space and that can easily be torn by a bone spicule resulting from cranial fracture. Because arterial blood fills the space, slowly separating the dura from the bone, it usually takes several hours before a large hematoma is formed. Once the hematoma reaches a volume of 50 to 60 mL, it is large enough to compress the brain and cause coma. If unrecognized, epidural hematoma is invariably lethal.

Subdural hematomas occupy the space between

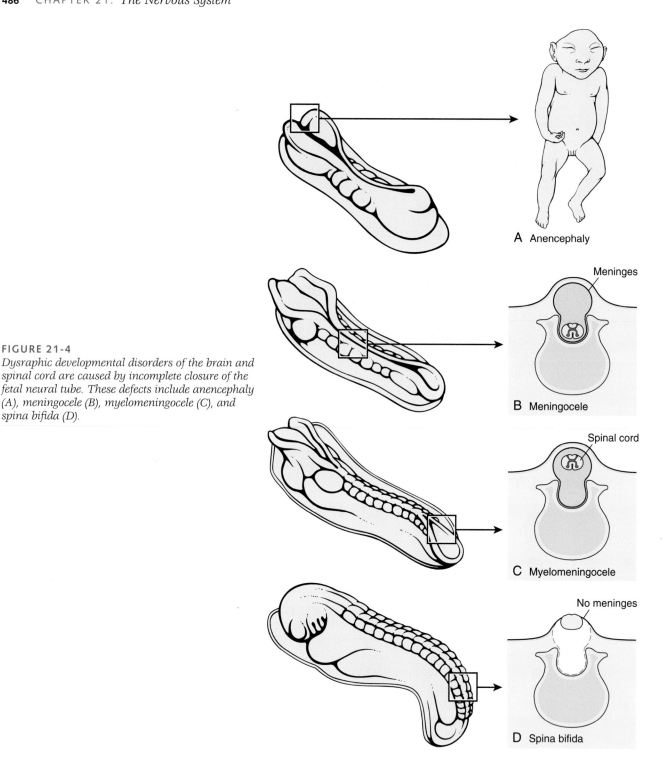

FIGURE 21-4
Dysraphic developmental disorders of the brain and spinal cord are caused by incomplete closure of the fetal neural tube. These defects include anencephaly (A), meningocele (B), myelomeningocele (C), and spina bifida (D).

A Anencephaly

Meninges

B Meningocele

Spinal cord

C Myelomeningocele

No meninges

D Spina bifida

the dura and the arachnoid. Under normal circumstances, this space is bridged by thin-walled veins that can easily be torn by trauma, especially the type of blunt trauma that causes sudden movement of the brain in one direction and the dura in another. Subdural hematomas are typically found in boxers or in unattended bedridden elderly patients who have fallen out of bed. Repeated trauma has a cumulative effect. It is thought that the sudden movement of the brain in one direction, if unaccompanied by a similar movement of the dura, has a tearing effect on the bridging veins and can rupture them. The coagulated blood typically covers the lateral hemispheres like a cap. The symptoms are usually nonspecific (e.g., headache), but tend to progress as the hematoma enlarges.

Subarachnoid hemorrhages are located in the space between the arachnoid and the pia (i.e., the brain surface). Most often, subarachnoid hemorrhages are caused by traumatic contusion of the

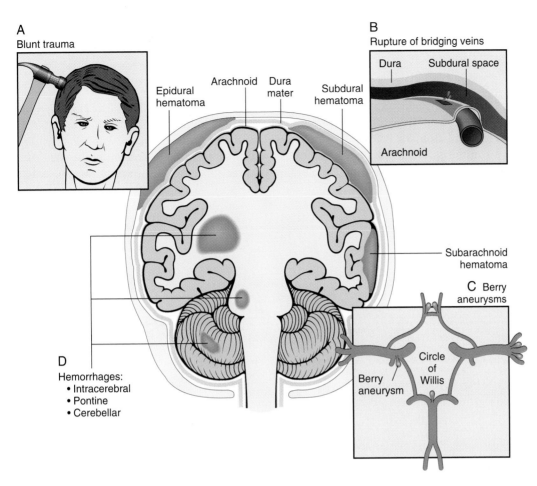

FIGURE 21-5

Intracranial hemorrhages. (A) Epidural hemorrhage is caused by trauma and rupture of the middle meningeal artery. (B) Subdural hemorrhage is caused by traumatic rupture of bridging veins. (C) Subarachnoid hemorrhage is typical of ruptured berry aneurysm of the circle of Willis at the base of the brain. (D) Intracerebral hemorrhage is a complication of hypertension. The most common sites of hypertensive hemorrhages are the basal ganglia, pons, and cerebellum.

brain, in which case the blood leaks into the subarachnoid space from the ruptured cerebral blood vessels at the base of the brain.

Ruptured congenital aneurysms of the circle of Willis are yet another important cause of subarachnoid hemorrhages. Congenital saccular aneurysms, called *berry aneurysms* because of their small size and shape, are found in 1 percent to 2 percent of the general population. Rupture can be precipitated by hypertension, but often occurs spontaneously, without any obvious cause. Bleeding into the subarachnoid space is associated with high mortality. If recognized, berry aneurysms can be treated surgically, usually by placing clips at the site of their origin, thereby preventing the entry of blood into the lumen of the aneurysm.

Intracerebral hemorrhage is a common complication of head trauma, regardless of the nature of the trauma. Blunt trauma caused by a club, or open trauma, such as that caused by a metal object, such

as a hammer, may cause contusion of the brain and bleeding from the ruptured intracerebral vessels. Gunshot wounds are also accompanied by intracerebral hemorrhage.

Among the nontraumatic forms of intracerebral hemorrhages, the most important are various forms of stroke. Intracerebral hemorrhage is also common in leukemia and other hematologic diseases associated with abnormal coagulation.

Cerebrovascular Diseases

Cerebrovascular disease (CVD) is the third most common cause of death and the most common crippling disease in the United States. The most important clinical manifestation of CVD is **stroke.** Typically, CVD is a disease of old age and, in most instances, is related to atherosclerosis of the cerebral arteries. Other important pathogenetic factors include arterial hypertension and thromboembolism, which often accompany atherosclerosis.

Atherosclerosis of the cerebral vessels has the same morphologic features as atherosclerosis in other sites. The lesions may involve the major blood arteries or their branches (Fig. 21-6). Narrowing of the arteries may be gradual, owing to progressive atherosclerotic fibrosis and calcification, or it may occur suddenly, as when an atherosclerotic plaque ruptures, provoking intravascular thrombosis and complete occlusion of the arterial lumen. Depending on the type of vascular lesions, CVD will cause either widespread or localized lesions.

Global Ischemia

Patients who have widespread atherosclerotic narrowing of the entire cerebrovascular system develop multiple foci of ischemic necrosis. Such *lacunar infarcts* cause minor neurologic deficits but, over time, result in slowly progressive mental deterioration (*multi-infarct dementia*).

FIGURE 21-6

Cerebral infarcts. Localized infarcts are caused by an occlusion of the internal or basilar artery or their major branches. Diffuse infarcts, caused by hypoperfusion of the brain, occur in watershed areas and in the form of laminar necrosis in the innermost layers of the cortex. Occlusion may be caused by thrombosis or emboli.

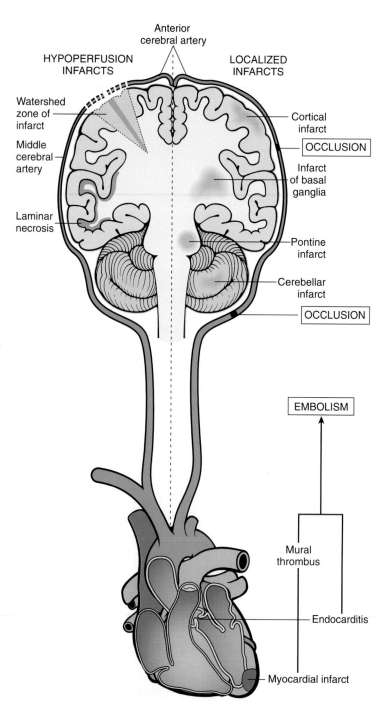

Cardiac failure or any other form of vascular collapse (e.g., hypotensive shock secondary to hemorrhage into the intestines of patients whose cerebral blood flow is marginal) will result in widespread infarcts. Such hypoperfusion infarcts are typically located in the parasagittal cortex, in the areas representing the marginal zones of arterial supply by the branches of the carotid artery on one side and the basilar artery on the other. Systemic hypotension lowers the perfusion from both sides, and the area in the border zone becomes hypoxic, resulting in so-called *"watershed infarcts."* Hypoperfusion also leads to *laminar necrosis* of the deeper zones of the gray matter. These zones receive blood from the short penetrator arteries entering the cortex from the surface. Owing to hypotension, the blood entering the cortex does not reach the deep cortex, and necrosis ensues. If heart function is restored, patients recover with only minor neurologic deficits. Nevertheless, these minor CVAs have a cumulative effect and ultimately cause mental deterioration.

Cerebral Infarct

An infarct or ischemic necrosis of a distinct anatomic part of the brain caused by CVD clinically presents as a stroke. Cerebral infarcts are most often caused by thrombotic occlusion of an atherosclerotic artery. Thromboemboli originating in the heart chambers (e.g., following a myocardial infarction) or on the cardiac valves (e.g., owing to endocarditis) are the second most common causes. Other diseases, such as arteritis, are rarely associated with stroke.

The pathologic changes in the brain vary depending on the time that has elapsed since the onset of occlusion. Ischemic brain liquefies, and the ischemic area undergoes necrosis, transforming into a putty-like mush. This focus of *encephalomalacia* ("softening of the brain") may remain pale (pale or bland infarct), or it may be perfused with blood from the collateral circulation and transform into a hemorrhagic infarct. White matter infarcts usually remain pale, whereas those in the gray matter tend to transform into red infarcts. Red infarcts are common following cerebral embolization because such infarcts are more readily perfused by arterial blood from adjacent, unoccluded blood vessels.

The brain tissue surrounding the infarcts, regardless of their color, is edematous. During this phase of maximal cerebral swelling, patients experience the most profound neurologic deficits and are at the greatest risk of dying. Within a few days after infarction, the cerebral edema subsides and the condition of patients surviving this critical period improves in most instances. The margins of the viable tissue surrounding the infarct become vascularized. The necrotic material is removed from the infarct by scavenger cells that invade the area from the newly formed blood vessels. Ultimately, the infarct transforms into a fluid-filled cavity (*"pseudocyst"*). Brain infarcts cannot heal, and the neurologic deficits caused by them are permanent.

The clinical presentation of cerebral infarction depends on the site of arterial occlusion. For example, occlusion of the middle cerebral artery, which is the most common cause of cerebral infarction, results in contralateral hemiplegia (loss of the capacity to move the extremities), sensory loss on the same side of the body, and bilateral symmetrical loss of vision in half of the visual fields, with the eyes deviating to the side of the lesion. Global aphasia (an inability to speak or write) develops if the infarct occurs in the dominant hemisphere. Drowsiness, stupor, and coma may develop depending on the extent of cerebral edema, but these symptoms, which are caused by brain edema, may recede in patients who survive.

Following a stroke, the treatment of unconscious patients includes intensive life-supporting measures. Brain edema, which is the most important life-threatening feature of an acute stroke, must be treated vigorously with corticosteroids and dehydrating hyperosmolar agents that drain the water fluid from the brain tissue into the circulation.

Physical therapy is important in the long-term rehabilitation of these patients, and occupational therapy may improve their general well-being and quality of life. Approximately 80 percent of patients survive the initial stroke, and 60 percent are alive 3 years thereafter.

Intracerebral Hemorrhage

In patients who have no vascular anomalies, such as aneurysms or hemangiomas, intracerebral hemorrhage or apoplexy is most often caused by arterial hypertension. Hemorrhage results from the rupture of small blood vessels that have been damaged mechanically by hypertension. The most common sites of hemorrhage are the basal ganglia, which are affected in about two thirds of cases. Cerebellar and pontine hemorrhage account for most of the remaining cases, whereas other sites are rarely involved.

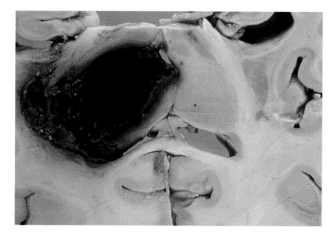

FIGURE 21-7
Hypertensive hemorrhage.

With recent improvements in the treatment of hypertension, intracerebral hemorrhages have become less common than before.

Intracerebral hemorrhage typically results in a well-circumscribed hematoma (Fig. 21-7). Like the infarcts, such hematomas are surrounded by edematous brain tissue. Cerebral edema subsides in patients who survive the apoplexy, with resorption of the extravasated blood and the necrotic tissue destroyed by the hemorrhage. Ultimately, the infarct transforms into a pseudocyst, which usually contains yellow fluid. The wall of the pseudocyst typically contains hemosiderin-laden macrophages.

The clinical features of intracerebral hemorrhage may resemble those of cerebral infarction. However, in most cases, the clinical picture is more dramatic, with about 30 percent of patients losing consciousness and appearing stricken. Other patients may complain of severe headache or may experience an urge to vomit. Hemorrhage into the basal ganglia is accompanied by a rapid onset of hemiplegia and hemiparesis, which are fully developed in most patients admitted to the hospital. Cerebellar hemorrhage typically presents with nausea and vomiting, loss of balance, and severe headache. The patient rapidly lapses into coma and most die within 48 hours. Pontine hemorrhages are almost invariably lethal, with most patients dying within hours of the onset of the first, usually nonspecific, symptoms.

Treatment of patients with hypertensive hemorrhages includes supportive measures. Recovery depends on the site and extent of the brain lesion.

Trauma of the Central Nervous System

Injuries of the head, neck, and spinal cord are major causes of disability and mortality worldwide. In the United States, head injuries occur at an estimated yearly rate of 200 per 100,000; neck injuries at a rate of 5 per 100,000; and spinal cord injuries at a rate of 3 per 100,000.

Brain Injury

Brain injuries vary in severity and are classified as concussion, contusion, or laceration. In addition, head trauma is often accompanied by hematomas, as discussed earlier in this chapter.

Brain concussion presents as a transient loss of consciousness, usually following blunt head trauma. Loss of consciousness is based on functional disturbances affecting the temporal lobes and the reticular activating system of the brain stem. There are no significant macroscopic or microscopic changes in the brain.

Brain contusion (bruise) is characterized by a disruption of cerebral and/or meningeal blood vessels by severe blunt trauma. The lesions are hemorrhagic and are typically located at the site of impact (*coup lesion*) and its diametrically opposite pole (*countercoup lesion*) (Fig. 21-8). A coup lesion is caused by direct force, whereas a countercoup lesion is a result of the deceleration of the moving brain caused by the skull bones that serve as shock absorbers. Rotation of the head upon impact causes even more damage. Contusions of the brain are serious injuries associated with considerable mortality. Survivors may have severe neurologic deficits, some of which may be permanent.

FIGURE 21-8
Spinal cord trauma. A coup lesion of the brain occurs at the site of impact, whereas a countercoup lesion is diametrically opposite to it. The spinal cord lesion depicted here is caused by hyperextension.

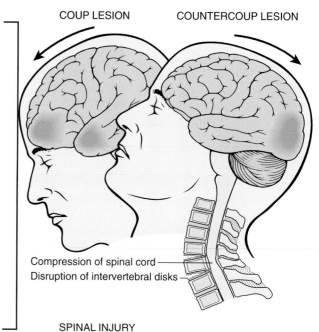

COUP LESION   COUNTERCOUP LESION

Compression of spinal cord
Disruption of intervertebral disks

SPINAL INJURY

Laceration of the brain is typically caused by open trauma that disrupts the integrity of the brain. Gunshot wounds also produce laceration of the brain tissue. Such wounds have high mortality. Death is related to acute expansion of the intracranial volume and the consequent compression of the vital centers in the brain stem. Patients who survive gunshot wounds of the brain usually have major neurologic deficits, and some of them may develop epilepsy (seizures).

Neck and Spinal Cord Injuries

Spinal cord injuries may occur anywhere along the spinal cord. The mobility of the neck accounts for the greatest vulnerability of the cervical spine, which is especially susceptible to injury during traffic accidents. "Backlash injury" of the neck is the most common. However, none of the segments of spinal cord is immune to injury.

Injuries of the cervical spine have traditionally been classified as either hyperextension or hyperflexion injuries. In *hyperextension injury,* an impact on the forehead will cause hyperextension and rupture of the anterior spinal ligaments, with subsequent compression of the posterior side of the spinal cord. In *hyperflexion injury,* the impact on the occiput causes extensive anterior flexion of the spinal cord and compression of the anterior portion of the spinal cord. Both hyperextension and hyperflexion injuries may cause complete transection of the spinal cord, resulting in a loss of both motor and sensory functions below the site of injury. Typically, the injured person experiences flaccid paralysis accompanied by a loss of sensation below the site of injury. Urination and defecation reflexes are also lost. With time, the reflex functions return and the paraplegia or quadriplegia becomes spastic. The reflexes governing the bladder and bowel functions may also be partially restored.

Infections of the Central Nervous System

Infections of the CNS are common. Any infectious pathogen can cause CNS disease, although in clinical practice, bacterial, viral, protozoal, and fungal infections are the primary culprits.

Etiology and Pathogenesis. Infections of the CNS can be acquired through several routes: by direct extension, hematogenously, or via the nerves.

Bacterial infections of the brain typically develop hematogenously during sepsis and bacteremia or from septic emboli (Fig. 21-9), as in infectious endocarditis. Open wounds of the brain are usually in-

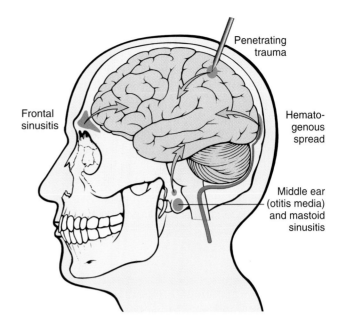

FIGURE 21-9
Bacterial infections of the central nervous system. Infectious organisms may reach the brain through several routes: hematogenously, by direct entry secondary to penetrating trauma, or by direct spread from adjacent structures, such as the inner ear or the nasal sinuses.

fected by bacteria that have gained direct entrance into the brain parenchyma. Bacterial infections of the paranasal sinuses or the middle ear also may spread into the cranium and cause CNS infection.

The most important bacterial pathogens are *Neisseria meningitidis* (meningococcus), and *Streptococcus pneumoniae,* which account for most cases of bacterial meningitis in adults. *Escherichia coli* is an important cause of bacterial meningitis in neonates, whereas *Haemophilus influenzae* is the predominant cause of meningitis in children aged 3 months to 3 years. Tuberculosis of the brain was important in the past, but is rare today. Syphilis is a late complication of infection with *Treponema pallidum.* Neurosyphilis is a feature of the third stage of this disease.

Viral infections are usually spread to the brain by a hematogenous route. Viral pathogens include common childhood viruses, such as the measles virus, rubella, or adenovirus. The ubiquitous viruses, such as herpesvirus or cytomegalovirus, may infect the brain of children or adults. Neurotropic viruses (i.e., viruses that infect exclusively neural tissue), which are known for their geographic provenance (e.g., St. Louis encephalitis), are transmitted by ticks and cause epidemic CNS infections.

Herpesvirus is the most common viral cause of encephalitis in the United States. *Japanese B encephalitis,* caused by an arthopode-borne virus, is the most common neurotropic virus associated with epidemic forms of encephalitis.

Among the neurotropic viruses, *rabies virus*

should also be mentioned. The rabies virus usually enters the human body through wounds inflicted by rabid dogs, foxes, or various other animals, such as raccoons and bats. In contrast to other viruses, the rabies virus reaches the CNS by traveling along the peripheral nerves from the site of inoculation through the spinal cord and specific neural path-ways. Intracytoplasmic viral inclusions, or so-called Negri bodies, are found most prominently in the neu-rons of the brain stem.

Prions are small infectious particles composed of protein. Previously classified as "slow viruses," prions seem to be distinct from viruses in that they do not contain DNA or RNA. Prions infect the nervous system selectively and are transmitted by direct exposure to infected material. For example, Creutzfeldt-Jakob disease has been transmitted by corneal transplants. Even human brains that are re-moved at autopsy are infectious.

Protozoal infections of the CNS are usually ac-quired hematogenously. The most important proto-zoal pathogen is *Toxoplasma gondii,* an important cause of encephalitis in neonates. Toxoplasmosis is also an important infection in patients with acquired immunodeficiency syndrome (AIDS).

Fungi reach the brain hematogenously. Fungal encephalitis or meningitis is usually found in im-munosuppressed patients and is especially common in those with AIDS. The most important pathogens are *Candida albicans, Aspergillus flavus,* and *Crypto-coccus neoformans.*

Pathology. Infections of the CNS may involve the brain and the spinal cord or the meninges. Such in-fections may present in several pathologic forms.

Encephalitis is a diffuse infection of the brain parenchyma. Typically, it is caused by viruses that invade neural or glial cells. Viral encephalitis is mor-phologically recognizable by the presence of lympho-cytic infiltrates that typically fill the perivascular Vir-

chow-Robin spaces (Fig. 21-10). Viral inclusions can be also recognized in the nuclei or the cytoplasm of infected cells.

Myelitis is a diffuse infection of the spinal cord. Like encephalitis, it is usually caused by viruses. Po-liomyelitis, a viral infection most prominently affect-ing the anterior horns of the spinal cord, was previ-ously a major crippling disease, but has been eradicated by immunization.

A *cerebral abscess* is a localized suppurative infec-tion of the brain. It presents as a mass lesion and may be mistaken for a tumor. The abscess consists of a cavity filled with pus and a capsule composed of glial cells and fibroblasts. Most abscesses are caused by pyogenic bacteria, but in immunosuppressed pa-tients, some abscesses may be of fungal origin or may contain mixed flora.

Meningitis is an inflammation of meninges. Viral meningitis, probably the most common and the most underdiagnosed infectious disease of the CNS, occurs in many viral diseases, such as the common flu. It is characterized by a lymphocytic exudate in the sub-arachnoid space. Viral encephalitis may also extend into the meninges. In such cases, CSF analysis will reveal lymphocytosis. Bacterial meningitis caused by pyogenic bacteria, such as *N. meningitidis,* will cause exudation of neutrophils. In severe cases, the entire surface of the brain is covered with pus that fills the subarachnoid spaces (Fig. 21-11). The CSF typically contains numerous neutrophils, a finding that is im-portant in establishing the diagnosis.

Neurosyphilis usually presents as chronic menin-gitis. The meninges are infiltrated with lymphocytes and plasma cells, which are typically centered around small blood vessels. In the healing stages of syphilitic infection, meningeal fibrosis predominates. Fibrosis of the spinal meninges may compress the dorsal

FIGURE 21-10
Viral encephalitis. The perivascular spaces contain prominent infiltrates of lymphocytes.

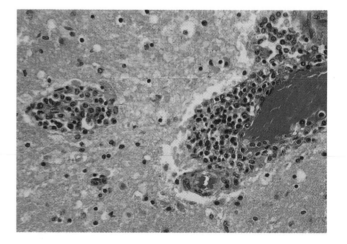

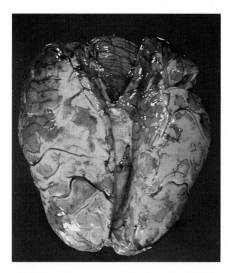

FIGURE 21-11
Bacterial meningitis. The surface of the brain is covered with pus. (Courtesy of Dr. John J. Kepes, Kansas City, Kansas.)

roots, resulting in atrophy of afferent, sensory axons entering the spinal cord. This causes the best-known complication of neurosyphilis: *tabes dorsalis.* Tabes dorsalis is pathologically recognized on cross sections of the spinal cord by the atrophy of the dorsal (sensory) columns. Syphilitic perivascular inflammation of the brain causes ischemic necrosis of the cortical centers. The loss of neurons correlates with motor and mental changes, collectively known as the *syphilitic general paresis of the insane.*

Various pathologic forms of AIDS-related CNS lesions are sometimes combined and found in the same patient. This is best illustrated by the so-called *AIDS-related encephalopathy,* a rather common finding in terminally ill patients infected with the human immunodeficiency virus (HIV). HIV infects macrophages and T lymphocytes, and these cells "import" the virus into the CNS. The infected "newcomers" secrete various cytokines, some of which appear to be toxic to brain cells. AIDS dementia seems to be a consequence of these adverse influences. In addition, the HIV-infected brain is less resistant to invasion by a variety of bacterial, viral, parasitic, and fungal pathogens which rarely enter the normal brain. Among these pathogens, the most prominent are Toxoplasma and Cryptococcus. Meningitis, encephalitis, or brain abscesses may develop. Most of these infections are resistant to treatment, and many patients die of CNS infection.

Autoimmune Diseases of the Central Nervous System

Autoimmune diseases of the CNS are poorly understood. Although it has been known for some time that such diseases exist, and despite the fact that there are several good animal models for studying such diseases, neuroimmunology is still a rather obscure field. An immune form of encephalitis has been described in patients immunized against various infectious diseases. Some late forms of postinfectious encephalitis may represent an immune disease. However, the most important of all immunologic disorders is multiple sclerosis.

Multiple Sclerosis

Multiple sclerosis (MS) is a demyelinating disease that is presumed to be of autoimmune origin. It is the most common immunologic CNS disease, affecting approximately 250,000 Americans, most of whom are 20 to 45 years of age. It has a prevalence of 1 in 1000 and is, thus, the leading neurologic disease in young adults. Women are affected twice as often as men.

Etiology and Pathogenesis. The cause of MS is not known. The search for possible causes has, however, revealed many interesting epidemiologic, genetic, and immunologic facts. One day, these leads may help us better understand the disease, uncover its etiology, and find a cure for it.

Epidemiologic data indicate that MS occurs predominantly in caucasians of Western and Northern European origin who live in temperate climate zones above the 40th parallel. The disease is uncommon in the tropics and among non-whites. However, if persons at risk live for the first 15 years of life in a moderate climate and move to the tropics, they have the same high risk as they would if they were in their original domicile.

Genetic studies have shown that MS affects certain families more often than others. The first degree relatives of an affected person have a 15 times higher risk of developing the disease than the general population living under the same conditions. If one monozygotic twin develops symptoms, the second twin will also become ill in 25 percent of cases.

Did You Know?

Many famous personalities of the past died of neurosyphilis. Because neurosyphilis causes both neurologic and psychiatric symptoms, many of these individuals were confined to asylums for the insane before they died. The blood-thirsty Russian czar Ivan the Terrible was thought to have gone mad from syphilis.

Genetic linkage studies have disclosed a high prevalence of certain human major histocompatibility antigens among the affected individuals, further supporting the theory of genetic predisposition.

Immunologic studies have shown that MS resembles allergic encephalitis, which can be experimentally induced in animals immunized with CNS myelin. T-helper and T-suppressor lymphocytes and macrophages have been demonstrated in early lesions in the human brain. T cells in the MS lesions belong to a few clones that have been immunized to some local antigen in the brain. In contrast to such oligoclonal T-cell populations in the brain, the peripheral T lymphocytes in the blood do not show any evidence of clonal expansion. This has led scientists to conclude that the T cells attracted to the brain play an important pathogenetic role, and that most likely, these cells have been sensitized to some component of myelin. The nature of this hypothetical antigen has not been elucidated. It is also not known whether the macrophages in the brain lesion are only secondary bystanders whose function is to remove the debris from damaged cells, or whether the macrophages are essential for the initial presentation of antigen to the T cells. Also, the role of B lymphocytes and plasma cells is enigmatic. These antibody-producing cells are usually found around the cerebral blood vessels in the vicinity of the lesion. Immunoglobulin G (IgG), secreted by these cells, is found in the CSF. By immunoelectrophoresis, it may be shown that the IgG in the CSF is composed of oligoclonal bands, suggesting that the B cells in the brain also represent selected clones that have been immunized to some unidentified antigen. Although the significance of these immunologic findings remains uncertain, oligoclonal IgG bands in the CSF are useful in the diagnosis of MS.

Clinical Features. Multiple sclerosis is a chronic disease characterized by episodes of exacerbation and remission of neurologic symptoms. Symptoms include both sensory and motor abnormalities. Among the sensory defects, the most common are loss of sensation of touch accompanied by tingling. Blurred vision is a frequent early symptom. Motor symptoms include muscle weakness, unsteady gait, incoordination of movements, and sphincter abnormalities, such as urinary incontinence. These symptoms usually appear to be unrelated to one another, and the diagnosis of MS may, therefore, be rather difficult.

The diagnosis of MS is made on clinical grounds. Current criteria require documentation of two separate sets of CNS symptoms which occur in at least two episodes, separated from one another by a period of 1 month or more. Magnetic resonance imaging (MRI) is a useful diagnostic technique. With this specialized x-ray technique, a brain lesion is evident in 80 percent of patients. Oligoclonal IgG bands are typically found in the CSF, and although this abnormality is not pathognomonic of MS, it strongly supports the diagnosis.

MS has an unpredictable course. Most patients become physically incapacitated over a period of 20 to 30 years. Patients who develop MS after the age of 40 years and those with marked motor disability early in the course of disease have a poor prognosis.

Pathology. MS is a demyelinating disease that typically involves the white matter. Demyelination of the axons leads to the formation of typical plaques (Fig. 21-12) that are usually found in the white matter of the brain, optic nerves, or spinal cord. Periventricular plaques in the lateral hemispheres of the brain are typical. Histologically, the early lesions are infiltrated with lymphocytes and macrophages. The older lesions consist of demyelinated axons surrounded by reactive astrocytes. Oligodendroglial cells—the cells responsible for the myelination of axons—are remarkably absent, as they were most likely destroyed in the acute stage of the disease.

FIGURE 21-12

Multiple sclerosis. Early lesions contain demyelinated axons surrounded by lymphocytes and foamy macrophages. Late lesions—that is, fully formed demyelinated plaques—consist of demyelinated axons and astrocytes.

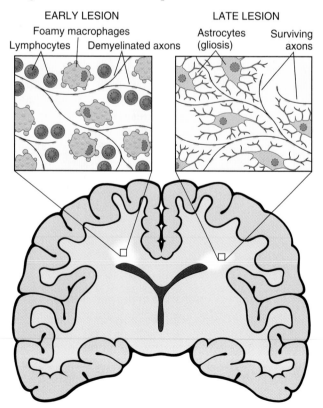

Metabolic and Nutritional Diseases of the Nervous System

Inborn Errors of Metabolism

Metabolic injury of the brain is a common feature of many inborn errors of metabolism. Diseases involving the enzymes essential for maintenance of myelin and cell membranes of neurons are accompanied by extensive lesions of the CNS. The best known among these incurable diseases are

- *Tay-Sachs disease,* a deficiency of the enzyme hexosaminidase A that leads to accumulation of gangliosides in neurons. The disease presents early in life and is characterized by progressive mental and motor deterioration and blindness.
- *Niemann-Pick disease,* a deficiency of sphyngomyelinase that leads to an accumulation of sphyngomyelin. This disease also begins in childhood and is characterized by progressive mental deterioration. The accumulation of sphyngomyelin in the cytoplasm damages the cells. Neuronal loss leads to profound atrophy of the brain.

Nutritional Diseases

Among the nutritional deficiencies affecting the brain, the most important are those related to an inadequate intake of vitamins. Some vitamin deficiencies occur because of gastrointestinal disorders that prevent normal absorption (e.g., pernicious anemia, which is marked by an inability to absorb vitamin B_{12}). The most important vitamin deficiencies that affect the brain are deficiencies of thiamine (vitamin B_1), vitamin B_{12}, and nicotinic acid.

Thiamine deficiency presents clinically as Wernicke's encephalopathy, or **Wernicke-Korsakoff syndrome,** a triad that includes disturbances in ocular function, gait, and mental function. Korsakoff's psychosis, manifested as mental deterioration whereby patients lose memory (amnesia) and make up incredible stories (confabulation), may also appear. Degenerative neuronal changes are typically found in the hypothalamus, the periacqueductal region of the midbrain, and mamillary bodies.

Vitamin B_{12} deficiency presents with uncoordinated movements and a sensorimotor peripheral neuropathy with signs of spinal cord disease. Typically, affected patients have an abnormal gait. Psychiatric symptoms are also present, but are highly variable. Some patients are demented, others delirious or depressed, and still others mentally slow.

Nicotinic acid deficiency results in pellagra, a clinical syndrome characterized by dermatitis, diarrhea, and delirium (the "three Ds"). The neurologic and psychiatric symptoms of pellagra are highly variable.

Alcoholism

Alcohol has profound effects on the brain. In small amounts, it stimulates the brain, causing euphoria and lack of inhibition. In larger amounts, alcohol induces sleep and depresses brain functions. Alcohol, when ingested in excessive amounts, may even act as a neurotoxin and cause death.

Chronic alcoholism affects the nervous system directly and indirectly. In addition to its direct neurotoxic effects, alcohol damages the liver and alters intermediary metabolism. These general metabolic changes are often combined with nutritional deficiencies, such as deficiencies of thiamine, folic acid, or nicotinic acid, all of which can affect the brain.

The neuropathologic changes related to chronic alcoholism usually reflect the complex nutritional and metabolic disturbances in these patients. Thiamine deficiency probably accounts for the Wernicke-Korsakoff syndrome and the variety of psychiatric and neurologic deficiencies encountered under these conditions. The pathologic lesions are located in the same regions of the midbrain as in thiamine deficiency (Fig. 21-13). Cerebellar atrophy accounts for uncoordinated movements during walking and

FIGURE 21-13
Pathologic changes in the nervous system caused by chronic alcoholism.

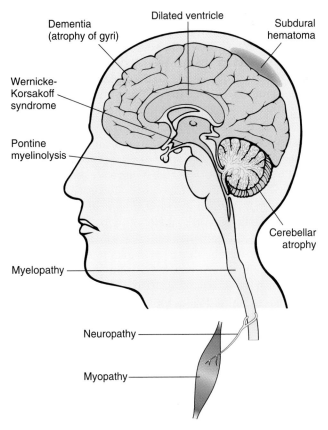

Dementia (atrophy of gyri)
Dilated ventricle
Subdural hematoma
Wernicke-Korsakoff syndrome
Pontine myelinolysis
Cerebellar atrophy
Myelopathy
Neuropathy
Myopathy

work. General cortical atrophy of the brain, probably related to a loss of neurons exposed to the neurotoxic effects of alcohol, results in progressive mental deterioration, loss of memory, an inability to concentrate, irritability, and many other symptoms. Myelopathy and sensory-motor neuropathy account for sensory deficiencies and the tremor and fatigability of muscles. Alcohol also has a direct adverse effect on the striated muscle cells.

Some of the pathologic changes encountered in chronic alcoholics are only indirectly related to alcohol abuse. For example, subdural hematoma, which is often found in such patients, may be related to repeated head trauma sustained in falling when inebriated. Pontine myelinolysis is a peculiar lesion in the pons that is related to vigorous correction of sodium imbalance in chronic alcoholics with cirrhosis. Withdrawal of alcohol, as in chronic alcoholics who are hospitalized, may induce an acute confusional state, known as delirium tremens (DT). DT develops suddenly and is characterized by agitation, confusion, and hallucinations. The patient cannot concentrate, pays no attention to others, and may hear strange voices or see objects that do not exist, like white mice or devils on the wall.

Neurodegenerative Diseases

The term **neurodegenerative disorders** is used (for lack of a better one) to describe a group of diseases of unknown etiology that are limited to the CNS. These diseases, which are unrelated to one another, present with a variety of neurologic and psychiatric symptoms. For example, Parkinson's disease presents with movement disorders, Huntington's disease is characterized by abnormal body movements and progressive mental deterioration, and Alzheimer's disease presents with only a loss of mental capacities, but no motor deficits.

The diagnosis of neurodegenerative disorders can readily be made in typical cases. However, many patients do not have all the typical clinical features, and the diagnosis may be made only by excluding all other brain diseases that could cause the same set of symptoms. Because these neurodegenerative diseases are incurable, one must be certain that the patient does not have a curable disease before establishing a diagnosis of neurodegenerative disease (Fig. 21-14).

Alzheimer's Disease

Alzheimer's disease is a form of dementia (loss of mental capacities) of unknown etiology. It is characterized pathologically by atrophy of the cortical parts of the frontal and temporal parts of the brain and typical histologic features. It affects older people,

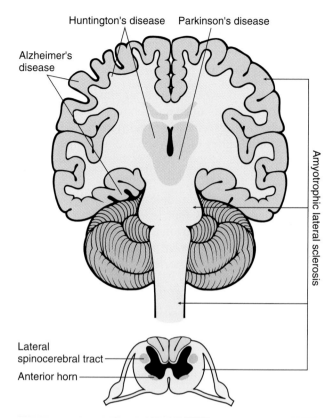

FIGURE 21-14
Degenerative diseases of the brain involve preferentially various parts of the brain. Alzheimer's disease causes atrophy of the frontal and occipital cortical gyri. Huntington's disease affects the frontal cortex and basal ganglia. Parkinson's disease is marked by changes in the substantia nigra. Amyotrophic lateral sclerosis affects the motor neurons in the anterior horn of the spinal cord, brain stem, and the frontal cortex of the brain.

most of whom are older than 70 years of age. The symptoms of Alzheimer's disease are seen only rarely in people younger than 60 years of age. The number of clinical cases increases progressively with age. Estimates are that 50 percent to 60 percent of people 85 years of age or older have dementia, and most of them have Alzheimer's disease. At the present time, there are approximately 600,000 people affected by Alzheimer's disease in the United States, and at least 60,000 new cases are diagnosed every year. As the population of the United States ages, the number of patients with Alzheimer's disease will increase, and one can expect that the number will exceed one million early in the 21st century.

Etiology and Pathogenesis. The causes of Alzheimer's disease and the pathogenesis of cerebral lesions are not known. Investigations have centered on possible genetic factors and the elucidation of the reasons for the degeneration of neurons that leads to atrophy of the cortex and mental deterioration.

Genetic factors play a role in the pathogenesis of

the familial form of Alzheimer's disease, but unfortunately, this form of disease is very rare and accounts for only a negligible number of cases. Familial Alzheimer's disease has been linked to genetic changes on chromosomes 21 and 19. In this context, it is of interest to mention that trisomy 21 is typical of Down syndrome, which shows identical neuropathologic changes to those of Alzheimer's disease. In both conditions, the brain has deposits of a special form of amyloid (amyloid beta protein), which could mediate brain injury. Chromosome 19 carries the gene for apolipoprotein E4 (apo E4), a plasma protein that is deposited in the brain lesions characteristic of Alzheimer's disease. It has been shown that the deposited apo E4 is actually a variant of normal plasma protein. The abnormal protein is produced by a mutated apo E4 gene. This mutated apo E4 gene is found in 3 percent of the normal population. The carriers of this abnormal gene develop Alzheimer's disease at an astounding rate (90 percent), which suggests that this gene may play an important pathogenetic role.

Neuronal loss in the brain of patients with Alzheimer's disease has been studied extensively. Existing evidence points to possible neurotoxic effects of amyloid, a fibrillar extracellular substance that is deposited in the brain lesions. Intracellular defects (e.g., abnormal function of a microtubule binding protein in neural cells) or the phosphorylation of neurofilaments have also been implicated. Neuronal loss may be related to decreased levels of nerve growth factor, which is essential for maintenance of normal nerve cells. None of these findings however, fully explains the pathogenesis of brain lesions in Alzheimer's disease, and so the search for its causes goes on.

Clinical Features. Alzheimer's disease presents clinically as a dementia. *Dementia* is defined as a progressive loss of cognitive functions and a functional decline that typically interferes with work and social activities. The loss of memory predominates; this loss is usually insidious, but tends to progress until the patient becomes completely dysfunctional and cannot perform any mental operations. As clinical function deteriorates, most patients also develop speech problems, must limit their daily activities, and finally become bedridden and completely dependent on nursing care. With adequate care, most patients with Alzheimer's disease live long lives. Death is not related to Alzheimer's disease itself, but usually reflects the decreased resistance to infection that normally occurs with advancing age.

The clinical diagnosis of Alzheimer's disease is based on the demonstration of progressive dementia. It should be remembered that dementia can result from a variety of cardiovascular, endocrine, and metabolic diseases, and that it may be induced by certain drugs. Brain tumors and infections also can cause dementia. The diagnosis of Alzheimer's disease should be made only after all these other possible causes of dementia have been excluded.

Specialized x-ray studies, such as computed tomography (CT) scans and MRIs, are useful for documenting atrophy of the cortex, but similar atrophy may be found in nondemented elderly people and those with multi-infarct dementia. Thus, the x-ray findings are not diagnostic. Laboratory findings are nonspecific and do not provide any direct support to the clinical diagnosis. Nevertheless, such studies may be useful in excluding other "organic" forms of dementia.

Pathology. The pathologic diagnosis of Alzheimer's disease is based on gross and microscopic neuropathologic findings. On gross examination, the brain appears atrophic and shows narrowing of the gyri and a widening of the sulci. Atrophy affects the frontal and temporal lobes most prominently. Histologic changes are most prominent in the cortex. Typical histologic features are neuritic (senile) plaques, neurofibrillary tangles, granulovacuolar degeneration, and deposition of amyloid in the neuritic plaques and the wall of the cerebral vessels. Some of these changes can be recognized on routine hematoxylin-eosin–stained slides, but they are more easily identified on slides prepared by special procedures. For example, neuritic plaques and neurofibrillary tangles are best seen after silver impregnation of tissue sections, whereas amyloid is best demonstrated by the Congo red stain or immunohistochemically, with specific antibodies.

Parkinson's Disease

Parkinson's disease (PD) is a subcortical neurodegenerative disorder characterized by movement disorders and pathologic changes of the extrapyramidal (involuntary) motor system nuclei of the midbrain. PD is relatively common, and it typically affects the elderly.

Etiology and Pathogenesis. The cause of PD is not known. The disease is characterized by a decreased number of dopaminergic neurons in the substantia nigra. These neurons release dopamine, a neurotransmitter, which is transported into another nucleus called striatum. The striatum and the substantia nigra form a functional unit. The substantia nigra of patients with PD is not dark (as is normal), but rather is depigmented owing to the loss of pigmented neurons. The amount of dopamine in the striatum is also reduced, which correlates with the retarded transmission of neuronal impulses between these nuclei. The loss of neurotransmitters correlates with the clinical appearance of movement disorders. The midbrain centers regulate and coordinate these movements and the impulses essential for the performance of such movements. L-dopa, a precursor of dopamine, and other drugs that increase the levels of dopamine in the brain may temporarily improve the symptoms in some patients. However, in most cases, PD is progressive and incurable.

Most patients with PD have the idiopathic form of the disease. In addition to this form, clinicians also recognize a secondary form, which is also called *parkinsonism*. The symptoms of parkinsonism are indistinguishable from those of PD except that, in the former group, the onset of symptoms can be traced to another pathologic event, such as encephalitis. Many drugs, especially those used in the treatment of psychiatric disease, can cause parkinsonism.

Clinical Features. PD presents with disturbances of movement, primarily tremor, rigidity, bradykinesia, and postural instability. Tremor or twitching of the muscles is most prominent in the hands or face and is typically enhanced by emotional stress. It is less prominent during voluntary movements. Rigidity and resistance to passive movements are increased. For example, if an affected patient is asked to move the arms against slight pressure exerted by the examiner, the movement has a staggering, cogwheel-like character. Bradykinesia refers to slowing of movements. Affected patients exhibit instability while walking. They walk bent forward, as if "chasing their point of gravity." A significant number of patients with PD become depressed, and about 10 percent develop dementia. The treatment of PD is symptomatic, as no cure is available.

Pathology. PD presents with rather consistent pathologic changes involving the striatonigral part of the brain stem. On gross examination, the substantia nigra appears pale. Histologically, this change is related to a loss of melanin-rich neurons in this subcortical nucleus. The remaining neurons contain typical round eosinophilic inclusions composed of neurofilaments, known as Lewy bodies. Similar inclusions are also seen in the cortical neurons, accounting for the development of depression and dementia in some of these patients.

Huntington's Disease

Huntington's disease is an autosomal dominant neurodegenerative disease characterized clinically by involuntary, gyrating movements (choreiform movements) and progressive dementia. The disease occurs in families and affects 1 in 20,000 people. The gene for the disease has been localized to chromosome 4.

Pathologically, Huntington's disease is characterized by atrophy of the cortex and subcortical nuclei, most prominently the caudate and putamen. Histologic changes are nonspecific and include atrophy, degeneration, and loss of neurons, accompanied by reactive gliosis.

Depite the hereditary nature of Huntington's disease, the first symptoms usually do not appear before mid-life. Once the symptoms appear, however, the patient's condition rapidly deteriorates. Most affected patients become completely mentally incapacitated by the age of 50 to 60 years, or even earlier.

Amyotrophic Lateral Sclerosis

Amyotrophic lateral sclerosis (ALS) is a neurodegenerative disease characterized by motor weakness and progressive wasting of muscles in the extremities, leading ultimately to generalized muscle loss and death. It is also known as Lou Gehrig disease, named after the famous baseball player who was afflicted by it. Although ALS is a rare disease, affecting 1 in 100,000 people, it has been of interest to scientists because of its unique features which could provide new insight into the pathogenesis of other, more common neurodegenerative diseases.

ALS affects older men and women. A familial form of ALS has been described in 10 percent of cases. The gene for this familiar form of the disease has been identified and localized to chromosome 21, the same chromosome that is involved in Down syndrome and Alzheimer's disease.

Clinically, ALS presents with weakness and wasting of the small hand muscles. Fasciculations (involuntary twitching) of muscles is typical. Such movements occur as fast, involuntary contractions that do not move the limbs. Speech becomes slurred in advanced cases, but the intellect is not affected. Most patients become immobile and ultimately die as a result of paralysis of the respiratory muscles. Pathologically, the disease is characterized by a loss of motor neurons in the spinal cord, midbrain, and finally, in the cerebral cortex. Most prominent is the loss of the lateral cerebrospinal pathways in the spinal cord (which prompted the name of the disease), as the lateral parts of the white matter are replaced by sclerosis. This change is related to the loss of motor axons and the skeletal muscle atrophy that is readily visible on muscle biopsy.

The diagnosis of ALS is made clinically. Electromyography shows typical denervation and muscular atrophy. Muscle biopsy can confirm this finding, but is rarely necessary. ALS is an incurable, progressive disease that inevitably leads to death over a period of a few years.

Neoplasms of the CNS

Neoplasms of the CNS are relatively rare, accounting for only 2 percent of all deaths secondary to cancer. Nevertheless, these tumors are important clinically for several reasons.

- Brain tumors have a very high mortality. This high mortality is partially related to the malignant nature of brain tumors and partially to their location. Any enlarging mass inside the cranial cavity could eventually kill a patient by compressing the vital centers!
- Brain tumors occur at any age, but are relatively prominent in younger age groups. In childhood, brain tumors account for 20 percent of all malignant diseases. In the 20- to 40-year age group, they are still among the most common cancers, accounting for 10 percent of cancer deaths. The occurrence of brain tumors does not decrease with age, but in that age group, tumors of the CNS do not stand out as such because they are overshadowed by the more common neoplasms.

Approximately 50 percent of brain tumors are primary neoplasms, whereas the other 50 percent represent metastases from other sites. Because there is a 50 percent chance that a tumor could be a metastasis, it is important to determine whether the patient has a malignant lesion elsewhere, before establishing a diagnosis of a primary malignant brain lesion. This approach also avoids unnecessary brain surgery.

Intracranial tumors can be histologically classified as benign or malignant. Malignant tumors have a tendency for infiltrative growth; therefore, it is almost impossible to remove them completely by surgery. Benign tumors are curable, but may also cause death owing to their inaccessibility or their location close to a vital center. Although histologically benign, such tumors could clinically be considered to be malignant.

Malignant tumors of the CNS differ from malignant diseases in other parts of the body in that they do not metastasize. Death occurs as a result of intracranial mass effects and the compression of vital centers. This can occur owing to the direct impingement of the tumor on vital centers or because of increased intracranial pressure and the compression of the brain stem by the herniated cerebellar tonsils or the uncal gyri of the hippocampus (see Fig. 21-3).

Classification. Tumors of the CNS can be classified, according to their derivation, into several groups, the most important of which are

- tumors of glial cells (75 percent)
- tumors of neural cell precursors (2 percent)
- tumors of the meninges (15 percent)
- tumors of the cranial and spinal nerves (5 percent)

Other tumors, such as hemangiomas and hemangioblastomas originating from cerebral blood vessels, primary cerebral lymphomas, or pinealomas (tumors of the pineal gland), are generally rare. An increased incidence of primary brain lymphoma has been noted in immunosuppressed patients with AIDS.

Tumors can occur in any part of the CNS. Various histologic tumor forms differ in their predilection for certain anatomic sites (Fig. 21-15). For exam-

FIGURE 21-15
Intracranial tumors. The sketch shows the most common anatomic sites of various tumors.

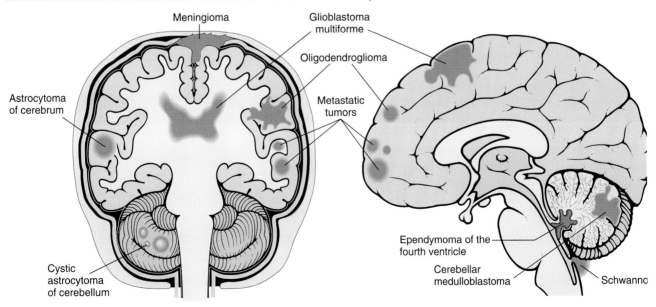

ple, medulloblastoma is always located in the cerebellum. Cystic astrocytomas of childhood are most often found in the cerebellum, whereas solid astrocytomas and glioblastoma multiforme occur most often in the cerebrum. Meningiomas arise from the meninges, most often along the falx cerebri, the midsagittal line between the two cerebral hemispheres.

Etiology and Pathogenesis. The causes of brain tumors are not known. No definitive risk factors have been identified for most CNS tumors. Nevertheless, there are several promising leads for future research that have been derived from the study of some less common forms of CNS tumors. For example, nerve sheath tumors involving cranial nerve VIII (acoustic schwannomas) are familial, and are a feature of the hereditary neurofibromatosis type II syndrome. These tumors have been linked to changes in a tumor suppressor gene typically found in affected families. An increased incidence of meningiomas has been noted in patients with familial neoplastic syndromes, such as neurofibromatosis type I and multiple endocrine adenomatosis type II, a syndrome characterized by the appearance of medullary carcinoma of the thyroid and adrenal medullary tumors (pheochromocytomas). Approximately 75 percent of meningiomas show a peculiar chromosomal change: deletion of the long arm of chromosome 22. This chromosomal segment carries the neurofibromatosis tumor suppressor gene. These findings link meningiomas to neurofibromatosis and provide evidence for the possible genetic etiology of these tumors. Cerebellar hemangioblastomas are also familial. These tumors are found in families affected by von Hippel-Lindau disease, a hereditary condition characterized by blood vessel tumors in the brain and retina; cysts in the kidney, liver, and pancreas; and a strong tendency for renal cell carcinoma. These patients carry a mutated suppressor gene that has been localized to chromosome 3.

The molecular biological and chromosomal changes in glial cell tumors, the most common CNS neoplasms, are more complex. Like colon cancer and several other malignant diseases, most glioblastomas show mutation of the p53 suppressor gene. A loss of alleles from chromosomes 17 and 19 is found at a high rate, but the significance of these genetic and chromosomal changes remains enigmatic. No genetic markers unique to brain tumors have yet been identified.

Gliomas

Tumors arising from glial cells can be classified as astrocytic, oligodendroglial, or ependymal. Tumors previously considered to be of microglial origin have been reclassified as cerebral lymphomas.

Astrocytic tumors, known as astrocytomas and glioblastoma multiforme, account for about 80 percent of these tumors. Oligodendrogliomas and ependymomas are less common, each accounting for 10 percent of all gliomas. All gliomas are malignant.

Astrocytic gliomas can be subdivided into two groups. The less malignant tumors are called astrocytomas, whereas the highly malignant variety is called glioblastoma multiforme.

Astrocytomas occur as solid cerebral tumors in adults and as cystic cerebellar tumors in children. On histologic examination, astrocytomas are composed of relatively well-differentiated astrocytes. Initially, these slow-growing tumors show low mitotic activity and no cellular anaplasia. However, with time, they tend to become more malignant and ultimately progress into lesions that are histologically indistinguishable from glioblastoma multiforme.

Glioblastoma multiforme is the most common CNS tumor. Its peak incidence occurs at 65 years of age, but it may occur in younger persons as well. Most of these tumors are found in the lateral hemispheres of the brain (Fig. 21-16). As its name implies, the tumor has a highly variegated gross appearance. Parts of the tumor are necrotic and yellow, parts are hemorrhagic red, and parts are white, like normal brain. Typically, the lesion is irregularly shaped and poorly demarcated from normal brain parenchyma, often extending through the corpus callosum from one cerebral hemisphere into the other. On cross-sectional examination of the brain at autopsy, or by CT scanning and MRI in living patients, such bilateral lesions have a butterfly-like appearance.

Histologic studies reveal that glioblastomas are composed of highly anaplastic astrocytic cells. These cells may retain a fetal appearance, in which case

FIGURE 21-16

Glioblastoma multiforme. Gross appearance of a bilateral "butterfly" tumor. (From Okazaki H, Scheithauer BW. Atlas of neuropathology. New York/London: Gower Medical Publishing, 1988. By permission of Mayo Foundation.)

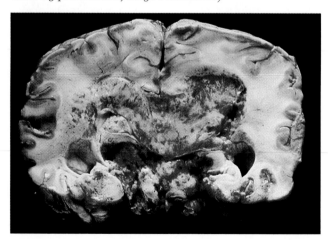

they have small blue nuclei and no cytoplasm. Alternatively, they may become enlarged, take on a bizarre shape, or be multinucleated with well-developed cytoplasm. Mitotic figures are numerous. Typically, the blood vessels in the tumor show marked proliferative changes. Invasive, rapid growth of cells and the vascular changes account for the common occurrence of necrosis and hemorrhage in the tumor.

Oligodendrogliomas are rare gliomas that usually involve the cerebral hemisphere of middle-aged adults. These tumors are usually well circumscribed, often partially cystic, and calcified. Histologically, these tumors are composed of well-differentiated oligodendroglial cells. The tumors can be classified histologically as low-grade or high-grade malignant lesions, but the correlation between histologic findings and survival is not perfect. The poor correlation between histology and prognosis is related to the fact that 50 percent of all oligodendrogliomas contain astrocytes, which may not be evident in a small brain biopsy. Because astrocytes proliferate at a higher rate than do oligodendroglial cells, mixed tumors (occasionally called oligoastrocytomas), grow faster than pure oligodendrogliomas. Such tumors may progress to glioblastoma multiforme. Pure, well-differentiated oligodendrogliomas have a more indolent course.

Ependymomas are derived from ependymal cells lining the ventricles and central canal of the spinal cord. Ventricular ependymomas are typically found in children. In adults, ependymomas are usually located in the spinal cord. On histologic examination, ependymoma cells have round or elongated nuclei and are enmeshed in a fibrillar background. Tumor cells line the papillary structures or form rosettes (i.e., structures reminiscent of ependymal canals and fetal neural tubes). Ependymomas of the filum terminale (i.e., the terminal part of the spinal cord) are often composed of papillae in loose myxomatous connective tissue (myxopapillary ependymoma).

The prognosis of gliomas depends on their location and their histologic composition. Glioblastoma multiforme is invariably fatal, regardless of its location. With modern surgical and radiation therapy, patients with astrocytomas may survive 5 years after diagnosis, but most die because the tumors cannot be removed in their entirety. Cerebral oligodendrogliomas and ependymomas have a somewhat more favorable prognosis, but even these tumors have a high mortality. Ependymomas of the filum terminale can be removed surgically and have a good prognosis.

Tumors of Neural Cell Precursors and Undifferentiated Cells

Terminally differentiated neurons cannot proliferate and are thus incapable of malignant transformation. Hence, it is thought that neuroectodermal tumors probably arise from undifferentiated, fetal precursors retained in the brain of infants and children. It has also been proposed that the neural cells may undergo reverse development, or "dedifferentiation," regressing to a fetal stage, becoming mitotic, and giving rise to neoplasms. There is no support for any of these theories and, thus, the source of neuroectodermal tumors remains obscure.

Approximately 10 percent to 15 percent of all brain tumors are composed of primitive neuroectodermal cells resembling those found in the fetal neural tube. The most important tumor in this group is *medulloblastoma,* a cerebellar childhood tumor of uncertain origin. It is generally assumed that medulloblastomas originate from fetal neural cell precursors, although it is not clear why such fetal cells would remain in the cerebellum. An alternative explanation, involving dedifferentiation of neurons or proliferation of the outer granular layer of cerebellum, is speculative and is not supported by solid evidence.

Medulloblastomas are composed of fetal-like neuroectodermal cells (i.e., cells that are reminiscent of those in fetal medulla spinalis). These tumors are limited to the cerebellum and are found only in children. The tumors grow quickly, and although they are sensitive to radiation therapy and chemotherapy, they have a poor prognosis. Medulloblastoma cells can enter the CSF and be carried by CSF. These cells may travel through the central canal of the spinal cord and form implantation metastases in the spinal cord.

Meningioma

Meningiomas arise from the meninges (Fig. 21-17). Most meningiomas are benign and are located in the midline, impinging from outside the cerebral hemispheres. However, meningiomas can also arise from the meninges at the base of the brain and along the spinal cord. Compression of the brain may cause

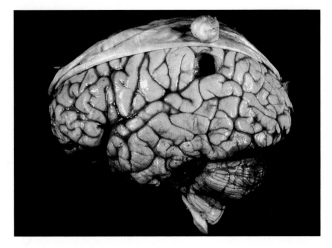

FIGURE 21-17
Meningioma. The round tumor has been shelled out from the hole that it has produced in the brain. (From Okazaki H, Scheithauer BW. Atlas of neuropathology. New York/London: Gower Medical Publishing, 1988. By permission of Mayo Foundation.)

epileptic seizures or motor deficits. These localized tumors can be removed surgically and, therefore, have an excellent prognosis.

Tumors of the Cranial and Spinal Nerves

Tumors originating from the nerves, collectively called *neuromas,* are composed of cells enveloping the axons. Those composed of schwann cells are called *schwannomas* or *neurilemomas,* whereas those composed of neurofibroblasts are termed *neurofibromas.*

Schwannomas can originate anywhere along the length of the cranial or spinal nerves. Because schwann cells envelop not only the peripheral portion of the nerves, but also the initial intradural parts, some schwannomas are intradural (i.e., located inside the vertebral canal or the cranial cavity). Intracranial schwannomas arise most often from the cranial nerve VIII and are located in the cerebellopontine angle.

Neuromas may be solitary or multiple. Multiple tumors of the peripheral nerves are a feature of neurofibromatosis type I, an autosomal dominant disease that affects approximately 100,000 Americans. Acoustic neuromas are typical of neurofibromatosis type II. These neuromas cause hearing loss and vertigo, and may compress the cerebellum and pons.

Most of the solitary and even the multiple neuromas are benign. Malignant neural tumors, called neurofibrosarcomas, are rare. Most neurofibrosarcomas are found in patients with neurofibromatosis. These tumors develop as a result of the malignant transformation of a preexisting benign nerve tumor. Sporadic neurofibrosarcomas are less common.

Metastases to the Brain

Approximately 50 percent of all brain tumors represent metastases from a malignant tumor involving some other site. Metastases may be solitary or multiple. Although any malignant tumor may metastasize to the brain, certain malignant tumors have a special predilection for spread to the brain, including lung cancer, breast cancer, and melanoma. Any part of the brain may be involved.

Review Questions

1. List the main components of the central and peripheral nervous system.
2. Describe the functions of the four major lobes of the brain.
3. Compare the functions of the midbrain, pons, and medulla oblongata with that of the cerebellum.
4. Describe the function of the spinal cord.
5. Describe the circulation of the cerebrospinal fluid.
6. List the main cells of the nervous system.
7. What are the most important diseases of the nervous system?
8. What are the sites of brain herniation caused by intracranial hypertension?
9. List the main dysraphic disorders of the central nervous system and describe their pathogenesis.
10. List the most important intracranial hemorrhages and describe their causes.
11. What is stroke?

12. What is global cerebral ischemia and what are its consequences?

13. What is the pathogenesis of "watershed infarcts" and laminar necrosis of the brain?

14. Describe the pathology of cerebral infarcts.

15. Correlate the pathology of intracerebral hemorrhage with the clinical features of this disease.

16. What are the main pathologic findings following brain injury?

17. Compare hyperextension and hyperflexion injuries of the cervical spine.

18. Compare bacterial and viral infections of the central nervous system.

19. What are prions?

20. List the most important protozoal and fungal causes of opportunistic diseases of the central nervous system.

21. Compare the pathology of encephalitis and meningitis.

22. Describe the features of neurosyphilis.

23. What are the most important AIDS-related CNS lesions?

24. What is multiple sclerosis?

25. Correlate the pathologic features of multiple sclerosis with the clinical signs and symptoms of this disease.

26. How do inborn errors of metabolism affect the central nervous system?

27. What is the cause and what are the signs of Wernicke-Korsakoff syndrome?

28. How does alcohol affect the brain?

29. What are the most important neurodegenerative diseases?

30. What is Alzheimer's disease and how is it diagnosed?

31. Describe the macroscopic and microscopic pathologic findings in Alzheimer's disease.

32. What is Parkinson's disease?

33. Correlate the pathology of Parkinson's disease with the clinical features of this disease.

34. What is amyotrophic lateral sclerosis?

35. Correlate the pathology of amyotrophic lateral sclerosis with the clinical features of this disease.

36. Classify brain tumors.

37. List the most common brain tumors and their predominant location.

38. Compare glioblastoma multiforme with other gliomas.

39. Which brain tumors occur most often in children?

40. Why to medulloblastomas metastasize?

41. What are meningiomas?

42. Which tumors originate from the peripheral nerves?

After reading this chapter, the student should be able to:

1. Describe the normal anatomy and physiology of the eye and its appendages.

2. Describe two developmental disorders affecting the eyes.

3. Discuss the adverse effects of ocular trauma.

4. Describe the various forms of infection of the eye and define conjunctivitis, keratitis, and endophthalmitis.

5. Describe the adverse effects of arterial hypertension and diabetes on the eye.

6. Describe the pathogenesis of glaucoma and its effect on vision.

7. Discuss the significance of cataracts.

8. Discuss eye tumors, with special emphasis on retinoblastoma and melanoma.

Additional Key Terms and Concepts

Blindness

Conjunctivitis

Papilledema

Retinitis pigmentosa

Retinopathy

Trachoma

Chapter Outline

The Eye
Chapter 22

The visual system consists of the eye, the optic nerve, the optic nerve pathways, and the visual centers in the occipital lobe of the brain.

NORMAL ANATOMY AND PHYSIOLOGY

The eyes are the primary organs of vision (Fig. 22-1). Each eyeball (the globe or bulbus) is located within the bony orbit of the skull, which provides protection and support from the posterior side. On the anterior side, the eyes are protected by the eyelids. The lacrimal glands, which are also located in the bony orbit, secrete tears which keep the anterior surface of the eye, the cornea, and the sclera moist. Tears also contain antibacterial substances and protect the eye from infections. The extraocular muscles attached to the posterior and lateral sides of the globe make eye movement possible.

The globes are composed of three layers: (1) the fibrous layer called the *sclera;* (2) the vascular layers, which are composed of three distinct parts: *choroid, ciliary body,* and *iris;* and (3) the inner layer called the *retina,* which is composed of pigmented and neural cells. On the anterior side, the sclera extends into a *cornea,* a translucent layer that allows the passage of light into the inside of the globe. The external surface of the cornea and sclera are covered with a thin, translucent layer called the conjunctiva, which also covers the inside of the eyelids. The space behind the cornea is called the anterior eye chamber. Posteriorly, this space is delimited by the lens and the iris. The lens is attached laterally by ligaments to the smooth muscles of the ciliary body. The space behind the lens, called the vitreous cavity, is filled with a gelatinous, clear, vitreous body. The posterior wall of the globe is multilayered. The innermost layer is the retina, lying on the uvea, which, in turn, is attached to the sclera. The neural part of the retina is composed of photoreceptor, bipolar, and ganglionic neurons. The axons of the ganglionic neurons form the optic nerve, which exits the eye posteriorly.

All of these components of the eye are important directly or indirectly in sustaining the sensory function of the eye—that is, the ability of the eye to receive visual stimuli. The light entering the eye through the anterior side of the globe is refracted through the cornea and the lens. Passing through the vitreous, it reaches the rods and cones of the retina. There are approximately 3 million cones and 100 million rods in the retina. Cones are especially prominent in the central uvea in the center of the retina, which is called the macula lutea (in Latin, "yellow spot") because of its yellow color. The fovea is the area of sharpest vision. All parts of the retina can receive light signals except the site at which the optic nerve leaves the globe, called the blind spot, or optic disc.

Vision depends on the proper function of all parts of the eye. The cornea, lens, aqueous humor, and vitreous body must be translucent to allow the passage of light. The cornea and the lens must also have a normal shape and must be able to accommodate so that rays of light are refracted properly. The lens is kept in place by connective tissue ligaments,

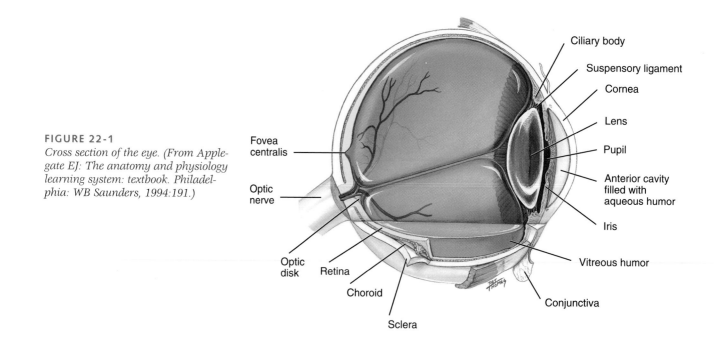

FIGURE 22-1

Cross section of the eye. (From Applegate EJ: The anatomy and physiology learning system: textbook. Philadelphia: WB Saunders, 1994:191.)

Fovea centralis

Optic nerve

Optic disk   Retina

Choroid

Sclera

Ciliary body

Suspensory ligament

Cornea

Lens

Pupil

Anterior cavity filled with aqueous humor

Iris

Vitreous humor

Conjunctiva

Table 22-1 Functions of the Major Parts of the Eye

Structure	Function
Sclera	External protection
Cornea	Light refraction
Choroid	Blood supply
Iris	Light absorption and regulation of pupillary width
Ciliary body	Secretion of vitreous fluid. In addition, its smooth muscles change the shape of the lens.
Lens	Light refraction
Retinal layer	Light receptor that transforms optic signals into nerve impulses
Rods	Means of distinguishing light from dark, and perceiving shape and movement
Cones	Color vision
Central fovea	Area of sharpest vision
Macula lutea	Blind spot
External ocular muscles	Movement of the globe
Optic nerve (cranial nerve II)	Transmission of visual information to the brain
Lacrimal glands	Secretion of tears
Eyelid	Eye protection

which must be firm and resilient to keep the lens in place. The shape of the lens is modified by the contraction of the smooth muscles in the ciliary body. The ciliary body also secretes the aqueous humor, the fluid that fills the anterior eye chamber. The iris contains pigment cells that prevent side entry of light into the globe. The iris can dilate (*mydriasis*) or constrict (*myosis*) under the influence of sympathetic or parasympathetic stimuli, respectively.

The most important functions of the various anatomic parts of the eye are listed in Table 22-1.

OVERVIEW OF MAJOR DISEASES

Diseases of the eye are very common. Minor visual problems, like shortsightedness, are not even considered to be "true" diseases, but rather represent cosmetic defects. Eyeglasses to correct for farsightedness can be bought in drug stores without a prescription. These functional disturbances have not been adequately explained in terms of pathologic anatomy, and so will not be discussed here.

Functional eye problems—that is, problems of diffraction—are treated by optometrists. Ophthalmologists (from the Greek *ophthalmos,* meaning eye) are the medical specialists who treat pathologically altered eyes using sophisticated surgical instruments, laser beams, and medications.

The most important diseases of the eye and its appendages are

- infections
- immunologic diseases
- traumatic lesions
- circulatory disturbances, including disorders of blood circulation or flow of aqueous humor
- degenerative diseases, such as cataracts
- neoplasms

Several facts important to an understanding of eye pathology are presented here, before a discussion of specific pathologic entities.

1. *Most functional visual problems do not have a defined pathology.* The most common reason people go to see an eye doctor is to get eyeglasses. One third of the population in the United States wears eyeglasses or contact lenses. Eyeglasses are an efficient means of correcting shortsightedness (*myopia*) or longsightedness (*hyperopia*). An irregular surface of the cornea or the lens may result in uneven refraction of light, leading to *astigmatism,* which can also be corrected with eyeglasses or contact lenses. Farsightedness of old age, or *presbyopia* (*presbys* meaning old in Greek), is thought to be related to the loss of elasticity of the lens in the elderly. The reasons for the high prevalence of difractory abnormalities in younger people are not known. The eyes of affected individuals do not show any pathologic changes.

2. *Eye problems occur at any age, but overall, their prevalence increases with advancing age.* Presbyopia, or old-age farsightedness, occurs predictably, and essentially all people older than 60 years of age require glasses for reading. The prevalence of other eye diseases also increases proportionally with age. The most prominent among these diseases are various circula-

Did You Know?

Reading in dim light does not damage the eye or cause shortsightedness. It is a common misconception that bookish people, especially those who read in inadequately lighted rooms, are at risk of damaging their eyesight. The cause of nearsightedness is not known, nor is the structural basis of shortsightedness understood.

tory disturbances related to atherosclerosis, diabetes mellitus, and hypertension. *Glaucoma,* a disease related to impeded circulation of vitreous fluid, is also very common in the elderly. *Cataracts* (i.e., opacification and blurring of the lens) are yet another very common cause of impaired vision in the elderly. *Macular degeneration,* an age-related disease affecting the pigmented cells in the macula lutea, is the leading cause of visual problems in the elderly. The pathogenesis of all these diseases of aging is not understood.

3. *Infections of the eyes and eye appendages are common because the eyes are exposed to the external world.* Eyes are prone to infections with bacteria, viruses, and many other pathogens that reach the eye in droplets by dirt on fingers or dust. Because the lacrimal canals drain into the upper respiratory tract, all flu-like infections of the nose, mouth, and pharynx often extend into the eye.

4. *Eyes are often affected by allergies.* Various antigens from the external world, such as pollen or organic components of house dust, are readily deposited on the conjunctiva; such substances may evoke an immunoglobulin E (IgE)–mediated, type I hypersensitivity reaction. Conjunctivitis is, therefore, a constant feature of hay fever and similar hypersensitivity reactions.

5. *Nutritional deficiencies and metabolic disturbances may affect a person's sight.* The best known among the nutritional deficiencies is avitaminosis A, which results in night blindness. Additionally, diabetic retinopathy is an important cause of blindness.

6. *Blindness, or complete loss of vision, may be caused by many diseases involving the eye, the optic nerve, or the brain.* Blindness is a very important health problem. In the United States, 4 of every 1000 persons are blind, but in other parts of the world, blindness is even more common. The most important causes of blindness in the United States are metabolic and developmental anomalies, eye trauma, diabetes, glaucoma, and cataracts. Senile macular degeneration, a disease of old age that is poorly understood, is an important cause of blindness in the elderly. In parts of Africa, infections with *Mycoplasma trachomatis* and a parasite *Onchocerca volvulus* still cause blindness among millions.

7. *Tumors of the eye originate most often from the melanocytes and retinal cells.* Overall, tumors of the eye globe are rare. However, these tumors have unique features because of their location and because they originate from highly specialized cells: the retinal melanocytes and specialized neural cells.

Skin tumors of the lids are 100 times more common than intraocular tumors. These neoplasms, which are usually diagnosed histologically as basal or squamous cell carcinomas, have all the features of histologically identical skin tumors, and so are not included here. Similarly, tumors of the lacrimal

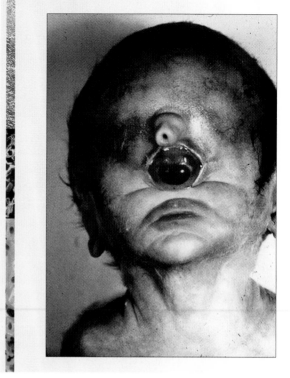

This congenitally deformed child has only one eye, resembling a Cyclops. Fortunately, such severe malformations are rare.

glands are histologically identical to those in the salivary glands, and so are not discussed here.

Developmental Disorders

Developmental disorders of the eye may occur in an isolated form and without an obvious cause, or they may be associated with other congenital defects. In addition, they are occasionally related to a well-defined cause, such as intrauterine rubella infection.

Congenital developmental disorders of the eye may present as numerical or structural abnormalities. Congenital lack of one eye is usually incompatible with life because it is associated with major brain malformations. The solitary eye of these babies is usually located in the middle of the forehead. The anomaly is called cyclopia, a term derived from the one-eyed monsters (Cyclops) in Greek mythology.

Structural congenital abnormalities of the eyes are common consequences of intrauterine infections with the pathogens that cause the TORCH syndrome (toxoplasmosis, rubella, cytomegalovirus, and herpesvirus). Maternal infection during pregnancy with any of these pathogens may result in one-sided or bilateral blindness, *congenital cataracts* (clouding of the lens), or *microphthalmia* (underdeveloped, small bulbus).

Many chromosomal abnormalities are associated with congenital eye abnormalities. The best known are the eye changes in Down syndrome, which include pigmentary abnormalities of the iris (so-called *Brushfield's spots*). The eyes are tilted laterally and have a medial palpebral rim known as epicanthus.

Not all congenital eye defects are as obvious as those described above. Some of them are just minor cosmetic defects, like *coloboma,* a slit-like defect in the iris. A pigmented nevus of the iris is nothing more than a beauty mark!

Retinitis pigmentosa is a hereditary disease affecting the retina. Although the disease is inherited, the symptoms, such as partial loss of the visual field, occur in adulthood. Retinitis pigmentosa ultimately leads to blindness.

Trauma

Trauma to the eyes may be induced mechanically by various objects or chemically by acids, alkali, or metals. Mechanical trauma can be classified as blunt, superficial, or penetrating. Chemical trauma may be classified as irritating or mordant. In some cases, the mechanical injury is combined with chemical after-effects. For example, a small sliver of iron lodged in the globe may oxidize and release potentially dangerous ferric ions which could propagate the injury.

Blunt trauma usually leads to intraocular hemorrhages. Such hemorrhages typically originate from disrupted small blood vessels. The bleeding from the conjunctiva usually leads to hematoma of the cornea, which is clearly visible on the white background on which it has occurred. Intraocular hematomas that are not readily recognized on external examination are typically reported by the patient as reddish blurring of the vision. Such hematomas can be documented by ophthalmoscopy.

Hemorrhages behind the retina, called retroretinal hemorrhages, are especially dangerous because they typically cause blindness. Retroretinal hemorrhages are characteristically found in battered children. In such cases, the bleeding occurs when the child's head is forcefully shaken by an adult. Histologic confirmation of retroretinal hemorrhage is important for legal documentation of battered child syndrome.

Superficial trauma causes minor defects on the eye surface, such as *corneal abrasion.* Typically, the trauma is caused by a sharp object (knife, needle), by scratching, or by a foreign body (speck of dust). The lesion presents with pain, redness of the cornea, and tearing. Healing occurs in most cases,

but occasionally, scarring may be an important late complication.

Penetrating trauma of the eye, usually inflicted with a sharp object like a knife or screwdriver, punctures the globe. Owing to the loss of intraocular fluid, the bulbus collapses and the eye may be irreparably damaged. Infections are important late complications.

Chemical trauma usually damages the cornea and sclera. Superficial ulcerations are prone to infection, but may heal without consequence. Scarring is an important complication of severe chemical burns of the cornea. Such injury may necessitate corneal transplantation.

Infections

Infections of the eye are common, and are designated according to the anatomic structure involved (Fig. 22-2). Fortunately, most infections are superficial and limited to the conjunctiva and eyelids. Endophthalmitis, an infection of the inside of the eye that is usually a complication of trauma, is rare.

Conjunctivitis (or "pinkeye"), an infection of the conjunctiva lining the anterior side of the globe and the inside of the palpebrae, is a very common disease. It is usually caused by viruses or bacteria. The inflamed eye shows marked redness owing to active hyperemia. An exudate may form and the palpebral pockets may be filled with pus. The disease heals spontaneously or it may respond to local antibiotic treatment. Its consequences are rarely serious.

Conjunctival inflammation may spread to adjacent structures. For example, it may involve the lacrimal glands (*dacryocystitis*). Stye involving the glands of the eyelids is called *hordeolum.* Inflammation of the eyelids (*blepharitis*) results in edema and redness of the eyelids, and may be so severe that the patient cannot open the eyes.

Keratitis develops when an infection extends into the cornea or when conjunctivitis presents as an ulcerating disease. In this country, this is usually a

Did You Know?

Pinkeye can be treated efficiently with nonprescription eye drops. Treatment should not be indiscriminate, however. Indeed, no treatment is usually the best treatment because pinkeye is most often caused by viruses, which do not respond to antibiotics. Bacterial infections, which can be treated with antibiotics, are less common. Allergy is a common but treatable cause of pinkeye.

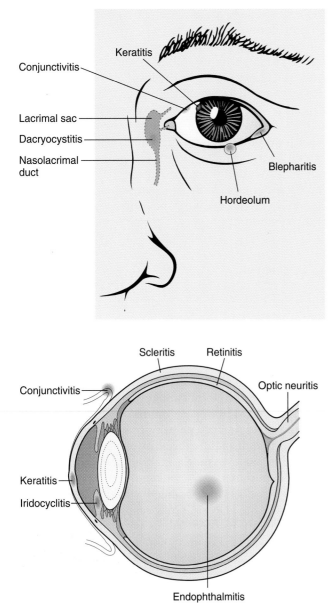

FIGURE 22-2
Infections of the eye: blepharitis, conjunctivitis, keratitis, dacryocystitis, iridocyclitis, and endophthalmitis.

feature of herpesvirus infection. Herpesvirus initially causes corneal vesicles, which ulcerate and then are covered with crusts. These lesions heal, but may cause permanent defects in the form of scars.

Trachoma is a conjunctivitis, caused by *Chlamydia trachomatis,* which is prevalent in underdeveloped countries of Africa and Asia. The infection is typically associated with corneal ulcers and scarring. Blindness is an important late complication in such cases.

Keratitis, uveitis, and retinitis are uncommon complications of superficial eye infections that have extended into the deeper layers of the eye. Nevertheless, they are a component of some chronic infectious diseases, such as syphilis. The infection may in-

volve the entire eye (**panophthalmitis**), or it may be localized to the inside of the eye (**endophthalmitis**). In many cases, only part of the globe inside is involved. For example, inflammation of the uveal tract can involve the entire structure (*uveitis*), or only one part (e.g., **iridocyclitis**).

All eye infections require prompt treatment because they may cause loss of eyesight. Superficial infections have a good prognosis. Ulcerating infections and those involving the deeper layers of the eye may result in blindness.

Immunologic Disease

Infectious diseases of the eye must be distinguished from allergies, which often present with the same clinical symptoms. Type I hypersensitivity reaction is the cause of allergic conjunctivitis, an itchy superficial inflammation that responds well to antihistamines and steroid treatment. Type III hypersensitivity reactions involving the ciliary body or the choroid are occasionally found in patients with systemic lupus erythematosus. Type IV hypersensitivity reactions (i.e., granulomas of the eye bulbus) are rare. The prototypical disease of this type—sarcoidosis—often presents with granulomas of the lacrimal glands.

Circulatory Disorders

The delicate, thin-walled blood vessels of the eye are susceptible to damage caused by **circulatory disorders** associated with several systemic diseases. Most notable among these are hypertension and diabetes.

Hypertensive Retinopathy

Sustained arterial hypertension or sudden bouts of arterial hypertension may damage retinal and choroidal blood vessels and cause damage on the eye background. Such arteriolar changes are readily seen by fundoscopy using an ophthalmoscope (Fig. 22-3). The extent of the changes can be graded, on a scale from I to IV, as mild, moderate, advanced, or severe. Prolonged hypertension, which is typically associated with arteriosclerosis, leads to reactive narrowing of the retinal arterioles. On ophthalmoscopic examination, such arterioles appear like copper wires. As the blood flow diminishes because of increasing arteriolar constriction, the arterioles become whitish, like silver wires. Elevated blood pressure leads to formation of microaneurysms and hemorrhages into the retinal nerve fiber layer, known as dot and flame-shaped hemorrhages. Exudates, known as hard exudates, soft exudates, macular star, and cotton-wool spots, are also found. In severe hypertensive retinop-

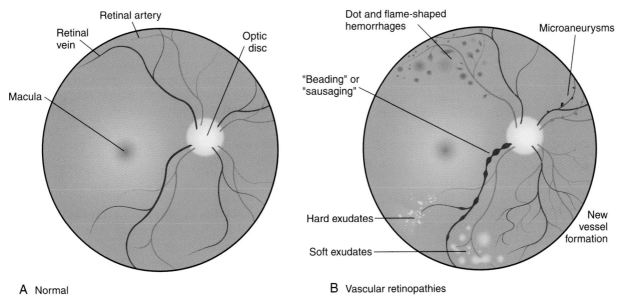

FIGURE 22-3
Vascular retinal diseases are most often caused by diabetes and hypertension. (A) Normal fundus of the retina, as seen with an ophthalmoscope. (B) Vascular and retinal lesions that can easily be diagnosed by ophthalmoscope.

athy, there is edema of the optic disc (papilledema). Because these changes are irreversible, it is clearly advisable to prevent them by treating the underlying hypertension rather than to wait passively until the retina has been damaged irreparably.

Diabetic Retinopathy

Diabetes mellitus is one of the major causes of blindness in the United States. Diabetes affects the eye in several ways, most notably by promoting the formation of cataracts and by causing diabetic retinopathy.

Pathology. Diabetic retinopathy occurs in two forms: background and proliferative retinopathy. Both forms of diabetic retinopathy can be explained in terms of changes in the basement membrane of the arterioles and capillaries of the choroid and retina. Diabetic microangiopathy manifests itself either as a narrowing of the vascular lumina or focal dilatation and formation of microaneurysms (Fig. 22-4). The diabetic blood vessels are more permeable than normal vessels, which leads to edema and hemorrhages into the eye (*background retinopathy*). Such serous exudates are recognized on fundoscopy as cotton-wool spots. Ischemia secondary to vascular changes results in degenerative changes and fibrous streaks. Reperfusion of ischemic areas is accomplished by neovascularization (*proliferative retinopathy*). In severe forms of the disease, there is retroretinal fibrosis and retinal detachment, typically associated with blindness.

FIGURE 22-4
Diabetic retinopathy. (A) Nonproliferative retinopathy shows edema, microaneurysm, and exudates. (B) Proliferative retinopathy shows new blood vessel formation.

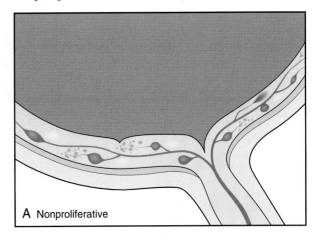

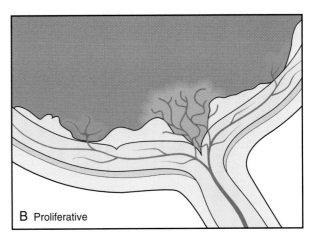

Glaucoma

Glaucoma is a term used to describe several eye diseases characterized by increased intraocular pressure and leading to atrophy of the optic nerve and retinal ganglion cells with consequent loss of peripheral as well as central visual fields. It is a very common disease, affecting 1 percent to 3 percent of all people older than 40 years of age. Early diagnosis and treatment can prevent progression of ocular changes and blindness.

Pathophysiology. Glaucoma is related to disturbances in the formation and circulation of the intraocular fluid. Under normal circumstances, the aqueous humor is secreted by the ciliary body into the posterior chamber. From there, it moves into the anterior chamber, passing through a narrow space delimited anteriorly by the iris and posteriorly by the lens and the zonular ligaments that hold the lens in place. From the anterior chamber, the fluid is resorbed into the small veins at the anterolateral margin of the iris. In glaucoma, the flow of fluid is disrupted, with the result that it accumulates inside the globe, causing intraocular hypertension.

Pathology. Glaucoma is considered to be *primary* when it occurs without any obvious cause. It is classified as *secondary* when it is related to a preexisting eye disease, such as iridocyclitis, intraocular hemorrhage, trauma, or tumors. Primary glaucoma is more common than the secondary form of this disease.

Primary glaucoma may be pathogenetically classified into two subtypes: open-angle and closed-angle glaucoma (Fig. 22-5). The etiology of primary open-

FIGURE 22-5
Glaucoma. (A) In open-angle glaucoma, the obstruction occurs in the trabecular meshwork. (B) In closed-angle glaucoma, the trabecular meshwork is covered by the root of the iris or adhesions between the iris and the cornea.

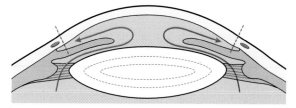

A Open-angle glaucoma

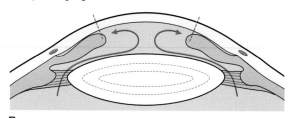

B Closed-angle glaucoma

Did You Know?

Sharp pain that is typical of acute closed-angle glaucoma most often occurs in dim light. As the pupil dilates in response to dim light, the iris folds, closing the lateral angle of the anterior chamber and impeding the outflow of aqueous humor from the eye. The sudden rise in intraocular pressure may cause sudden blindness and pain.

angle glaucoma, the most frequent form of disease, is unknown. As implied by its name, the angle of the anterior chamber through which the aqueous humor is resorbed is open. The disease develops insidiously and is characterized by a progressive, slowly evolving elevation of intraocular pressure. This can be measured using an ophthalmic tonometer applied to the anterior side of the eye globe. There are no obvious histologic abnormalities, and the reasons for impeded resorption of aqueous humor are not known. If left untreated, the disease leads to optic nerve and retinal atrophy and blindness. Although the disease is bilateral, one eye is usually affected to a greater degree than the other.

Primary closed-angle glaucoma is characterized by a visible obstruction of the angle, typically produced by the iris during contraction. This form of glaucoma often presents with an acute onset of intraocular pain and loss of vision, as well as redness of the eye. The intraocular pressure is elevated, but only during the attacks.

Glaucoma is, in most cases, a slowly progressive disease. It causes loss of peripheral sight, which often remains unnoticed by the patient. The diagnosis is made by measuring the intraocular pressure. Early diagnosis and treatment are essential for preventing irreversible eye lesions. Glaucoma can be medically treated with drugs that decrease the production of aqueous humor or reduce intraocular pressure. If left untreated, glaucoma leads to blindness.

Cataract

Cataract, an opacification or clouding of the crystalline lens of the eye, is the most common cause of decreased vision in the United States. However, cataracts also represent one of the most successfully treated chronic eye ailments. More than a million cataracts are removed surgically every year.

On the basis of etiology, cataracts can be classified as either senile or secondary.

- *Senile cataracts* are the most common form of cataracts. Approximately 60 percent of all people older than 70 years of age have some evidence of clouding of the lens. It is considered to be a disease of aging that has no obvious causes except for wear-and-tear of the material that makes up the lens.

- *Secondary cataracts* are the result of lens opacification that is a consequence of trauma, inflammation, or radiation injury. Metabolic diseases, such as diabetes, also predispose individuals to cataracts. Some secondary cataracts are congenital, and are found in infants.

Cataracts usually develop slowly over a period of years. Patients typically complain of blurry vision. As the disease progresses, the visual acuity diminishes and eventually, the vision may be lost entirely. The symptoms depend on the extent of changes and their location in the lens. Axial opacities—that is, those affecting the nucleus of the lens or the central subscapular area—are more troublesome than peripheral opacities.

Early cataracts are readily diagnosed only on the basis of an ophthalmoscopic examination. As the cataract "matures," the lens becomes progressively more cloudy and the cataract becomes visible by naked eye inspection. Surgical removal of the cataract will usually improve the patient's vision, but the patient will require glasses or contact lenses.

Neoplasms

Except for skin tumors of the eyelids, all other neoplasms of the eye are rare. The most important intraocular tumors are retinoblastoma and melanoma. The incidence of retinoblastoma is 1:25,000, whereas the incidence of intraocular melanoma is 1:100,000. Lymphomas are the most common retrobulbar neoplasms.

Retinoblastoma

Retinoblastoma is a rare tumor of infancy and childhood. Nevertheless, it has generated considerable interest among researchers for several reasons. In about 5 percent of cases, the tumor is hereditary. In about 25 percent of sporadic cases and almost all hereditary forms, the retinoblastoma is bilateral. Long-term survivors of retinoblastoma are at a risk for developing other neoplasms, most notably, osteosarcoma. All of these facts were instrumental in the discovery of the retinoblastoma supressor gene (Rb), the first tumor suppressor gene that was fully characterized.

Retinoblastomas grow as intraocular masses that ultimately fill the entire globe and extend into the optic nerve (Fig. 22-6). Clinically, the tumor is recognized as a white pupil. Vision progressively deterio-

FIGURE 22-6

Retinoblastoma. (A) The tumor occupies a large portion of the inside of the eye bulbus. (Courtesy of Dr. Walter Richardson and Dr. Jamsheed Khan, Kansas City, Kansas.) (B) Histologically, the tumor is composed of cells resembling fetal retinal cells ("retinoblasts").

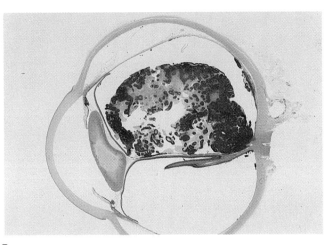

B

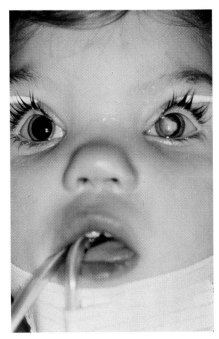

A

rates until it is lost. If untreated, retinoblastoma is almost always lethal, but with modern therapy, more than 90 percent of affected children survive.

Melanoma

Melanomas are the most common primary intraocular tumors affecting adults. Most tumors originate from the pigmentary cells of the uveal tract (i.e., the iris ciliary body or the choroid). The tumors grow as pigmented masses and ultimately fill the entire globe. If diagnosed early and treated adequately, they have a good prognosis, especially if the tumor is composed of spindle cells. Tumors composed of "nonspindle cells" with areas of necrosis and high mitotic activity have a less favorable outcome. Spindle cell melanomas of the iris tend to grow slowly and are amenable to local resection. Melanomas of the choroid usually require removal of the entire globe (enucleation). Approximately 50 percent of patients undergoing enucleation of an eye involved by melanoma survive more than 15 years. Peculiarly, some patients develop metastases many years after the removal of the original tumor.

Review Questions

1. What is the function of the sclera, cornea, choroid, iris, ciliary body, lens, and retina?
2. Compare myopia with hyperopia.
3. What is presbyopia?
4. How do metabolic and circulatory disorders affect the eyes?
5. What causes microphthalmia?
6. What is retinitis pigmentosa?
7. Describe the effects of trauma on the eyes.
8. What are the causes of "pink eye"?
9. Compare conjunctivitis, keratitis, and iridocyclitis.
10. Describe the pathology of hypertensive and diabetic retinopathy.
11. What is glaucoma and what are its causes?
12. Compare open-angle and closed-angle glaucoma.
13. What are cataracts?
14. Compare senile and secondary cataracts.
15. List the most important eye neoplasms.
16. What is retinoblastoma?
17. What is ocular melanoma?

Learning Objectives

After reading this chapter, the student should be able to:

1. Describe the normal anatomy and physiology of the ear.
2. List the most common diseases involving the external ear.
3. Discuss the causes and the symptoms of otitis media.
4. Discuss the causes and pathogenesis of vertigo.
5. Discuss the causes of deafness.

Additional Key Terms and Concepts

Labyrinthitis

Otosclerosis

Vertigo

Chapter Outline

The Ear
Chapter 23

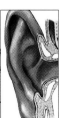

NORMAL ANATOMY AND PHYSIOLOGY

The ears are the primary auditory organs. Each ear consists of three major anatomic parts: the external ear, the middle ear, and the inner ear (Fig. 23-1).

The *external ear* comprises the cartilaginous auricle and the external auditory canal. The auricle is attached to the lateral side of the head. It is composed of elastic cartilage covered with skin. Its main function is to collect the sound waves and direct them toward the eardrum, which is located on the internal side of the auditory canal. The auditory canal is an extension of the auricle that forms as an S-shaped tube inside the temporal bone of the skull. The auditory tube ends blindly on the tympanic membrane, which separates it from the middle ear.

The *middle ear* consists primarily of the air-filled tympanic cavity, which is laterally delimited by the tympanic membrane and medially delimited by the partially fenestrated petrous bone. The openings on the petrous bone are known as the oval window and the round window. The oval window separates the middle ear from the semicircular canals. The middle ear ossicles, malleus, incus, and stapes represent a link between the tympanic membrane and the semicircular canals. These ossicles are essential for the transmission of sound impulses.

The *inner ear* comprises the bone and the membranous labyrinth. The membranous labyrinth, which is filled with endolymph, is enclosed by the bone that forms the chambers of the osseous labyrinth. The inner ear has three parts: the vestibule; the semicircular canals, which are organs of equilibrium; and the cochlea, which is the primary auditory organ. The inner ear is linked to cranial nerve VIII, which transmits the signals from the cochlea, vestibule, and semicircular canals to the auditory centers in the temporal lobes.

OVERVIEW OF MAJOR DISEASES

Diseases of the ear are very important because they impair hearing and can cause deafness. Hearing is essential for many social functions, and loss of hearing can impair the normal social interaction of affected persons, as well as their function in society. Loss of the sense of equilibrium may also be incapacitating.

Diseases of the ear are treated by specialists, known as ear-nose-throat (ENT) surgeons or otorhinolaryngologists.

The most important diseases affecting the ear are

- diseases of the auditory canal
- otitis media
- disturbances of the sense of equilibrium
- deafness

Several facts important to an understanding of ear pathology are presented here, before a discussion of specific pathologic entities.

1. *The external ear is covered with skin and thus is affected by the same diseases that occur on the skin.* External ear allergies, infections, and tumors are indistinguishable from those on other parts of the face. In

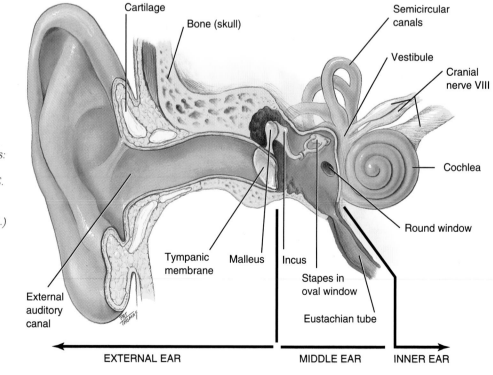

FIGURE 23-1
The ear consists of three parts: the external ear, middle ear, and inner ear. (From Jarvis C. Physical examination and health assessment. Philadelphia: WB Saunders, 1992:365.)

Cartilage

Bone (skull)

Semicircular canals

Vestibule

Cranial nerve VIII

Cochlea

Round window

Tympanic membrane

Malleus

Incus

Stapes in oval window

Eustachian tube

External auditory canal

EXTERNAL EAR

MIDDLE EAR

INNER EAR

other words, the skin covering the outer ear has no unique features. Infection of the cartilage of the ear lobes is rare.

2. *The shape of the external ear varies in human populations.* Some people have small ears, whereas others have disproportionately large ears. Ear dimensions and shapes may be of importance to cosmetic surgeons, but they have no significance in terms of auditory functions of the ear.

3. *The external auditory canal contains ceruminous glands that secrete cerumen, a greasy substance also known as earwax.* Cerumen may form a firm plug that occludes the auditory canal, causing temporary deafness. Impacted earwax can easily be removed by nurses or physicians. If patients attempt removal themselves, using forceps or some other instrument, the eardrum could be perforated or unnecessary irritation of the ear could result.

4. *The tympanic membrane serves as a resonator for sound while also protecting the middle ear.* Rupture of the tympanic membrane could be caused by earpicking with a sharp instrument, barotrauma caused by increased pressure or by an explosion, or following a purulent inflammation. Such holes will impair hearing. The defect in the tympanic membrane also facilitates the entry of bacteria into the middle ear, predisposing the individual to recurrent infections.

5. *The ear is connected to the nasopharynx by the eustachian tube.* The function of this tube is to equalize the pressure in the middle ear cavity and the outer world. At the same time, this anatomic passageway may serve as a conduit for the spread of infections from the nasopharynx into the middle ear. Otitis media is, therefore, a common complication of upper respiratory tract infections.

6. *The auditory ossicles in the middle ear function properly only if mobile.* The malleus, incus, and stapes are tiny ossicles that transmit the sound vibrations of the tympanic membrane to the oval window of the semicircular canals. If one or all of the ossicles become immobile (sclerotic), as in *otosclerosis,* their function is lost, resulting in deafness.

7. *The function of the semicircular canals is to process stimuli that are essential for the maintenance of equilibrium.* Diseases involving this part of the inner ear result in *vertigo*—that is, a sensation of whirling motion or rotation and dizziness.

8. *Diseases of the ear, cranial nerve VIII, or the auditory centers in the brain may cause deafness.* There are several forms of deafness, and it is up to the ENT physician or an audiologist to determine the site of injury.

9. *Tumors of the middle ear and the inner ear are rare.* Although neoplasms may arise in the middle and inner ear, these lesions are uncommon and are rarely a clinical problem. Tumors of cranial nerve VIII, which are also rare, actually account for most tumor-related hearing losses.

Diseases of the External Ear

Diseases of the external ear can be caused by trauma, infection, or allergies. Tumors also occur in the external ear.

Trauma of the ear may result in rupture, hematoma, or complete loss (avulsion) of the ear lobe. Major laceration of the ear or repeated hematoma caused by boxing can result in a deformity known as a cauliflower ear.

Infections of the outer ear may be caused by bacteria, viruses (e.g., herpesvirus), or other pathogens. Infection of the external auditory canal, called swimmer's ear, is a well-known disease affecting athletes who spend long hours in water.

Allergic otitis externa is most often found in children suffering from atopic dermatitis (eczema).

Tumors are usually found on the auricles of the elderly. On histologic examination, such tumors most often prove to be squamous cell or basal cell carcinomas.

Diseases of the Middle Ear

Like the diseases of the external ear, **diseases of the middle ear** may be related to trauma or infection. Allergies and tumors are less important. Some middle ear diseases, such as otosclerosis, are considered to be idiopathic because their cause is unknown.

Perforation of the tympanic membrane is the most important consequence of middle ear trauma. The tympanic membrane may rupture as a result of direct injury with a sharp object (such as a toothpick used to remove impacted cerumen), explosive acoustic trauma, barotrauma secondary to high air pressure caused by an explosion, or infections. Small defects usually heal spontaneously. Infection prevents healing and may result in deafness. The defects can be repaired by microsurgery.

Otitis Media

Otitis media occurs in two forms: acute or chronic infection. *Acute otitis media* is typically caused by bacteria that invade the cavity of the middle ear (Fig. 23-2). The disease is most common in children and is often precipitated by a viral upper respiratory tract infection. Such infection causes edema of the eustachian tube and accumulation of fluid in the inner ear, which becomes infected with bacteria. The patient often complains of pain and hearing loss. The ear is typically sensitive to touch. On otoscopic ex-

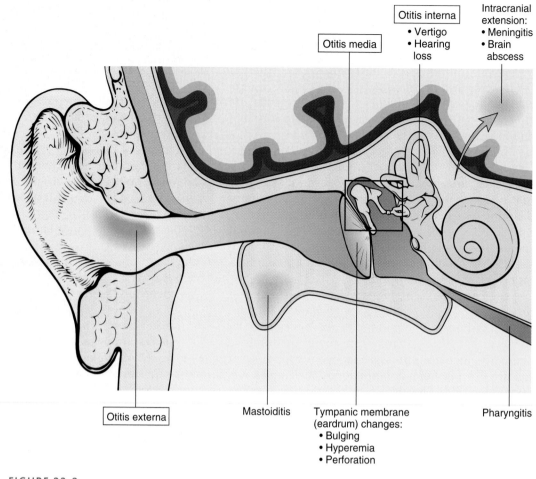

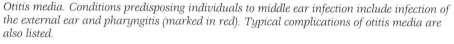

FIGURE 23-2
*Otitis media. Conditions predisposing individuals to middle ear infection include infection of
the external ear and pharyngitis (marked in red). Typical complications of otitis media are
also listed.*

amination, the tympanic membrane appears red and
bulging and, if left untreated, may perforate. In such
cases, pus pours out of the ear canal. Bacterial otitis
media usually responds well to antibiotic treatment.
Tympanocentesis—that is, puncture of the tympanic
membrane with a needle to drain the exudate—may
occasionally be indicated in resistant cases for typing
of pathogens. Myringotomy—that is, surgical incision
of the tympanic membrane to drain the pus—is only
rarely indicated.

The complications of acute purulent otitis media
include chronic otitis media, extension of the infec-

At least 50 percent of all children aged 1 to 3 years
have a middle ear effusion once a year. In most
cases, the effusion regresses on its own, and few
children develop serious ear infections.

tion into the mastoid (mastoiditis), and spread of infections into the inner ear and the brain.

Chronic otitis media is usually a consequence of
recurrent acute infections, but it also may follow traumatic rupture of the tympanic membrane. Clinically,
the hallmark of the disease is a chronic purulent
ear discharge. The disease is accompanied by chronic
pain and loss of hearing. The tympanic membrane is
usually ruptured or entirely missing. Treatment is directed at eradicating the bacterial infection. After resolution of the infection, the eardrum and the middle
ear structures can be reconstructed surgically.

Cholesteatoma, an epidermal inclusion cyst, is a
common complication of chronic otitis media. This
tumor-like growth results from invagination of the
squamous epidermis, which continues growing from
the auditory canal through the defect of the tympanic
membrane into the middle ear and the mastoid bone.
The epidermis forms keratin layers which accumulate in the lumen of the cyst and resemble pearly
white material. Cholesteatoma is treated surgically.

Glue ear is a special form of nonbacterial chronic

otitis media. A consequence of acute otitis in children, it is characterized by a persistent viscous effusion in the middle ear cavity. At least 5 of every 1000 children younger than 5 years of age are treated surgically for this condition. The treatment often includes insertion of grommets or plastic tubes into the eustachian tubes, or adenoidectomy to improve the drainage of fluids from the middle ear.

Otosclerosis

Otosclerosis is the most common cause of conductive hearing loss in middle-aged Americans. This disease of unknown etiology is inherited as an autosomal dominant trait, affecting approximately 10 percent of all whites and 1 percent of all blacks in the United States. It is twice as common among women than among men.

The disease affects both ears, although one ear seems to incur more damage than the other. Pathologically, it is characterized by the deposition of newly formed bones on both sides of the oval window. The sclerotic bone first encases the foot of the stapes, impeding its movements. As the sclerosis progresses, the entire stapes is replaced by new bone. Treatment involves stapedectomy, or removal of the sclerotic stapes, and replacement of the sclerotic stapes by a plastic prosthesis.

Diseases of the Inner Ear

Meniere's Disease

Meniere's disease is a disease of unknown etiology that affects adults. Its peak incidence occurs in those who are 40 to 60 years of age. The disease is associated with hydrops of the endolymphatic system of the cochlea.

Clinically, its presents with the following triad:

1. Episodic vertigo that lasts 1 to several hours. The vertigo typically subsides, but then recurs after a few hours or days.

Did You Know?

Noise monitoring in the workplace has been instituted by governmental regulatory agencies to prevent hearing loss secondary to noise trauma. All sounds exceeding 85 dB are potentially harmful to the cochlea. As an example, at takeoff, jet engines have a loudness of 150 dB. Thus, earplugs and protective gear should be worn while working on the tarmac.

Did You Know?

Vertigo is a common complaint, and one should not immediately consider it to be a sign of inner ear disease. Vertigo may be induced by alcohol, and is a typical feature of motion sickness, height sickness, or sea sickness.

2. Sensorineural hearing loss for low-frequency sound
3. Tinnitus, or ringing in the ears

The cause of increased endolymphatic pressure is not known, but a low-salt diet and diuretic therapy, aimed at lowering endolymphatic pressure, have yielded good results.

The diagnosis of Meniere's disease requires that other causes of vertigo be excluded. The differential diagnosis includes

- viral labyrinthitis, which usually follows upper respiratory tract infections
- vestibular neuronitis, an idiopathic form of vertigo thought to be of neuronal origin. It occurs as a solitary event and does not recur.
- traumatic vertigo, which is a consequence of head trauma
- peripheral vertigo, migraine-associated vertigo, and other functional diseases that are not associated with inner ear pathology
- vertigo of central neural origin, secondary to a neuroma involving cranial nerve VIII or a brain lesion

Deafness

Deafness, or hearing loss, is a very common disease with multiple causes (Fig. 23-3). More than 28 million Americans have a hearing impairment, and 2 million of these are profoundly deaf.

Deafness can be classified as

- conductive
- sensory
- neural

Conductive hearing loss is caused by external or middle ear lesions. In the auditory canal, the cause of hearing loss may be obstruction, such as with impacted cerumen. Loss of the tympanic membrane or its perforation by trauma or infection also causes conductive hearing loss. Effusion in the middle ear, cholesteatoma, or hemorrhage into the middle ear cavity can also cause hearing loss. Otosclerosis causes deafness by impeding the transmission of signals from the tympanic membrane to the oval window.

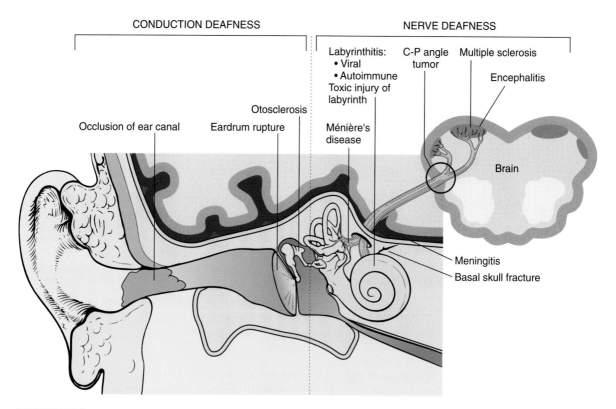

FIGURE 23-3

Causes of deafness. Conductive deafness may be caused by occlusion of the ear canal, rupture of the eardrum, otosclerosis, or diseases affecting the labyrinth. By contrast, nerve deafness is caused by injury of the acoustic nerve and auditory centers in the brain. C-P, cerebellopontine.

Sensory hearing loss results from cochlear abnormalities. Noise trauma at the workplace is an mportant cause of sensory hearing loss. Ototoxic drugs, such as streptomycin, antimalarial drugs, and certain diuretics, may also cause deafness. Presbycusis, the hearing loss of unknown etiology that affects elderly people, is also classified as a sensory defect.

Neural hearing loss results from lesions of cranial nerve VIII or of the central nervous system. This is the least common form of hearing loss. Typical causes include neuromas of cranial nerve VIII, multiple sclerosis, and cerebrovascular accidents.

The diagnosis of deafness is based on clinical data, but must be documented by audiologic techniques. Some causes of hearing loss can be treated surgically, whereas others require the use of permanent hearing aids.

Review Questions

1. Describe the principal anatomic components of the external, middle, and inner ear.
2. What are the main functions of the ear?
3. List the most important diseases of the external ear.
4. List the most important diseases of the middle ear.
5. Compare acute and chronic otitis media.
6. What is cholesteatoma?
7. What is otosclerosis?
8. What is Meniere's disease?
9. Compare conductive, sensory, and neural deafness.

Glossary

abortion Interruption of pregnancy; may be spontaneous or induced.

abscess Localized collection of pus.

achalasia Failure of the lower esophageal sphincter to relax.

achlorhydria Absence of hydrochloric acid in gastric secretions.

achondroplasia Hereditary disorder of cartilage formation resulting in dwarfism.

acne An inflammatory skin disease involving the hair follicles and sebaceous glands.

acromegaly Abnormal enlargement of the terminal parts of the extremities, jaws, and nose owing to an excess of growth hormone.

acute disease Disease of sudden onset and short duration of symptoms.

Addison's disease Adrenocortical insufficiency secondary to destruction of the adrenal glands.

adenocarcinoma Malignant tumor composed of glandular or ductal epithelium.

adenoma Benign tumor composed of glandular or ductal epithelium.

agenesis Developmental disorder in which an organ or structure is not formed.

AIDS Acquired immunodeficiency syndrome, a disease caused by the human immunodeficiency virus.

albinism Congenital absence of skin pigmentation.

alkaline phosphatase An enzyme that is found in the cell membrane of many cells and is released into serum and body fluids.

allergy Immunologic hypersensitivity reaction to an antigen (allergen).

alopecia Baldness or loss of hair; may be diffuse or focal.

amylase An enzyme that is produced by the pancreas and salivary glands and that catalyzes the hydrolysis of starch into simpler compounds.

amyloidosis Disease caused by the deposition of amyloid, an aggregate of insoluble fibrillar proteins.

anaphylaxis A form of hypersensitivity (allergic) reaction that is usually mediated by histamine.

anaplasia Abnormal differentiation of cells found in malignant tumors.

anasarca Generalized edema marked by the accumulation of fluid in organs and body cavities.

anastomosis A communication between blood vessels or tubular organs (like the intestines).

anemia A decrease in the number of circulating red blood cells or hemoglobin to below-normal levels.

anencephaly A congenital defect characterized by incomplete formation of the cranium and destruction or loss of the brain.

aneurysm A localized dilatation of an artery.

angina A severe pain in the chest (angina pectoris) that is usually a sign of heart disease.

angiography A radiographic technique for visualizing blood vessels following an injection of contrast medium.

ankylosis Stiffening and reduced mobility of a joint that has been obliterated by fibrous tissue.

anomaly Marked deviation from the normal; may be congenital or acquired.

anorexia Loss of appetite.

anoxia Oxygen deficiency.

antibody An immunoglobulin produced by the body in response to antigenic stimulation.

antigen Allergen, immunogen; i.e., any substance that can induce an immune response of the body.

aphthae Superficial mucosal ulcerations covered with exudate.

apoplexy Stroke caused by cerebral hemorrhage.

apoptosis Programmed cell death that occurs normally in developing and adult tissues, but that can also be induced by various drugs and viruses.

appendicitis Inflammation of the appendix.

arachnodactyly Spider-like, long, and slender fingers and toes (typically found in Marfan syndrome).

arrhythmia Abnormal heart rhythm.

arteriosclerosis Hardening or calcification of arterial walls.

arthritis An inflammation of one or more joints; may be infectious or immunologic (as in rheumatoid arthritis).

asbestosis A lung disease caused by the inhalation of asbestos fibers.

ascites An abnormal accumulation of serous fluid in the abdomen, as may occur in end-stage liver disease.

ascorbic acid Vitamin C.

aseptic necrosis of bone Localized death of bone tissue in the absence of an infection.

aspiration Entry of foreign material into the larynx, trachea, or lungs.

asthma Allergic pulmonary disease marked by bronchospasm, wheezing, and excessive mucus formation.

astrocytoma A brain or spinal cord tumor composed of astrocytes.

asymptomatic Devoid of symptoms.

atelectasis Collapse of all or part of a lung; characterized by an absence of air in the pulmonary alveoli.

atherosclerosis A systemic disease characterized by fibrosis, an accumulation of lipids in arterial walls and calcification of arteries.

atresia Absence of a lumen in a tubular organ, such as the intestines.

atrophy A decrease in the size of cells, tissues, or organs.

autolysis Postmortem dissolution and disintegration of cells or tissues by the enzymes present in those tissues.

basophil A white blood cell containing bluish (basophilic) granules; it is a precursor of tissue mast cells.

bronchiectasis Dilatation of bronchi secondary to chronic inflammation.

bulla A blister or large skin vesicle.

cachexia A state of general ill health and poor nutrition that typically occurs in chronic diseases (e.g., cancer).

calcification Deposition of calcium salts in tissue.

calculus A stone or abnormal accumulation of mineral salts that usually forms in the lumen of the gallbladder or urinary tract.

callus New bone formation that occurs following fractures.

carcinoid A malignant tumor of neuroendorine cells.

carcinoma A malignant tumor composed of epithelial cells.

cardiomyopathy A term used to describe a variety of diseases affecting the myocardium.

cardiovascular Pertaining to the heart and blood vessels.

cartilaginous Consisting of cartilage.

caseous Pertaining to a form of necrosis resembling cheese; typical of tuberculosis, but may be found in some fungal granulomas as well.

cerebral palsy Congenital weakness or paralysis of muscles owing to intrauterine brain damage.

chemotaxis Movement of inflammatory cells toward a chemical attractant.

chemotherapy Treatment of disease with chemical agents.

cholecystitis Inflammation of the gallbladder.

cholelithiasis Presence of stones in the gallbladder.

chondroma Benign cartilaginous tumor.

chondrosarcoma Malignant cartilaginous tumor.

chronic disease Disease of long duration.

cicatrization Scarring, i.e., formation of a cicatrix (scar).

cirrhosis Chronic disease of the liver characterized by liver cell damage, nodular regeneration, and fibrosis and resulting in a loss of normal liver architecture; synonym for end-stage liver failure.

coagulation Clotting of blood.

colitis Inflammation of the large intestine.

collagen A collective term for a group of mostly fibrous structural proteins found in connective tissues. Type I collagen is the most abundant structural protein in the body.

complement A group of serum proteins that mediate inflammation.

congenital Present at birth; a term used to describe a trait or anomaly with which one is born.

congestion Engorgement of vessels with blood.

contusion Mechanical injury resulting in extravasation of blood into tissue; a bruise.

Creutzfeldt-Jakob disease Infectious dementia and spongiform encephalopathy caused by prions.

Crohn's disease Regional enteritis; an ulcerative disease of unknown origin characterized by inflammation of the terminal ileum or colon.

croup Spastic laryngitis characterized by a bark-like cough.

cryptorchidism Congenital absence of a testis from the scrotum.

curettage The scraping or cleaning of a diseased surface or the internal surface of an organ for diagnosis or treatment, as in uterine curettage.

Cushing's syndrome A disease caused by an excess of corticosteroids secondary to tumors of the adrenal cortex or exogenously injected synthetic hormones.

cyanosis Bluish discoloration of the skin indicating a lack of oxygen.

cyst A closed, usually fluid-filled sac lined by epithelium.

cystic fibrosis An autosomal recessive disorder characterized by abnormal secretion by sweat and mucous glands and complicated by pancreatic and pulmonary insufficiency.

cystitis Inflammation of the urinary bladder.

cytology The study of cells.

degeneration The deterioration of cell function following nonlethal cellular injury.

dehydration Loss of water from the body or from body tissue.

demineralization Excessive elimination or loss of minerals (calcium and phosphates) from the bones.

dermatitis Skin inflammation.

desmoplasia Proliferation of connective tissue within a carcinoma.

diabetes mellitus A metabolic disease caused by a lack of insulin or by tissue resistance to insulin that adversely affects the metabolism of glucose and results in hyperglycemia.

diapedesis Exit of blood cells from a blood vessel into the tissue (as occurs in inflammation).

diastole The resting phase of the heart, characterized by the dilation of ventricles.

differentiation The process by which cells acquire specialized functions and tissue- or organ-specific features.

diffuse Widespread; not limited or localized.

dilatation Widening of a hollow organ or orifice, such as the heart chambers.

diverticulum Saccular outpouching of the wall of a hollow organ, such as the large intestine.

Down syndrome Congenital disease caused by trisomy of chromosome 21.

Duchenne muscular dystrophy X-linked recessive muscle disease causing generalized muscle weakness and death in early adulthood.

dwarfism Abnormally short stature.

dysphagia Difficulty in swallowing.

dysplasia Abnormal differentiation or maturation of tissue; refers also to preneoplastic changes in the epithelium (e.g., cervical dysplasia).

dysuria Painful urination (as occurs in cystitis).

ecchymoses Hemorrhagic spots on the skin and mucosae that are larger than petechiae.

ectopia Congenital displacement of an organ or structure.

eczema Chronic skin inflammation (dermatitis) caused by various mechanisms; often caused by allergy.

edema An abnormal accumulation of fluid in tissues of body cavities.

embolus Blood clot or foreign matter in the circulation that may produce obstruction of blood flow.

emphysema Loss of pulmonary parenchyma resulting in widening of the terminal respiratory spaces.

empyema Collection of pus in a body cavity, as in the pleural cavity.

encephalitis Inflammation of the brain.

endocarditis Inflammation of the inner heart lining and cardiac valves.

endocrinology The study of the endocrine system and hormonal disturbances.

endometriosis A condition in which foci of endometrium are located outside the uterine cavity.

enteritis Inflammation of the intestine.

eosinophil A white blood cell, usually binucleated, that contains red (eosinophilic) cytoplasmic granules.

ependymoma A tumor arising from the ependymal cells lining the ventricles and central canal of the spinal cord.

epididymo-orchitis Inflammation of the epididymis and testis.

epidural hematoma A blood clot in the space between the dura mater and the bone of the skull.

epilepsy A neurologic disease characterized by convulsions.

epiphysis The secondary center of ossification in the proximal and distal ends of long bones.

epistaxis Nosebleed.

epithelial cell One of the basic cells forming (1) all solid internal organs except the heart and brain; (2) the epidermis of the skin; and (3) the internal lining of the hollow organs.

erosion Destruction of tissue surface; ulceration.

erythrocyte Red blood cell.

erythropoietin A hormone produced by the kidneys that promotes red blood cell production (erythropoiesis).

esophagitis Inflammation of the esophagus.

estrogen Female sex hormone produced by the ovaries and adrenals.

etiology The study of the origin of disease; also used as synonym for cause of disease.

Ewing's sarcoma A malignant bone tumor involving the shaft of the long bones. It is composed of small, undifferentiated cells, the origin of which is unknown.

exacerbation An increase in the severity of a disease.

exophthalmos Abnormal protrusion (bulging) of the eyeball.

exudate Protein-rich fluid in the interstitial spaces or body cavities that contains leukocytes and is usually caused by inflammation.

fibrin An insoluble fibrillar protein found in clots formed from fibrinogen in the plasma during blood coagulation.

fibroadenoma A benign tumor composed of glandular epithelium and fibroblastic stroma; typically found in the breast.

fibroblast A connective tissue cell that synthesizes collagen.

fibrocystic changes Changes in the breast that occur in many women as part of the normal aging process.

fibroma A benign connective tissue tumor composed of fibroblasts.

fibrosis Hardening of tissues secondary to deposition of collagen; excessive fibrosis may cause scarring.

fissure A groove or slit-like tissue defect, especially in the skin, anus, and mouth.

fistula A channel, caused by inflammation or tumor, that connects two hollow organs (e.g., loops of intestines or rectum and vagina).

gastrin A hormone that stimulates gastric acid secretion.

gastritis Inflammation of the mucosa of the stomach.

glioma A malignant brain tumor composed of glial cells.

glomerulonephritis A kidney disease characterized by inflammation of the glomeruli.

glucosuria Excretion of glucose in urine.

goiter Enlargement of the thyroid.

gonorrhea Sexually transmitted disease caused by *Neisseria gonorrhoeae*.

gout A hereditary form of arthritis related to hyperuricemia and deposition of uric acid crystals in joints.

granulation tissue Newly formed tissue composed of blood vessels, macrophages, and fibroblasts; typically forms during the healing stages of inflammation or healing of wounds and fractures.

granuloma An inflammatory lesion that is composed of macrophages, lymphocytes, and/or giant cells and that forms microscopic aggregates or nodules.

Graves' disease Immunologically mediated hyperthyroidism.

gynecologic Pertaining to the study of the female genital tract.

gynecomastia Enlargement of the male breast.

hamartoma A nodule composed of an abnormal accumulation or overgrowth of mature cells and tissues that are normally present in the affected organ. It results from abnormal development and is, in most instances, congenital, although not necessarily diagnosed at birth and infancy.

hemangioma A benign vascular tumor.

hematemesis The vomiting of blood.

hematochezia The passage of bright red blood in the stool.

hematocrit Relative volume of red blood cells in whole blood, expressed as a percentage.

hematogenous Disseminated by or derived from blood.

hematology The study of blood and blood-forming tissues.

hematoma Coagulated blood located outside a blood vessel.

hematuria Blood in the urine.

hemiparesis Muscle paralysis on one side of the body.

hemolysis Red blood cell destruction.

hemophilia An X-linked hereditary bleeding disorder caused by a deficiency of factor VIII or IX.

hemorrhage The escape of blood from a ruptured blood vessel.

hemothorax A collection of blood in the thoracic cavity.

hepatitis Inflammation of the liver.

hepatomegaly Liver enlargement.

hernia Protrusion of a part of an organ or the entire organ through an abnormal opening in the structure normally containing it, such as the abdominal wall.

Hirschsprung's disease Congenital megacolon (widening of the large intestine) caused by incomplete development of colonic neurons (ganglia).

hirsutism Excess of hair on the face or the body.

histamine A biogenic amine, released from mast cells, that mediates inflammation in type I hypersensitivity reactions.

Hodgkin's disease A malignant neoplastic disease involving the lymph nodes.

homeostasis Maintenance of stability or equilibrium between cells and fluids in the human body.

Huntington's disease Autosomal dominant hereditary dementia that becomes evident only in adulthood.

hydrocephalus Accumulation of cerebrospinal fluid in the ventricles of the brain.

hydronephrosis Distention of the renal pelvis with urine.

hydrothorax A collection of clear fluid (transudate) in the thoracic cavity.

hyperplasia Enlargement of an organ owing to an increased number of cells.

hypertension Elevation of arterial blood pressure.

hypertrophy An enlargement in an organ or body part caused by an increase in cell size; usually pertains to skeletal muscles or heart.

hyperuricemia An excess of uric acid in the blood.

hypoplasia Underdevelopment of an organ or structure.

hypotension Low arterial blood pressure.

hypoxia A reduction in oxygen supply to the tissues.

iatrogenic Resulting from intervention by physicians.

icterus Jaundice.

idiopathic Of unknown cause.

immunity The body's defense mechanism against infection or foreign substances; may be mediated by antibodies or cells.

immunoglobulin A protein that is produced by the plasma cells and that is capable of reacting with antigens and acting as an antibody.

impetigo Superficial bacterial skin infection.

incidence The number of newly diagnosed cases of a disease in a given time period, usually a year.

infarct Localized area of ischemia or necrosis.

infertility An inability to conceive or have children.

inflammation The body's reaction to injury, characterized by a typical cellular, humoral, and circulatory response.

insulin A hormone secreted by the beta cells of the pancreatic islets of Langerhans that mediates uptake and utilization of glucose in cells.

insulinoma An endocrine tumor of the pancreas composed of neoplastic beta cells that secrete insulin.

interleukin A biologically active substance secreted by activated cells (most notably, leukocytes and macrophages).

invasion The spreading of cancer into normal tissues.

ischemia Inadequate blood flow in the tissues.

jaundice Yellowish discoloration of the skin or mucous membranes due to hyperbilirubinemia; synonymous with icterus.

Kaposi's sarcoma Malignant tumor composed of blood vessels; often found in patients with AIDS.

keloid A nodular, hyperplastic scar.

keratin A fibrillar protein forming the intermediate filaments in the cytoplasm of epithelial cells.

leiomyoma A benign tumor involving smooth muscle.

lesion An abnormal structural change in tissues or organs resulting from injury or disease.

leukemia Cancer of the blood-forming organs characterized by the appearance of malignant white blood cells in circulation.

leukocytes White blood cells.

leukocytosis An increased number of circulating white blood cells.

lipase A fat-splitting enzyme secreted by the pancreas.

lipid Fat.

lipoma A benign tumor composed of fat cells.

liposarcoma A malignant tumor composed of fat cells.

liquefaction A form of necrosis characterized by the transformation of solid tissue into fluid.

lithiasis Formation of calculi (stones), as may occur in the gallbladder (cholelithiasis) or urinary tract (urolithasis).

lymphadenopathy An enlargement of lymph nodes that is caused by inflammation or neoplasia.

lymphoma Malignant neoplasm involving lymphoid tissue.

lysis Destruction or decomposition.

macrophage Mononuclear phagocytic cells in tissues.

malabsorption Impaired intestinal absorption of nutrients.

malnutrition Any disorder caused by inadequate nutrition.

MALT Mucosa-associated lymphoid tissue; found in the gastrointestinal and respiratory tract.

mammography X-ray examination of the breast for the detection of tumors.

Marfan's syndrome A hereditary disorder of the connective tissue that is characterized by weakness of connective tissue, tendons, and blood vessels.

mast cell A tissue cell derived from circulating basophils.

mastectomy Surgical removal of the breast.

mastitis Inflammation of the breast.

measles A contagious viral disease of childhood, also called rubeola.

medulloblastoma A brain tumor affecting the cerebellum of children.

megacolon A congenital or functional dilatation of the colon.

megaloureter Congenital ureteral dilatation without obvious cause.

melanoma A pigmented malignant tumor, composed of melanocytes, that most often arises in the skin or the eye.

melena Black, tarry stools resulting from gastrointestinal bleeding.

meningioma A benign tumor of the meninges.

meningitis Inflammation of the meninges of the brain and spinal cord.

metaphysis The part of bone where the diaphysis and epiphysis meet.

metaplasia A change from one cell type to another.

metastasis The transfer or spread of cancer cells from one site to another.

morbidity The frequency of disability within a population.

multiple sclerosis An incurable immunologic disease of the central nervous system that causes progressive muscle weakness.

myasthenia gravis An autoimmune disease involving the neuromuscular junction and presenting as muscle weakness.

mycosis Infectious disease caused by a fungus.

myelomeningocele Herniation of the meninges and spinal cord.

myocardial infarct Ischemic necrosis of the heart muscle.

myocarditis Inflammation of the myocardium.

myopathy A term for muscle diseases of various etiologies; may be congenital or acquired.

necrosis The morphologic changes in tissue caused by cell death.

neoplasm Tumor tissue mass resulting from abnormal cells.

nephritis Inflammation of the kidney.

nephrolithiasis Formation of renal calculi.

neuroblastoma A tumor composed of neuroblasts (i.e., immature neural cell precursors).

nevus A mole or localized, benign, and pigmented skin lesion.

obstruction Blockage of a tube-like organ, such as the intestines.

occlusion Blockage of vessels.

occult Hidden or inapparent.

oligodendroglioma A malignant brain tumor composed of oligodendroglia.

oliguria Excretion of a reduced amount of urine.

opsonization The coating of bacteria with opsonins, which are substances that facilitate phagocytosis.

osteogenesis imperfecta A hereditary bone disease resulting in fractures.

osteoid The soft, organic part of the bony matrix.

osteolytic Relating to osteolysis or dissolution of bone.

osteoma A benign bone tumor.

osteomalacia A condition marked by softening of the bones.

osteomyelitis An infection of bone, usually caused by bacteria.

osteopetrosis A hereditary disorder resulting in abnormally dense bone ("marble-bone disease").

osteoporosis Increased thinning and fragility of bones owing to atrophy and loss of bone substance.

osteosarcoma A malignant bone-forming tumor composed of neoplastic osteoblasts.

Paget's disease Osteitis deformans; a bone disease marked by bone densities and deformities.

pancreatitis Inflammation of the pancreas.

pannus The presence of granulation tissue in a joint as a result of rheumatoid arthritis.

paralysis A loss or impairment of motor function of a body part.

paraplegia Paralysis of the lower extremities.

Parkinson's disease A neurologic disease characterized by movement disorders.

pathogenesis The sequence of events that precedes the development of disease.

pathophysiology Physiology in abnormal conditions or disease states.

pelvic inflammatory disease Bacterial infection of the internal female genital organs, often abbreviated as PID.

peptic ulcer A defect in the mucosa of the stomach or duodenum that is caused by pepsin and hydrochloric acid.

perforation A hole in the wall of a hollow organ, such as the intestine.

pericarditis Inflammation of the pericardium.

periodontal Pertaining to the gums or the area surrounding the teeth.

peritonitis Inflammation of the peritoneum.

pernicious anemia A form of anemia related to the body's inability to absorb vitamin B_{12}.

petechia A pinpoint intradermal or subcutaneous skin hemorrhage.

phagocytosis The ingestion of microorganisms by leukocytes or macrophages.

pheochromocytoma A tumor of the adrenal medulla that usually secretes epinephrine and norepinephrine, causing hypertension.

plasma cell A cell derived from B-cell lymphocytes that secretes immunoglobulins.

pneumoconiosis A pulmonary disease characterized by the accumulation of dust and particulate matter in the lungs.

pneumonia A bacterial or viral infection of the lungs.

pneumothorax Air in the thoracic cavity.

poliomyelitis An acute viral disease that attacks the central nervous system; it has almost completely been eradicated by vaccination.

polyarteritis nodosa An immunologic disease involving the arteries.

polycystic kidney disease A hereditary kidney disease characterized by multiple cysts.

polycythemia An increase in the total red cell mass in the blood.

polymyositis An immunologic muscle disease affecting several muscle groups.

polyuria Excretion of a large amount of urine.

portal hypertension Increased pressure in the portal vein, usually caused by cirrhosis.

postmenopausal After menopause.

prevalence The total number of cases of a disease at any one place and time.

prognosis The predicted outcome of a disease.

prostaglandins Substances derived from lipids that mediate inflammation, smooth muscle cell contraction, and vascular permeability. Abbreviated as PGs.

proteinuria Excretion of increased amounts of protein in the urine.

purulent Associated with pus formation.

pus A yellow inflammatory discharge composed of exudated neutrophils.

pyelonephritis Infection of the kidney and renal pelvis, usually caused by bacteria.

pyothorax Collection of pus in the thoracic cavity.

pyrogens Substances that cause fever.

regeneration The preferred method of body repair by which the original function of the cell is restored.

renin An enzyme, produced by the kidneys, that increases blood pressure by acting on angiotensinogen.

retinoblastoma A malignant eye tumor of infancy and childhood.

rhabdomyosarcoma A malignant tumor of skeletal muscle.

rheumatic fever An immunologic reaction to streptococci that affects the joints and the heart.

rheumatoid arthritis An immune-mediated, chronic, systemic disease producing inflammatory changes in the joints.

rhinitis Inflammation of the mucous membranes of the nose resulting in a nasal discharge.

rickets A disease caused by a deficiency of vitamin D that results in softening and deformity of bones and that usually affects children.

rupture Forcible tearing of tissue or organs.

sarcoidosis Immune-mediated disease characterized by the formation of noncaseating granulomas.

sarcoma A malignant tumor of connective tissue cells.

scar The formation of fibrous tissue following healing of inflammation or injury of certain organs, such as skin or intestines.

scirrhous Pertaining to or of the nature of a hard cancer, usually with abundant fibrous tissue stroma.

scleroderma Systemic sclerosis; a systemic disease characterized by excessive deposition of collagen and causing stiffening of affected tissues.

scoliosis A lateral curvature of the spine, causing a deformity of the body.

scurvy A disease caused by a deficiency of vitamin C.

seminoma A germ cell tumor of the testis, equivalent to dysgerminoma of the ovary.

senile Pertaining to old age.

septicemia Bacteremia; the presence of bacteria in the blood.

serum The clear, straw-colored, liquid part of plasma that contains no cells or coagulation factors.

sexually transmitted diseases Diseases acquired by sexual intercourse (e.g., syphilis, gonorrhea).

silicosis Fibrotic lung disease caused by the inhalation of silica particles.

spasm An involuntary, usually painful, muscle contraction.

spina bifida A congenital defect in the posterior part of the vertebrae that exposes the spinal cord to injury.

splenomegaly Enlargement of the spleen.

squamous cell carcinoma A malignant epithelial tumor composed of epidermoid (squamous) cells.

steatorrhea Fatty stool resulting from intestinal malabsorption of fats.

subdural hematoma A blood clot between the dura and arachnoid.

syphilis A contagious venereal disease caused by *Treponema pallidum.*

systemic lupus erythematosus A systemic autoimmune disease most often affecting the skin, joints, and kidneys.

tachycardia Excessively rapid heartbeat.

teratoma A tumor, usually of germ cell origin, which is composed of haphazardly arranged tissues not normally found at the site of origin of the tumor.

tetralogy of Fallot A congenital heart disease characterized by four specific defects.

thrombus A blood clot or mass of clotted blood, usually within a blood vessel.

tophus A urate deposit occurring in gout.

trauma An injury caused by an external force.

tuberculosis An infectious, inflammatory disease, usually of the lungs, caused by *Mycobacterium tuberculosis.*

tumor Neoplasm; a mass resulting from the abnormal growth of cells.

ulcer A superficial defect in the mucosa of a hollow organ or the skin.

ulcerative colitis A disease of unknown origin affecting the large intestine and causing widespread ulceration.

uremia End-stage kidney disease.

urolithiasis Stone formation in the urinary tract.

varicella Chickenpox; a viral childhood disease characterized by a vesicular skin eruption.

varices Dilated veins.

volvulus The twisting of one part of the bowel upon itself.

Wegener's granulomatosis An immunologic disease of unknown etiology that typically affects the upper respiratory tract, lungs, and kidneys.

Wernicke-Korsakoff syndrome A neuropsychiatric disorder caused by thiamine deficiency; most often associated with chronic alcoholism.

Wilms' tumor A malignant renal tumor of infancy and childhood.

xenograft A transplant of tissues or organs from one species to another (e.g., pig skin to humans).

zoonosis A disease that affects both humans and animals.

Index

Note: Page numbers in *italics* refer to illustrations; page numbers followed by t refer to tables.